Essentials of
Practical Microbiology

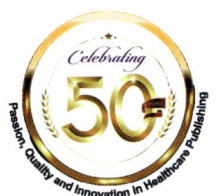

Essentials of
Practical Microbiology

SECOND EDITION

Apurba S Sastry MD (JIPMER) DNB MNAMS PDCR
Hospital Infection Control Officer
Officer In-charge, HICC
Antimicrobial Stewardship Lead
Associate Professor
Department of Microbiology
Jawaharlal Institute of Postgraduate Medical Education and Research (JIPMER), Puducherry, India

Sandhya Bhat (Gold medalist) MD DNB MNAMS PDCR
Professor
Department of Microbiology
Pondicherry Institute of Medical Sciences (PIMS)
(A Unit of Madras Medical Mission)
Puducherry, India

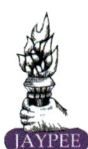

JAYPEE BROTHERS MEDICAL PUBLISHERS
The Health Sciences Publisher
New Delhi | London

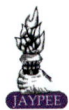 **Jaypee Brothers Medical Publishers (P) Ltd**

Headquarters
Jaypee Brothers Medical Publishers (P) Ltd
EMCA House, 23/23-B
Ansari Road, Daryaganj
New Delhi - 110 002, INDIA
Landline: +91-11-23272143,+91-11-23272703, +91-11-23282021,+91-11-23245672
Head Office : 011-43574357
@E jaypee@jaypeebrothers.com: www.jaypeebrothers.com

Corporate Office
Jaypee Brothers Medical Publishers (P) Ltd
4838/24, Ansari Road, Daryaganj
New Delhi 110 002, India
Phone: +91-11-43574357
Fax: +91-11-43574314
Email: jaypee@jaypeebrothers.com

Overseas Office
J.P. Medical Ltd
83 Victoria Street, London
SW1H 0HW (UK)
Phone: +44 20 3170 8910
Fax: +44 (0)20 3008 6180
Email: info@jpmedpub.com

Website: www.jaypeebrothers.com
Website: www.jaypeedigital.com

© 2021, Jaypee Brothers Medical Publishers

The views and opinions expressed in this book are solely those of the original contributor (s)/author (s) and do not necessarily represent those of editor (s) of the book.

All rights reserved. No part of this publication may be reproduced, stored or transmitted in any form or by any means, electronic, mechanical, photocopying, recording or otherwise, without the prior permission in writing of the publishers/ editors.

All brand names and product names used in this book are trade names, service marks, trademarks or registered trademarks of their respective owners. The publisher is not associated with any product or vendor mentioned in this book.

Medical knowledge and practice change constantly. This book is designed to provide accurate, authoritative information about the subject matter in question. However, readers are advised to check the most current information available on procedures included and check information from the manufacturer of each product to be administered, to verify the recommended dose, formula, method and duration of administration, adverse effects and contraindications. It is the responsibility of the practitioner to take all appropriate safety precautions. Neither the publisher nor the author (s)/editor (s) assume any liability for any injury and/or damage to persons or property arising from or related to use of material in this book.

This book is sold on the understanding that the publisher is not engaged in providing professional medical services. If such advice or services are required, the services of a competent medical professional should be sought.

Every effort has been made where necessary to contact holders of copyright to obtain permission to reproduce copyright material. If any have been inadvertently overlooked, the publisher will be pleased to make the necessary arrangements at the first opportunity. The **CD/DVD-ROM** (if any) provided in the sealed envelope with this book is complimentary and free of cost. **Not meant for sale.**

Inquiries for bulk sales may be solicited at: jaypee@jaypeebrothers.com

Essentials of Practical Microbiology

First Edition: 2018

Second Edition: **2021**

ISBN: 978-81-948028-2-2

Printed at Samrat offset Pvt. Ltd.

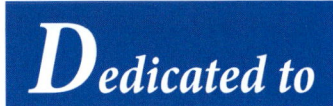

Our Beloved Parents, Family Members
And, above all, the Almighty

"Life is the most difficult exam. Many fail because they tend to copy others, not realizing that everyone has a different question paper."

"Gold medalists are not made up of gold. They are made up of determination and hard work and ready to kill themselves to achieve their goals."

"Success is not the key to happiness. Happiness is the key to success. If you love what you are doing, you will be successful."

"You can succeed only if the fire inside you burns brighter than the fire around."

Golden Rules of Goal Setting

Dear Students

Here are some important tips which will help you in setting your goals in studies:

1. Set Goals That Motivate You: This means making sure that they are important to you, and that there is value in achieving them
2. Set SMART Goals
   - Specific: Your goal must be clear and well defined, not vague or generalized
   - Measurable: Goals must have measurable objectives
   - Attainable : Make sure that your goals are achievable and within your limit
   - Relevant: Will take you to the direction you want your life and career to go
   - Time Bound: You must know when you have the deadline and can celebrate success
3. Set Goals in Writing: Written commitment in presence of your close people (parents, close friends) will always push and remind you whenever you tend to deviate from your goal
4. Make an Action Plan: Do not focus only on the outcome, but make planning of all small steps that collectively take to the outcome. This is especially important if your goal is big and demanding, or long-term
5. Monitor Yourself: Compliance to the action plan should be monitored at least weekly (for one month goal) or monthly (for a yearly goal), depending upon your goal size.

Remember,

"Success is not final; failure is not fatal: It is the courage to continue that counts."
—*Winston S Churchill*

"There are two types of people who will tell you that you cannot make a difference in this world: those who are afraid to try and those who are afraid you will succeed."
—*Ray Goforth*

"Success ke piche mat bhago. Kabil bano kabil. Kamyabi toh sali jhak maar ke peeche ayegi."
—*Aamir Khan*

Preface to the Second Edition

It gives us immense pleasure to announce the release of second edition of *Essentials of Practical Microbiology.* This book is prepared according to competency based medical education (CBME) MBBS curriculum and the content of the book is modified from the traditional organism-based teaching to system-based teaching. The content has been **updated, concised and reshuffled**—the three major types of changes incorporated in this edition. The uniqueness of this book is the Problem Solving Exercises. Each chapter starts with a problem solving exercise, i.e., clinical case scenario. The book is categorized into two sections.

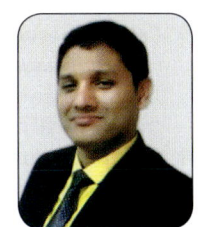

Apurba S Sastry

Section I: General Microbiology, Immunology and Hospital Infection Control

- ❖ **General microbiology** chapters are meticulously restructured with the inclusion of general virology, general parasitology and general mycology chapters. **General bacteriology** is reorganized into a single chapter with several subchapters.
- ❖ **Immunology** chapters are thoroughly updated. Various topics have been updated such as MAC ELISA, Elek's gel precipitation test, etc. have been updated.
- ❖ **Hospital infection control (HIC)** chapters need a special mention. We must say that this section underwent a major update. In the era of COVID-19 pandemic, the practical application of hospital infection control is being increased to thousand folds. Every healthcare personnel is supposed to be well verse with the finer details of HIC. Therefore, the updated version of this section will be a key in making of a skilled Indian medical graduate. The content has been thoroughly updated with the inclusion of new topics such as hand hygiene, personal protective equipment with special emphasis on donning/doffing and transmission-based precautions, needle stick injury, and biomedical waste management. The **sterilization and disinfection** chapter is completely revised based on hospital use of sterilizers and disinfectants rather than traditional 'Microbiology use' and aptly shifted from general microbiology section to HIC section.

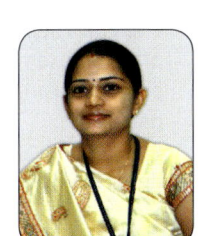

Sandhya Bhat

Section II: Systemic Microbiology (Infectious Diseases)

It comprises of several chapters; each chapter comprises of several infective syndromes pertaining to system. Each infective syndrome starts with a problem solving exercise, followed by the detailed information about the etiological agent(s) and covers the important practical aspects of the topic.
- ❖ **Bloodstream and cardiovascular system infections chapters** cover topics such as infective endocarditis, acute rheumatic fever, sepsis, enteric fever, scrub typhus, brucellosis, leptospirosis HIV/AIDS, dengue, malaria, visceral leishmaniasis, lymphatic filariasis and systemic candidiasis
- ❖ **Gastrointestinal tract infections chapters** cover topics such as shigellosis, nontyphoidal salmonellosis, cholera, *Clostridioides difficile* diarrhea, rotavirus gastroenteritis, intestinal amoebiasis, giardiasis, cryptosporidiosis, intestinal taeniasis, hymenolepiasis, *Schistosoma mansoni* infection, trichuriasis, enterobiasis, ascariasis, hookworm infection and strongyloidiasis
- ❖ **Hepatobiliary system infections chapters** cover topics such as viral hepatitis, amoebic liver abscess and hydatid disease

- ❖ **Respiratory tract infections chapters** cover topics such as streptococcal pharyngitis, diphtheria, pneumococcal pneumonia, *Haemophilus influenzae* pneumonia, *Klebsiella pneumoniae* pneumonia, pulmonary tuberculosis, *Pseudomonas* infections, influenza, COVID-19, infectious mononucleosis, paragonimiasis, zygomycosis, aspergillosis and pneumocystosis
- ❖ **Skin, soft tissue and musculoskeletal system infections chapters** cover topics such as staphylococcal and streptococcal skin and soft tissue infections, gas gangrene, leprosy, cutaneous anthrax, mucocutaneous herpes, measles, rubella, dermatophytoses and mycetoma
- ❖ **Central nervous system infections chapters** cover topics such as pneumococcal meningitis, *Haemophilus influenzae* meningitis, meningococcal meningitis, viral meningitis, HSV encephalitis, Japanese encephalitis, rabies encephalitis, neurocysticercosis, *Toxoplasma* encephalitis and cryptococcal meningitis.
- ❖ **Genitourinary system infections chapters** cover topics such as urinary tract infection (UTI) (*Escherichia coli* UTI, *Klebsiella pneumoniae* UTI, *Proteus mirabilis* UTI, and enterococcal UTI), urinary schistosomiasis, syphilis, gonorrhea, non-gonococcal urethritis, trichomoniasis, vaginal candidiasis
- ❖ **AETCOM module** has been added as a new annexure, which covers several case scenarios pertaining to confidentiality in disclosing laboratory reports and demonstration of respect for patient samples
- ❖ There is a separate chapter for '**university practical examination**' showing the model university practical examination pattern and mark distribution. This will help the students to prepare for their practical examination. This will also help the teacher to modify or update the practical examination pattern.

As you know, human errors are inevitable; and no book is immune to it. We would request all the readers to provide any errata found and also valuable suggestions and updates via e-mail.

This is probably the first practical book in India on 'Clinical Microbiology', in true sense. We are confident and hoping that you all will fall in love with this edition of the book.

Apurba S Sastry
drapurbasastry@gmail.com

Sandhya Bhat
sandhyabhatk@gmail.com

Preface to the First Edition

When there is a dozen of books available in the literature on the same subject, is it required to bring another book? The idea to bring yet another book on Practical Microbiology was born after many discouraging and unsatisfying experiences from several existing books, that did not fulfill the needs of the enthusiastic students on the subject and also a strong desire to make medical microbiology more interesting, up to date, and clinically relevant. This book has several unique approaches which make it different from the existing books.

It is a clinical microbiology practical book. After reading this book, the students will have a bird's eye view on how to diagnose infectious diseases clinically followed by how to go about laboratory investigations.

It is the first microbiology book which is written in class-wise pattern according to MBBS practical class schedule. This will help the teacher know what to teach during a practical class, what to keep for demonstration during the practical class and also will give the teacher a holistic approach to make the yearly practical schedule. This will also help the students to know what to read during a practical class, what to write in the records and what to read during MBBS university practical examination.

There is a separate chapter for university practical examination providing the pattern for various universities. This will help the students prepare for their practical examination. This will also help the teacher to modify or update the practical examination pattern.

The uniqueness of this book is the Problem-based Exercises. Each chapter starts with a problem-based exercise, i.e. clinical case scenario. The whole chapter is about solving the problem covering the important practical aspects of the topic.

There are more than 600 images, kept according to the demonstrations of practical classes, which will help the teachers know what is needed to demonstrate in practical classes. If facility is not available, they can just keep the image itself during the practical class. Images will help the students coordinate and read about the items demonstrated in the class with what is given in the practical book.

Like our other books, this one also has followed the same principle, e.g. more content accommodated in less pages so as to give handy look and saving student's time, written in a concise, bulleted format and to-the-point text and simple and lucid language.

Several new practical class topics are covered in this book which are essential for MBBS graduates to learn, but are often missed in practical classes of most colleges, such as demonstration of automated culture and molecular methods; antimicrobial susceptibility testing (reading of disk diffusion and minimum inhibitory concentration)—interpretation with reference to Clinical and Laboratory Standards Institute (CLSI); sterilization and disinfection—according to hospital practice with special note on Central Sterile Services Department (CSSD), enzyme-linked immunosorbent assay (ELISA) and immunofluorescence, Western blot and rapid test; laboratory diagnosis of leptospirosis and scrub typhus and dengue; hepatitis viruses (understanding the interpretation of algorithms of markers); human immunodeficiency virus [understanding the interpretation of tests according to National AIDS Control Organization (NACO) guideline]; bacteriology of water, air and surface—importance of environmental surveillance; hospital-acquired infection—methods to perform hand hygiene and WHO's five moments of hand hygiene; biomedical waste—concept of segregation of waste in appropriate color-coded bags according to 2016 rule; vaccines and tables in parasitology chapters to make understanding easy.

We believe that this book would bring revolution in microbiology and help in modifying the pattern of undergraduate teaching in practical classes across the country by incorporating newer diagnostics and essential topics with the clinical touch.

Apurba S Sastry
drapurbasastry@gmail.com

Sandhya Bhat
sandhyabhatk@gmail.com

Acknowledgments

We take this opportunity to extend our sincere gratitude and appreciation to the following people without whom it would not have been possible to release the second edition of *Essentials of Practical Microbiology*.

Hearty acknowledgments to our teachers, departmental staff, family members and others, for their blessings and support.

1. We would like to sincerely thank **Dr Deepashree R,** Assistant Professor, Department of Microbiology, JSS Medical College, Mysuru, Karnataka and **Dr Anand B Janagond,** Professor, Department of Microbiology, S Nijalingappa Medical College, Bagalkot, Karnataka for their constant inputs during manuscript preparation.
2. We express heart-felt gratitude to **Dr Sujatha Sistla**, Professor, Department of Microbiology, JIPMER, for her guidance during manuscript preparation. I (Dr Apurba) am greatly indebted to you mam for your timely support and guidance.
3. We are extremely thankful to **Dr Rakesh Aggarwal,** Director, JIPMER, Puducherry for giving the permission to revise this textbook.
4. We are grateful to **Dr Renu G Boy Varghese**, Director-Principal, Pondicherry Institute of Medical Sciences (PIMS), Puducherry, for giving permission to revise this textbook.
5. We are extremely thankful to **Dr Jharna Mandal**, Additional Professor and Head, Department of Microbiology, JIPMER, for her constant encouragement and support during the preparation of the manuscript.
6. We would like to express our special word of thanks to **Dr Reba Kanungo**, Dean Research, Professor and Head, Department of Microbiology, Pondicherry Institute of Medical Sciences (PIMS). I (Dr Sandhya) am truly grateful to you mam for your wholehearted support.
7. **Other Faculty of Department of Microbiology, JIPMER**—Dr Rakesh Singh (Additional Professor), Dr Rahul Dhodapkar (Additional Professor), Dr Noyal M Joseph (Associate Professor), Dr Rakhi Biswas (Associate Professor), Dr Nonika Rajkumari (Associate Professor) and Dr Maanasa Bhaskar (Assistant Professor).
8. **Other Faculty of Department of Microbiology, PIMS**—Dr Shashikala (Professor), Dr Sheela Devi (Professor), Dr Johny Asir (Professor), Dr Vivian Joseph P (Professor), Dr Sujitha E (Associate Professor), Dr Anandhalakshmi (Associate Professor), Dr Arthi E (Associate Professor), Mrs Patricia Anita (Associate Professor), Dr Meghna (Assistant Professor) and Mrs Desdemona Rasitha (Tutor).
9. **Residents and postgraduates, JIPMER**—Dr Ketan Priyadarshi, Dr Mugundan, Dr Sindhu, Dr Gopichand, Dr Radha, Dr Rachna, Dr Sarumathi, Dr Anitha, Dr Kalpana, Dr Monika, Dr Lakshmi, Dr Soundarya, Dr Kowshalya, Dr Lullu, Dr Imola, Dr Symphonia, Dr Pheba, Ms Rosemary, Ms Lakshmishree, Ms Gopika and Ms Neeshma.
10. **HICC, JIPMER**—Infection control nurses and other office staff such as Ms Ilaveni, Ms Ramya and Mr Venkat.
11. **For providing photographs**—We are extremely thankful to all people/institutes/companies who have agreed to provide valuable photographs.
12. **Dr Abhishekh Mitra,** Senior Resident, AIIMS, Raipur, for his inputs during manuscript preparation of COVID-19 Chapter.
13. **Dr Anand Sastry**, Department of Neuromedicine, Banaras Hind University (BHU), Varanasi, Uttar Pradesh. For giving inputs during manuscript preparation of various CNS infections.

14. **Ex-residents from JIPMER: Dr Haritha M** and others—for giving inputs in the correction of content errors of first edition.
15. **Each and every reader** (faculty and students) from various parts of the country—for communicating to us by email and other electronic media about the content correction and updates from time to time.
16. **Our friends**—Dr Godfred, Dr Sadia, Dr Ramakrishna, Dr Mridula, Dr Srinivas Acharya, Dr Chaya, Dr Manisha, Dr Ira, Dr Sreeja, Dr Wajid, Dr Kumudavathi and others.
17. **Family**—Parents, brother, sister and other family members, maternal and paternal cousins and all other well-wishers.

Special Acknowledgments to My Publishers
Jaypee Brothers Medical Publishers (P) Ltd, New Delhi, India
- Shri Jitendar P Vij (Group Chairman)
- Mr Ankit Vij (Managing Director)
- Mr MS Mani (Group President)
- Dr Madhu Choudhary (Publishing Head–Education): She has been a great support throughout the manuscript preparation
- Ms Pooja Bhandari (Production Head)
- Ms Seema Dogra (Cover Visualizer)
- Dr Astha Sawhney (Development Editor): Extremely dynamic, have lot of patience and available 24x7 to address to our queries
- **The Development Team:** Mr Deepak Saxena (Typesetter), Mr Nitin Bhardwaj (Graphic Designer), Ms Neelam, Mr Laxmidhar and Mr Vakil Khan (Proofreaders). These guys are simply outstanding in their work. A special mention for Mr Deepak Saxena, we must say that he is the best operator of India in medical publishing. The way Nitin Bhardwaj does the designing of photographs is extraordinary. It is a treat for us to work with all of them. These guys are extremely workaholic and have a very good team spirit. We salute them, for their professionalism.
- **Marketing heads from various zones:** Mr Narendra Shekhawat (Vice President–Sales), Mr Venugopal V (South Head), Mr Rishi Sharma (North Region Head), CS Gawde (Western Head) and Sandip Gupta (Eastern Head).
- **Branch managers and Sales manager from various branches:** Bengaluru branch (Ravi Kumar, A Palani, E Venkatesh, Vivek Bhagawan), Chennai branch (Maran A [Adoption Head for South], Dharani Kumar P, RK Dharani, Dharanidaran), Kochi branch (Sujeesh VS, Diffin Robin, Arun Kumar), Hyderabad branch (Parimal Guha Neogy, Marthanda Sarma, Rajesh Malothu, Hamza Ali), Mumbai branch (Sameer S Mulla), Nagpur branch (Rajesh Shrivas), Ahmedabad branch (Ms Priyanka Kansara, Dinesh Waghade), Delhi branch (Sujatha Puri), and Kolkata branch (Sanjoy Chakraborthy).

Lastly, we would like to keep in record that without the support of our son, parents (of both Dr Sandhya and Dr Apurba) and other family members, it would have been impossible to continue the spirit on, during the journey of the current edition. A special mention to our son (Master Adarsh), who really helped us being very much cooperative. In fact, he was encouraging us to work for the book. We deeply apologize to you as well as our parents (Mr Anooj Sastry and Ms Tarini Purohit), as we could not give enough time and care during the manuscript preparation.

Apurba S Sastry
Sandhya Bhat

Contents

	Competency Number (MCI Curriculum)	Pages

Section 1: General Microbiology, Immunology and Hospital Infection Control

General Microbiology
1. Introduction to Microbiology Department — MI 1.1 — 3
2. Microscopy — MI 1.1, **1.2** — 5
3. General Bacteriology
    - 3.1. Morphology and Physiology of Bacteria — MI 1.1 — 12
    - 3.2. Specimen Collection and Transport — MI 8.9, **8.10** — 17
    - 3.3. Direct Detection 1: Simple Staining — MI 1.1, **1.2** — 23
    - 3.4. Direct Detection 2: Gram Staining — MI **1.2** — 25
    - 3.5. Direct Detection 3: Special Staining (Acid-Fast Stain, Albert Stain) and Other Methods — MI 1.1, **1.2**, 8.15 — 28
    - 3.6. Culture Media (Including Automated Culture) and Culture Methods — MI 1.1, 8.15 — 32
    - 3.7. Identification of Bacteria (Conventional and Automated) — MI 1.1, 8.15 — 42
    - 3.8. Antimicrobial Susceptibility Test — MI 1.6 — 49
    - 3.9 Molecular Diagnosis — MI 8.15 — 56
4. Laboratory Diagnosis of Viral Diseases — MI 1.1, **8.10**, 8.15 — 59
5. Laboratory Diagnosis of Parasitic Diseases — MI **1.2**, **8.10**, 8.15 — 68
6. Laboratory Diagnosis of Fungal Diseases — MI 1.1, **8.10**, 8.15 — 74

Immunology
7. Precipitation and Agglutination — MI 8.15 — 77
8. ELISA, ELFA and Immunofluorescence — MI 8.15 — 83
9. Western Blot, Rapid Tests and CLIA — MI 8.15 — 88

Hospital Infection control
10. Standard Precautions: Hand hygiene and PPE — MI **8.7** — 92
11. Transmission-based Precautions — MI 8.6, **8.7** — 101
12. Sterilization and Disinfection — MI 1.5 — 108
13. Biomedical Waste Management — MI 8.6 — 117
14. Needle Stick Injury — MI 8.6, **8.7** — 121
15. Environmental Surveillance — MI 8.8 — 125

Note: Competency numbers **highlighted bold** are skill based competencies.

Section 2: Systemic Microbiology (Infectious Diseases)

Bloodstream and Cardiovascular System Infections

16. Cardiovascular System Infections: Infective Endocarditis and Acute Rheumatic Fever — MI **2.3** — 133
17. Bloodstream Infections — MI **2.3**, 8.15 — 138
18. Bacterial Infections of Bloodstream: Enteric Fever, Scrub Typhus, Brucellosis, and Leptospirosis — MI **3.4**, **8.10**, 8.15 — 142
19. Viral Infections of Bloodstream: HIV/AIDS and Dengue — MI 2.7, 8.15 — 153
20. Parasitic Infections of Bloodstream: Malaria, Visceral Leishmaniasis and Lymphatic Filariasis — MI **2.6** — 162
21. Fungal Infections of Bloodstream: Systemic Candidiasis and Systemic Mycoses — MI 1.1, 8.15 — 172

Gastrointestinal Infections

22. Bacterial Diarrhea: Shigellosis, Cholera and Others — MI **3.2** — 176
23. Viral Gastroenteritis: Rotaviruses and Others — MI **3.2** — 184
24. Intestinal Protozoan Infections: Intestinal Amoebiasis, Giardiasis and Coccidian Parasitic Infections — MI **1.2**, **3.2**, 8.15 — 186
25. Intestinal Helminthic Infections — MI **1.2**, **3.2**, 8.15 — 192
    - Intestinal Cestode Infections: Intestinal Taeniasis, Hymenolepiasis and Others
    - Intestinal Trematode Infections: *Fasciolopsis buski*, *Schistosoma mansoni* and Others
    - Intestinal Nematode Infections: Trichuriasis, Enterobiasis, Ascariasis, Hookworm Infection, Strongyloidiasis

Hepatobiliary System Infections

26. Viral Hepatitis — MI 3.8 — 203
27. Parasitic Infections of Hepatobiliary System: Amoebic Liver Abscess, Hydatid Disease and Others — MI 3.1, **3.2** — 208

Skin, Soft Tissue and Musculoskeletal System Infections

28. Staphylococcal Infections — MI 4.2, 4.3, **1.2** — 211
29. Beta-hemolytic Streptococcal Infections — MI 4.3, **1.2** — 215
30. Miscellaneous Bacterial Infections of Skin and Soft Tissues: Anaerobic Infections including Gas Gangrene, Leprosy and Anthrax — MI 4.3, **1.2**, **8.10**, 8.15 — 220
31. Viral Exanthems and Other Cutaneous Viral Infections: Herpes Simplex, Measles, Rubella and Others — MI 4.3, **8.10**, 8.15 — 227
32. Superficial and Subcutaneous Fungal Infections — MI 4.3, **8.10**, 8.15 — 236

Respiratory Tract Infections

33. Bacterial Pharyngitis: *Streptococcus pyogenes* Pharyngitis and Diphtheria — MI 6.2, **8.10**, 8.15 — 243

Note: Competency numbers **highlighted bold** are skill based competencies.

34. Bacterial Pneumonia: Pneumococcal Pneumonia, *Haemophilus influenzae* Pneumonia, *Klebsiella pneumoniae* Pneumonia and Others	MI 6.3, **1.2**, **8.10**, 8.15	250
35. Tuberculosis	MI **6.3**, 8.15	260
36. *Pseudomonas* and *Acinetobacter* Infections	MI **6.3**	268
37. Viral Infections of Respiratory Tract: Influenza, COVID-19, Infectious Mononucleosis, and Others	MI **6.2**, **6.3**	272
38. Parasitic and Fungal Infections of Respiratory Tract: Paragonimiasis, Zygomycosis, Aspergillosis, Pneumocystosis and Others	MI **6.2**, **6.3**	281

Central Nervous System Infections

39. Bacterial Meningitis	MI **5.3**, **1.2**, **8.10**, 8.15	288
40. Viral Meningitis and Viral Encephalitis (Enteroviruses including Polio, Rabies, Japanese Encephalitis and Others)	MI 1.1, **5.3**, 8.15	295
41. Parasitic and Fungal Infections of Central Nervous System: Neurocysticercosis, Free-living Amoebae Infections, Toxoplasmosis, Cryptococcal Meningitis and Others	MI 1.1, 5.1, **5.3**, 8.15	302

Urogenital Tract Infections

42. Urinary Tract Infections	MI 7.3, 8.10, 8.15	307
43. Infective Syndromes of Genital Tract (Sexually-transmitted Infections) : Syphilis, Gonorrhoea, Non-gonococcal Urethritis (*Chlamydia trachomatis*), Vulvovaginitis (Trichomoniasis, Vaginal Candidiasis) and Others	MI 7.1, 7.2, **8.10**, 8.15	316

Miscellaneous

44. AETCOM in Microbiology	MI **8.11**, **8.14**	324
45. University Practical Examination		330

Index   *333*

Note: Competency numbers **highlighted bold** are skill based competencies.

Further Reading

1. Bailey & Scott's Diagnostic Microbiology, 14th Edition.
2. Harrison's Principles of Internal Medicine, 20th Edition.
3. Indian Council of Medical Research, New Delhi, India.
4. Jawetz Melnick and Adelbergs' Medical Microbiology, 28th Edition.
5. Koneman's Color Atlas and Textbook of Diagnostic Microbiology, 7th Edition.
6. Kuby's Immunology, 8th Edition.
7. Mackie and McCartney's Practical Medical Microbiology, 14th Edition.
8. National AIDS Control Organisation (NACO), India.
9. Revised National Tuberculosis Control Program (RNTCP), India.
10. Garcia's Diagnostic Medical Parasitology, 6th edition.
11. Various national and international journals and other internet sources.
12. World Health Organization (WHO).
13. Centers for Disease Control and Prevention, Atlanta, USA.

SECTION 1

General Microbiology, Immunology and Hospital Infection Control

SECTION OUTLINE

1. Introduction to Microbiology Department
2. Microscopy
3. General Bacteriology
   3.1. Morphology and Physiology of Bacteria
   3.2. Specimen Collection and Transport
   3.3. Direct Detection 1: Simple Staining
   3.4. Direct Detection 2: Gram Staining
   3.5. Direct Detection 3: Special Staining (Acid-Fast Stain, Albert Stain) and Other Methods
   3.6. Culture Media (Including Automated Culture) and Culture Methods
   3.7. Identification of Bacteria (Conventional and Automated)
   3.8. Antimicrobial Susceptibility Test
   3.9. Molecular Diagnosis
4. Laboratory Diagnosis of Viral Diseases
5. Laboratory Diagnosis of Parasitic Diseases
6. Laboratory Diagnosis of Fungal Diseases
7. Precipitation and Agglutination
8. ELISA, ELFA and Immunofluorescence
9. Western Blot, Rapid Tests and CLIA

10. Standard Precautions: Hand Hygiene and PPE
11. Transmission-based Precautions
12. Sterilization and Disinfection
13. Biomedical Waste Management
14. Needle Stick Injury
15. Environmental Surveillance

Introduction to Microbiology Department

CHAPTER 1

This is the first practical class in the department of Microbiology. In this class, a formal interaction between students and teachers (faculty/post-graduate students) takes place where:

- **Introduction:** The students and the teachers introduce themselves
- **Batch distribution:** Students are divided into batches and table teachers are allotted for each batch
- **Departmental tour:** Students are taken for the departmental tour. Activities/investigations carried out in each section are briefed to the students
- General instructions to be followed (see below).

General Instructions
The following instructions to be followed during the practical classes are conveyed to the students:
1. Students should wear clean ironed white coat
2. Students are warned about the importance of attendance and coming to the class on time
3. Practical record: Students must get the practical record to the class every time; which must be filled and signed by the table teacher on time
4. Girls should put their hair inside the white coat to avoid infection
5. Nails should be kept clean and short. No artificial nails should be worn
6. Personal belongings and bags should not be kept near work benches
7. No eatables should be brought into the student's practical laboratory
8. Do not put your fingers into your mouth during the practical class hours
9. Care of the microscope: Students are instructed how to handle and take care of the microscope (explained in Chapter 2)
10. All the slides must be stained on staining rod over the wash basin
11. Cap all the reagent bottles and place them in order in the rack after use
12. In case of accidental spillage of reagents, inform the table teacher immediately
13. In case of accidental contact of cultures or infectious materials, wash hands with the hand-wash solution immediately and inform the table teacher
14. While leaving the hall: Switch off the microscope, clean the lenses and discard the slide in the discarding jar after use
15. Handwashing: Students must perform handwashing at the end of every practical class before leaving the hall. Students are demonstrated how to perform handwash. The steps of handwashing are demonstrated and explained to them (Fig. 1.1)

Problem Solving Exercise

Rohan, a 2nd year MBBS student has attended a Microbiology practical session on Gram staining. After the class got over, he wanted to do handwashing. However, as there was a long queue of 70 students at the hand wash station, he decided to go to hostel and perform handwashing.
1. Opine, if the decision of Rohan was correct?
2. What are the steps to perform handwashing?
3. List the instructions to be followed by a 2nd year MBBS student who has attended a Microbiology practical session?

Explanation
No, Rohan's decision of going to hostel and then performing hand wash was wrong. As hands are contaminated with potential microorganisms in the Microbiology laboratory, students must immediately perform handwashing after the practical class. For answers to the other questions, refer text.

SECTION 1 ◈ General Microbiology, Immunology and Hospital Infection Control

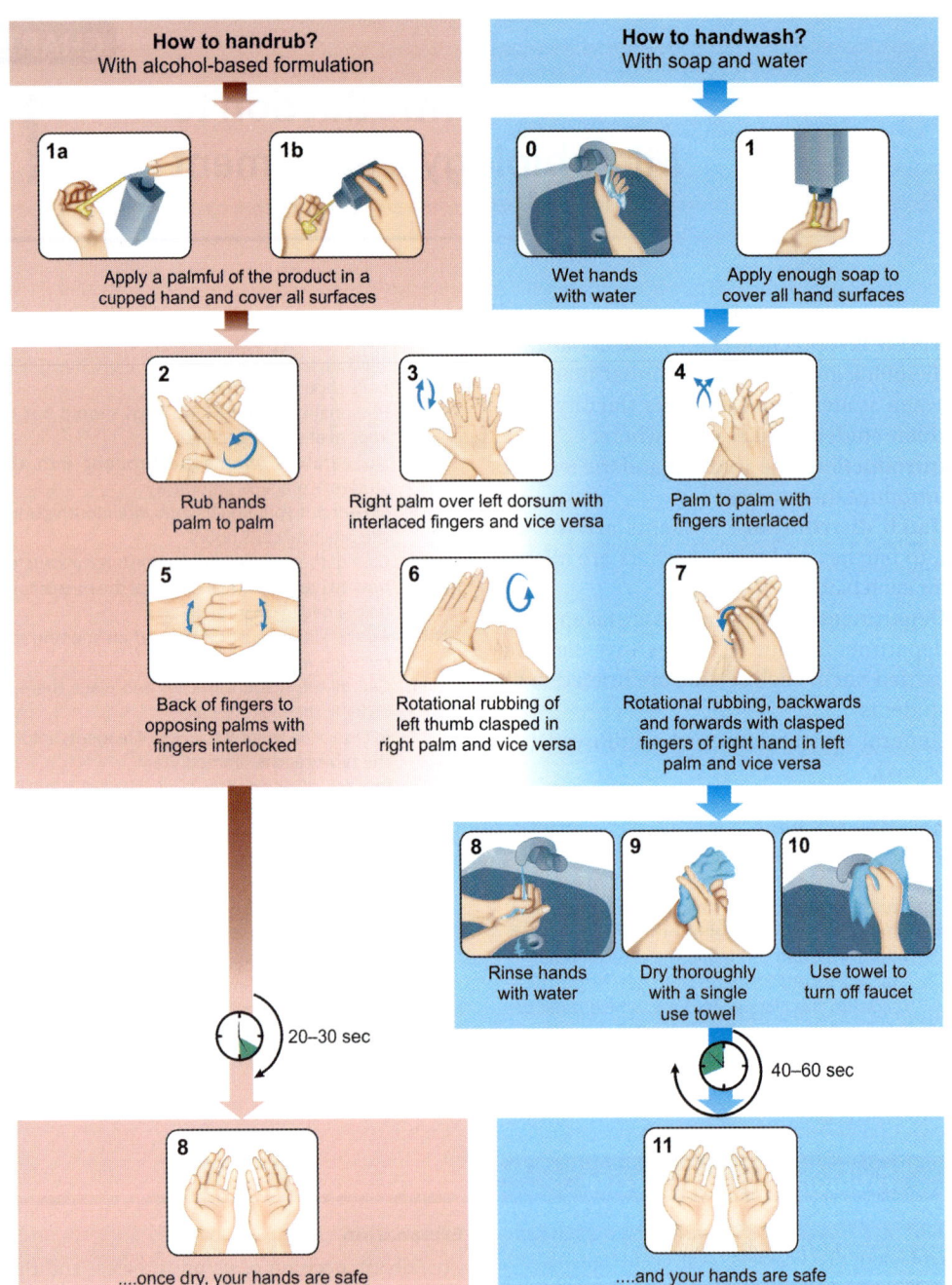

Fig. 1.1: Steps of handrub and handwash.
Source: World Health Organization.

Microscopy

CHAPTER 2

A microscope is an instrument used to see objects that are too small to be seen by the naked eye.

MICROSCOPE CARE

Proper care and maintenance of microscope can extend its life by many years.
- ❖ **Handle with care:** While carrying the microscope, hold it in both the hands, one hand supporting the base and the other holding the metal support arm. Do not pick it up by the stage, as this can cause misalignment
- ❖ **Keep lenses clear of slides:** While adjusting the microscope, lower the objective lens down carefully till the focus plane, without allowing the lens to touch the slide
- ❖ **Clean lenses:** Ensure the lenses are cleaned immediately after use, especially if using immersion oil. Use only lens paper and lens cleaner (not solvents). Rub the lens gently in a circular motion to remove sticky residue
- ❖ **Care of the bulb:** Turn off the bulb after use. When turning the microscope on and off, use the switch; not directly the power source. Do not switch the microscope on/off while using full light intensity. Never touch the bulb
- ❖ **Store:** Cover when not in use and store in a clean, dry place preferably in a cabinet. Do not remove eyepieces.

PROPERTIES OF A MICROSCOPE

A good microscope should have at least three properties:
1. **Good resolution:** Resolution power refers to the ability to produce separate images of closely placed objects so that they can be distinguished as two separate entities. The resolution power of:
    - Unaided human eye is about 0.2 mm (200 µm)
    - Light microscope is about 0.2 µm
    - Electron microscope is about 0.5 nm.

    Resolution depends on **refractive index** of the medium. Oil has a higher refractive index than air; hence use of oil enhances the resolution power of a microscope.
2. **Good contrast:** This can be further improved by staining of the specimen
3. **Good magnification:** This is achieved by use of lenses:
    - **Objective lenses:** Scanning (4X), low power (10X), high power (40X) and oil immersion (100X)
    - Ocular lens with a magnification power of 10X.

    Total magnification of a field is the product of the magnification of objective lens and ocular lens.
    - Scanning field (40X)
    - Low power field (100X)
    - High power field (400X)
    - Oil immersion field (1000X).

MICROMETRY

Micrometry refers to the measurement of dimensions of the microorganisms under a microscope by using micrometers. There are two micrometers, namely (1) ocular micrometer, and (2) stage micrometer (Figs 2.1A and B).
- ❖ **Ocular micrometer** is a circular glass disk that fits into the eyepiece of the microscope. It has 100 equally spaced divisions (Marked as 0–10, at every 10 division interval) (Fig. 2.1A)
- ❖ The **stage micrometer** is clipped to the stage of the microscope. In the center of the stage micrometer, a known 1 mm distance is divided

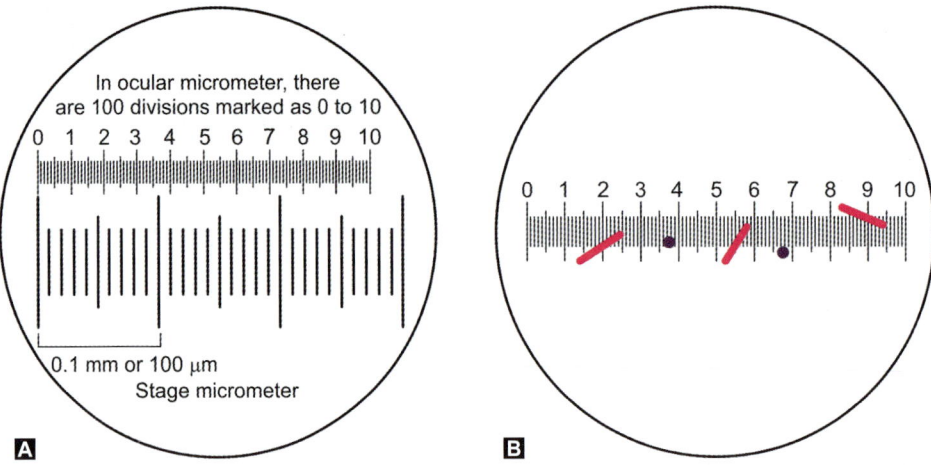

Figs 2.1A and B: (A) Principle of micrometry [The divisions of ocular micrometer are superimposed on graduations of stage micrometer. Distance between two graduations of stage micrometer equals to 37 divisions of ocular micrometer. Therefore, one division of ocular micrometer (i.e., calibration factor) measures to 100/37 = 2.7 µm]; (B) Stage micrometer is removed. Slide containing bacteria is focused. Size of the bacteria is determined by number of divisions of ocular micrometer it corresponds × 2.7 µm.

into 10 divisions (0.1 mm); each is further divided into 10 graduations of 0.01 mm or 10 µm each
- **Calibration:** The graduations on both micrometers are superimposed on each other. Then the graduations on the ocular microscope are calibrated against the standard graduations on the stage micrometer as given below (Fig. 2.1A):

> **Calibration factor** for one division on ocular micrometer (in µm) =
> $$\frac{\text{Known distance between two lines on stage micrometer, i.e., 100 µm}}{\text{Number of divisions on ocular micrometer that lies between two lines of stage micrometer}}$$
>
> Therefore in the above example (Fig. 2.1), one division of ocular micrometer (i.e., calibration factor) measures to 100/37 = 2.7 µm.
> Hence size of the bacteria = The number of divisions of ocular micrometer it corresponds to × 2.7 µm

- **Measurement:** After calibration, the ocular micrometer is used to measure the size of various microbes, such as length, breadth, and diameter. First, count the number of divisions occupied in ocular micrometer by the organism. Then, multiply this number by the calculated calibration factor. This value indicates the size of the organism (Fig. 2.1B).

TYPE OF MICROSCOPES

The following types of microscopes are in use now:
- Bright-field or light microscope
- Dark-field microscope
- Phase-contrast microscope
- Fluorescence microscope
- Electron microscope.

Bright-Field or Light Microscope

The bright-field or light microscope forms a dark image against a brighter background, hence the name.

Structure

The parts in a bright-field microscope are divided into three groups (Fig. 2.2):

Mechanical Parts
- **Base:** It holds various parts of microscope, such as the light source, the fine and coarse adjustment knobs
- **C-shaped arm:** It is used for holding the microscope and it connects the eyepiece to the objective lens
- **Mechanical stage:** The arm bears a stage with stage clips to hold the slides and the stage control knobs to move the slide

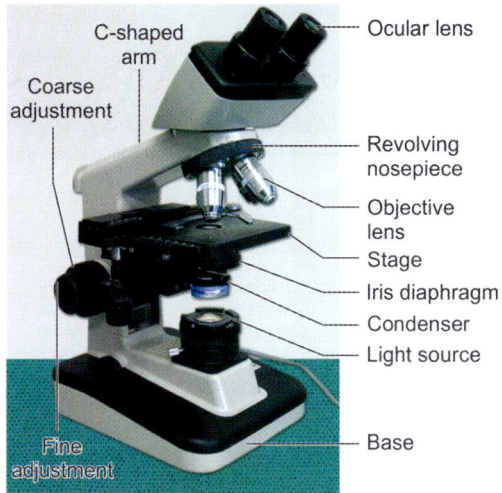

Fig. 2.2: Bright-field microscope.
Source: Nikon Alphaphot (*with permission*).

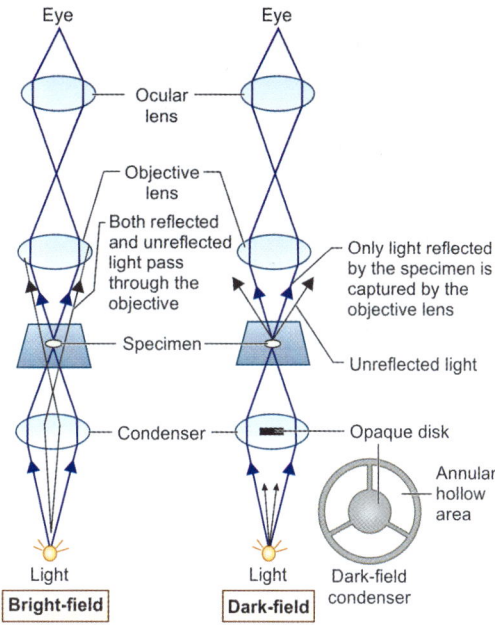

Fig. 2.3: Light pathways of bright-field microscopes and dark-field microscopes.

during viewing. It has an aperture at the center to permit light to reach the object from the bottom.

Magnifying Parts
- **Ocular lens:** The arm contains an eyepiece that bears an ocular lens of 10X magnification power. Microscopes with two eyepieces are called as binocular microscopes
- **Objective lens:** The arm also contains a revolving nosepiece that bears three to five objectives with lenses of differing magnifying power (4X, 10X, 40X and 100X).

Illuminating Parts
- **Condenser:** It is mounted beneath the stage which focuses a cone of light on the slide
- **Iris diaphragm:** It controls the light that passes through the condenser
- **Light source:** It may be a mirror or an electric bulb
- **Fine and coarse adjustment knobs:** They sharpen the image.

Working Principle
The rays emitted from the light source pass through the iris diaphragm and fall on the specimen. The light rays passing through the specimen are gathered by the objective and a magnified image is formed. This image is further magnified by the ocular lens to produce the final magnified virtual image (Fig. 2.3).

Dark-field Microscope

Principle
In dark-field microscope, the object appears bright against a dark background. This is made possible by use of a special dark-field condenser (Fig. 2.3).
- The dark-field condenser has a central opaque area that blocks light from entering the objective lens directly and has a peripheral annular hollow area which allows the light to pass through and focus on the specimen obliquely
- Only the light which is reflected by the specimen enters the objective lens, whereas the unreflected light does not enter the objective. As a result, the specimen is brightly illuminated, but the background appears dark.

Applications
Dark-field microscope is used to:
- Identify the living, unstained cells

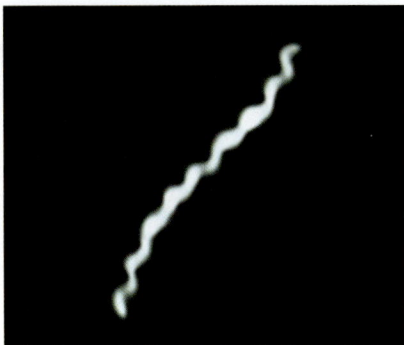

Fig. 2.4: Dark ground microscopic picture demonstrating spirally coiled bacteria (spirochete).
Source: Public Health Image Library, ID# 2043; Centers for Disease Control and Prevention (CDC), Atlanta (*with permission*).

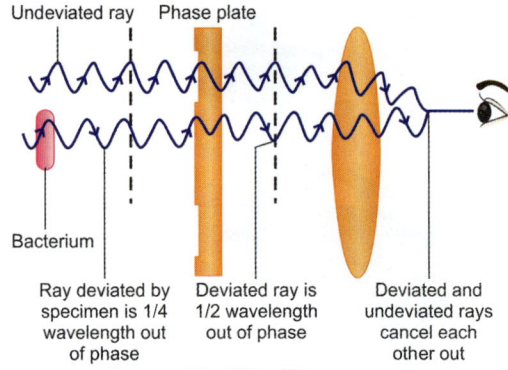

Fig. 2.5: Principle of phase-contrast microscope.

- Identify thin bacteria like spirochetes which cannot be visualized by light microscopy (Fig. 2.4).

Phase-contrast Microscope

Contrast is an important property of a microscope to visualize the objects. Contrast can be enhanced by staining the specimen. However, as staining kills the microbes, the properties of living cells cannot be studied.

The phase-contrast microscope is used to visualize the living cells by creating difference in contrast between the cells and water. It converts slight differences in refractive index and cell density into easily detectable variations in light intensity.

Principle

The condenser is similar to that of dark-field microscope, consists of an opaque central area with a thin, transparent ring which produces a hollow cone of light.
- As this cone of light passes through a cell, some light rays are bent due to variations in density and refractive index within the specimen and are retarded by about one-fourth of a wavelength (Fig. 2.5)
- The undeviated light rays strike a *phase ring* in the phase plate, (a special optical disk located in the objective), while the deviated rays miss the ring and pass through the rest of the plate

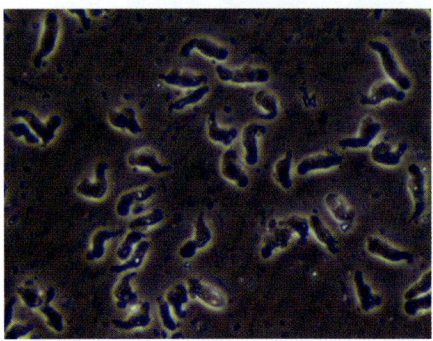

Fig. 2.6: Phase-contrast microscopic picture demonstrating *Naegleria fowleri* trophozoites (free-living amoeba)
Source: Centers for Disease Control and Prevention (CDC), Atlanta (*with permission*).

- The phase ring is constructed in such a way that the undeviated light passing through it is advanced by one-fourth of a wavelength, the deviated and undeviated waves will be about half wavelength out of the phase and will cancel each other when they come together to form an image (Fig. 2.5)
- The background, formed by undeviated light, is bright, while the unstained object appears dark and well-defined (Fig. 2.6).

The light rays go through → condenser → specimen (e.g., bacterium) → phase ring → objective lens → ocular lens.

Applications

Phase-contrast microscopy is especially useful for studying:

- Microbial motility
- Determining the shape of living cells
- Detecting microbial internal cellular components, such as the cell membrane, nuclei, mitochondria, spindles, chromosomes, Golgi apparatus, endospores and inclusion bodies; which become clearly visible because they have refractive indices markedly different from that of water.

Fluorescence Microscope

The "fluorescence microscope" refers to any microscope that uses fluorescence property to generate an image.

Principle

When fluorescent dyes are exposed to ultraviolet (UV) rays, they become excited and are said to fluoresce, i.e., they convert this invisible, short wavelength rays into light of longer wavelengths (i.e., visible light) (Fig. 2.7).
- The source of light may be a mercury-vapor lamp, which emits rays that pass through an excitation filter
- The excitation filter is so designed that it allows only short wavelength UV light (about 400 nm) to pass through, blocking all other long wavelength rays
- The exciting rays then get reflected by a dichromatic mirror in such a way that they fall on the specimen, which is stained with fluorescent dye
- The fluorescent dye absorbs the exciting rays of short wavelength, gets activated and in turn emits fluorescent rays of higher wavelength
- A barrier filter positioned after the objective lens removes any remaining UV light, which could damage the viewer's eyes, or blue and violet light, which would reduce the image's contrast.

Applications of Fluorescence Microscopy

Epifluorescence microscope: It is the simplest form of fluorescence microscope, which has the following applications:
- **Auto-fluorescence:** Certain microbes directly fluoresce when placed under UV lamp, e.g., *Cyclospora* (a protozoan parasite)
- **Microbes coated with fluorescent dye:** Certain microbes fluoresce when they are stained by fluorochrome dyes
  - Acridine orange dye is used for the detection of parasites, such as *Plasmodium* and filarial nematodes by a method called as quantitative buffy coat (QBC) examination
  - Auramine phenol is used for the detection of tubercle bacilli (Fig. 2.8).
- **Immunofluorescence:** It uses fluorescent dye-tagged immunoglobulins to detect cell surface antigens or antibodies bound to cell surface antigens. There are two types—

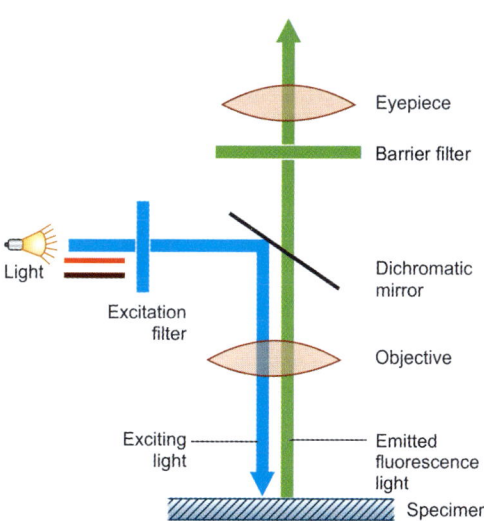

Fig. 2.7: Principle of fluorescence microscope.

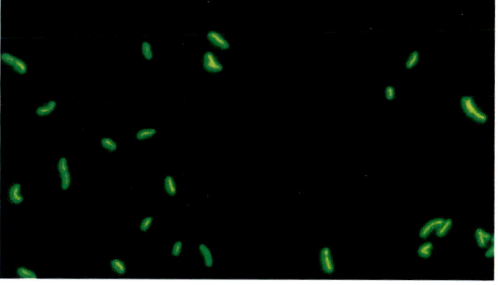

Fig. 2.8: Tubercle bacilli seen under fluorescence microscope.
Source: Department of Microbiology, JIPMER, Puducherry (*with permission*).

direct and indirect immunofluorescence test (described in detail in Chapter 8).

Electron Microscope

An electron microscope (EM) uses accelerated electrons as a source of illumination. It has a much better resolving power than a light microscope; hence, it can reveal the details of flagella, fimbriae and intracellular structures of a cell. EMs are of two types:
1. Transmission electron microscope (most common type) (Fig. 2.9)
2. Scanning electron microscope (SEM).

Differences between light microscope and EM are listed in Table 2.1.

Transmission Electron Microscope

Specimen Preparation

Very thin specimens (20–100 nm thickness) are suitable for EM. To prepare the thin specimen, cells are first fixed by using glutaraldehyde or osmium tetroxide, then dehydrated with organic solvents (e.g., acetone) and then finally embedded in plastic polymer to form a solid block. Followed which specimen is cut into thin slices by ultramicrotome knife and mounted on a metal slide (copper).

Electron Pathway

Electrons are generated by electron gun, which travel in high speed. The medium of travel in EM should be a fully vacuum path because in air path, electrons can get deflected by collisions with air molecules.
- Electron pass through a magnetic condenser and then bombard on the thin-sliced specimen mounted on the copper slide
- The specimen scatters electrons passing through it, and then the electron beam is focused by magnetic lenses to form an enlarged, visible image of the specimen on a fluorescent screen (Figs 2.10 and 2.11).

Various measures are followed to increase the contrast of EM, such as:
- **Staining with** heavy metal salts, such as lead citrate and uranyl acetate
- **Negative staining** with heavy metals, such as phosphotungstic acid

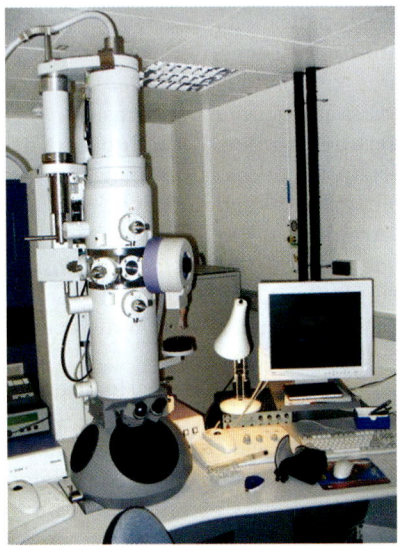

Fig. 2.9: Transmission electron microscope.
Source: David J Morgan/Wikipedia.

Table 2.1: Differences between light microscope and electron microscope.

Features	Light microscope	Electron microscope
Highest practical magnification	About 1,000–1,500	Over 100,000
Best resolution	0.2 µm	0.5 nm
Radiation source	Visible light	Electron beam
Medium of travel	Air	High vacuum
Specimen mount	Glass slide	Metal grid (usually copper)
Type of lens	Glass	Electromagnet

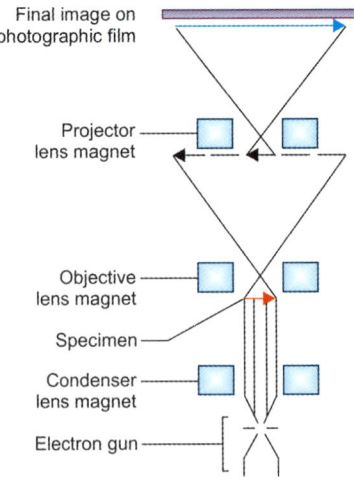

Fig. 2.10: Principle of transmission electron microscope.

CHAPTER 2 ◆ Microscopy

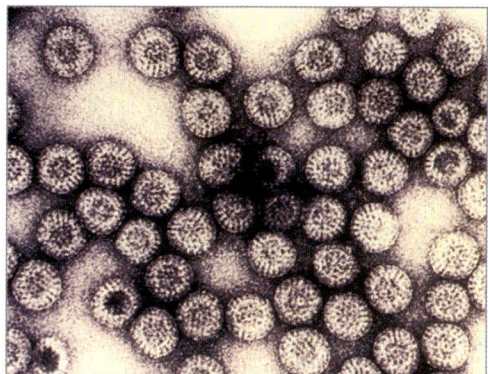

Fig. 2.11: Rotavirus (electron micrograph).
Source: Public Health Image Library, /ID# 15194/Dr Erskine L Palmer/Centers for Disease Control and Prevention (CDC), Atlanta (*with permission*).

- ❖ **Shadowing:** Specimen is coated with a thin film of platinum or other heavy metal at 45° angle so that the metal strikes the microorganism on only one side
- ❖ **Freeze-etching technique** is used to view internal organelles within the organisms giving a *three-dimensional* view.

Scanning Electron Microscope

Scanning electron microscope has been used to examine the surfaces of microorganisms in great detail. It has a resolution of 7 nm or less. The SEM differs from other EM in producing an image from electrons emitted by an object's surface rather than from transmitted electrons.

Problem Solving Exercise

1. A microscopic photograph has been provided (Fig. 2.8). Which microscope is used for visualization? Discuss its principle and applications.
2. List the various parts of bright-field microscope and discuss their functions.
3. How will you take care of a microscope?

Explanation
The microscopic photograph provided in Figure 2.8 belongs to an image visualized under fluorescence microscope. For answer to the other questions, refer text.

General Bacteriology: Morphology and Physiology of Bacteria

CHAPTER 3.1

■ MORPHOLOGY OF BACTERIA

Problem Solving Exercise 1

Morphology of Bacteria

Gram stained smears of the organisms have been focused in Figs 3.1.2A, 3.1.3A and 3.1.4A. Identify the probable organism based on the morphological appearance in the Gram stain.

Explanation

❑ Figure 3.1.2A: Reveals Gram-positive cocci arranged in cluster (e.g., *Staphylococcus*).
❑ Figure 3.1.3A: Reveals Gram-negative cocci arranged in pair, lens-shaped, capsulated (e.g., meningococcus).
❑ Figure 3.1.4A: Reveals Gram-positive bacilli: (A) arranged in chain, sporing (e.g., *Bacillus*).

Size and Shape of Bacteria

Bacteria are measured in micrometer (1 μm = 10^{-3} mm). Most of the bacteria of medical importance generally measure 0.2–1.5 μm in diameter and 3–5 μm in length. Depending on their shape, bacteria are classified into:

- Cocci (singular coccus, from kokkos, meaning berry) are oval or spherical cells
- Bacilli (singular *Bacillus*, meaning rod-shaped).

Cocci are arranged in groups (clusters), pair or chains. Similarly, bacilli can be arranged singly or in chain or pair; some bacilli are curved, comma shaped, cuneiform shaped (Table 3.1.1 and Fig. 3.1.1).

Both cocci and bacilli are further classified based on Gram-staining property into (Table 3.1.1 and Figs 3.1.1 to 3.1.5):

- Gram-positive cocci (Figs 3.1.2A to C)
- Gram-negative cocci (Figs 3.1.3A and B)
- Gram-positive bacilli (Figs 3.1.4A to C)
- Gram-negative bacilli (Figs 3.1.5A to C)

However, there are some bacteria that are weakly Gram stained and hence need special stains for their demonstration, such as:

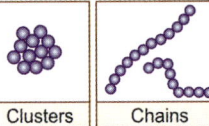 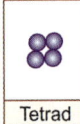  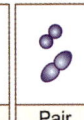

Clusters | Chains | Tetrad | Octate | Pair

Gram-positive cocci

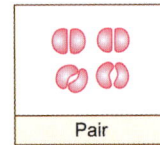 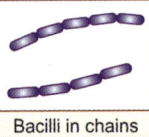 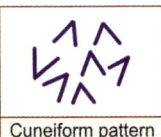

Pair | Bacilli in chains | Cuneiform pattern

Gram-negative cocci | **Gram-positive bacilli**

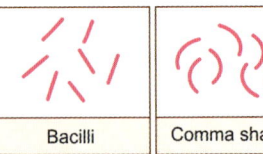 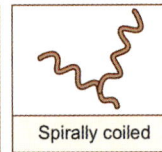

Bacilli | Comma shaped | Spirally coiled

Gram-negative bacilli | **Spirochete**

Fig. 3.1.1: Different morphology of bacteria and Gram-staining property.

- Spirochetes (*Treponema* and *Leptospira*): Thin spirally coiled bacilli (Fig. 3.1.5D)
- *Mycoplasma* (cell wall-deficient free living bacteria)
- Rickettsiae and chlamydiae are obligate intracellular bacteria.

CHAPTER 3.1 ◆ General Bacteriology: Morphology and Physiology of Bacteria

Table 3.1.1: Classification of bacteria depending on their morphology and Gram-staining property.

Bacteria	Example
Gram-positive cocci arranged in	
Cluster	Staphylococcus
Chain	Streptococcus
Pairs, lanceolate shaped	Pneumococcus
Pair or in short chain, spectacle shaped	Enterococcus
Tetrads	Micrococcus
Octate	Sarcina
Gram-negative cocci arranged in	
Pairs, lens shaped	Meningococcus
Pairs, kidney shaped	Gonococcus
Gram-positive bacilli arranged in	
Chain (bamboo stick appearance)	Bacillus anthracis
Chinese letter or cuneiform pattern	Corynebacterium diphtheriae
Palisade pattern	Diphtheroids
Branched and filamentous form	Actinomyces and Nocardia
Gram-negative bacilli arranged in	
Pleomorphic (various shapes)	Haemophilus, Proteus
Thumb print appearance	Bordetella pertussis
Comma shaped (fish in stream appearance)	Vibrio cholerae
Curved	Campylobacter and Helicobacter
Others	
Chain	Streptobacillus
Spirally coiled, flexible	Spirochetes
Rigid spiral forms	Spirillum
Bacteria that lack cell wall	Mycoplasma

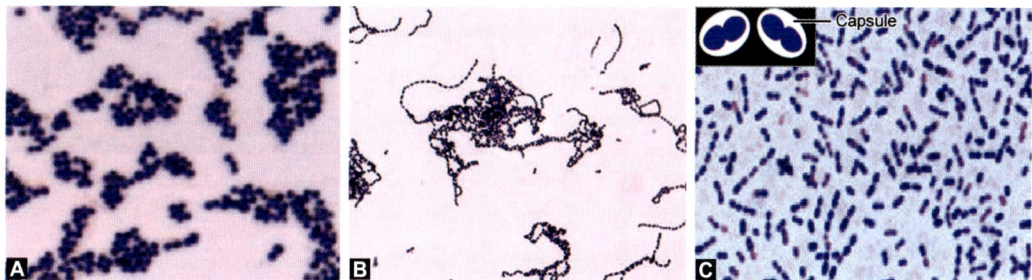

Figs 3.1.2A to C: Gram-positive cocci arranged in: (A) Cluster (e.g., *Staphylococcus*); (B) Chain (e.g., *Streptococcus*); (C) Pair, lanceolate-shaped (e.g., pneumococcus).
Source: Department of Microbiology, Pondicherry Institute of Medical Sciences, Puducherry (*with permission*).

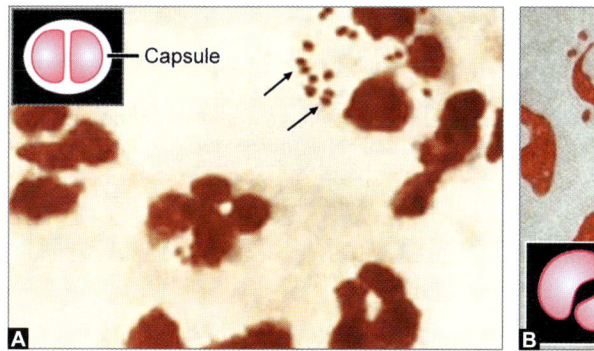
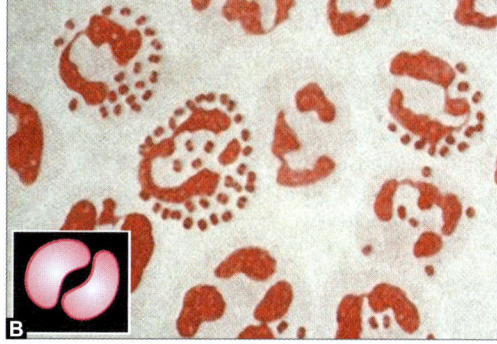

Figs 3.1.3A and B: Gram-negative cocci arranged in: (A) Pair, lens-shaped, capsulated (e.g., Meningococcus); (B) Pair, kidney-shaped (e.g., Gonococcus).
Source: (A) Centers for Disease Control and Prevention (CDC), Atlanta; (B) Public Health Image Library, ID# /2108, Centers for Disease Control and Prevention (CDC), Atlanta (*with permission*).

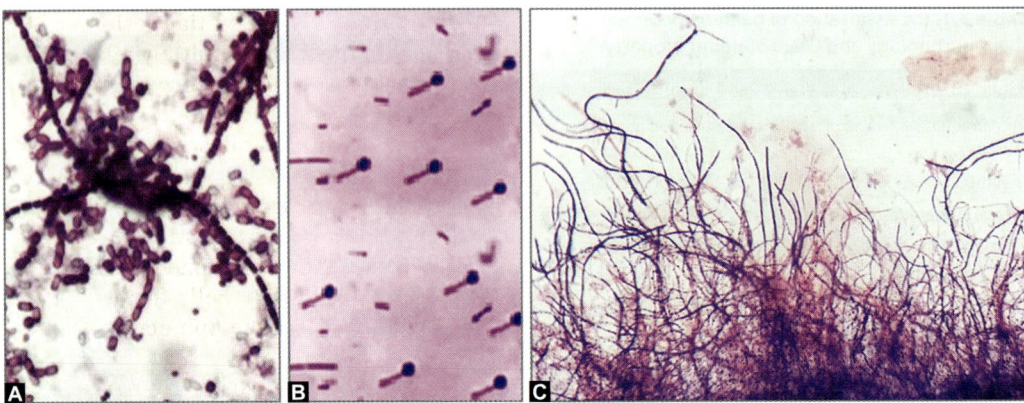

Figs 3.1.4A to C: Gram-positive bacilli: (A) Arranged in chain, sporing (e.g., *Bacillus*); (B) With terminal spore, drumstick appearance (e.g., *Clostridium tetani*); (C) Branching, filamentous (e.g., *Actinomycetes*).
Source: (A) Department of Microbiology, JIPMER, Puducherry (*with permission*); (B) Public Health Image Library, ID# 6373, Centers for Disease Control and Prevention (CDC), Atlanta (*with permission*); (C) Dr Isabella Princess, Apollo Hospitals, Chennai (*with permission*).

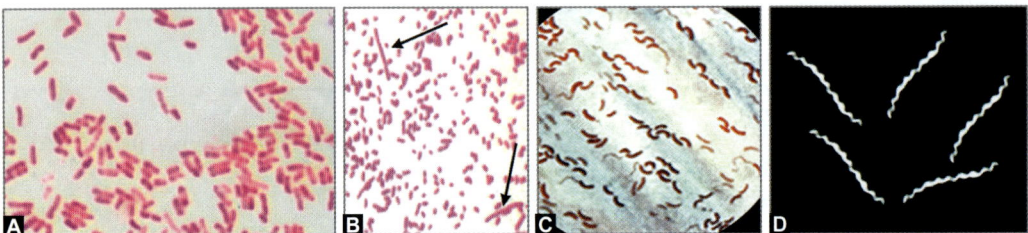

Figs 3.1.5A to C: Gram-negative bacilli: (A) Arranged singly (e.g., *Escherichia coli*); **Fig. 3.1.5D:** Spirochete (spirally (B) Pleomorphic (e.g., *Haemophilus influenzae*); (C) Comma-shaped (e.g., *Vibrio cholerae*). coiled bacilli) in dark ground microscopy.
Source: (A and B) Department of Microbiology, Pondicherry Institute of Medical Sciences, Puducherry (*with permission*); (C and D) (C) ID#:5324; (D) ID#:2043, Public Health Image Library, Centers for Disease Control and Prevention (CDC), Atlanta (*with permission*).

PHYSIOLOGY OF BACTERIA

Problem Solving Exercise 2

Bacterial Growth Curve

A bacterium is inoculated into a suitable liquid culture medium and incubated. The bacterial count of the liquid culture is determined at different intervals and plotted in relation to time (Fig. 3.1.6). Answer the following questions.
1. In which phase of this curve, the bacterium obtains maximum size?
2. Which phase of this curve is ideal for performing Gram staining?
3. In which phase, the bacterium undergoes sporulation?
4. In which phase of this curve, involution forms are seen?

Explanation

Fig. 3.1.6 depicts a bacterial growth curve, which is obtained when bacterial count of the liquid culture is determined at different intervals and plotted in relation to time. It has four phases—lag, log, stationary and decline phases.
1. The bacterium obtains maximum size at the end of lag phase.
2. Log phase is ideal for performing Gram staining.
3. The bacterium undergoes sporulation in stationary phase.
4. Involution forms are seen in decline phase.

Bacterial Growth Curve

When a bacterium is inoculated into a suitable liquid culture medium and incubated, its growth follows a definite course. When bacterial count of such culture is determined at different intervals and plotted in relation to time, a *bacterial growth curve* is obtained comprising of four phases (Fig. 3.1.6 and Table 3.1.2).

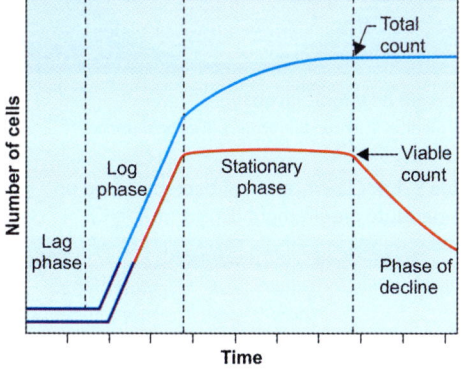

Fig. 3.1.6: Bacterial growth curve.

1. **Lag phase:** It is the initial period, where bacteria do not start multiplying, but take some time to build-up enzymes and metabolites
2. **Log phase:** In this phase, bacteria divide exponentially
3. **Stationary phase:** Here, the bacteria start dying due to exhaustion of nutrients and accumulation of toxic products. The number of progeny cells formed is just enough to replace the number of cells that die
4. **Decline phase:** Gradually, the bacteria stop dividing completely, while the cell death continues.

Factors Affecting Growth of Bacteria

There are several environmental factors that affect the growth of the bacteria:

Oxygen

On the basis of their oxygen requirements, classification of bacteria is shown in Table 3.1.3.

Table 3.1.2: Various phases of bacterial growth curve.

	Lag	Log	Stationary	Decline
Bacteria divide	No	Yes	Yes	No
Bacterial death	No	No	Yes	Yes
Total count	Flat	Raises	Raises	Flat
Viable count	Flat	Raises	Flat	Falls
Special features	Accumulation of enzymes and metabolites, attains maximum size	Uniformly stained, Metabolically active, Small size	Gram variable Produce: Granules, spores, exotoxin, antibiotics, bacteriocin	Produce involution forms

Table 3.1.3: Classification of bacteria based on their oxygen requirement.

Types	Definition	Examples
Obligate aerobes (Figs 3.1.7A and B-1)	Grow only in the presence of oxygen	*Pseudomonas, Mycobacterium, Bacillus, Nocardia*
Facultative anaerobes (Figs 3.1.7A and B-2)	They are aerobes that can also grow anaerobically	*Escherichia coli, Staphylococcus aureus*
Microaerophilic bacteria	Grow in presence of low oxygen tension (5–10% O_2)	*Campylobacter, Helicobacter, Mycobacterium bovis*
Obligate anaerobes (Figs 3.1.7A and B-3)	Grow only in the absence of oxygen	Most of the clostridia spp.
Aerotolerant anaerobes	Tolerate oxygen for some time, but do not use it	*Clostridium histolyticum*

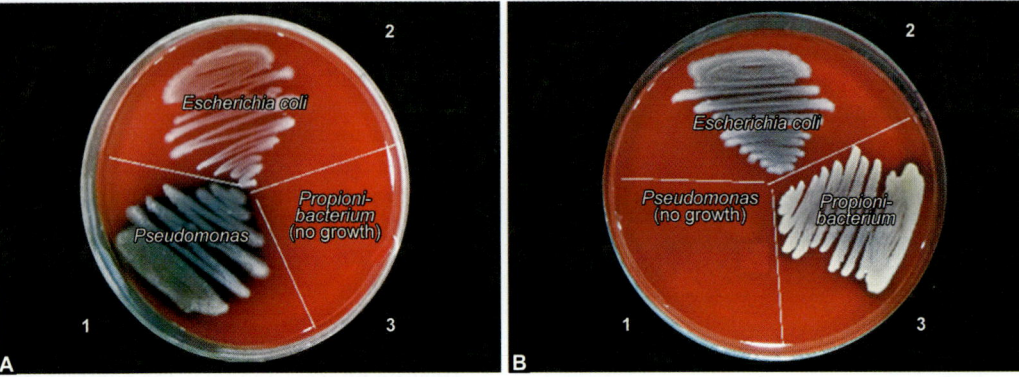

Figs 3.1.7A and B: (A) Aerobic incubation; (B) Anaerobic incubation.
Source: Department of Microbiology, Pondicherry Institute of Medical Sciences, Puducherry (*with permission*).

Carbon Dioxide

Organisms that require higher amounts of carbon dioxide (5–10%) for growth are called as **capnophilic bacteria**. Examples include *Brucella abortus, Streptococcus pneumoniae*, etc.

Temperature

Most of the pathogenic bacteria grow optimally at 37°C. However, the optimal temperature range varies with different bacterial species. According to temperature requirements, bacteria can be grouped as given in Table 3.1.4.

pH

Most pathogenic bacteria grow between pH 7.2 and pH 7.6. Very few bacteria (lactobacilli) can grow at acidic pH (below pH 4), while bacteria, such as *Vibrio cholerae* are capable of growing at alkaline pH (8.2–8.9).

Table 3.1.4: Classification of bacteria based on temperature requirement (Figs 3.1.8A to C).

Types	Definition	Examples
Psychrophiles	Grow best at temperatures below 20°C	Most of the saprophytes (e.g., *Pseudomonas*)
Mesophiles	Grow within a temperature range 25°C and 40°C	Most of the pathogenic bacteria (e.g., *Staphylococcus aureus*)
Thermophiles	Grow at a high temperature range of 55–80°C	*Geobacillus stearothermophilus*

Light

Bacteria (except phototrophs) grow well in darkness. Photochromogenic mycobacteria produce pigments only on exposure to light.

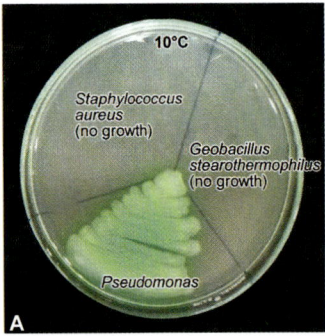
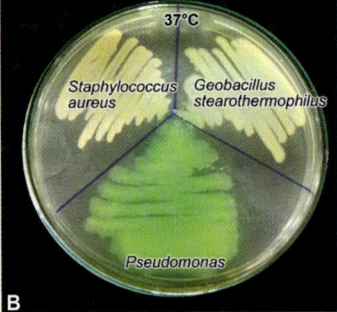
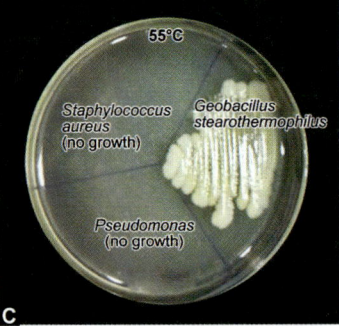

Figs 3.1.8A to C: (A) Psychrophiles (10°C); (B) Mesophiles (37°C); (C) Thermophiles (55°C).
Source: Department of Microbiology, Pondicherry Institute of Medical Sciences, Puducherry (*with permission*).

CHAPTER 3.2
General Bacteriology: Specimen Collection and Transport

■ INTRODUCTION

Laboratory diagnosis of bacterial infections is useful for the following purposes:
- **Identification:** To identify the causative bacterial agent responsible for the disease
- **Treatment:** To provide accurate antimicrobial therapy
- **Surveillance purpose:** To assess the disease burden in the community by estimating the prevalence and incidence of the infections
- **For outbreak investigation,** e.g., diphtheria outbreaks in the community, MRSA (methicillin-resistant *S. aureus*) outbreaks in the hospitals
- **To start PEP** (post-exposure prophylaxis): Useful in infectious diseases, such as, anthrax and plague
- **To initiate appropriate infection control measures:** For example, contact precaution for MRSA infection, droplet precaution for diphtheria and airborne precaution for tuberculosis (Chapter 11).

Laboratory diagnosis of bacterial infections comprises of several steps—specimen collection, direct detection, culture, identification and antimicrobial susceptibility test, serology and molecular methods (Table 3.2.1).

Table 3.2.1: Overview of laboratory diagnosis of bacterial infections.

1. **Specimen collection**
2. **Direct detection**
   - Microscopy: Gram stain, acid-fast stain, Albert stain, histopathological staining, dark ground, phase-contrast and fluorescence microscopy
   - Antigen detection from clinical specimen
   - Molecular diagnosis: Detecting bacterial DNA or RNA from clinical specimen
3. **Culture**
   - Culture media
   - Culture methods
   - Colony morphology, smear and motility testing
4. **Identification**
   - Biochemical identification
   - Automated identification methods
5. **Antimicrobial susceptibility testing**
6. **Serology**
7. **Molecular methods**
8. **Typing methods**

■ SPECIMEN COLLECTION

Problem Solving Exercise

Specimen Collection

A young patient with history of high grade fever with chills for two days, presents to the out patient department. Upon detailed clinical examination, clinician decides to admit him and requests for his blood and urine culture and susceptibility testing. After two days of hospitalization he develops diarrhea with two episodes of vomiting. His stool specimen was collected and sent for culture. Discuss the method of collection of the following specimens for culture.
- Blood for blood culture
- Urine specimen for microscopy and culture
- Stool specimen for microscopy and culture

Explanation

The specimen collection has been explained in the following Chapters
- Blood collection for culture: Refer Chapter 17
- Urine specimen collection for microscopy and culture: Refer this Chapter and Chapter 42
- Stool specimen collection for microscopy and culture: Refer this Chapter and Chapters 5 and 22.

Specimen collection depends upon the type of underlying infections (Table 3.2.2). The proper collection of specimen is of paramount importance for the isolation of the bacteria in culture.

General Principles

The following general principles should be followed while collecting the specimen:
- **Standard precautions** should be followed for collecting and handling all specimens (Chapter 10 for details)
- **Before antibiotics start:** Whenever possible, culture specimens should be collected prior to administration of any antimicrobial agents
- **Contamination** with indigenous flora should be avoided, especially when collecting urine and blood culture specimens
- **Swabs** are though convenient but considered inferior to tissue, aspirate and body fluids
- **Container:** Specimens should be collected in sterile, tightly sealed, leak proof, wide-mouth, screw-capped containers
- **Labeling:** All specimens must be appropriately labeled with name, age, gender, name of the treating physician, clinical diagnosis, antibiotic history, type of specimen, and desired investigation name
- **Rejection:** Specimens grossly contaminated or compromised or improperly labeled may be rejected (see highlight box)
- If **anaerobic culture** is requested, proper anaerobic collection containers with media should be used
- Specimen should not be sent in container containing **formalin** for microbiological analysis.

> **Specimen rejection criteria**
> Microbiology samples that do not meet the *appropriate sample* and the *test request requirements* need to be rejected, so as to prevent inaccurate data and to ensure the safety of patients and laboratory personnel. Reasons for sample rejection may include the following:
> ❑ Improperly labeled or unlabeled sample
> ❑ Incomplete specimen-related or clinical information on the sample and/or on the requisition form
>
> *Contd...*

Table 3.2.2: Types of infections and various specimens collected.

Type of infections	Specimens collected
Bloodstream infection, sepsis, endocarditis	Paired blood culture specimens • Collected aseptically by two-step disinfection of skin; first with alcohol followed by chlorhexidine • 8–10 mL of blood (for adults) collected in blood culture bottles
Infectious diseases requiring serology	• Blood (2 mL/investigation) • Collected by minimal asepsis (one-step skin disinfection with alcohol) • Collected in vacutainer
Diarrheal diseases	Stool (mucus flakes), rectal swab
Meningitis	Cerebrospinal fluid (CSF)
Infections of other sterile body area	Sterile body fluids, e.g., pleural fluid, synovial fluid, peritoneal fluid
Skin and soft tissue infections	Pus or exudate, wound swabs, aspirates from abscess and tissue bits
Anaerobic infections	Aspirates, tissue specimens, blood and sterile body fluids, bone marrow (swabs, sputum not satisfactory)
Upper respiratory tract infections	Throat swab with membrane over the tonsil, nasopharyngeal swab, pernasal swab
Lower respiratory tract infections	Sputum, endotracheal aspirate, bronchoalveolar lavage (BAL), protected specimen brush (PSB) and lung biopsy
Pulmonary tuberculosis	• Sputum—early morning and spot • Collected in well-ventilated area • Gastric aspirate for infants
Urinary tract infections	Midstream urine Suprapubic aspirated urine Catheterized patient—collected from the catheter tube, after clamping distally and disinfecting; not from urobag
Genital infections	Urethral swab, cervical swab—for urethritis Exudate from genital ulcers
Eye infections	Conjunctival swabs Corneal scrapings Aqueous or vitreous fluid
Ear infections	Swabs from outer ear Aspirate from inner ear

Contd...

- Sub-optimal sample, i.e., leaking urine and/or stool containers, insufficient quantity or inappropriate sample for the test requested
- Duplicate microbiology samples received on the same day, i.e., multiple stool, sputum samples
- Sample delayed in transit more than the accepted limit.

COLLECTION TECHNIQUE OF VARIOUS SPECIMENS

Blood Specimen

In clinical microbiology laboratories, blood collection is indicated either for blood culture or for serological tests.

Collection of Blood Specimen for Culture

Blood culture is regarded as one of the most important culture investigation performed by clinical microbiology laboratory. As there is a high risk of contamination with skin flora, sterile aseptic precautions must be taken for collection and skin is disinfected with two agents—70% alcohol followed by chlorhexidine. It is discussed in detail in Chapter 17.

Collection of Blood Specimen for Serology

Collection of blood specimen for serological (e.g., virology or immunology) diagnostic tests is similar to as done for culture; except that skin disinfection is performed by only one agent i.e., 70% isopropyl alcohol. This is because contamination with skin flora is not an issue while performing these investigations.

- The blood sample is collected in clean sterile tubes (Vacutainers)
- Tube is filled 3/4th full and then allowed to stand at room temperature for a few hours to allow a solid clot to form and retract
- Then the tube is centrifuged, serum is separated, placed in another clean tube, which can be used for further diagnostic testing.

CSF and Other Sterile Body Fluids

CSF and other sterile body fluids should be collected before the starting of antimicrobial therapy, in sterile screw capped container, under adequate aseptic precautions.

- **CSF:** CSF is collected by lumbar puncture at interspace L3-L4, or L4-L5. The site is first disinfected with antiseptics similar to that used for blood culture. After collection, CSF is then divided into three sterile tubes (2 mL each) for three diagnostic laboratories
  - Biochemistry (for total protein and glucose)
  - Bacteriology (culture and susceptibility, Gram staining, antigen detection)
  - Cytology (for cell count).
- **Body fluids from other sterile sites** such as ascitic fluid, pleural fluid, peritoneal fluid, and synovial fluid specimens are collected by percutaneous aspiration under aseptic precautions with syringe and needle
- **Body fluid specimens** can also be inoculated at bedside directly on to BacT/ALERT bottles for culture. In these case, a portion of the specimen should be aliquoted separately for Gram stain
- **Transport:** Specimens should be transported immediately (within 15 min) to the laboratory; If any delay is expected, body fluid specimens can be stored at 37°C (in incubator) or at room temperature; ***but never refrigerated.***

Sterile Universal Specimen Container (Fig. 3.2.1)

These are designed for collecting biological specimens, including urine, stool, sputum, peritoneal exudate, joint fluid, biopsy specimen, sterile body fluids and aspirates for microbiological culture and susceptibility testing. It is very convenient for sample collection at the bed side. These containers should have the following specifications:

- They should be sterile, leak-proof, wide mouthed and screw capped.
- Each container should bear the name of the patient, from whom the specimen was collected and his hospital register number.
- Specimen type and date and time of collection
- A completely filled investigation requisition form should always accompany the specimen indicating the investigation requested along with the probable clinical diagnosis and current antibiotic therapy.

Fecal Specimens

A small quantity of semisolid/solid stool or one third of the container in case of liquid stool

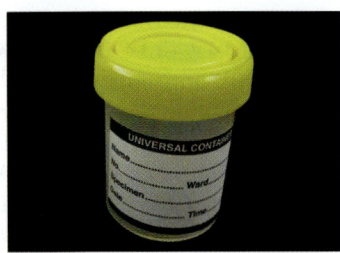

Fig. 3.2.1: Sterile universal container.

specimen is collected in a wide mouthed, sterile screw capped, leak proof container (Fig. 3.2.1); preferably prior to initiation of antibiotics.
- ❖ **Rectal swabs** may be collected in case of asymptomatic carriers
- ❖ **Transport:** Sample should be immediately transported to the laboratory. In case of delay suitable transport media may be employed such as Cary Blair medium or Venkatraman Ramakrishnan (VR) medium.

Respiratory Specimens

Respiratory specimens are categorized into two groups.
- ❖ Upper respiratory tract specimens such as throat swab, nasopharyngeal swabs, bits of membrane from tonsil
- ❖ Lower respiratory tract specimens such as sputum, endotracheal aspirate (ETA) and bronchoalveolar lavage (BAL), protected specimen brush (PSB) and lung biopsy.

Sputum

Sputum cultures are indicated to identify the pathogens causing pneumonia.
- ❖ Sputum specimen that results following a deep cough is preferable and is collected in a sterile screw capped, wide-mouthed, leak proof container (Fig. 3.2.1). Patient should be instructed to place the rim of the container under the lower lip to catch entire expectorated mucopurulent sputum
- ❖ **Early morning sputum** samples should be obtained as they contain pooled overnight secretions, as they may contain increased concentration of pathogens
- ❖ **For suspected tuberculosis**
  - ■ **Two sputum** specimens are collected- spot and early morning. Sputum collection booths should be located away from other people, outside in an open well ventilated space
  - ■ **Gastric aspirate** may be collected for infants in suspected case of tuberculosis. Early morning specimen is ideal before eating/getting up. Transport time should be < 15 minutes.
- ❖ Collected specimen has to be transported to the laboratory as soon as possible (within two hours); as delicate pathogens may otherwise die, if there is a delay.

ETA, BAL, PSB and Lung Biopsy Specimens

Collection of endotracheal aspirate (ETA), bronchoalveolar lavage (BAL), protected specimen brush (PSB) and lung biopsy specimens is technically demanding and requires specialized techniques. These specimens should be transported immediately to the laboratory and cultured within one hour of collection.

Throat Swab

Throat swab samples for bacterial culture is collected by depressing the tongue with a tongue depressor. The oropharyngeal swab is rubbed on the back of the throat, over the tonsils, and in any other area where there is redness or pus. Whenever possible, a portion of pseudomembrane may be collected.

Nasopharyngeal Secretions

Nasopharyngeal specimens are the best specimens which may be obtained by:
- ❖ **Nasopharyngeal aspiration** (best method): Collected by inserting flexible swab through nose into posterior nasopharynx and rotating for 5 seconds; specimen of choice for *Bordetella pertussis*
- ❖ **Per-nasal swab**: Collected by using a sterile swab on a flexible wire.

Note: For culture in a suspected case of pertussis, alginate swabs are the best followed by dacron swabs. Cotton swabs are not satisfactory. It is recommended to collect six swabs, at 1–2 days intervals to achieve maximum yield.

Exudate Specimens

Wound swabs (sterile cotton swab, Fig. 3.2.2) are recommended to identify the etiological agents causing deep-seated wound infection.

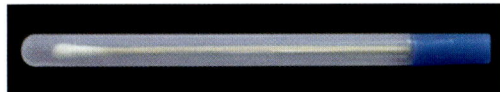

Fig. 3.2.2: Sterile cotton swab.

- Wound swabs are ideally collected prior to starting of antibiotic therapy and only for clinically infected wounds or that fail to heal even after a long period
- **For closed wounds** disinfect with 70% alcohol or 2% chlorhexidine followed by 10% povidone-iodine. Remove iodine with alcohol just prior to specimen collection
- **Open wounds** are first debrided and then thoroughly rinsed with sterile saline prior to collection
- Preferably sample the **viable tissue** and not the superficial debris
- A portion of the sample also must be placed in Robertson's Cooked Meat (RCM) medium, if anaerobic culture is indicated
- For collection of pus in the form of **abscess**, aspirate the deepest portion of the lesion with a syringe and needle
- **For burn wound** swab collection, consider sampling different areas of the burn, as organisms may not be evenly distributed in a burn wound
- **Aspirates and tissue specimens** should be delivered to the laboratory for further processing within 30 minutes of collection for best recovery. Tissue specimens must be kept moist to preserve viability of organisms
- **For anaerobic culture,** aspirates or tissue specimens are recommended. Specimen which are not suitable include swab, urine, sputum etc.
- **Discharging sinus:** In case of actinomycetoma, **granules** present in the discharge are collected in sterile gauze or loop by pressing the sinuses from the periphery to express them out.

Urine Specimen

It is extremely important to collect the urine specimens carefully to avoid the contamination with normal urethral flora. The various type of collection of urine specimen for culture has been described below.
- **Midstream clean catch urine:** It is the most common type of urine specimen collected for culture. After properly cleaning the urethral meatus or glans with soap and water, urine specimen is collected in a sterile, wide mouthed, screw capped, leak proof container by voiding the first portion (which is likely to be contaminated with normal urethral flora) (Fig. 3.2.1)
- **Indwelling catheter:** Urine specimen should be collected from the catheter tubing (after clamping and disinfecting a portion of the catheter tubing with alcohol), by inserting a sterile syringe and needle directly into the catheter tubing. Urine *must not be* collected from the drainage bag
- **Suprapubic aspiration:** It is the **most ideal** urine specimen, as it avoids the risk of contamination with urethral flora
  - However it is invasive and therefore is recommended only for patients in coma or infants
  - The skin above the bladder is disinfected and then urine is collected needle aspiration above the symphysis pubis through the abdominal wall into the full bladder.

Urine specimen must be transported to the microbiology laboratory as soon as possible and should be processed immediately. If delay is expected for more than two hours, then it can be stored in refrigerator or stored by adding boric acid, glycerol or formate for maximum 24 hours before plating.

Genital Specimens

Common genital specimens include urethral discharge for urethritis and exudate from genital ulcers

Urethral Discharge

Urethral swab in men and cervical swab in women are the preferred specimens. Vaginal swab is not satisfactory.
- **Method:** The urethral meatus is cleaned with gauze soaked in saline. The purulent discharge is expressed out by pressing at the base of the penis and collected directly on to slides or swabs
- **Swab:** Dacron or rayon swabs are preferred, as cotton and alginate swabs are inhibitory to many urethral pathogens such as gonococci
- **In chronic urethritis:** As discharge is minimal, prostatic massage is done to collect

the secretion; alternatively, the morning drop of secretion may also be collected
- **Transport Media:** Specimens should be transported immediately. If not possible, then charcoal containing Stuart's or Amies transport medium can be used.

Exudate from Genital Ulcers

Surface of the genital ulcer is cleaned with saline, gentle pressure is applied at the base of the lesion, and a drop of exudate is collected on a slide.

Endometrial specimens: Collected by surgical biopsy or trans-cervical aspirate via sheathed catheter.

Other Specimens

- **Ocular specimens**: They are precious specimens, should be transported to laboratory within 15 min. Bedside inoculation onto blood agar may be considered if delay is unavoidable
  - **Conjunctival swab:** Swabs should be pre-moistened with sterile saline and samples should be collected from both the eyes
  - **Corneal scrapings:** Clinicians should instill local anesthetics before collection
  - **Aqueous or vitreous fluid** for endophthalmitis cases.
- **Ear specimens:**
  - **External ear:** Specimen is collected by firmly rotating the swab into the outer ear (Fig. 3.2.2)
  - **Inner ear specimens:** If ear drum is intact, material behind the drum is aspirated with syringe; if ear drum is ruptured, swab is used to collect material from the inner ear. Ear canal should be cleaned with mild soap solution before aspiration.

Specimen Transport

The specimens should reach the laboratory for further processing as soon as possible after the collection. If required appropriate transport media should be used (discussed subsequently in this chapter).

For most of the specimens, transport time should not exceed **two hours**. However, there are some exceptions.

- Specimens such as CSF and body fluids, ocular specimens, tissue specimens, suprapubic aspirate and bone specimen should be **transported immediately** (<15 minutes)
- **Urine (midstream)** added with preservative (boric acid) is acceptable up to 24 hours, otherwise should be transported within 2 hours
- **Stool culture:** Stool specimen should be transported within 1 hour, but with transport media such as Cary-Blair medium or Venkatraman Ramakrishnan (VR) medium, is acceptable up to 24 hours
- **Rectal swabs**—up to 24 hours is acceptable
- **For anaerobic culture**: Specimens should be put into Robertson's cooked meat broth or any specialized anaerobic transport system and transported immediately to the laboratory.

Specimen Storage before Processing

Most specimens can be stored **at room temperature** immediately after receipt, for **up to 24 hours**. However, there are some exceptions.
- **Blood cultures**—should be incubated at 37°C immediately upon receipt
- Sterile body fluids, bone, vitreous fluid, suprapubic aspirate—should be immediately plated upon receipt and incubated at 37°C
- **Corneal scraping**—should be immediately plated at bed-side on to blood agar and chocolate agar
- **Stool culture**—stool specimen for culture can be stored up to 72 hours at 4°C
- **Urine** (mid-stream and from the catheter), **lower respiratory** tract specimen, **gastric biopsy** (for *Helicobacter pylori*)—can be stored up to 24 hours at 4°C

Prioritizing the Specimen for Processing

Certain precious specimens such as CSF and sterile body fluids, ocular specimens, tissue specimens, suprapubic aspirate and bone specimen should be processed immediately as soon as received, not more than 15 min delay. Similarly, blood culture bottles should be immediately incubated upon receipt.

CHAPTER 3.3

General Bacteriology: Direct Detection 1: Simple Staining

Direct detection of bacteria in the clinical specimen plays a very important role in early institution of antimicrobial therapy. These methods include microscopic demonstration of bacteria—staining techniques and other methods, such as detection of antigen or nucleic acid in the clinical specimen.

■ STAINING TECHNIQUES

Structural details of bacteria cannot be seen under a light microscope due to lack of contrast. Hence, it is necessary to use staining methods to produce color contrast and thereby increase the visibility. Before staining, the fixation of the smear to the slide is done.

Fixation

Fixation is the process by which the internal and external structures of cells are preserved and fixed in position. There are two types of fixation as follows:
1. **Heat fixation** is usually done for *bacterial smears* by gently flame heating an air-dried smear of bacteria. This preserves overall morphology of cells
2. **Chemical fixation** is done by using chemicals, such as ethanol, acetic acid, formaldehyde, methanol and glutaraldehyde. This is useful for examination of blood smears. They protect the fine internal structure of cells.

The fixed smear is stained by appropriate staining techniques.

Common Staining Techniques Used in Microbiology Laboratory

Simple Staining

Here, only one stain is used which imparts only one color to all the bacteria present in the smear. Basic dyes, such as methylene blue or basic fuchsin are used as simple stains (explained subsequently in this chapter).

Differential Staining

Here, two stains are used which impart different colors to different bacteria. Gram staining is most commonly employed staining technique in diagnostic microbiology laboratory. It differentiates bacteria into gram-positive and gram-negative groups (discussed in detail in Chapter 3.4).

Special Staining

Special stains used are:
- **Acid-fast stain:** Differentiates bacteria into acid-fast and nonacid-fast groups
- **Albert stain:** Differentiates bacteria having metachromatic granules from other bacteria that do not have
- **Negative staining:** Example, India ink stain for demonstration of capsule
- **Impregnation methods:** Example, silver impregnation method for demonstration of thin organisms, such as spirochetes.

These special staining techniques are discussed in Chapter 3.5.

■ SIMPLE STAINING

Basic dyes, such as methylene blue or basic fuchsin are used as simple stains (Figs 3.3.1 and 3.3.2). They provide a quick and easy way to determine cell shape, size, and arrangement.

Procedure

Bacterial smear is stained with one of the simple stains for one minute and then the slide is rinsed with water and allowed to air dry and focused under oil immersion objective.

Problem Solving Exercise

Simple Staining

Smear made from a bacterial colony is provided.
1. Perform simple stain of the smear provided.
2. Draw your observations with the help of a diagram and give your interpretation.
3. What are the uses of simple staining?

Explanation

For answers to these questions, refer text.

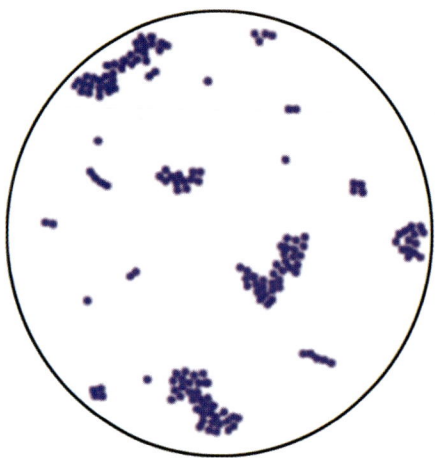 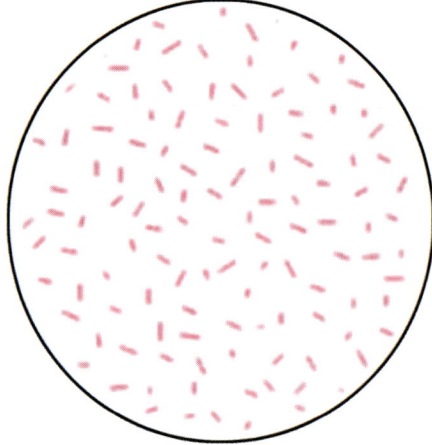

Fig. 3.3.1: Methylene blue stained smear demonstrating blue-colored cocci in cluster.
Source: Department of Microbiology, JIPMER, Puducherry (*with permission*).

Fig. 3.3.2: Basic fuchsin stained smear demonstrating pink-colored bacilli in scattered arrangement.
Source: Department of Microbiology, JIPMER, Puducherry (*with permission*).

Result and Interpretation

They provide the color contrast, but impart the same color to all the bacteria in a smear.

- Methylene blue stain imparts blue color (Fig. 3.3.1).
- Basic fuchsin stain imparts pink color (Fig. 3.3.2).

General Bacteriology: Direct Detection 2: Gram Staining

CHAPTER 3.4

Problem Solving Exercise

Gram Staining

Case Scenario 1: A smear is provided, made from a sputum specimen of a 5-year-old child with acute onset of fever, productive cough and dyspnea for the past two days. Physical examination revealed dull note on percussion.

Case Scenario 2: A smear is provided, made from a CSF specimen of a two year old baby presented with high grade fever, vomiting and excessive crying for past three days.

Case Scenario 3: A smear is provided, made from a pus discharge of a postoperative wound infection of a 65-year-old man who has undergone an abdominal surgery.

Case Scenario 4: A smear is provided, made from a wound swab specimen of a foot ulcer of a diabetic patient.

1. Perform Gram stain of the smear provided.
2. Draw your observations with the help of a neat labeled diagram and give your interpretation.
3. Suggest which antibiotic can be started empirically for the treatment of this case?
4. What are various theories of Gram staining?
5. What are the various uses of Gram staining?

Explanation

The above clinical presentations are suggestive of a case of:
- Lobar pneumonia (case scenario 1)
- Pyogenic meningitis (case scenario 2)
- Surgical site infection (case scenario 3)
- Diabetic foot ulcer (case scenario 4)

The answers to the above questions are explained in this chapter.

Gram Staining technique was originally developed by Hans Christian Gram (1884) and it is the most widely used stain in diagnostic bacteriology.

■ PROCEDURE

Fixation

The smear is made on a clean glass slide from bacterial culture or clinical specimen. It is then air dried and heat fixed.

Step 1 (Primary Stain)

The smear is stained with pararosaniline dyes, such as crystal violet (or gentian violet or methyl violet) for one minute. Then the slide is rinsed with water. Crystal violet stains all the bacteria violet in color (irrespective of whether they are gram-positive or gram-negative).

Step 2 (Mordant)

Gram's iodine (dilute solution of iodine) is poured over the slide for one minute. Then the slide is rinsed with water. Gram's iodine acts as a mordant, binds to the dye to form bigger dye-iodine complexes in the cytoplasm.

Step 3 (Decolorization)

Next step is pouring of few drops of decolorizer to the smear, such as acetone (for 2–3 sec) or ethyl alcohol (20–30 sec) or acetone alcohol (for 10 sec). Slide is immediately rinsed with water. Decolorizer removes the primary stain from gram-negative bacteria while the gram-positive bacteria retain the primary stain.

Note: Decolorization is the most crucial step of Gram staining. If the decolorizer is poured for more time,

Contd...

Contd...

even gram-positive bacteria lose color *(over decolorization)* and if poured for less time, the gram-negative bacteria do not lose the color of primary stain properly *(under decolorization).*

Step 4 (Counterstain)

Secondary stains, such as dilute carbol fuchsin or safranin are added for 30 seconds. They impart pink to red color to the gram-negative bacteria. Alternatively, neutral red may also be used as counterstain especially for gonococci. The slide is rinsed in tap water, dried, and then examined under oil immersion objective.

The steps of Gram staining and the color of gram-positive and gram-negative bacteria after each step are depicted in Figure 3.4.1.

■ INTERPRETATION

Smear is examined under oil immersion objective (Fig. 3.4.2).
- Gram-positive bacteria resist decolorization and retain the color of primary stain, i.e., violet
- Gram-negative bacteria are decolorized and, therefore, take counterstain and appear pink.

■ MECHANISM OF GRAM STAINING

Though the exact mechanism is not understood, the following theories have been put forward.

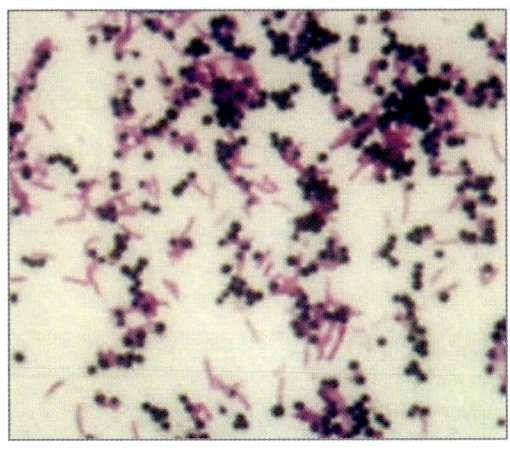

Figs 3.4.2: Gram staining demonstrating violet-colored gram-positive cocci in clusters and pink-colored gram-negative bacilli in scattered arrangement.
Source: Department of Microbiology, Pondicherry Institute of Medical Sciences, Puducherry (*with permission*).

pH Theory

Cytoplasm of gram-positive bacteria is more acidic, hence can retain the basic dye (e.g., crystal violet) for longer time. *Iodine* serves as mordant, i.e., iodine combines with the primary stain to form a dye-iodine complex which gets retained inside the cell.

Cell Wall Theory

This is believed to be the most important postulate to describe the mechanism of Gram staining.

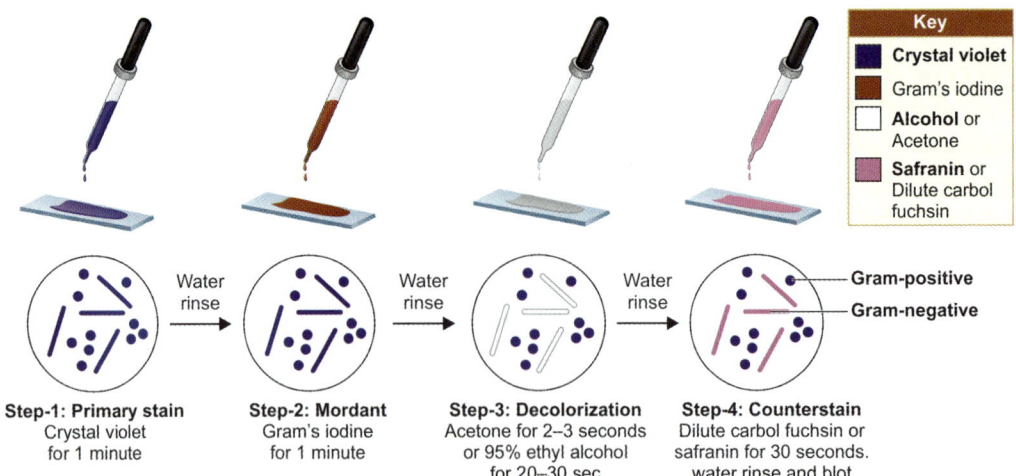

Fig. 3.4.1: Principle and procedure of Gram staining.

Table 3.4.1: Differences between gram-positive and gram-negative cell wall.

Characters	Gram-positive cell wall	Gram-negative cell wall
Peptidoglycan layer	Thicker (15–80 nm), 50–100 layers, cross linked by pentaglycine bridge	Thinner (2 nm), 1–2 layers, directly linked, no pentaglycine bridge
Lipid content	Nil or scanty (2–5%)	Present (15–20%)
Lipopolysaccharide	Absent	Present (endotoxin)
Teichoic acid	Present	Absent
Variety of amino acids	Few	Several
Aromatic amino acids	Absent	Present

- Gram-positive cell wall has a thick peptidoglycan layer (50–100 layers thick), which are tightly cross linked to each other
- The peptidoglycan itself is not stained; instead it seems to act as a permeability barrier preventing loss of crystal violet (Table 3.4.1)
- Gram-negative cell wall is more permeable, thus allowing the outflow of crystal violet easily (Table 3.4.1). This is attributed to:
    - The thin peptidoglycan layer in gram-negative cell wall which is not tightly cross linked
    - Presence of lipopolysaccharide layer in the cell wall of gram-negative bacteria gets disrupted easily by the action of acetone or alcohol, thus allowing the primary stain to come out of the cytoplasm.
- After mordanting with Gram's iodine, bigger dye-iodine complexes are formed in the cytoplasm. Following decolorization, gram-negative bacterial cell wall (as more lipid content) gets dissolved leading to formation of larger pores through which the dye-iodine complexes escape. Due to less lipid in gram-positive bacterial cell wall, smaller pores are formed and dye-iodine complexes are retained.

MODIFICATIONS OF GRAM STAINING

There are few minor modifications of Gram staining which vary slightly from the method described earlier:
- **Kopeloff and Beerman's modification:** Primary stain and counterstain used are methyl violet and basic fuchsin, respectively
- **Jensen's modification:** This method involves use of absolute alcohol as decolorizer and neutral red as counterstain. It is useful for detection of meningococci and gonococci
- **Weigert's modification:** This modification is useful for staining tissue sections. Here, aniline-xylol is used as a decolorizer
- **Preston and Morrell's modification:** Here, iodine-acetone is used as decolorizer
- **Brown and Brenn modification:** This is used for Actinomycetes.

USES OF GRAM STAIN

Gram staining has the following uses:
- **Differentiation of bacteria into gram-positive and gram-negative:** It is the first step towards identification of bacteria
- **To start empirical treatment:** Gram staining of clinical specimen gives preliminary clue about the bacteria present (based on the shape and Gram staining property of the bacteria) so that the empirical treatment with broad spectrum antibiotics can be started early, before the culture and susceptibility report is available
- **For identification:** Gram staining from bacterial culture gives an idea to put the required biochemical tests for further identification of bacteria
- **For fastidious organisms,** such as *Haemophilus* which takes time to grow in culture, Gram staining helps in early presumptive identification based on their morphology (pleomorphic gram-negative bacilli)
- **Anaerobic organisms**, such as *Clostridium* do not grow in routine culture. Therefore, organisms detected in Gram stain, but aerobic culture-negative gives a preliminary clue to perform an anaerobic culture of the specimen
- **Yeasts:** In addition to stain the bacteria, Gram staining is useful for staining certain fungi, such as *Candida* and *Cryptococcus* (appear gram-positive budding yeast cells)
- **Quality of specimen:** Gram staining helps in screening the quality of the **sputum specimen** before processing it for culture. Presence of more pus cells and less epithelial cells indicates good quality specimen.

General Bacteriology: Direct Detection 3: Special Staining (Acid-Fast Stain, Albert Stain) and Other Methods

CHAPTER 3.5

ACID-FAST STAIN

Problem Solving Exercise 1

Acid-fast Staining

A smear is provided, made from a sputum specimen of a 15-year-old boy presented with fever, productive cough and hemoptysis for past two weeks.
1. Perform acid-fast staining of the smear provided.
2. Draw your observations with the help of a neat labeled diagram and give your interpretation.
3. Suggest the treatment regimen given in this case.
4. What is RNTCP grading and its implications?
5. Which is the conventional culture medium used and describe the colonies grown?
6. What is the recommended molecular method available for rapid and accurate identification? Mention its advantages?

Explanation

The above clinical presentation is suggestive of a case of pulmonary tuberculosis. The answers to the above questions have been explained in this chapter and also in Chapter 35.

The acid-fast staining was discovered by Paul Ehrlich and subsequently modified by Ziehl and Neelsen. This staining is done to identify acid-fast organisms, such as *Mycobacterium tuberculosis* and others (Table 3.5.1). Acid-fastness is due to presence of mycolic acid in the cell wall.

Ziehl-Neelsen Technique (Hot Method)

Smear Preparation

Smear measuring 2 × 3 cm in size is prepared in a new clean grease free, scratch free slide from the yellow, purulent portion of the sputum.

Heat Fixation

The smear is air dried and then heat fixed by passing over the flame. Coagulation of the proteinaceous material in the sputum will facilitate fixing of the smear.

Step 1 (Primary Stain)

Smear is poured with carbol fuchsin (1%) for 5 minutes. Intermittent heating is done by flaming the underneath of the slide until the fumes appear. Heating helps in better penetration of the stain.

Table 3.5.1: Acid-fast organisms or structures and percentage of sulfuric acid suitable for staining (for decolorization).

Acid-fast organisms/structures	Sulfuric acid (%) needed for decolorization
Mycobacterium tuberculosis	25
Mycobacterium leprae	5
Nocardia	1
Acid-fast parasites, such as *Cryptosporidium, Cyclospora, Cystoisospora,* Microsporidia*, *Taenia saginata* segments, hooklets of hydatid cyst	0.5–1
Bacterial spore	0.25–0.5

*Microsporidia are now considered to be evolved from fungi.

- ❖ Care must be taken to ensure that the smear does not dry out. To prevent drying, more carbol fuchsin stain is added to the slide and then the slide is reheated
- ❖ Rinse the slide with tap water, until all free carbol fuchsin stain is washed away. At this point, the smear on the slide looks red in color (Fig. 3.5.1).

CHAPTER 3.5 ❖ General Bacteriology: Direct Detection 3: Special Staining and Other Methods

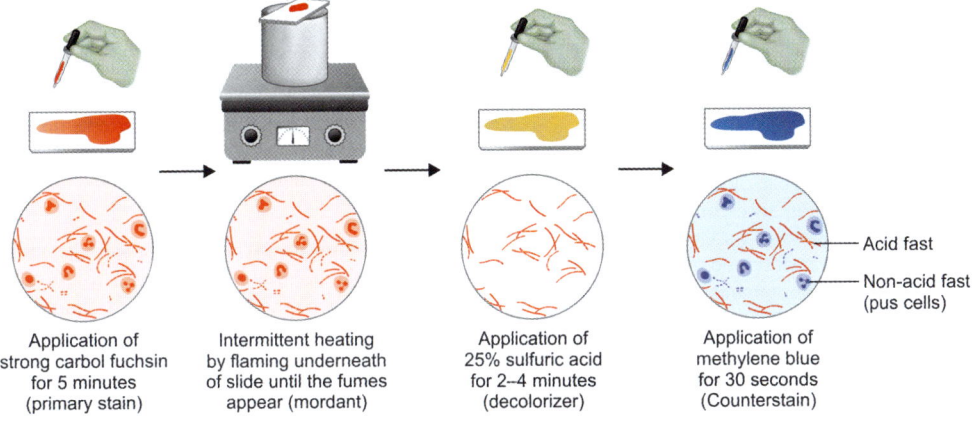

Fig. 3.5.1: Ziehl-Neelsen technique.

Step 2 (Decolorization)

It is done with 25% sulfuric acid for 2–4 minutes. Repeat decolorization for 1–3 minutes if the slide is still red. Then the slide is gently rinsed with tap water and tilted to drain off the water. The back of the slide is wiped clean with a swab dipped in sulfuric acid.

Step 3 (Counterstaining)

It is done with methylene blue (0.1%) for 30 seconds. Slide is rinsed in tap water, dried, and then examined under the binocular microscope using low power objective (10×) to select a suitable area and then screened under oil immersion field (100×). Contaminated materials/slide should be discarded in jar containing 5% phenol.

Interpretation

Mycobaterium tuberculosis appears as long slender, straight or slightly curved, beaded, less uniformly stained, red-colored acid-fast bacillus. Other non-acid fast organisms present in the smear, pus cells and the background take up the counterstain and appear blue (Fig. 3.5.2).

Modifications of Acid-fast Staining

Hot method (Ziehl-Neelsen technique) is the most commonly done acid-fast staining technique. Other modifications include:
- ❖ Cold method *(Kinyoun's method)*: It differs from Ziehl-Neelsen stain in that—
  - Heating is not required

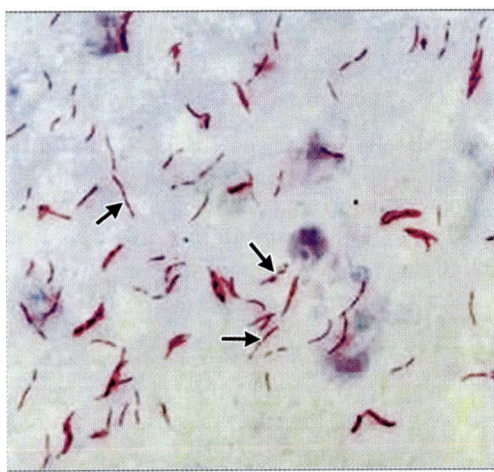

Fig. 3.5.2: Ziehl-Neelsen staining of sputum smear showing long slender, straight or slightly curved, beaded red colored acid–fast bacilli.

Source: Department of Microbiology, JIPMER, Puducherry (*with permission*).

- Phenol concentration in carbol fuchsin is increased
- Duration of carbol fuchsin staining is more.
- ❖ Decolorization can be done with acid-alcohol (3 mL of HCl and 97 mL of ethanol)
- ❖ Malachite green can be used as counterstain
- ❖ Concentration of sulfuric acid may vary depending on the acid-fastness of the structure to be demonstrated. More the content of mycolic acid in the cell wall, more is the acid-fastness, hence more is the percentage of sulfuric acid needed (Table 3.5.1).

ALBERT STAIN

> ### Problem Solving Exercise 2
>
> **Albert Staining**
> A smear is provided, made from a throat swab specimen of a 15-year-old boy presented to an ENT OPD with fever, sore throat and difficulty in swallowing for past two days. On examination, a dirty grey membrane was observed over the tonsils.
> 1. Perform a suitable staining of the smear provided.
> 2. Draw your observations with the help of a neat labeled diagram and give your interpretation.
> 3. Suggest which antibiotic can be started empirically for treatment in this case
> 4. How can this clinical condition be prevented?
>
> **Explanation**
> The above clinical presentation is suggestive of a case of faucial diphtheria. The answers to the above questions have been explained in this chapter and also in Chapter 33.

Albert stain is used to demonstrate the metachromatic granules of *Corynebacterium diphtheriae*.

Composition of Albert Stain

Includes:
- Albert I: Comprises of toluidine blue, malachite green, glacial acetic acid, alcohol (95% ethanol), and distilled water
- Albert II: Contains iodine in potassium iodide.

Procedure

1. *Fixation*: The smear is heat fixed
2. Smear is covered with Albert I (Albert's stain) for 5 minutes, then the excess stain is drained out
3. Albert II is poured over the smear so as to cover it completely for 1 minute
4. Slide is washed in water, blotted dry and examined under oil immersion field.

Interpretation

Corynebacterium diphtheriae appears as green-colored bacilli arranged in Chinese letter or cuneiform pattern, with bluish-black metachromatic granules at polar ends (Fig. 3.5.3). These can be differentiated from diphtheroids which do not show granules and are arranged in palisade pattern. However, certain bacteria, such as *Corynebacterium xerosis* and *Gardnerella vaginalis* also possess metachromatic granules.

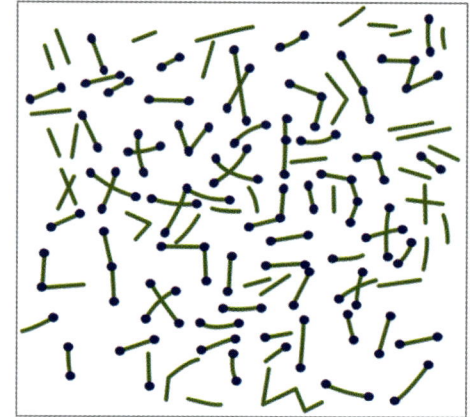

Fig. 3.5.3: Albert stained smear of *Corynebacterium diphtheriae* showing green bacilli with blue-black metachromatic granules (schematic).

NEGATIVE STAINING

A drop of bacterial suspension is mixed with dyes, such as India ink or nigrosin. The background gets stained black whereas unstained bacteria stand out in contrast. This is very useful in the demonstration of bacterial or yeast capsules which do not take up simple stains (Refer Fig. 41.3A, Chapter 41).

IMPREGNATION METHODS

Bacterial cells and structures that are too thin to be seen under the light microscope are thickened by impregnation of silver on their surface to make them visible, e.g.,

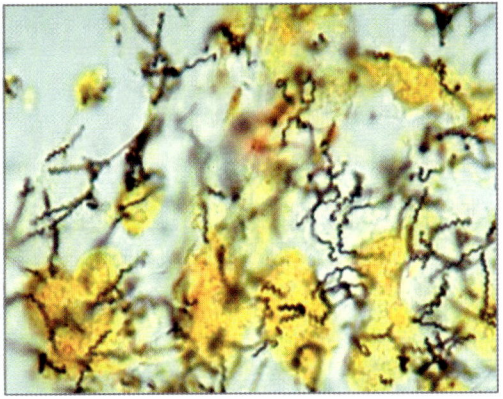

Fig. 3.5.4: Silver impregnation staining demonstrating spirochetes.
Source: Public Health Image Library, ID# 836, Centers for Disease Control and Prevention (CDC), Atlanta (*with permission*).

demonstration of bacterial flagella and spirochetes (Fig. 3.5.4).

OTHER METHODS OF DIRECT DETECTION

Other Microscopic Techniques

Other microscopic techniques include:
- **Dark-ground and phase-contrast microscopy**—for demonstration of spirochetes in genital specimens (Refer Fig. 2.4, Chapter 2)
- **Hanging drop preparation for stool specimen**—for demonstration of darting motility; gives a clue about *V. cholerae* (discussed in Chapter 3.7).

Antigen Detection

Various immunological methods, such as latex agglutination test, immunochromatographic test are available which detect antigens directly from the clinical specimens.
- The classical example includes detection of capsular antigen of pneumococci, meningococci, *H. influenzae* in CSF specimen
- Urinary antigen detection for pneumococci and *Legionella*
- Direct fluorescent antibody test—for detection of *Treponema pallidum* from tissue sections or exudates.

Details about these antigen detection methods are discussed in Chapters 7 to 9.

Molecular Diagnosis

Bacterial DNA or RNA can be directly detected in the clinical specimens by various molecular methods, such as polymerase chain reaction (PCR). It is discussed in detail in Chapter 3.9.

# General Bacteriology: Culture Media (Including Automated Culture) and Culture Methods

CHAPTER 3.6

Culture investigation is the most common diagnostic method used for the detection of bacterial infections. It involves several steps—(i) specimens are inoculated on to various culture media and incubated, (ii) colonies grown are subjected to identification (Chapter 3.7) and (iii) antimicrobial susceptibility testing (Chapter 3.8).

■ CULTURE MEDIA

Culture media are required to isolate the bacteria from the clinical specimens. The basic constituents of culture media are enlisted in Table 3.6.1. Various types of culture media used in the laboratory are as follows:

Simple or Basal Media

They contain minimum ingredients that support the growth of nonfastidious bacteria (Table 3.6.2). The basal media are used for:
❖ Testing the nonfastidiousness of bacteria

Table 3.6.1: Basic constituents of culture media.

Constituents	Uses
Water	Distilled water or potable water
Electrolytes	Sodium chloride or other electrolytes
Peptone	It is a complex mixture of partially digested proteins
Agar	Used for solidifying the culture media • Prepared from seaweeds • It is bacteriologically inert • It melts at 98°C and usually solidifies at 42°C • Concentration of agar used for solid agar preparation (1–2%)
Others	Meat extract, yeast extract and malt extract
Blood and serum	Usually 5–10% of sheep blood is used for enriched media to provide extra nutrition to fastidious bacteria

Table 3.6.2: Basal media and their properties.

Basal media	Properties
Peptone water (Fig. 3.6.1A)	It contains peptone (1%) + NaCl (0.5%) + water
Nutrient broth	It is made up of peptone water + meat extract (1%)
Nutrient agar (Fig. 3.6.1B)	It is made up of nutrient broth + 2% agar

❖ They serve as the base for the preparation of many other media
❖ Nutrient broth is used for studying the bacterial growth curve
❖ Nutrient agar is the preferred medium for:
  ▪ Performing the biochemical tests, such as oxidase, catalase and slide agglutination test, etc.
  ▪ To study the colony character
  ▪ Pigment demonstration.

Enriched Media

When a basal medium is added with additional nutrients, such as blood, serum or egg, it is called as enriched medium. In addition to nonfastidious organisms, they also support the growth of fastidious nutritionally exacting bacteria (Table 3.6.3, Figs 3.6.1C and D).

Enrichment Broth

They are the liquid media added with some inhibitory agents which selectively allow certain organism to grow and inhibit others. This is important for isolation of the pathogens from clinical specimens which also contain normal flora (e.g., stool and sputum specimen) (Table 3.6.4).

Selective Media

They are solid media containing inhibitory substances that inhibit the normal flora present

CHAPTER 3.6 ◆ General Bacteriology: Culture Media and Culture Methods

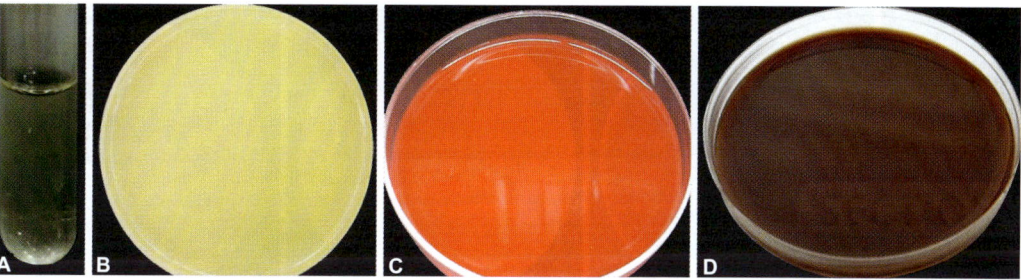

Figs 3.6.1A to D: (A) Peptone water; (B) Nutrient agar; (C) Blood agar; (D) Chocolate agar.
Source: (A to D) Department of Microbiology, JIPMER, Puducherry (*with permission*).

Table 3.6.3: Enriched media and their properties.

Enriched media	Properties
Blood agar (Fig. 3.6.1C)	It is the most commonly used media It is used to test the hemolytic property of the bacteria
Chocolate agar (Fig. 3.6.1D)	It is the heated blood agar, more nutritious than blood agar It supports certain highly fastidious bacteria, such as *Haemophilus influenzae* that does not grow on blood agar
Loeffler's serum slope	It is used for isolation of *Corynebacterium diphtheriae*
Blood culture media	They are used for culture of blood specimen. They are either monophasic or biphasic media • *Monophasic medium* is made up of brain-heart infusion (BHI) broth (Fig. 3.6.2C) • *Biphasic medium* has a liquid phase containing BHI broth and a solid agar slope made up of BHI agar (Fig. 3.6.2D)

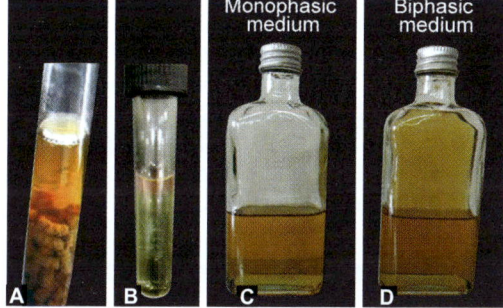

Figs 3.6.2A to D: (A) Robertson's cooked meat medium; (B) Thioglycollate broth; (C) Brain-heart infusion broth; (D) Biphasic medium (Brain-heart infusion broth/agar).
Source: (A, C and D) Department of Microbiology, JIPMER, Puducherry; B. Department of Microbiology, Pondicherry Institute of Medical Sciences, Puducherry (*with permission*).

Table 3.6.4: Enrichment broth and their uses.

Enrichment media	Used for isolation of
Tetrathionate broth	*Salmonella* Typhi
Gram-negative broth	*Shigella, Salmonella*
Selenite F broth	*Shigella*
Alkaline peptone water	*Vibrio cholerae*

Table 3.6.5: Selective media and their uses.

Selective media	Used for isolation of
Lowenstein-Jensen (LJ) medium (Fig. 3.6.3A)	*Mycobacterium tuberculosis* from sputum
Thiosulfate citrate bile salt sucrose (TCBS) agar	*Vibrio cholerae* from stool (Fig. 3.6.3B)
Deoxycholate citrate agar (DCA) (Fig. 3.6.3C)	Enteric pathogens, such as *Salmonella* and *Shigella* from stool
Xylose lysine deoxycholate (XLD) agar (Fig. 3.6.3D)	
Potassium tellurite agar (PTA)	*Corynebacterium diphtheriae* from throat swab

in the specimen and allow the pathogens to grow (Table 3.6.5).

Transport Media

They are used for the transport of the clinical specimens suspected to contain delicate organism or when the delay is expected while transporting the specimens from the site of

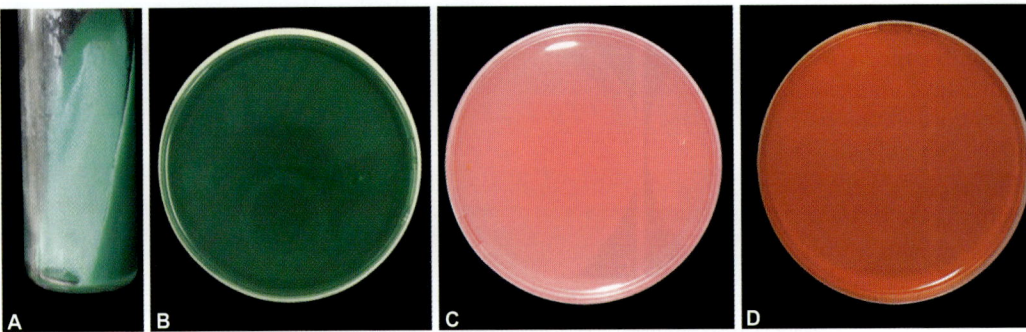

Figs 3.6.3A to D: (A) Lowenstein-Jensen medium; (B) Thiosulfate citrate bile salt sucrose agar; (C) Deoxycholate citrate agar; (D) Xylose lysine deoxycholate agar.
Source: Department of Microbiology, JIPMER, Puducherry (*with permission*).

Table 3.6.6: Transport media used for common bacteria.

Organism	Transport media
Streptococcus	Pike's medium
Neisseria	Amies medium, Stuart's medium
Vibrio cholerae	VR (Venkatraman-Ramakrishnan) medium Cary-Blair medium
Shigella, Salmonella	Buffered glycerol saline Cary-Blair medium

collection to the laboratory (Table 3.6.6). Bacteria do not multiply in the transport media; they only remain viable.

Differential Media

These media differentiate between two groups of bacteria by using an indicator, which changes the color of the colonies of a particular group of bacteria but not the other group.

❖ **MacConkey agar:** It is a differential and low selective medium commonly used for the isolation of enteric gram-negative bacteria (Fig. 3.6.4A)
 ▪ It differentiates organisms into LF or lactose fermenters (produce pink-colored colonies, e.g., *Escherichia coli*) and NLF or nonlactose fermenters (produce colorless colonies, e.g., *Shigella*) (Fig. 3.6.4B)
 ▪ Most microbiology laboratories use combination of blood agar and MacConkey agar for routine bacterial culture.
❖ **CLED agar** (Cysteine lactose electrolyte-deficient agar): This also differentiates between LF and NLF; used for the processing of urine specimens (Fig. 3.6.4C).

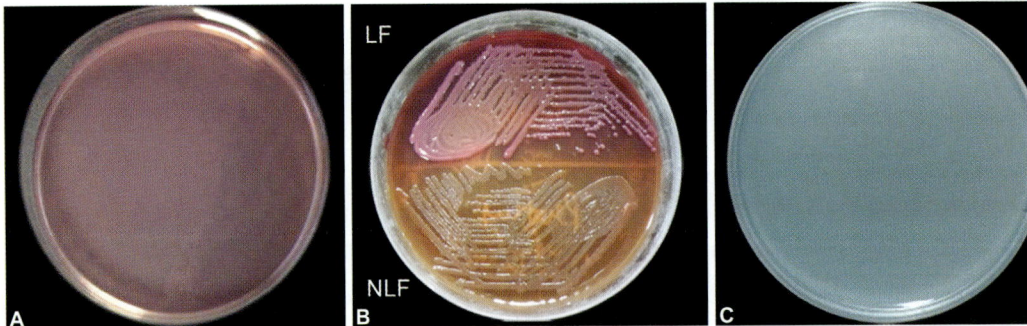

Figs 3.6.4A and B: (A) MacConkey agar; (B) Lactose fermenters (LF) and nonlactose fermenters (NLF) colonies on MacConkey agar; (C) Cysteine lactose electrolyte-deficient (CLED) agar.
Source: (A and C) Department of Microbiology, JIPMER, Puducherry (*with permission*); (B) Department of Microbiology, Pondicherry Institute of Medical Sciences; Puducherry (*with permission*).

Anaerobic Culture Media

Anaerobic media contain reducing substances which take up oxygen and create lower redox potential and thus permit the growth of obligate anaerobes, such as *Clostridium*. Examples are:

Robertson's cooked meat (RCM) broth: It contains chopped meat particles (beef heart), which provide glutathione (a sulfhydryl group containing reducing substance) and unsaturated fatty acids. It is the most widely used anaerobic culture medium (Fig. 3.6.2A).

Other anaerobic media include:
- Thioglycolate broth (Fig. 3.6.2B)
- BHIS agar (Brain-heart infusion agar) with supplements (vitamin K and hemin)
- *Bacteroides* bile esculin agar (BBE agar).
- Anaerobic blood agar
- Neomycin blood agar
- Egg yolk agar
- Phenylethyl agar.

Blood Culture Media

Recovery of bacteria from blood is difficult as they are usually present in lesser quantity in the blood and many of the blood pathogens are fastidious. Therefore, enriched media are used for isolating microorganisms from blood. Blood culture media are available either as conventional or automated media.

Conventional Blood Culture Media

The conventional blood culture media are of two types.
1. **Monophasic medium:** It contains brain–heart infusion (BHI) broth (Fig. 3.6.2C)
2. **Biphasic medium:** It has a liquid phase containing BHI broth and a solid agar slope made up of BHI agar (Fig. 3.6.2D).

The recovery of organisms in the blood is enhanced by mixing the blood in the broth periodically. If any growth occurs, it can be detected by subcultures.

Disadvantages

In conventional blood culture, subcultures are made manually.
- **From monophasic BHI broth,** subcultures are made onto blood agar and MacConkey agar periodically for 1 week. There is a higher risk of contamination due to opening of the cap of the bottle every time when subcultures are made
- **From biphasic BHI broth,** subcultures can be made just by tilting the bottles so that the broth runs over the agar slope. There is lower risk of contamination as it obviates the opening of the cap of the bottle.

Automated Blood Culture Techniques

Automated blood culture techniques are revolutionary, offer several advantages over conventional blood cultures.
- **Continuous automated monitoring:** Following inoculation, the culture bottles are loaded inside the automated culture system
  - The incubated bottles are periodically tilted automatically every 10 minutes, which allows mixing of blood with broth which fastens the recovery
  - Bottles are periodically monitored for the microbial growth once in every 10 minutes by the instrument. Once positive for microbial growth, the instrument gives a signal (producing beep or color change on the screen).
- **Composition:** Automated blood culture bottles contain:
  - Tryptic soy broth and/or brain heart infusion broth (as enriched media) added with
  - Polymeric resin beads which adsorb and neutralize the antimicrobials present in blood specimen.
- **Specimens:** In addition to blood, these bottles can also be used for culture of bone marrow, sterile body fluids, such as CSF, peritoneal, pleural and synovial fluid
- **More sensitive:** It gives a higher yield of positive cultures from clinical specimens
- **Rapid:** It takes less time than conventional methods
- **Less labor intensive,** as fully-automated.

Automated Systems

There are three automated systems commercially available.
1. **BacT/ALERT 3D** (Figs 3.6.5A and B): Its principle is based on colorimetric detection of growth. When bacteria multiply, they produce CO_2 that increases the pH, which in

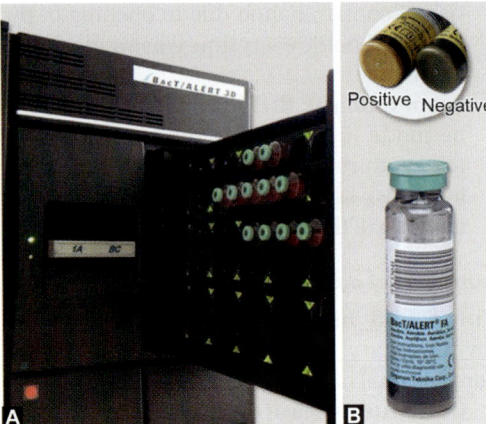

Figs 3.6.5A and B: (A) BacT/ALERT automated blood culture system; (B) BacT/ALERT blood culture bottle.
Source: Department of Microbiology, JIPMER, Puducherry (with permission).

turn changes the color of a blue-green sensor present at the bottom of the bottle to yellow, i.e., detected by colorimetry

2. **BacT/ALERT VIRTUO** (Fig. 3.6.6): It is an advanced form of BacT/ALERT which offers several advantages, such as (i) automatic loading and unloading of bottles, (ii) faster detection of growth, (iii) can determine the volume of blood present in the bottle
3. **BACTEC:** Its principle is based on fluorometric detection of growth; uses an oxygen-sensitive fluorescent dye present in the medium.

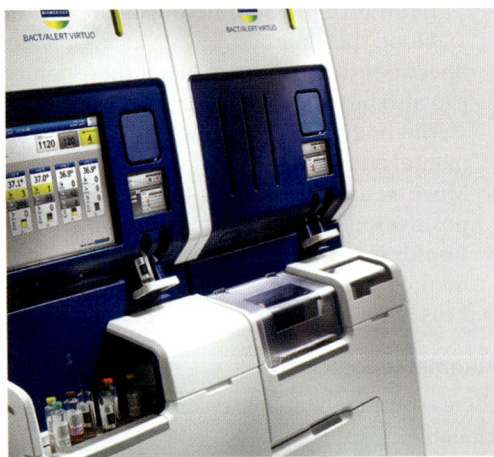

Fig. 3.6.6: BacT/ALERT VIRTUO automated blood culture system.
Source: Department of Microbiology, JIPMER, Puducherry (with permission).

Note: There is an automated culture system available for culture of *Mycobacterium tuberculosis* from various pulmonary and extrapulmonary specimens; called as Mycobacteria Growth Indicator Tube (**MGIT**, Chapter 35). This works on fluorometric principle of detection, similar to BACTEC.

Disadvantages
Automated culture methods do have several disadvantages, such as (1) high cost of the instrument and culture bottles, (2) inability to observe the colony morphology as liquid medium is used.

CULTURE METHODS

Culture methods involve inoculating the specimen on to appropriate culture media, followed by incubating the culture plates in appropriate conditions.

Selection of Media

The first step of a culture investigation is selection of appropriate media, which in turn depends upon the type of specimen to be processed. In general, combination of blood agar and MacConkey agar is commonly used for processing of most specimens. However, there are few specimens for which additional or alternative media are used (Table 3.6.7).

Inoculation of the Specimens

Inoculation of the specimens onto the culture media is carried out with the help of bacteriological loops made up of platinum or nichrome wire (Fig. 3.6.7A).

❖ The inoculating loop is first heated in the Bunsen flame by making it red hot (Fig. 3.6.7B) and then made cool waiting for 10 seconds
❖ The entire process of bacteriological culture method should be carried out in a biological safety cabinet and wearing appropriate personal protective equipment, such as gloves, laboratory coat or gown and mask (for respiratory specimens).

Biosafety Cabinet (BSC)
It is an enclosed, ventilated laboratory work station, used to protect the laboratory personnel while working with potential infectious clinical specimens.

Contd...

Contd...

- They are especially designed in a way that the air is blown into the cabinet away from the worker and then exhausted outside through a duct lined with HEPA filters (Fig. 3.6.8)
- There are various types of BSCs, depending upon air velocity and percentage of air recirculated. Most of the microbiology laboratories require Class 2A BSC. A higher class of BSCs may be required for certain high-risk pathogens.

Table 3.6.7: Selection of media for various specimen types.

Specimens	Recommended culture media
Exudate specimens*	Blood agar plus MacConkey agar
Sterile body fluids	Blood agar, plus MacConkey agar, plus chocolate agar or Automated blood culture bottles
Blood	Blood culture bottles (Conventional or automated)
Urine	Blood agar plus MacConkey agar CLED agar can be used alternatively
Stool	Selenite-F broth plus MacConkey agar plus DCA and/or XLD agar (if cholera is suspected—add TCBS agar)
Respiratory specimens	Blood agar, plus MacConkey agar, plus chocolate agar (if diphtheria is suspected—add LSS and PTA)

*Exudate specimens include pus, wound swab, aspirates, and tissue bits.

Abbreviations: CLED, cysteine lactose electrolyte deficient agar; DCA, deoxycholate citrate agar; XLD, xylose lysine deoxycholate; TCBS, thiosulfate-citrate-bile salts-sucrose agar; LSS, Loeffler serum slope; PTA, potassium tellurite agar.

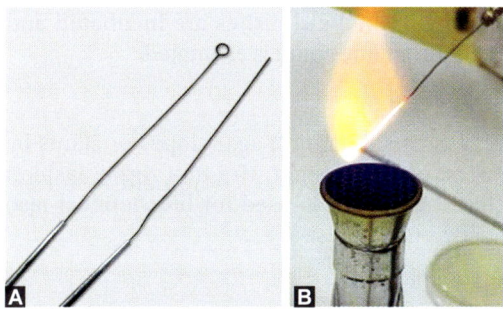

Figs 3.6.7A and B: (A) Bacteriological loop and straight wire; (B) Flaming the loop (red hot).
Source: (A) Department of Microbiology, JIPMER, Puducherry (*with permission*).

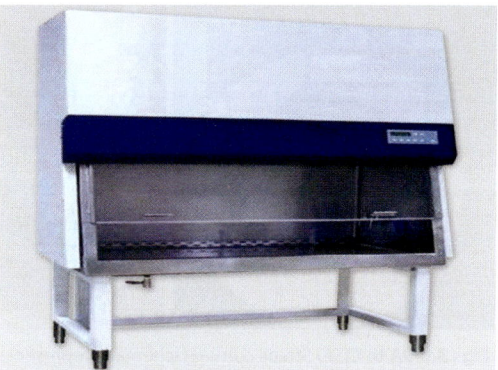

Fig. 3.6.8: Biological safety cabinet.
Source: Department of Microbiology, Pondicherry Institute of Medical Sciences, Puducherry (*with permission*).

Inoculation Methods

Inoculation methods are of two types:
1. Methods used for inoculating clinical specimens on to the culture media
2. Methods used for inoculating colonies on to various media for further processing.

Streak Culture

It is the most common inoculation method; used for the inoculation of the specimens on to the solid media. It is also used for obtaining individual isolated colonies from a mixed culture of bacteria.

- **Streaking:** A loopful of the specimen is smeared onto the solid media to form round-shaped primary inoculum, which is then spread over the culture plate by streaking parallel lines to form the secondary, tertiary inoculum and finally a feathery tail end (Fig. 3.6.9A)
- **Intermittent heating:** The loop is flamed and cooled in between the different set of streaks to get isolated colonies on the final streaks (Fig. 3.6.9B). Obtaining isolated colonies is the prerequisite to perform tests for identification and AST.

Liquid Culture

Liquid culture is used for culture of specimens, such as blood or body fluids, which are inoculated by directly adding the specimen into the liquid medium or with the help of a syringe or pipette.

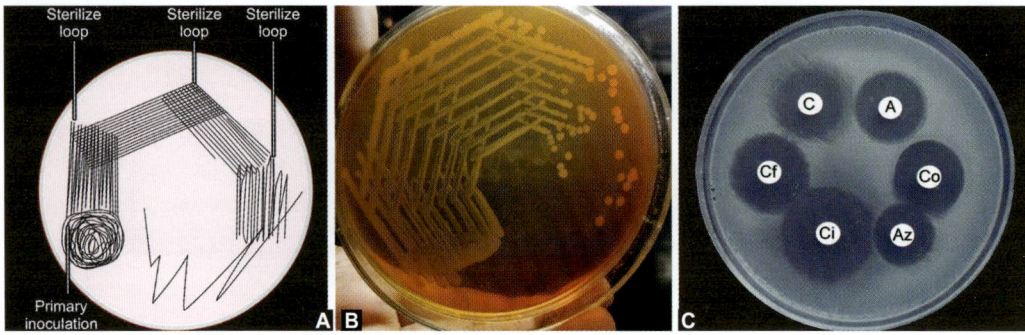

Figs 3.6.9A to C: (A) Streak culture (schematic representation); (B) Isolated colonies grown by following streak culture; (C) Lawn culture of a bacterial isolate to perform the antimicrobial susceptibility testing.
Source: Department of Microbiology, JIPMER, Puducherry (*with permission*).

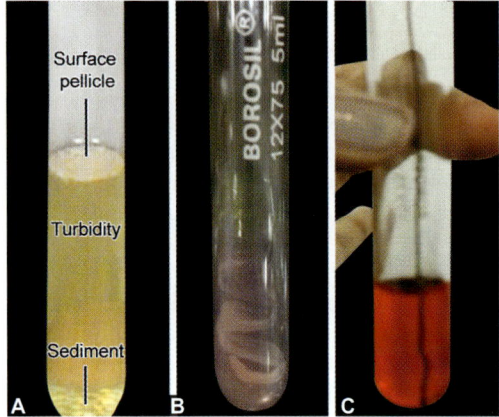

Figs 3.6.10A to C: (A) Liquid culture in test tube (turbidity indicates growth); (B) Stroke culture; (C) Stabbing with inoculation wire (stab culture).
Source: Department of Microbiology, Pondicherry Institute of Medical Sciences, Puducherry (*with permission*).

- ❖ **Bacterial growth** is detected by observing the turbidity in the medium. Some aerobic bacteria form surface pellicles (Fig. 3.6.10A)
- ❖ **Uses:** Liquid cultures are useful for—(1) blood, or body fluids culture, (2) automated culture for mycobacteria (MGIT, i.e., mycobacteria growth indicator tube), (3) water analysis
- ❖ **Advantages:** Liquid cultures are preferable for culture of—(1) specimens containing small quantity of bacteria, (2) specimens (e.g., blood) containing antibiotics and other antibacterial substances, as they get neutralized by dilution in the medium, (3) it is also preferred when large yields of bacteria are required
- ❖ **Disadvantages:** (1) Liquid cultures do not provide a pure culture from a mixed inoculum, (2) there is no visible colonies, therefore unlike solid media, it does not give any preliminary clue about the bacteria.

Lawn or Carpet Culture

Lawn culture is useful to carry out antimicrobial susceptibility testing (AST) by disk diffusion method (Fig. 3.6.9C). Here, the uniform lawn of bacterial growth is obtained by either swabbing or flooding with a bacterial broth onto the culture plate (discussed in detail in Chapter 3.8).

Pour Plate Technique

Seldom used for quantifying the bacterial load present in the specimens, such as urine or blood. Here, serial dilutions of the specimen are added on to the molten agar. After being cooled and solidified, the Petri dishes are incubated and then the colony count is estimated.

Stroke Culture

This is carried out on agar slopes or slants by streaking the straight wire in a zigzag fashion (Fig. 3.6.10B). It is used for biochemical test, such as urease test.

Stab Culture

It is made by stabbing the semisolid agar butt by a straight wire. It is used for motility testing using mannitol motility medium (Fig. 3.6.10C), and triple sugar iron agar test (here, both stroke and stab cultures are made).

Incubatory Conditions

Most of the pathogenic bacteria are aerobes or facultative anaerobes; grow best at 37°C, i.e., body temperature of human beings. Therefore, the inoculated culture plates are incubated at 37°C aerobically overnight in an incubator.

> **Bacteriological Incubator**
> It is an equipment used to incubate the culture plates, biochemical tests and AST plates (Fig. 3.6.11). The incubator maintains optimal temperature. Some incubators are especially designed to maintain other conditions, such as humidity and CO_2.

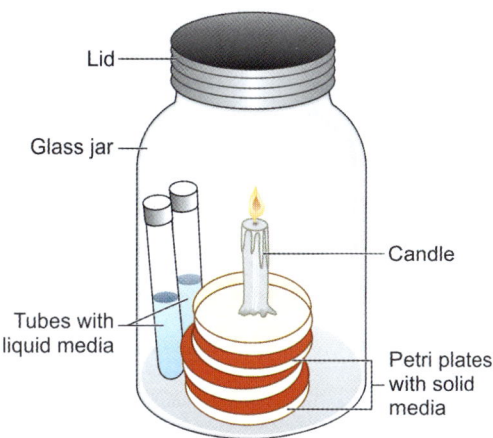

Fig. 3.6.12: Candle jar.

Other Incubatory Conditions

The incubatory conditions may vary depending upon the bacteria to be isolated.

- **For capnophilic bacteria:** Candle jar is used. Here, inoculated media are placed inside a jar, along with a lighted candle and then jar is sealed
  - The burning candle reduces oxygen to a point where the flame goes off (Fig. 3.6.12). This provides an atmosphere of approximately 3–5% CO_2
  - This is useful for capnophilic bacteria, such as *Brucella*, *Streptococcus*, pneumococcus and gonococcus.
- **For microaerophilic bacteria,** such as *Campylobacter* and *Helicobacter* require 5% oxygen for optimum growth
- **For obligate anaerobes,** anaerobic culture methods are used (see below).

Anaerobic Culture Methods

Obligate anaerobic bacteria can grow only in the absence of oxygen, hence for the growth of such bacteria, anaerobic environment is needed. The following are the methods used to create anaerobiosis.

Evacuation and Replacement

This involves evacuation of the air from jar and replacement with inert gas, such as hydrogen followed by removal of the residual oxygen by use of a catalyst. It is carried out either by:

- **Manual method** by using McIntosh and Filde's anaerobic jar (Fig. 3.6.13A): It was the most popular method for creating anaerobiosis in the past, now not in use
- **Automated system (Anoxomat):** It automatically evacuates air and replaces by hydrogen gas from a cylinder (Fig. 3.6.13B)
  - The catalyst used to combust residual oxygen is a sachet containing aluminum pellets coated with palladium
  - It is easier to operate than McIntosh jar method and claims to be highly effective for creating anaerobiosis.

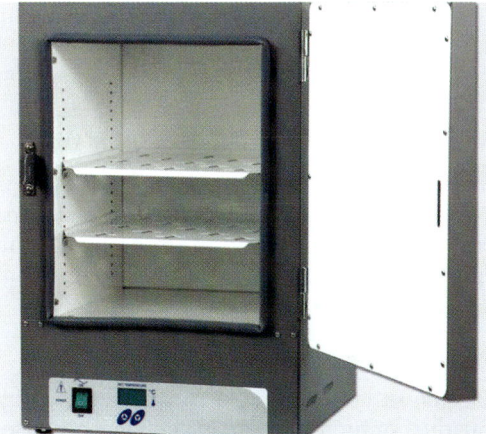

Fig. 3.6.11: Bacteriological incubator.
Source: Department of Microbiology, JIPMER, Puducherry (with permission).

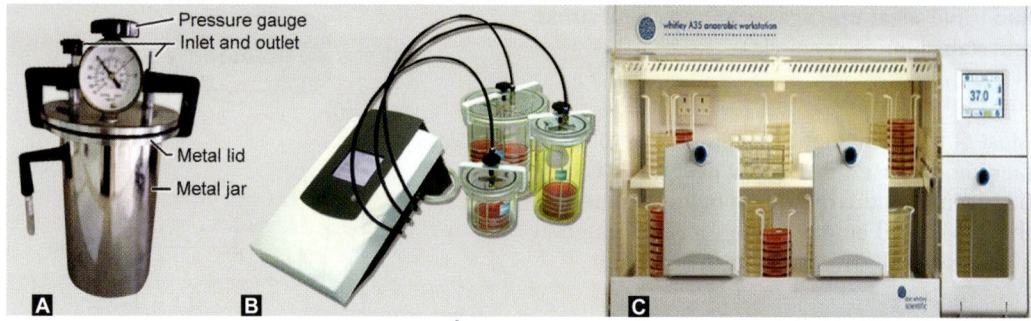

Figs 3.6.13A to C: (A) McIntosh and Filde's anaerobic jar; (B) Anoxomat anaerobic system; (C) Anaerobic work station (Whitley Pvt Ltd).

Source: (A) Department of Microbiology, Pondicherry Institute of Medical Sciences, Puducherry; (B) Department of Microbiology, JIPMER, Puducherry; (C) Dr Padmaja A Shenoy, Department of Microbiology, Kasturba Medical College, Manipal, Karnataka (*with permission*).

Absorption of Oxygen by Chemical Methods

GasPak system (BD diagnostics) works on this principle. It is the the most commonly used method for anaerobiosis, especially for laboratories with less sample load.

- Here, the oxygen is removed by chemical reactions, instead of evacuation and replacement technique used in Anoxomat
- It uses a sachet containing sodium bicarbonate and sodium borohydride which react chemically in presence of water, to produce hydrogen and CO_2 gas
- The traces of oxygen is removed by using the same catalyst used for Anoxomat (aluminum pellets coated with palladium) placed below the jar lid (Fig. 3.6.14)
- **Indicator of anaerobiosis:** The effectiveness of anaerobiosis can be checked by:
  - **Chemical indicator:** Reduced methylene blue remains colorless in anaerobic conditions, but turns blue on exposure to oxygen
  - **Biological indicator** using obligate aerobe, such as *Pseudomonas:* Absence of its growth indicates that complete anaerobiosis has been achieved.

GENbag (bioMérieux): It consists of an airtight transparent bag with a generator sachet, which rapidly produces carbon dioxide and creates an anaerobic environment. Its application is similar to that of GasPak system.

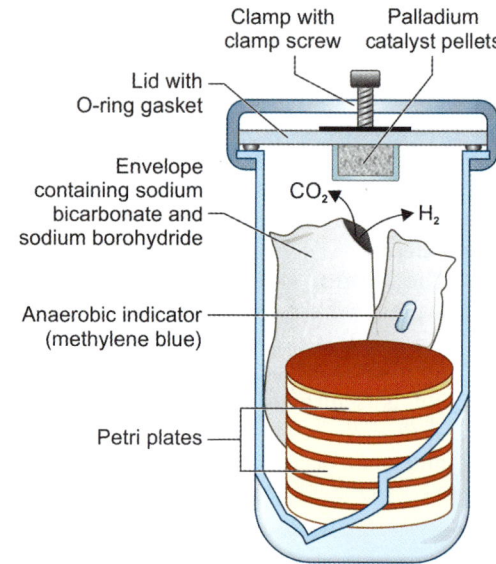

Fig. 3.6.14: GasPak anaerobic system.

Anaerobic Glove Box and Anaerobic Work Station

These systems provide facility for easy processing, incubation and examination of the specimens without exposure to oxygen (Fig. 3.6.13C).

Reducing Agents

Oxygen in culture media can be reduced by various reducing agents, such as glucose, thioglycollate, cooked meat pieces, cysteine and

CHAPTER 3.6 ◆ General Bacteriology: Culture Media and Culture Methods

ascorbic acid. **Robertson cooked meat broth** is the most widely employed anaerobic culture medium which uses chopped meat particles (beef heart) as reducing agent (Fig. 3.6.2A).

Pre-reduced Anaerobically Sterilized (PRAS)
PRAS media are prepared entirely under oxygen-free conditions from initial sterilization to packaging in sealed foil packets.

Problem Solving Exercise

Culture Media and Culture Methods

Case scenario 1: A 72-year-old female presented with fever (104°F), heart rate of 116 beats/minute and respiratory rate of 25 breaths/minute. A provisional diagnosis of sepsis is made and blood cultures were collected. Discuss the culture medium and culture method required for processing of blood culture. What is automated blood culture? Discuss with examples.

Case scenario 2: A 21-year-old female was admitted with increased frequency and burning micturition for the past 2 days. The urine specimen was collected and sent to the laboratory. What are the culture media required for processing of urine specimen. What is differential media, discuss with examples?

Case scenario 3: A 2-year-old baby was admitted with complain of passing liquid stool for 10-12 times since one day. The stool specimen was collected and sent for culture. What are the culture media required for processing of stool specimen. What is selective medium; how it is different from enrichment medium?

Case scenario 4: A 12-year-old boy was admitted with fever, productive cough and dyspnoea. Sputum specimen was collected and sent to the laboratory. What are the culture media required for processing of sputum specimen. What is enriched media, discuss with examples?

Case scenario 5: Following a penetrating trauma to his right thigh, a construction laborer developed discolored tissue and fowl smelling discharge. Anaerobic infection was suspected. How will you collect specimen for anaerobic culture? What are the methods used to achieve anaerobiosis. What are the common culture media used for processing anaerobic culture?

Explanation
The following are the recommended culture media used.

Case scenario 1: For blood culture—Conventional blood culture (monophasic media, such as brain heart infusion broth and biphasic media, such as brain heart infusion broth/agar) or automated blood culture (BACTEC or BacT/ALERT) media can be used.

Case scenario 2: For urine culture—Combination of blood agar plus MacConkey agar is used. CLED agar can be used alternatively.

Case scenario 3: For stool culture—Selenite-F broth plus MacConkey agar plus DCA and/or XLD agar is recommended. If cholera is suspected, alkaline peptone water and TCBS agar are used in addition.

Case scenario 4: For culture of respiratory specimens—Blood agar plus MacConkey agar plus chocolate agar is recommended. If diphtheria is suspected and throat swab is sent, Loeffler's serum slope (LSS) and potassium tellurite agar (PTA) are used in addition.

Case scenario 5: For anaerobic culture—Robertson's cooked meat (RCM) broth is used. Other culture media are brain-heart infusion agar with supplements (vitamin K and hemin), *Bacteroides* bile esculin agar (BBE agar), neomycin blood agar, egg yolk agar and phenylethyl agar. The common methods to achieve anaerobiosis include Anoxomat and GasPak system. For the answers to other questions (of all the case scenarios), refer the text in this chapter.

General Bacteriology: Identification of Bacteria (Conventional and Automated)

CHAPTER 3.7

Problem Solving Exercise

Identification of Bacteria

Case scenario 1: A 3 year old boy presents to OPD with watery diarrhea resembling rice water. Stool specimen is sent to the laboratory. Perform a test for the presumptive identification of *Vibrio cholerae* directly from the stool specimen?

Case scenario 2: Urine specimen collected from a patient suffering from burning micturition, and increased urinary frequency is sent to the laboratory. Culture on MacConkey agar revealed lactose fermenting pink colonies with colony count >10^5/mL. Perform the conventional biochemical tests for identification of the etiological agent.

Case scenario 3: Sputum specimen of a 25 old man presented with productive cough, fever and dyspnoea is sent to the laboratory. Culture on blood agar revealed α-hemolytic colonies. What is the automated identification system that can identify the organism from the colony within minutes. Discuss its principle?

Explanation

Case scenario 1: The presumptive identification of *Vibrio cholerae* directly from stool specimen is made by performing motility testing.
- Hanging drop is the most common method used for demonstrating motility (refer text, for detail).
- *Vibrio cholerae* exhibits highly active motility, described as darting motility.

Case scenario 2: Patient suffering from burning micturition and increased urinary frequency is suggestive of urinary tract infection (UTI).
- Lactose fermenting pink colonies on MacConkey agar is suggestive of either *Escherichia coli* (most common cause of UTI), or *Klebsiella*
- The conventional biochemical tests performed for their identification are indole test, citrate test, urease test and triple sugar iron test (refer text and Chapter 42, for detail)

Case scenario 3: α-hemolytic colonies on blood agar is suggestive of either pneumococcus (pathogen in sputum) or viridans streptococci (commensal in sputum). **MALDI-TOF** is the automated identification system that can identify the organism from the colony within minutes. Its principle is discussed in the text.

Accurate identification of bacteria is necessary as it helps in choosing the appropriate panel of antibiotics for performing antibiotic susceptibility test. This in turn will guide in instituting the accurate antimicrobial therapy.
- The **presumptive identification** of bacteria is made by observing their colony appearance in culture media, followed by performing culture smear (by Gram stain) and motility testing
- The **final identification** can be confirmed by performing either conventional biochemical tests or by automated identification systems.

■ COLONY MORPHOLOGY

After overnight incubation, the culture media are removed from the incubator and are examined under bright illumination. The appearance of bacterial colony on culture medium is characteristic for many organisms; which helps in their preliminary identification. The following features of the colony are studied:
- Size—in millimeters; e.g., pinhead size is characteristic of staphylococcal colony, whereas pinpoint size is characteristic of streptococcal colony

- Shape—circular or irregular
- Consistency—dry, moist or mucoid
- Density—opaque, translucent or transparent
- Hemolysis on blood agar (see below)
- **Color of the colony:** Colonies may be colored due to certain properties of the media or organisms. For example, pink colonies produced by lactose fermenters on MacConkey agar and black colonies by *Corynebacterium diphtheriae* on potassium tellurite agar due to the reduction of tellurite. Color of the colonies may also be due to pigment production by the bacteria
- **Pigment production:** Bacteria may produce two types of pigments:
  1. **Diffusible pigments**, e.g., blue-green pigments produced by *Pseudomonas aeruginosa*
  2. **Non-diffusible pigments:** They do not diffuse into surrounding media, hence only the colonies are colored, not the surrounding media; e.g., *S. aureus* producing golden-yellow colonies.

Hemolysis on Blood Agar

Certain bacteria produce hemolysin enzymes that lyse the red blood cells surrounding the colonies on blood agar, forming a zone of hemolysis (Fig. 3.7.1). Hemolysis may be:

- ❏ **Partial or α hemolysis:** Partial clearing of blood around the colonies occurs with green discoloration of the surrounding medium; outline of the RBCs is intact (e.g., pneumococci, viridans streptococci)

Contd...

Contd...

- ❏ **Complete or β hemolysis:** Zone of complete clearing of blood around the colonies due to complete lysis of the RBCs (e.g., *Staphylococcus aureus* and *Streptococcus pyogenes*)
- ❏ **No hemolysis (γ hemolysis, a misnomer):** There is no color change surrounding the colony (e.g., *Enterococcus*)

CULTURE SMEAR AND MOTILITY TESTING

Culture Smear

The colonies grown on the culture media are subjected to Gram staining and motility testing by hanging drop method.

- Culture smear is prepared by emulsifying a bacterial colony with a drop of saline on a slide
- Then the smear is allowed to air-dry and then subjected to Gram staining (Refer Chapter 3.4)
- The morphological appearance of the bacterium on Gram staining of culture smear may sometimes give a preliminary clue about the identification of the organism (Table 3.1.1, Chapter 3.1).

Demonstration of Bacterial Motility

Bacteria can be further differentiated based on whether they are motile or nonmotile (Table 3.7.1). Even motile bacteria can be further differentiated based on the type of motility they produce (Table 3.7.2). Bacterial motility can be tested by various methods.

- Cragie tube method
- Semisolid medium, e.g., mannitol motility medium
- Swarming of the bacteria on agar plate
- Dark-ground microscopy
- Phase-contrast microscopy.

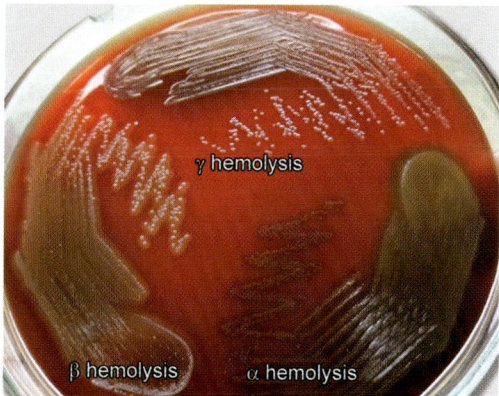

Fig. 3.7.1: Hemolysis on blood agar.
Source: Department of Microbiology, Pondicherry Institute of Medical Sciences, Puducherry (*with permission*).

Table 3.7.1: Examples of motile and nonmotile bacteria.

Motile bacteria	Nonmotile bacteria
Escherichia coli	*Klebsiella*
Proteus	*Shigella*
Salmonella	*Acinetobacter*
Vibrio	
Pseudomonas	

Table 3.7.2: Various types of motility.

Types of motility	Bacteria shown
Tumbling motility	Listeria
Gliding motility	Mycoplasma
Stately motility	Clostridium
Darting motility	Vibrio cholerae
Swarming motility	Proteus, Clostridium tetani
Corkscrew motility	Spirochete

Hanging Drop Method

Hanging drop preparation is one of the most common and easiest method to demonstrate bacterial motility. The procedure is explained in Figure 3.7.2. After the drop is prepared on a coverslip and kept over the cavity slide, the edge of the drop is focussed. The edge is focused because:

- **Better contrast at the edge:** Due to difference in the refractive index of the drop and the cover slip
- As the drop hangs, it thins towards the edge, containing less number of bacteria and less overcrowding; hence motility can be clearly appreciated
- Live aerobic bacteria come towards the edge to get more oxygen for respiration.

Types of Bacterial Motility

Three types of movements can be noticed in a hanging drop preparation. Active movement is the true motility exhibited by motile bacteria which needs to be differentiated from passive and Brownian movements shown by nonmotile bacteria.

- **Active movement:** Organism move in different directions and change their positions in the field
- **Passive movement:** Drifting of the organisms in the same direction along the convectional current in the fluid
- **Brownian movement:** It is an oscillatory movement about a nearly fixed point possessed by all small bodies suspended in fluid and due to irregularities in their bombardments by molecules of water.

CULTURE IDENTIFICATION

Identification of bacteria from culture is confirmed by performing either by conventional biochemical tests or by automated identification systems.

Biochemical Identification

Based on the type of colony morphology and Gram staining appearance observed in culture smear, the appropriate biochemical tests are employed.

1. **Initially,** catalase and oxidase tests are done on all types of colonies grown on the media
2. **For gram-negative bacilli:** The following are the common biochemical tests done routinely, abbreviated as 'ICUT':
   - Indole test
   - Citrate utilization test
   - Urea hydrolysis test
   - Triple sugar iron test (TSI).
3. **For gram-positive cocci:** The useful biochemical tests are as follows:
   - Coagulase test (for *Staphylococcus aureus*)
   - CAMP (Christie-Atkins-Munch-Petersen) test for group B *Streptococcus*
   - Bile esculin hydrolysis test (for *Enterococcus*)
   - Inulin fermentation test and bile solubility test (for pneumococcus)
   - Antimicrobial susceptibility tests done for bacterial identification are as follows:
     - Optochin susceptibility test—done to differentiate pneumococcus (sensitive) from viridans streptococci (resistant)

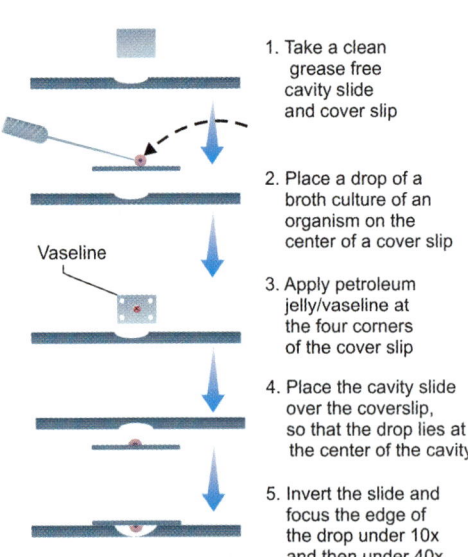

Fig. 3.7.2: Hanging drop method (procedure).

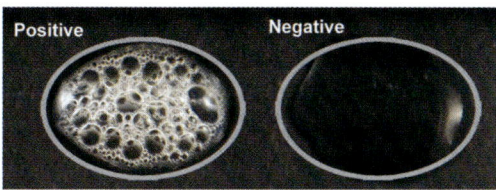

Fig. 3.7.3: Catalase test.
Source: Department of Microbiology, JIPMER, Puducherry *(with permission).*

- Bacitracin susceptibility test—done to differentiate group A (sensitive) from group B (resistant) *Streptococcus.*

Some of the important biochemical tests are described below. Coagulase test and other biochemical reactions for gram-positive cocci are described in the respective chapters.

Catalase Test

When a colony of any catalase producing bacteria is mixed with a drop of hydrogen peroxide (3% H_2O_2) placed on a slide, effervescence or bubbles appear due to breakdown of H_2O_2 by catalase to produce oxygen (Fig. 3.7.3).
- ❖ Catalase test is primarily used to differentiate between *Staphylococcus* (catalase positive) from *Streptococcus* (catalase negative)
- ❖ It is also positive for members of the families Enterobacteriaceae, Vibrionaceae, Pseudomonadaceae, etc.

Oxidase Test

It detects the presence of cytochrome oxidase enzyme in bacteria, which catalyzes the oxidation of reduced cytochrome by atmospheric oxygen.
- ❖ When a filter paper strip or disk, soaked in oxidase reagent is smeared with a bacterial colony producing cytochrome oxidase enzyme, the smeared area turns deep purple within 10 seconds due to oxidation of the dye to form a purple-colored compound indophenol blue
- ❖ Interpretation (Fig. 3.7.4A) and examples:
  - **Oxidase positive (deep purple):** Examples include *Pseudomonas, Vibrio, Neisseria, Bacillus, Haemophilus,* etc.
  - **Oxidase negative (no color change):** Examples include; members of family Enterobacteriaceae, *Acinetobacter,* etc.

Indole Test

It detects the ability of certain bacteria to produce an enzyme tryptophanase that breaks down amino acid tryptophan present in the medium into indole.
- ❖ When Kovac's reagent is added to an overnight incubated broth of a bacterial colony, it complexes with indole to produce a cherry red color ring near the surface of the medium
- ❖ **Indole positive** (Fig. 3.7.4B): A red-colored ring is formed near the surface of the broth. Examples include *Escherichia coli, Proteus vulgaris, Vibrio cholerae,* etc.
- ❖ **Indole negative** (Fig. 3.7.4B): Yellow-colored ring is formed near the surface of the broth, e.g., *Klebsiella pneumoniae, Proteus mirabilis, Pseudomonas, Salmonella,* etc.

Citrate Utilization Test

It detects the ability of a few bacteria to utilize citrate as the sole source of carbon for their growth, with production of alkaline metabolic products. Test is performed on Simmon's citrate medium. Citrate utilizing bacteria produce growth and a color change, i.e., original green color changes to blue (Fig. 3.7.5A).
- ❖ Citrate test is positive for *Klebsiella pneumoniae, Citrobacter, Enterobacter,* etc.
- ❖ The test is negative for *Escherichia coli, Shigella,* etc.

Urea Hydrolysis Test

Urease producing bacteria can split urea present in the medium to produce ammonia that makes the medium alkaline.
- ❖ Test is done on Christensen's urea medium, which contains phenol red indicator that

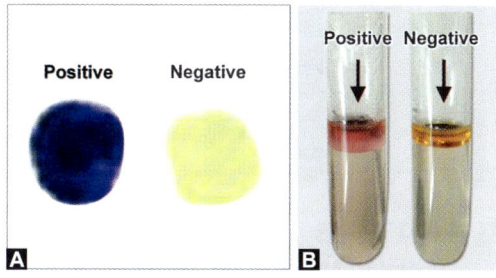

Figs 3.7.4A and B: (A) Oxidase test; (B) Indole test.
Source: Department of Microbiology, Pondicherry Institute of Medical Sciences, Puducherry *(with permission).*

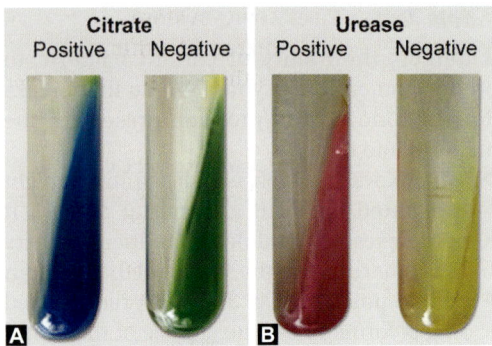

Figs 3.7.5A and B: (A) Citrate utilization test; (B) Urea hydrolysis test.
Source: Department of Microbiology, Pondicherry Institute of Medical Sciences, Puducherry (*with permission*).

changes to pink color in alkaline medium (Fig. 3.7.5B)
- **Urease test is positive for:** *Klebsiella pneumoniae, Proteus* species, *Helicobacter pylori, Brucella,* etc.
- **Urease test is negative for:** *Escherichia coli, Shigella, Salmonella,* etc.

Triple Sugar Iron (TSI) Agar Test

TSI is a very important medium employed widely for identification of gram-negative bacteria. TSI medium contains three sugars—glucose, sucrose and lactose in the ratio of 1:10:10 parts. Uninoculated TSI medium is red in color; has a slant and a butt (Fig. 3.7.6A). After inoculation, the medium is incubated at 37°C for 18–24 hours.

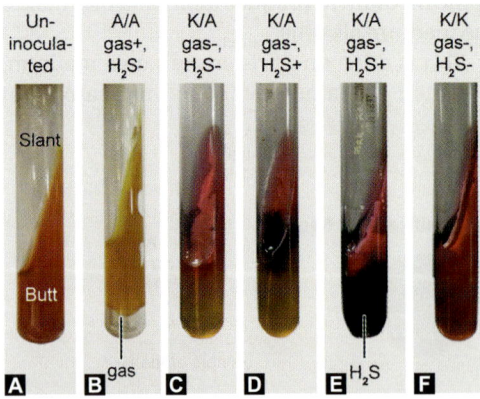

Figs 3.7.6A to F: Triple sugar iron test.
Source: Department of Microbiology, JIPMER, Puducherry (*with permission*).

Interpretation

TSI detects three properties of bacteria, which includes fermentation of sugars to produce acid and/or gas and production of H_2S (Figs 3.7.6A to F and Table 3.7.3).

- **Acid production:** If acid is produced, the medium is turned yellow from red. Accordingly the organisms are categorized into three groups:
  1. **Nonfermenters:** They do not ferment any sugars, hence the medium (both slant and butt) remain red, producing Alkaline slant/Alkaline butt (K/K) reaction (Fig. 3.7.6F); e.g., *Pseudomonas* and *Acinetobacter*
  2. **Glucose only fermenters:** They ferment only glucose and produce little acid only at the butt, whereas the slant remains alkaline giving rise to Alkaline slant/Acidic butt (K/A) reaction (Fig. 3.7.6C); e.g., *Salmonella* and *Shigella*
  3. **≥2 sugars fermenters:** They ferment glucose and also ferment lactose and/or sucrose to produce large amount of acid so that the medium (both slant and butt) change to yellow giving rise to Acidic

Table 3.7.3: Various reactions in TSI with examples.

Reactions in TSI	Examples
Acidic slant/acidic butt	**≥2 sugars fermented** (1) glucose, (2) lactose or/ and sucrose
A/A, gas produced, no H_2S (Fig. 3.7.6B)	*Escherichia coli* *Klebsiella pneumoniae*
Alkaline slant/acidic butt	**Only glucose-fermenter group**
K/A, no gas, no H_2S (Fig. 3.7.6C)	*Shigella*
K/A, no gas, H_2S produced (small amount) (Fig. 3.7.6D)	*Salmonella* Typhi
K/A, no gas, H_2S produced (abundant) (Fig. 3.7.6E)	*Proteus vulgaris*
K/A, gas produced, H_2S produced (abundant)	*Salmonella* Paratyphi B
K/A, gas produced, no H_2S	*Salmonella* Paratyphi A
Alkaline slant/alkaline butt	**Non-fermenters group**
K/K, no gas, no H_2S (Fig. 3.7.6F)	*Pseudomonas, Acinetobacter*

slant/Acidic butt (A/A) reaction (Fig. 3.7.6B); e.g., *E. coli* and *Klebsiella*.
- **Gas production:** If gas is produced, the medium is lifted up or broken with cracks (Fig. 3.7.6B); examples, *E. coli* and *Klebsiella*
- **H$_2$S production:** If H$_2$S is produced, the medium changes color to black (Figs 3.7.6D and E); e.g., *Salmonella* Typhi and *Proteus vulgaris*.

Automated Systems for Bacterial Identification

Automated identification systems are revolutionary in diagnostic microbiology. They have several advantages—(i) produce faster result, (ii) can identify a wide range of organisms with accuracy, which are otherwise difficult to identify (e.g., anaerobes) through conventional biochemical tests.

- **MALDI–TOF** (Matrix-assisted laser desorption/ionization time-of-flight), e.g., VITEK MS (bioMérieux): Refer the highlight box and Fig. 3.7.7 for details
- **VITEK 2** (bioMérieux) for automated identification and antimicrobial susceptibility test: Refer the highlight box and Figure 3.7.8 for details
- **Phoenix** (BD Diagnostics) for automated identification and antimicrobial susceptibility test
- **MicroScanWalkAway system** (Beckman Coulter) for automated identification and antimicrobial susceptibility test.

MALDI-TOF

MALDI-TOF technology (Matrix Assisted Laser Desorption Ionization Time-of-Flight) has revolutionized the identification of organisms in clinical microbiology laboratories.
- It can identify bacteria, fungi, and mycobacteria with a turnaround time of few minutes and with absolute accuracy
- Two systems are commercially available: VITEK MS (bioMérieux) and Biotyper system (Bruker).

Principle (Fig. 3.7.7)
MALDI-TOF examines the pattern of ribosomal proteins present in the organism.

Sample preparation: The colony of an organism is smeared onto a well of the slide and one drop of matrix solution (composed of cyano-hydroxy-cinnamic acid) is added to the same well and mixed; then the slide is loaded in the system.

Steps after loading: Overall, mass spectrometry can be divided into three steps occurring in three chambers of the system.
1. **Ionization chamber:** Here, the wells are irradiated with the laser beam. The matrix absorbs the laser light causing desorption and ionization of bacterial ribosomal proteins, generating singly protonated ions
2. **Analyzer:** These ions are then accelerated into an electric field which directs them to the analyzer

Contd...

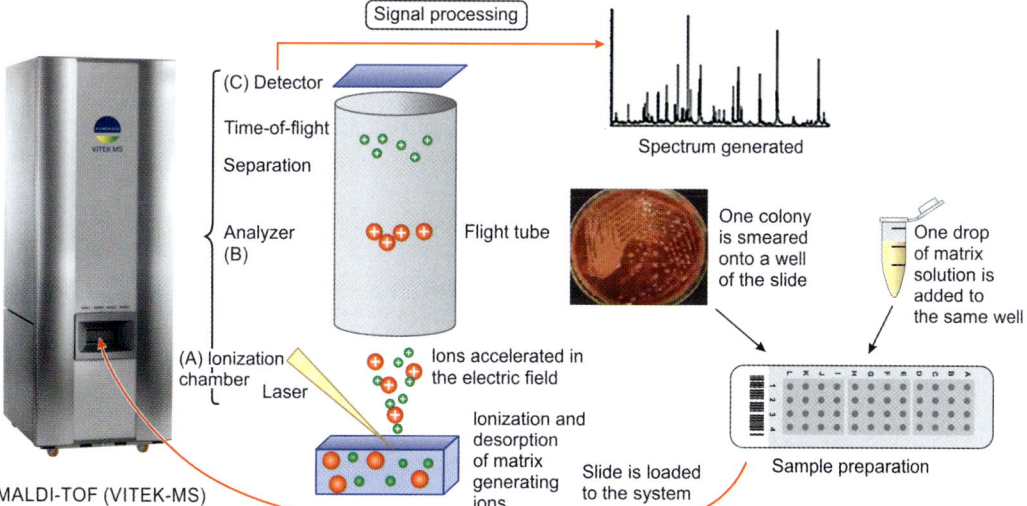

Fig. 3.7.7: MALDI-TOF and its working principle.
Source: Department of Microbiology, JIPMER, Puducherry (*with permission*).

Contd...

chamber. The analyzer (mass spectrometer) separates them according to their time-of-flight (TOF) in the flight tube. The smaller molecules travel faster, followed by the bigger, according to the mass to charge (m/z) ratio

3. **Detector:** It converts the received ion into an electrical current which is then amplified and digitized to generate a characteristic spectrum that is unique to a species due to its conserved ribosomal proteins. The test isolate is identified by comparing its spectrum with a known database.

VITEK 2 Automated System

VITEK 2 is the most widely used automated system in India; can perform both identification and antimicrobial susceptibility testing (AST) of bacteria and yeast. Principle of VITEK for identification is discussed below, VITEK for AST is discussed in Chapter 3.8.
- It uses colorimetric reagent card containing 64 wells; each well contains an individual test substrate
- Separate cards are available for gram-negative, gram-positive bacteria, fastidious bacteria and yeasts (Fig. 3.7.8)
- Substrates in the well measure various metabolic activities, such as acidification, alkalinization, enzyme hydrolysis, etc., which helps in identification of the organism

Contd...

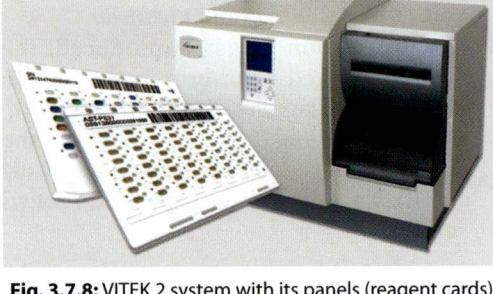

Fig. 3.7.8: VITEK 2 system with its panels (reagent cards) for identification and antimicrobial susceptibility test.
Source: Department of Microbiology, JIPMER, Puducherry (*with permission*).

Contd...

- The reaction pattern obtained from the test organism is compared with the database and the identification is reported with a confidence level of matching (excellent matching to the unidentified organism)
- **Incubation:** The cards are incubated in the system at 35.5 ± 1°C. The reading is taken once every 15 minutes by the optical system of the equipment, which measures the presence of any colored products of substrate metabolism (by advanced colorimetry method)
- The result of identification is usually available within 4–6 hours.

General Bacteriology: Antimicrobial Susceptibility Test

CHAPTER 3.8

ANTIMICROBIAL SUSCEPTIBILITY TEST

Antimicrobial susceptibility test (AST) is the most important investigation carried out by a Microbiology Laboratory.
- ❖ Bacteria exhibit great strain variations in susceptibility to antimicrobial agents. Therefore, AST plays a vital role to guide the clinician for tailoring the empirical antibiotic therapy to pathogen-directed therapy
- ❖ AST is performed only for pathogenic bacteria isolated from the specimen, and not for the commensal bacteria. For example, *E. coli* isolated from urine specimen should be subjected to AST, whereas *E. coli* isolated from stool is a commensal; hence, AST is not performed.

CLASSIFICATION OF AST METHODS

AST methods are classified into phenotypic and genotypic methods.
- ❖ The phenotypic methods are further grouped into:
  - Disk diffusion method, e.g., Kirby–Bauer's disk diffusion (DD) test
  - Dilution tests: Broth dilution and agar dilution methods
  - Epsilometer or E-test
  - Automated AST, e.g., Vitek, Phoenix and Microscan systems.
- ❖ Genotypic methods, such as PCR detecting drug-resistant genes.

DISK DIFFUSION METHOD

Problem Solving Exercise 1

Disk Diffusion Test

Urine culture of a 23-year old female with increased frequency and burning micturition yielded lactose-fermenting colonies which was identified as Escherichia coli. The antimicrobial susceptibility test (AST) performed is demonstrated in Figure 3.8.1. The zone size diameter recorded by using an instrument (Fig. 3.8.2) revealed ceftriaxone (23 mm), ciprofloxacin (8 mm), gentamicin (10 mm), amikacin (16 mm), meropenem (28 mm). Interpret the result according to CLSI zone interpretation criteria as mentioned in Table 3.8.1.
1. Name the AST method performed, the medium used and the instrument used to measure zone diameter?
2. Interpret the test result and suggest the antimicrobials recommended for treatment.

Explanation

1. Antimicrobial susceptibility test (AST) performed here is Kirby–Bauer's disk diffusion (DD) test and the medium used is Mueller Hinton agar (Fig. 3.8.1). The zone diameters were measured using Vernier caliper (Fig. 3.8.2).
2. The observed zone when compared with CLSI's zone interpretation chart (Table 3.8.1) revealed that the causative urinary pathogen is resistant to gentamicin and ciprofloxacin, intermediate to amikacin and sensitive to ceftriaxone and meropenem.

Ceftriaxone is a first-line (narrow spectrum) antibiotic whereas meropenem is a restricted antimicrobial agent (extended spectrum). Therefore, ceftriaxone would be the antibiotic of choice.

Kirby–Bauer's disk diffusion (DD) test is the most widely used AST method. They are suitable for rapidly growing pathogenic bacteria; however, they are not suitable for slow growing bacteria. It is mostly performed from colony (called colony-DD), or performed directly from the specimens (called direct DD).

Procedure (Colony Disk Diffusion)

Antibiotic disks are impregnated on to a suitable medium lawn cultured with the test isolate.

- **Antibiotic disks:** Antibiotic disks are available commercially or prepared in-house. Sterile filter paper disks of 6 mm diameter are impregnated with standard quantity of antibiotic solution
- **Medium:** Mueller–Hinton agar (MHA) is the standard medium used for AST. For certain fastidious organisms, such as *S. pyogenes* and *S. pneumoniae*, Mueller–Hinton blood agar (MHBA) containing 5% of sheep blood is used
- **Inoculum:** The inoculum is prepared by—(1) directly suspending the colony in the normal saline or (2) by inoculating into a suitable broth and incubating at 37°C for 2 hours
- **Turbidity:** The turbidity of the inoculum is adjusted to 0.5 McFarland opacity standard, which is equivalent to approximately 1.5×10^8 CFU/mL of bacteria
- **Lawn culture:** The broth is then inoculated on to the medium by spreading with sterile swabs
- **Disks impregnation:** After MHA plate is dried (3–5 min), the antibiotic disks are placed and gently pressed on its surface. Disks should be placed atleast 24 mm (center to center) apart on the MHA plate. Ordinarily, maximum up to 6 disks can be applied on a 100 mm plate (Fig. 3.8.1)
- **Incubation:** The plates are then incubated at 37°C for 16–18 hours and then interpreted.

Interpretation

The antibiotic in the disk diffuses through the solid medium, so that the concentration is highest near the site of application of the antibiotic disk and decreases gradually away from it
- Susceptibility to the drug is determined by the zone of inhibition of bacterial growth around

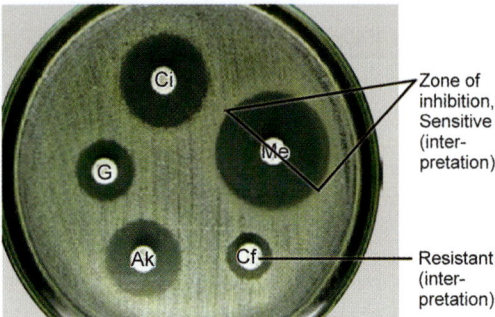

Fig. 3.8.1: Kirby–Bauer disk diffusion method.
Source: Department of Microbiology, Pondicherry Institute of Medical sciences, Puducherry (*with permission*).

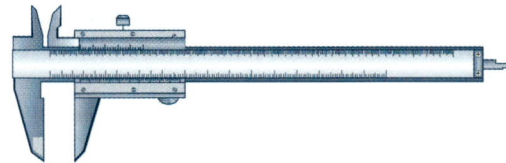

Fig. 3.8.2: Vernier caliper.

the disk, which can be measured by using Vernier caliper (Fig. 3.8.2)
- The interpretation of zone size into sensitive, intermediate or resistant is based on the standard zone size interpretation chart, provided by CLSI or EUCAST guidelines (Table 3.8.1).

Note: CLSI (Clinical and Laboratory Standards Institute) and EUCAST (European Committee on Antimicrobial Susceptibility Testing) are international agencies, which provide guidelines for zone size interpretation (Table 3.8.1), and are updated annually.

Direct Disk Diffusion Test

The direct DD (or direct susceptibility test, i.e., DST) test can be performed when results are required urgently and single pathogenic bacterium is suspected in the specimen (for positively-flagged blood culture bottle, sterile body fluids or urine).
- Here, the specimen is directly inoculated uniformly on to the surface of an agar plate and the antibiotic disks are applied
- The results of the direct-DD test should always be verified by performing AST from the colony subsequently

Table 3.8.1: Commonly used disk concentrations and interpretation of disk diffusion test (as per CLSI 2020 guideline).

Breakpoints for Enterobacteriaceae (CLSI 2020)							
Antimicrobial agents	Disk strength (µg)	Zone diameter breakpoints (mm)			MIC breakpoints (µg/mL)		
		Sensitive	Intermediate	Resistant	Sensitive	Intermediate	Resistant
Ceftazidime	30	≥ 21	18–20	≤ 17	≤ 4	8	≥ 16
Ceftriaxone	30	≥ 23	20–22	≤ 19	≤ 1	2	≥ 4
Ciprofloxacin	5	≥ 26	22–25	≤ 21	≤ 0.25	0.5	≥ 1
Piperacillin-tazobactam	100/10	≥ 21	18–20	≤ 17	≤ 16	32–64	≥ 128
Amikacin	30	≥ 17	15–16	≤ 14	≤ 16	32	≥ 64
Meropenem	10	≥ 23	20–22	≤ 19	≤ 1	2	≥ 4
Colistin	–	–	–	–	–	≤ 2	≥ 4
Breakpoints for gram-positive organisms (CLSI 2020)							
Antimicrobial agents	Disk strength (µg)	Zone diameter breakpoints (mm)			MIC breakpoints (µg/mL)		
		Sensitive	Intermediate	Resistant	Sensitive	Intermediate	Resistant
Cefoxitin (*S. aureus*)	30	≥ 22	–	≤ 21	≤ 4	–	≥ 8
Levofloxacin (*S. aureus*)	5	≥ 19	16–18	≤ 15	≤ 1	2	≥ 4
Cotrimoxazole (*S. aureus*)	1.25/23.75	≥ 16	11–15	≤ 10	≤ 2/38	–	≥ 4/76
Tetracycline (*S. aureus*)	30	≥ 19	15–18	≤ 14	≤ 4	8	≥ 16
Linezolid (*S. aureus*)	–	≥ 21	–	≤ 20	≤ 4	–	≥ 8
Vancomycin (*S. aureus*)	–	–	–	–	≤ 2	4–8	≥ 16
Ampicillin (*Enterococcus*)	10	≥ 17	–	≤ 16	≤ 8	–	≥ 16
Linezolid (*Enterococcus*)	30	≥ 23	21–22	≤ 20	≤ 2	4	≥ 8
Vancomycin (*Enterococcus*)	30	≥ 17	15–16	≤ 14	≤ 4	8–16	≥ 32

Abbreviation: CLSI, Clinical and Laboratory Standards Institute.

- This test is of no use when mixed growth is suspected in the specimen, e.g., pus, stool, sputum, etc.

DILUTION TESTS

Here, the antimicrobial agent is serially diluted, each dilution is tested with the test organism for antimicrobial susceptibility test and the MIC is calculated.
- MIC (minimum inhibitory concentration) is the lowest concentration of an antimicrobial agent that will inhibit the visible growth of a microorganism after overnight incubation
- Depending upon whether the dilutions of the antimicrobial agent are made in agar or broth, there are two types of dilution tests.

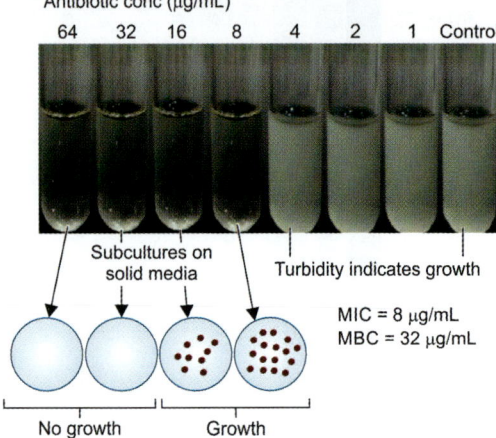

Fig. 3.8.3: Macrobroth dilution method.
Source: Department of Microbiology, Pondicherry Institute of Medical Sciences, Puducherry (*with permission*).

Broth Dilution Method

It is of two types: macrobroth dilution (performed in tubes) and microbroth dilution (performed in microtiter plate). The procedure of macrobroth dilution is explained below:
- Serial dilutions of the antimicrobial agent in Mueller-Hinton broth are taken in tubes and each tube is inoculated with a fixed amount of suspension of the test organism. A control organism of known sensitivity should also be tested. Tubes are incubated at 37°C for 18 hours
- The MIC is determined by noting the lowest concentration of the drug at which there is no visible growth, i.e., broth appears clear (Fig. 3.8.3)
- The minimum bactericidal concentration (MBC) can be obtained by subculturing from each tube (showing no growth) on to a nutrient agar plate without any antimicrobial agent. The tube containing the lowest concentration of the drug that fails to show growth, on subculture, is the MBC of the drug for that test strain (Fig. 3.8.3).

Problem Solving Exercise 2

Broth Dilution Test

Blood culture of a 77 years old man with fever, hypotension, increased respiratory rate and altered mentation yielded *Klebsiella pneumoniae*. Antimicrobial susceptibility test by macro broth dilution was performed for amikacin (Fig. 3.8.3). Observe the finding and interpret the result using CLSI interpretation criteria (Table 3.8.1).

Explanation

History of fever, hypotension, increased respiratory rate and altered mentation suggests that it is suspected case of sepsis. Blood culture yielded *Klebsiella pneumoniae*.
- AST of amikacin by macro broth dilution test (Fig. 3.8.3) revealed that the test isolate has grown (turbidity) in the test tubes containing amikacin ≤4 µg/mL; whereas it did not grow in test tubes containing amikacin ≥8 µg/mL (no turbidity). Therefore, the MIC of amikacin for the test isolate is 8 µg/mL. MIC (minimum inhibitory concentration) is the minimum concentration of the drug that inhibits the growth of the test isolate
- CLSI interpretation criteria for amikacin as given in Table 3.8.1 shows that MIC of ≥64 µg/mL is considered resistant, 32 µg/mL is taken as intermediate and ≤16 µg/mL is considered susceptible. Therefore, the result of amikacin susceptibility test by macro broth dilution is susceptible (MIC 8 µg/mL).

Problem Solving Exercise 3

Agar Dilution Test

Antimicrobial susceptibility test of vancomycin was performed by **agar dilution method** for four isolates of *Staphylococcus aureus* (Fig. 3.8.4). Observe the findings and interpret the result using CLSI interpretation criteria (Table 3.8.2).

Explanation

Fig. 3.8.4 shows agar dilution for MIC detection of four isolates of *Staphylococcus aureus* against vancomycin. The MIC (minimum drug concentration which inhibited the growth of the organism) and the AST interpretation (according to CLSI interpretation criteria, Table 3.8.2) is as follows.

- Isolate 1: The MIC is <2 µg/mL (sensitive)
- Isolate 2: The MIC is 16 µg/mL (resistant)
- Isolate 3: The MIC is 8 µg/mL (Intermediate)
- Isolate 4: The MIC is >16 µg/mL (resistant).

Agar Dilution Method

Here, the serial dilutions of the drug are prepared in molten Mueller–Hinton agar (MHA) and poured into Petri dishes. The test strain is spot inoculated. If growth occurs at the area of spot inoculum in a MHA plate added with a particular concentration of an antibiotic, suggests that the strain is resistant to the antibiotic at that concentration (Fig. 3.8.4, Table 3.8.2). This method is more convenient than broth dilution and has the added advantage of:

- Several strains can be tested at the same time by using the same plate
- It directly measures the MBC; there is no need of sub-culturing as it is done with broth dilution method.

■ EPSILOMETER OR E-TEST

This is a quantitative method of detecting MIC by using the principles of both dilution and diffusion of antibiotic into the medium.

- It uses an absorbent strip containing pre-defined gradient (serial dilution) of antibiotic concentration immobilized along its length
- It is applied to a lawn inoculum of a bacterium. Following incubation of the test organism, an elliptical zone of inhibition is produced surrounding the strip
- The antibiotic concentration at which the ellipse edge intersects the strip, is taken as MIC value (Fig. 3.8.5).

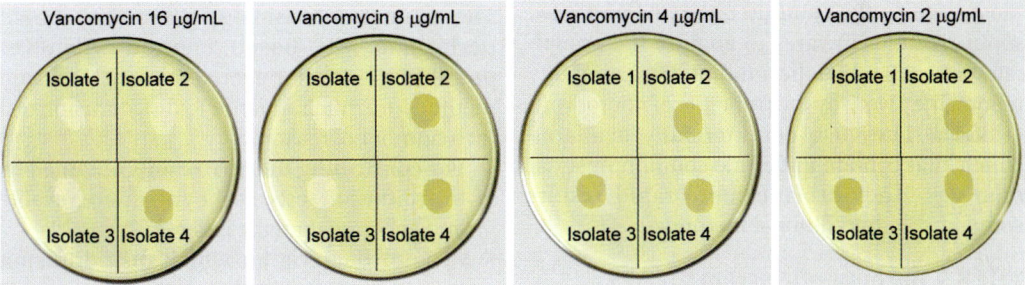

Fig. 3.8.4: Agar dilution for minimum inhibitory concentration (MIC) detection of *Staphylococcus aureus* against vancomycin. [Isolate 1: MIC- <2 µg/mL (sensitive); Isolate 2: MIC-16 µg/mL (resistant); Isolate 3: MIC-8 µg/mL (Intermediate); Isolate 4: MIC >16 µg/mL (resistant); Interpretation is based on Clinical and Laboratory Standards Institute (CLSI) guideline (Table 3.8.2)].

Table 3.8.2: Clinical and Laboratory Standards Institute (CLSI) interpretative categories and breakpoints for vancomycin susceptibility for *Staphylococcus aureus*.

Minimum inhibitory concentration	Interpretation	Organism is labeled as
≤2 µg/mL	Sensitive	Vancomycin-sensitive *Staphylococcus aureus*
4–8 µg/mL	Intermediate	Vancomycin-intermediate *Staphylococcus aureus*
≥16 µg/mL	Resistant	Vancomycin-resistant *Staphylococcus aureus*

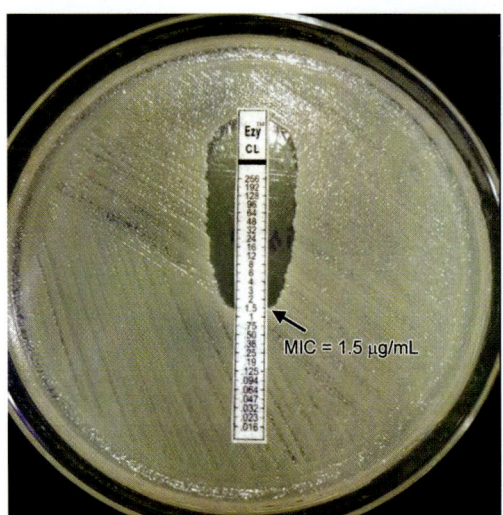

Fig. 3.8.5: Epsilometer or E-test.
Source: Department of Microbiology, Pondicherry Institute of Medical Sciences, Puducherry (*with permission*).

AUTOMATED ANTIMICROBIAL SUSCEPTIBILITY TESTS

Several automated systems are available now, such as:
- VITEK 2 identification and antimicrobial sensitivity system (bioMerieux)
- Phoenix System (Becton Dickinson)
- Micro Scan Walk Away system.

Most systems are computer assisted and have sophisticated softwares to analyze the growth rates and determine the antibiotic susceptibility report. They work by the principle of microbroth dilution. They use commercially available panels that contain antibiotic solution in serial dilutions. They provide more rapid results compared with traditional methods.

VITEK 2 Automated System for AST

VITEK 2 is the most widely used automated AST system in India; can perform AST of bacteria and yeasts; whereas other automated AST systems can perform AST of bacteria only, not for yeasts.
- It works on the principle of microbroth dilution
- It uses a reagent card containing 64 wells, which contain doubling dilution of antimicrobial agents. The organism suspension (of 0.5 McFarland turbidity) is added to the wells (Fig. 3.7.8, Chapter 3.7 and Table 3.8.3)

Table 3.8.3: Antibiotic panel used in VITEK AST card for Enterobacteriaceae.

Enterobacteriaceae	Antimicrobial agent used in VITEK
First line	Ampicillin, Amoxicillin-clavulanic acid, Ciprofloxacin, Ceftriaxone, Ceftazidime, Gentamicin, Cotrimoxazole
Second line	Cefoperazone-sulbactam, Piperacillin-tazobactam, Cefepime, Amikacin
Restricted	Meropenem, Doripenem, Ertapenem, Imipenem, Colistin, Tigecycline

- The cards are incubated in the system at 35.5 ±1°C. The reading is taken once in every 15 minutes by the optical system of the equipment. It measures the presence of any turbidity (by nephelometry) which indicates the organism has grown in that antibiotic well
- The MIC is determined as the highest dilution of the antimicrobial agent which inhibits the growth of organism and there is no turbidity in the well
- The results are available within 8–10 hours for gram-negative bacilli and 16–18 hours for gram-positive cocci.

Role of MIC-based Methods

The clinical microbiology laboratory should perform a MIC-based method whenever possible. This is because the MIC-based methods are much superior to disk diffusion test for a number of reasons.
- **For confirming the AST results** obtained by disk diffusion tests, as they are more reliable and accurate than the latter
- AST for bacteria for which disk diffusion test is not standardized should only be performed by MIC testing (e.g., vancomycin for *S. aureus*)
- For performing AST for slow growing bacteria, such as tubercle bacilli
- **To select the most appropriate antibiotic:** Lower is the MIC, better is the therapeutic efficacy
- **MIC-guided therapy:** There are certain situations (e.g., endocarditis), where the antibiotic treatment is MIC-guided.

INTERPRETATION OF AST

The result of AST (whether disk diffusion or MIC-based methods) is always expressed in four interpretative categories.
- **Susceptible (S):** Indicates that the antibiotic is clinically effective when used in standard therapeutic dose
- **Intermediate (I):** Indicates that the antibiotic is not clinically effective when used in standard dose; but may be active when used in increased dose. Antibiotics reported as 'I' should be avoided for treatment if alternative agents are available
- **Resistant (R):** Indicates that the antibiotic is NOT clinically effective when used in either standard dose or increased dose; and therefore should not be included in the treatment regimen.

CHOICE OF ANTIBIOTICS TO BE INCLUDED IN PANEL

The panel of the drugs to be tested against an isolate depends upon various factors:
- **Clinically indicated:** Include only those antibiotics for testing which are clinically indicated either as a first-line agent or alternative-agent for the suspected infective syndrome and the organism isolated
- **Organism isolated**, for which the AST is going to be performed, and its **local resistance pattern** (as per hospital antibiogram)
- **Intrinsic resistance:** The antibiotics to which the isolate is intrinsically resistant must be excluded from the test panel
- **Antimicrobial agent:** Both oral and parenteral antibiotics should be included in the testing panel, as they can be administered based on clinical severity (i.e parenteral drugs for severe and oral for mild illness)
- **Locally available** antibiotic at the hospital
- **Site of action:** Only those antibiotics should be tested which are active in the site. For example, the following antibiotics should be EXCLUDED from testing, depending upon the clinical specimen. For e.g., clindamycin, macrolides, tetracyclines should be excluded from testing.

Selective or cascade reporting aims at encouraging the clinicians to use narrow spectrum antimicrobials if found susceptible and to reserve the overuse of broad and extended spectrum antimicrobials (Table 3.8.3).

General Bacteriology: Molecular Diagnosis

CHAPTER 3.9

In the modern era of diagnostic microbiology, the molecular methods play a very important role in the diagnosis of infectious diseases. They can be used for the detection of the nucleic acid of the organism either directly from the clinical specimen or from the culture.

Molecular methods commonly used in diagnostic microbiology laboratory are:

- Polymerase chain reaction (PCR)
- Real-time polymerase chain reaction (rt-PCR)
- Automated PCR, such as Biofire FilmArray
- Automated real-time PCR, such as cartridge-based nucleic acid amplification test (CBNAAT): Used for tuberculosis, described in Chapter 35.

■ POLYMERASE CHAIN REACTION (PCR)

Problem Solving Exercise

Polymerase Chain Reaction

CSF specimen of four patients with suspected tuberculous meningitis are sent for PCR for *M. tuberculosis*. The results of which have been depicted in Fig. 3.9.1C.
1. Interpret the result.
2. What are the steps involved in PCR?
3. What is the modification needed to carryout dengue PCR?
4. Which modification of PCR is useful for the diagnosis of the infectious syndromes (e.g., pneumonia) that can be caused by more than one organism?

Explanation

1. Figure 3.9.1C is a photograph of gel electrophoresis of the PCR amplified products. It reveals that visible bands of amplified DNA in line 1 and 2; whereas line 3 and 4 did not show any bands. Therefore, test specimens 1 and 2 are positive for gene specific for *M. tuberculosis*.
2. For steps involved in PCR refer the text.
3. As dengue virus is an RNA virus, **reverse transcriptase PCR** needs to be performed to detect dengue virus specific RNA in clinical specimen.
4. **Multiplex PCR** is useful for the diagnosis of the infectious diseases that are caused by more than one organism.

Contd...

PCR is a technology in molecular biology used to amplify a single or few copies of a piece of DNA to generate millions of copies of DNA.

Principle of PCR

PCR involves three basic steps.
1. **DNA extraction from the organism:** This involves lysis of the organisms and release of the DNA which may be done by various methods—boiling, adding enzymes (e.g., proteinase K) or by DNA extraction kit.
2. **Amplification of extracted DNA:** This is carried out in a special PCR machine called thermocycler

Contd...

(Fig. 3.9.1A). The extracted DNA is subjected to repeated cycles (30–35 numbers) of amplification which takes about 3–4 hours. Each amplification cycle has three steps, such as (1) Denaturation at 95°C (2) Primer annealing (55°C) (3) Extension of the primer (72°C) by Taq Polymerase enzyme.

3. **Gel electrophoresis of amplified product:** The amplified DNA is electrophoretically migrated according to their molecular size by performing agarose gel electrophoresis (Fig. 3.9.1B). The amplified DNA forms clear band, which can be visualized under ultraviolet (UV) light (Fig. 3.9.1C).

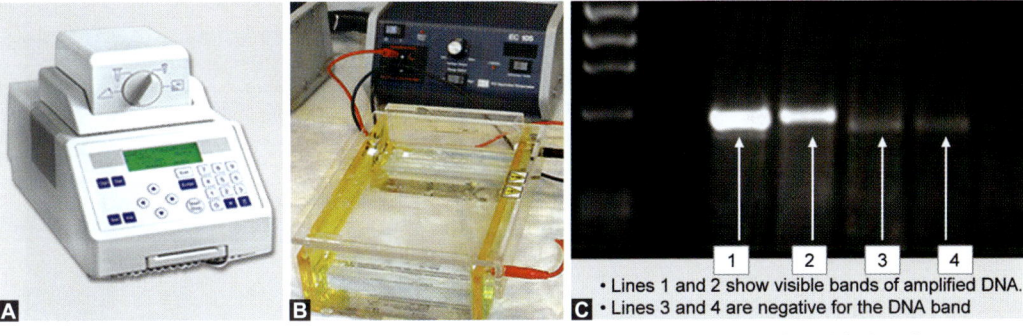

Figs 3.9.1A to C: (A) Thermocycler machine (Eppendorf); (B) Gel electrophoresis of amplified product; (C) Visualization of amplified DNA under UV light.
Source: Department of Microbiology, JIPMER, Puducherry (with permission).

Applications of PCR

PCR is now a common and often indispensable technique used in medical diagnostics and research laboratories for a variety of applications. It has the following advantages compared to the conventional culture methods:

- **More sensitive:** It can amplify very few copies of a specific DNA, so it is more sensitive
- **More specific:** Use of primers targeting specific DNA sequence of the organism makes the PCR assays highly specific
- PCR can be done to amplify the DNA of the organism: (1) either directly from the sample, or (2) to confirm the organism grown in culture
- PCR can also detect the organisms that are highly fastidious or noncultivable by conventional culture methods
- PCR can be used to detect the genes in the organism responsible for drug resistance (e.g., *mec* A gene detection in *Staphylococcus aureus*).

Disadvantages of PCR

Conventional PCR detects only the DNA, but not the RNA (latter can be detected by reverse transcriptase PCR).

- **Qualitative, not quantitative:** Conventional PCR can only detect the presence or absence of DNA. It cannot quantitate the amount of DNA of the organism present in the sample. This is possible by real time PCR
- **Viability:** PCR cannot differentiate between viable or nonviable organisms. It only detects the presence of DNA in the sample which may be extracted from viable or nonviable organism
- **False-positive amplification:** It may occur due to contamination with environmental DNA. Hence, strict asepsis should be maintained in the PCR laboratory
- **False-negative:** The PCR inhibitors present in some specimens, such as blood, feces, etc., may inhibit the amplification of target DNA.

Modifications of PCR

1. **Reverse transcriptase PCR (RT-PCR):** It is useful for for amplifying RNA. After RNA extraction, the first step is addition of reverse transcriptase enzyme that coverts RNA into DNA. Then, the remaining steps are similar as that for conventional PCR. It is useful for detection of RNA viruses from clinical specimen
2. **Nested PCR:** In nested PCR two rounds of PCR amplification are carried out by using two primers that are targeted against two different DNA sequences of the same organism
   - It is more sensitive (yields high quantity of DNA), more specific (uses two primers targeting two regions of DNA of the same organisms)
   - **Application:** It is used for detection of *Mycobacterium tuberculosis* (targeting IS6110 gene) in samples.
3. **Multiplex PCR:** It uses more than one primer which can detect many DNA sequences of several organisms in one reaction
   - Syndromic approach: Multiplex PCR is useful for the diagnosis of the infectious

diseases that are caused by more than one organism
- For example, for the etiological diagnosis of pyogenic meningitis, different primers targeting the common agents of pyogenic meningitis, such as pneumococcus, meningococcus and *H. influenzae* can be added simultaneously in the same reaction tube.

Biofire FilmArray

Biofire FilmArray (bioMérieux) is a completely automated multiplex nested PCR system where all the steps from sample preparation to amplification, detection and analysis are performed automatically by the system; giving result in about one hour. It has excellent sensitivity and specificity.

▌REAL-TIME PCR (RT-PCR)

It is based on PCR technology, which is used to amplify and simultaneously detect or quantify a targeted DNA molecule on a real-time basis. Reverse transcriptase real-time PCR formats can detect and quantify RNA molecules of the test organism in the sample on a real-time basis.

It uses a different thermocycler (Fig. 3.9.2) than the conventional PCR. It is very expensive, 5–10 times more than the cost of conventional PCR.

Advantages: Real-time PCR has many advantages over a conventional PCR, such as:
- ❖ **Quantitative:** rt-PCR can quantitate the DNA or RNA present in the specimen; hence can be used for monitoring the disease progression in response to treatment, e.g., viral load monitoring in HIV or hepatitis B viral infection
- ❖ **Takes less time:** In rt-PCR, the amplification can be visualized simultaneously during the process of amplification unlike the conventional PCR where there is an extra-step of gel electrophoresis to detect the amplicons

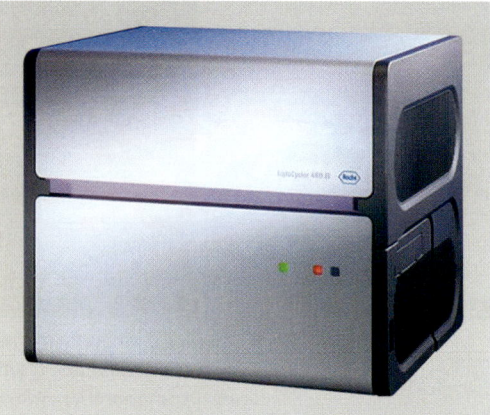

Fig. 3.9.2: Real-time PCR.
Source: Department of Microbiology, JIPMER, Puducherry *(with permission).*

- ❖ **Contamination rate** is extremely less
- ❖ **Sensitivity and specificity** of rt-PCR assays are much more than the conventional PCR.

Detection of amplification products of real-time PCR: The detection of amplified nucleic acid in a real-time PCR reaction is carried out by using a variety of fluorogenic molecules which may be either nonspecific or specific.
- ❖ **Nonspecific methods:** They use SYBR green dye that stains any nucleic acid nonspecifically
- ❖ **Specific methods:** They use fluorescent labeled oligonucleotide probe which binds (i.e., hybridizes) only to a particular region of amplified nucleic acid. Three types of hybridization probes are commonly used:
  - TaqMan or hydrolysis probe
  - Molecular beacon
  - Fluorescence resonance energy transfer (FRET) probe.

Post-amplification melting curve analysis is used for quantitation of the nucleic acid load. Problem based exercise on Real time PCR (for influenza and COVID-19) has been explained in detail in Chapter 37.

CHAPTER 4

Laboratory Diagnosis of Viral Diseases

■ INTRODUCTION

Laboratory diagnosis of viral infections is useful for the following purposes:

- ❖ **To start antiviral drugs** for those viral infections for which specific drugs are available, such as herpes, CMV, HIV, influenza and respiratory syncytial virus (RSV)
- ❖ **Screening of blood donors** for HIV, hepatitis B and hepatitis C helps in the prevention of transfusion-transmitted infections
- ❖ **Surveillance purpose:** To assess the disease burden in the community by estimating the prevalence and incidence of viral infections
- ❖ **For outbreak or epidemic investigation**, e.g., influenza epidemics, dengue outbreaks—to initiate appropriate control measures
- ❖ **To start post-exposure prophylaxis** of antiretroviral drugs to the healthcare workers following needle stick injury (Refer Chapter 14)
- ❖ **To initiate certain measures:** For example, if rubella is diagnosed in the first trimester of pregnancy, termination of pregnancy is recommended.

The various methods available for laboratory diagnosis of viral diseases are enlisted in Table 4.1.

■ SAMPLE COLLECTION

Specimen collection has to be done early in the patient's illness as possible, as viruses can be recovered only for a few days after the onset of illness. The following steps should be kept in mind during specimen collection:

Appropriate time: Specimens should be collected as soon as possible, preferably within 3 days after onset of symptoms
- ❖ From the correct site (Table 4.2)

Table 4.1: Methods available for laboratory diagnosis of viral diseases.

1. Direct Demonstration of Virus • Electron microscopy • Fluorescent microscopy • Light microscopy: ➢ Histopathological staining: To demonstrate inclusion bodies ➢ Immunoperoxidase staining
2. Detection of Viral Antigens By various formats, such as ELISA, direct IF, ICT, flow through assays
3. Detection of Specific Antibodies • Conventional techniques, such as HAI and neutralization test • Newer diagnostic formats, such as ELISA, ICT, flow through assays
4. Molecular Methods to Detect Viral Genes • Nucleic acid probe—for detection of DNA or RNA by hybridization • PCR—for DNA detection by amplification • Reverse transcriptase-PCR—for RNA detection • Real time PCR—for DNA quantification • Real time RT-PCR—for RNA quantification
5. Isolation of Virus by • Animal inoculation • Embryonated egg inoculation • Tissue cultures: Cell line culture using primary, secondary or continuous cell lines

Abbreviations: ELISA, enzyme-linked immunosorbent assay; ICT, immunochromatographic test; PCR, polymerase chain reaction; HAI, hemagglutination inhibition test; IF, Immunofluorescence assay.

- ❖ In the correct method of collection
- ❖ In adequate volume (Fig. 4.1)
- ❖ In suitable containers (sterile and chemical free)—e.g., viral transport media
- ❖ Transport in correct temperature: Specimen to be kept at 4°C for 3–5 days, after which the sample should be kept at –70°C (Fig. 4.1)
- ❖ Correctly labeled (patient details and specimen details).

Table 4.2: Various types of viral infections and specimen of choice.

Systemic infections	Causative viral agents	Specimens to be collected
Respiratory infections	• Influenza virus • Parainfluenza virus • Respiratory syncytial virus • Rhinovirus • Adenovirus • Coronavirus	• Swabs (nasal, throat, nasopharyngeal) • Bronchoalveolar lavage • Nasal washings • Gargles • Aspirates (nasal or sinus) • Serum
Viral encephalitis	• Herpes simplex virus • Japanese encephalitis virus • Rabies virus	• Cerebrospinal fluid • Tissue by brain biopsy (postmortem) • Throat washings • Stool • Serum
Viral gastroenteritis	• Rotavirus • Adenovirus-40, 41 • Calicivirus • Astrovirus	• Stool • Serum
Exanthematous infections	• Herpes simplex virus • Varicella zoster virus • Human papillomavirus • Molluscum contagiosum virus	• Vesicle aspirate • Skin scrapping • Skin biopsy
Poliomyelitis	• Polioviruses (I, II, III)	• Throat swabs • Stool • Rectal swabs • Serum
Sexually-transmitted infections	• Herpes simplex virus • Human papillomavirus • Human immunodeficiency virus	• Serum
Teratogenic viruses	• Rubella virus • *Cytomegalovirus* (CMV) • Herpes simplex virus • Varicella-zoster virus • Parvovirus	• Serum
Conjunctivitis	• Adenovirus • Enterovirus 70 • Coxsackie virus A-24	• Conjunctival swab
Vector-borne diseases	• Dengue virus • Chikungunya virus • Japanese encephalitis virus	• Serum

Note: Blood sample is collected for serological tests and for molecular diagnostic tests (e.g., real time polymerase chain reaction for estimation of viral load).

Viral Transport Medium

Viral transport medium (VTM) is a specially formulated medium for collection, transport and long-term freeze storage of viruses. Uses of VTM are given in Figure 4.2.

Composition of VTM: Viral transport consists of modified Hanks' balanced salt solution supplemented with:
- Phosphate-buffered saline (PBS) for adequate ion concentration—NaCl, KCl, $CaCl_2$, Na_2HPO_4, KH_2PO_4, Mg_2PO_4. It is used to control the pH
- Protective proteins (bovine serum albumin)
- Antibiotics and fungicides to control microbial contamination, such as streptomycin, amphotericin B, vancomycin, etc.
- Phenol red: It is used as a pH indicator
- Distilled water to make 1 liter.

DIRECT DEMONSTRATION OF VIRUS

Electron Microscopy

Detection of viruses by electron microscopy (EM) is increasingly used nowadays. Specimens

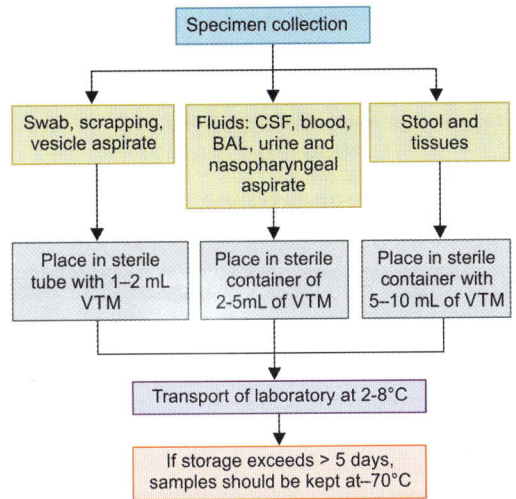

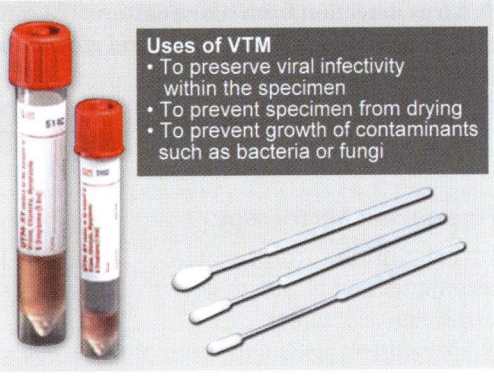

Fig. 4.1: Process of specimen collection and transport.
Abbreviations: VTM, viral transport medium; CSF, cerebrospinal fluid; BAL, bronchoalveolar lavage.

Fig. 4.2: Viral transport medium and rayon-tipped swabs used for sample collection.

are negatively stained by potassium phosphotungstate and scanned under EM.
- ❖ **Shape:** Viruses can be identified based on their distinct appearances; for example:
  - Rabies virus—bullet-shaped (Fig. 4.3A)
  - Rotavirus—wheel-shaped (Fig. 4.3B)
  - Ebola virus—filamentous (Fig. 4.3C)
  - Poxvirus—contains dumbbell-shaped capsid (Fig. 4.3D)
  - Adenovirus—space vehicle-shaped (Fig. 4.3E)
  - Hepatitis B virus—occurs in three forms: spherical form, tubular form and Dane particle (Fig. 4.3F).
  - Corona virus—possesses petal-shaped peplomers (Fig. 4.3G)
  - Astrovirus—possesses star-shaped peplomers.
- ❖ **Direct detection from specimens:** This is useful for viruses that are difficult to cultivate; e.g., rotavirus, hepatitis A and E viruses from feces and CMV from urine

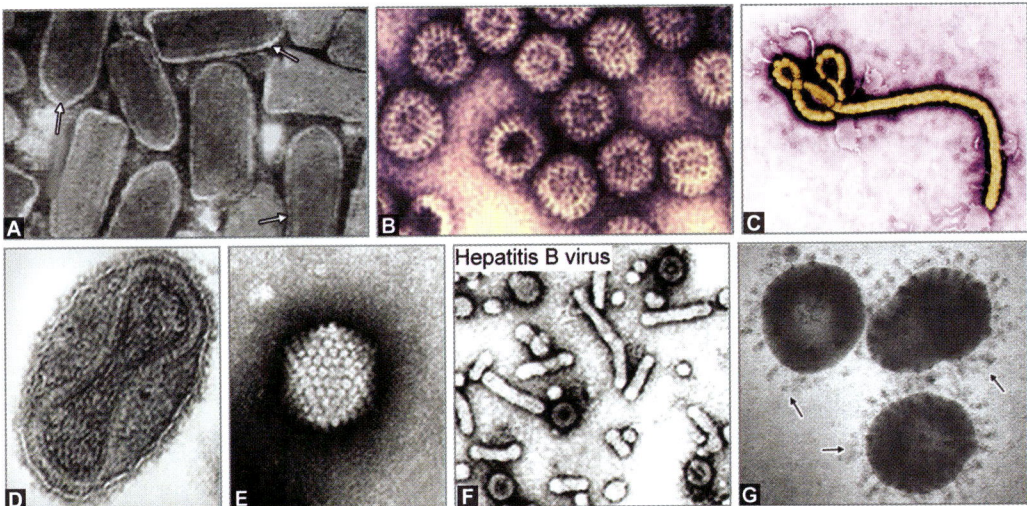

Figs 4.3A to G: Electron microscopy picture of: (A) Rabies; (B) Rotavirus; (C) Ebola virus; (D) Poxvirus; (E) Adenovirus; (F) Hepatitis B; (G) Corona virus.
Source: Public Health Image Library, Centers for Disease Control and Prevention, Atlanta. (A) ID #5611; (B) ID #15194; (C) ID #10815; (D) ID #1849; (E) ID #237; (F) ID #5631; (G) ID #10270.

- **Virus detection from tissue culture:** EM can also be used for detection of viral growth in tissue cultures
- **Drawbacks:** EM is highly expensive, has low sensitivity with a detection threshold of 10^7 virions/mL. The specificity is also low.

Fluorescent Microscopy

Direct immunofluorescence (Direct-IF) technique is employed to detect viral particles in the clinical samples.
- **Procedure:** Specimen is mounted on slide, stained with specific antiviral antibody tagged with fluorescent dye and viewed under fluorescent microscope
- **Clinical applications:**
  - Diagnosis of rabies virus antigen in skin biopsies, corneal smear of infected patients
  - Syndromic approach: Rapid diagnosis of respiratory infections caused by influenza virus, rhinoviruses, respiratory syncytial virus, adenoviruses and herpesviruses can be carried out by adding specific antibodies to each of these viruses
  - Detection of adenovirus from conjunctival smears.

Light Microscopy

Light microscopy is useful in the following situations.
- **Inclusion bodies:** Histopathological staining of tissue sections may be useful for detection of inclusion bodies which helps in the diagnosis of certain viral infections (Table 4.3)
- **Immunoperoxidase staining:** Tissue sections or cells coated with viral antigens are stained using antibodies tagged with horseradish peroxidase following which hydrogen peroxide and a coloring agent (benzidine derivative) are added. The color complex formed can be viewed under a light microscope.

> **Inclusion Body**
> Certain viruses induce characteristic changes in the host cells, called **inclusion body**, which can be detected by histopathological staining. They are the aggregates of virions or viral proteins and other products of viral replication that confer altered staining property to the host cell.
>
> *Contd...*

Table 4.3: Inclusion bodies and viruses producing them.

Intracytoplasmic inclusion bodies
Negri bodies—rabies virus (Fig. 4.4A)
Paschen body—variola virus
Guarnieri bodies—vaccinia virus
Bollinger bodies—fowlpox virus
Molluscum bodies—molluscum contagiosum virus (Fig. 4.4B)
Intranuclear inclusion bodies
Cowdry type A inclusions
Torres body—yellow fever virus
Lipschultz body—herpes simplex virus (Fig. 4.4D)
Cowdry type B inclusions
Poliovirus
Adenovirus
Intracytoplasmic and intranuclear inclusion bodies
Owl's eye appearance—cytomegalovirus (Fig. 4.4E)
Measles virus (Fig. 4.4C)

Contd...

Role in Laboratory Diagnosis
Inclusion bodies are characteristic of specific viral infections. They have distinct size, shape, location and staining properties by which they can be demonstrated in virus infected cells under the light microscope.

Location
They may be present either in the host cell cytoplasm or nucleus or both (Table 4.3 and Figs 4.4A to E).
- **Intracytoplasmic inclusion bodies:** They are generally acidophilic and can be seen as pink structures when stained with Giemsa or eosin methylene blue stains (e.g., most poxviruses and rabies)
- **Intranuclear inclusion bodies:** They are basophilic in nature. Cowdry (1934) had classified them into:
  - Cowdry type A inclusions: They are variable in size and have granular appearance
  - Cowdry type B inclusions: They are more circumscribed, amorphous or hyaline spheres; multiple in number.
- **Both intracytoplasmic and intranuclear inclusions.**

DETECTION OF VIRAL ANTIGENS

Various formats are available for the detection of viral antigens in serum and other samples, such as enzyme-linked immunosorbent assay (ELISA), immunochromatographic test

CHAPTER 4 ◆ Laboratory Diagnosis of Viral Diseases

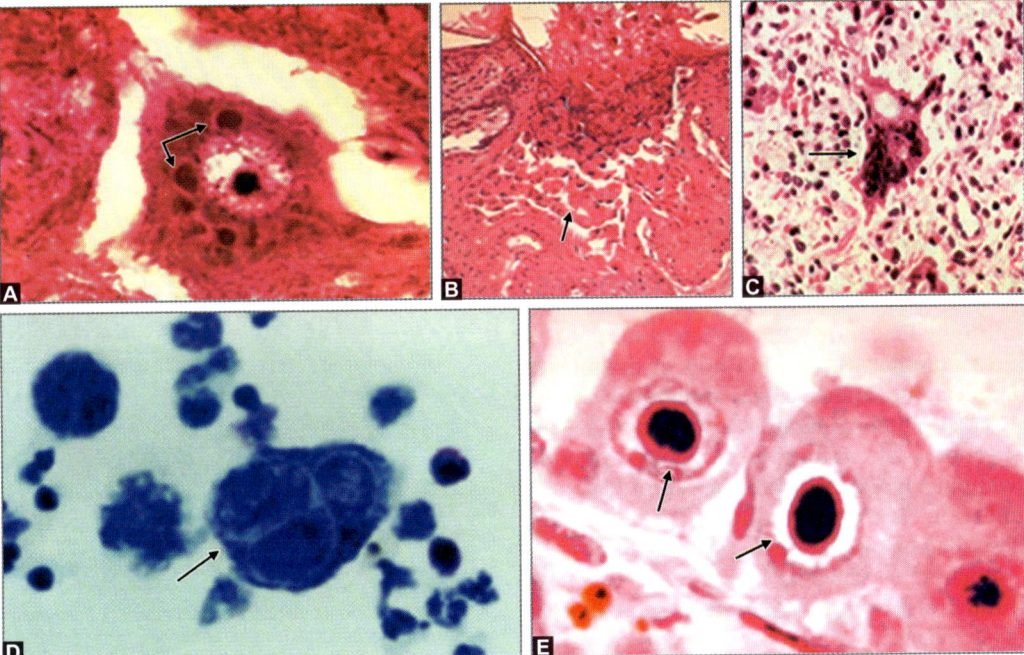

Figs 4.4A to E: (A) Negri bodies seen in brain infected with rabies; (B) Histopathology of skin showing molluscum bodies; (C) Multinucleated giant cell of measles; (D) Tzanck smear showing multinucleated giant cell of herpes simplex virus; (E) Histopathology of kidney showing cytomegalic host cell with owl's eye inclusion.
Source: Public Health Image Library, Centers for Disease Control and Prevention, Atlanta. (A) ID #3377; (B) ID #860; (C) ID #859; (D) ID #14428; (E) ID #1155.

(ICT), flow through assays, enzyme-linked fluorescence assay (ELFA), etc. Some important antigen detection tests include:
- HBsAg and HBeAg antigen detection for hepatitis B virus infection from serum
- NS1 antigen detection for dengue virus infection from serum
- SARS-CoV-2 antigen (nucleocapsid protein) detection in nasopharyngeal swabs by immunochromatographic assay
- p24 antigen detection for HIV infected patients from serum
- Rotavirus antigen detection from diarrheic stool
- CMV specific pp65 antigen detection in peripheral blood leukocyte.

Direct Immunofluorescence for Viral Antigen Detection

Direct immunofluorescence technique is employed to detect viral particles in the clinical samples.

Procedure

Specimen is mounted on slide, stained with specific monoclonal or polyclonal antibody tagged with fluorescent dye and viewed under fluorescent microscope.

Clinical Applications

Direct-IF has the following applications.
- Diagnosis of rabies in skin biopsies, corneal smear of infected patients (Fig. 4.5)

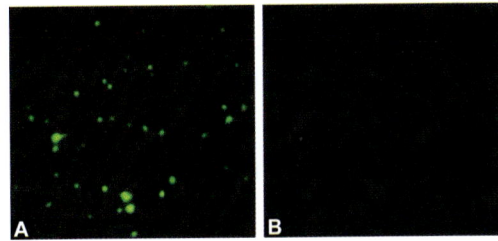

Figs 4.5A and B: Direct fluorescent antibody test for rabies antigen detection: (A) positive; (B) negative.
Source: Centers for Disease Control and Prevention, Atlanta (*with permission*).

- **Syndromic approach:** Rapid diagnosis of respiratory infections caused by influenza, rhinoviruses, respiratory syncytial virus, adenoviruses and herpes viruses can be carried out by adding specific antibodies to each of these viruses
- Detection of adenovirus from conjunctival smears.

DETECTION OF VIRAL ANTIBODIES

Antibody detection from serum is one of the most commonly used method in diagnostic virology. Appearance of IgM antibody or a four-fold rise of titer of IgG antibody indicates recent infection; whereas the presence of IgG antibody (without a recent rise) indicates chronic or past infection. Various techniques available are described below:

Techniques, such as ELISA, ELFA, ICT, flow through assays are widely used for antibody detection against most of the viral infections, for example:
- Anti-HBc, Anti-HBs and Anti-HBe antibodies in serum for hepatitis B infection
- Anti-hepatitis C antibodies in serum
- Antibodies against HIV-1 and HIV-2 antigens from serum
- Anti-dengue IgM/IgG antibodies from serum.

MOLECULAR METHODS

Advent of molecular techniques has eased the diagnosis of viral infections. They have revolutionized the diagnostic virology. They are more sensitive, specific and yield quicker results than culture.
- **Polymerase chain reaction (PCR):** It is the simplest molecular assay; used to detect viral DNA in clinical specimens (e.g., HSV DNA in CSF). It involves three basic steps:
  1. Viral DNA extraction from the specimen
  2. Amplification of specific region of viral DNA to 10^7 folds
  3. Detection of amplified products by gel electrophoresis.
- **Reverse transcriptase-PCR (RT-PCR):** It is used for the detection of RNA viruses (e.g., HIV and dengue RNA in blood). After RNA extraction, the viral RNA is reverse transcribed

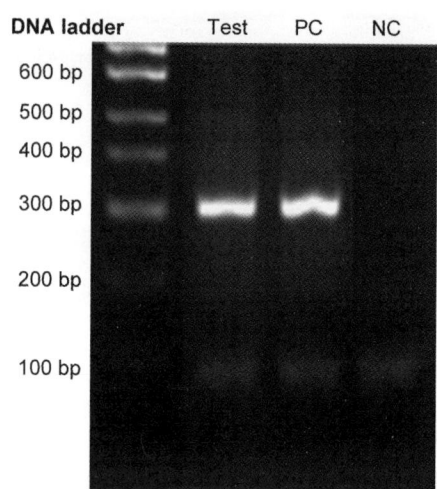

Fig. 4.6: PCR for dengue virus from serum sample. Band of 290 bp appeared for the test and positive control indicates presence of dengue virus serotype-3, in the test specimen.
Abbreviations: NC, negative control; PC, positive control.
Source: Department of Microbiology, Pondicherry Institute of Medical Sciences, Puducherry (*with permission*).

into DNA, which is then subjected to amplification similar to that followed in PCR (Fig. 4.6)
- **Multiplex PCR formats** are available that can simultaneously detect genes of common organisms responsible for a clinical syndrome; for example, multiplex PCR for upper respiratory syndromes simultaneously detects genes of adenovirus, influenza virus, parainfluenza virus and respiratory syncytial virus in respiratory specimen
- **BioFire FilmArray:** It is an automated nested multiplex PCR commercially available. It has various syndrome specific panels, such as respiratory, gastrointestinal, meningitis-encephalitis; each panel comprises of primers targeting 20–25 common pathogens infecting the respective systems
- **Real time-PCR (rt-PCR):** It is revolutionized the diagnostic virology; considered as the gold standard method for diagnosis of several viral infections, such as influenza, COVID-19, etc. It has several advantages over conventional PCR, such as:
  - Quantifying viral nucleic acid in the samples, hence used to monitor the treatment response and estimating viral load, e.g., HIV, hepatitis B virus

- Takes lesser time than PCR
- More sensitive and specific than PCR.

ISOLATION OF VIRUS

Viruses cannot be grown on artificial culture media. They are cultivated by animal inoculation, embryonated egg inoculation or tissue cultures.
❖ Being labor-intensive, technically demanding and time consuming, virus isolation is not routinely used in diagnostic virology
❖ The specimen should be collected properly and transported immediately to the laboratory. Refrigeration is essential during transportation as most viruses are heat labile. Type of specimen collected depends on the virus suspected.

Animal Inoculation

Because of the ethical issues related to use of animals, animal inoculation is largely restricted only for research purpose.
❖ **Research use:** To study viral pathogenesis or viral oncogenesis or for viral vaccine trials
❖ **Diagnostic use:** Primary isolation of certain viruses which are difficult to cultivate otherwise;, such as arboviruses and coxsackieviruses.

Egg Inoculation

Use of embryonated eggs for viral diagnostics is limited now. Embryonated hen's egg has four sites that are specific for the growth of certain viruses (Fig. 4.7).
❖ **Yolk sac inoculation:** Used for arboviruses (e.g., JE virus) and some bacteria, such as *Rickettsia*, *Chlamydia* and *Haemophilus ducreyi*

❖ **Amniotic sac:** Used for the isolation of influenza virus
❖ **Allantoic sac:** It is a larger cavity, hence is used for better yield of viral vaccines, such as influenza vaccine, yellow fever (17D) vaccine
❖ **Chorioallantoic membrane:** Used for the isolation of poxviruses (e.g., vaccinia and variola). They produce visible lesions over the chorioallantoic membrane called as pocks.

Tissue Culture

Cell line cultures are used for viral isolation.
❖ **Preparation of the cell lines:** Tissues are completely digested by treatment with proteolytic enzymes followed by mechanical shaking to completely dissociate them into individual cells. Then cells are suspended in viral growth medium containing balanced salt solution added with essential amino acids, vitamins, fetal calf serum and antibiotics. Then cells are in tissue culture flasks (Fig. 4.8)
  - On incubation, the cells adhere to the glass surfaces of the flask, divide and form a confluent monolayer sheet of cells within a week covering the floor of the tissue culture flask
  - Tissue culture flasks are incubated horizontally in presence of CO_2, either as a stationary culture or as a roller drum culture (for rotavirus isolation).
❖ **Types of cell lines:** Three types of cell lines are available.
  1. **Primary cell lines:** They are derived from normal cells freshly taken from the organs and cultured. They are capable of maximum up to 5–10 divisions. They have a diploid karyosome. Common examples include:

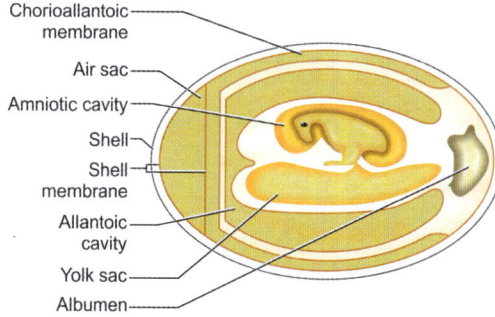

Fig. 4.7: Schematic diagram of embryonated egg.

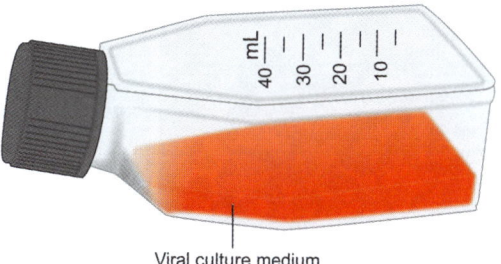

Fig. 4.8: Tissue culture flask.

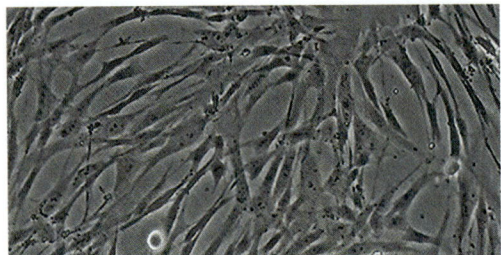

Fig. 4.9: Human lung fibroblast cell line (normal).
Source: American Type Culture Collection (ATCC), USA (*with permission*).

- Monkey kidney cell line—useful for isolation of myxoviruses, enteroviruses and adenoviruses
- Human amnion cell line and chick embryo cell line.

2. **Secondary or diploid cell lines:** They can divide maximum up to 10–50 divisions before they undergo death. They are also derived from the normal host cells and they maintain the diploid karyosome. Common examples include:
   - Human fibroblast cell line for recovery of CMV (Fig. 4.9)
   - MRC-5 and WI-38 (human embryonic lung cell strain): Used for preparation of various viral vaccines (rabies, chickenpox, MMR vaccines)
3. **Continuous cell lines** (*see* the box below).

Continuous Cell Lines
They are derived from cancerous cell lines, hence are immortal (capable of indefinite growth). They also possess altered haploid chromosome.

Contd...

Contd...

They are easy to maintain in the laboratories by serial subculturing for indefinite divisions. This is the reason why continuous cell lines are the most widely used cell lines.

Common examples include (Figs 4.10A to C)
- HeLa cell line (Human carcinoma of cervix cell line)
- HEp-2 cell line (Human epithelioma of larynx cell line)—widely used for RSV, adenoviruses and HSV
- KB cell line (Human carcinoma of nasopharynx cell line)
- McCoy cell line (Human synovial carcinoma cell line)—useful for isolation of viruses, as well as *Chlamydia*
- Vero cell line (Vervet monkey kidney cell line)—used for rabies vaccine production
- BHK cell line (Baby hamster kidney cell line).

Detection of Viral Growth in Cell Cultures

Following methods are used to detect the growth of the virus in cell cultures.

Cytopathic Effect (CPE)

It is defined as the morphological change produced by the virus in the cell line detected by a light microscope.

Cytopathic viruses: Not all, but few viruses can produce CPE and those are called as cytopathic viruses. The type of CPE is unique for each virus and that helps for their presumptive identification (Table 4.4).

Other Methods to Detect Viral Growth

Other methods to detect viruses in the cell line include:
- **Detection of viral antigens** on the surface of infected cells by direct immunofluorescence assay
- **Viral genes** detection by using PCR

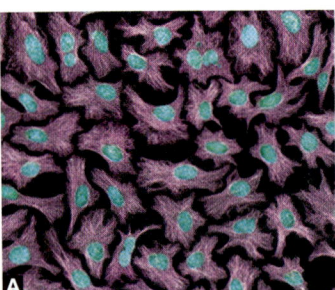 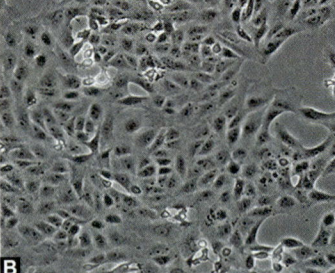 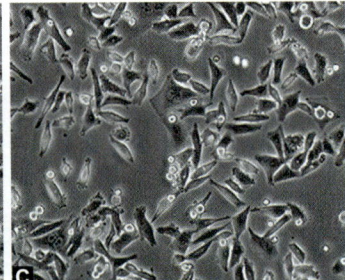

Figs 4.10A to C: Continuous cell lines (normal, uninfected): (A) HeLa cell line; (B) Vero cell line; (C) HEp-2 cell line.
Source: American Type Culture Collection (ATCC), USA (*with permission*).

Table 4.4: Viral cytopathic effects (CPE).

Types of cytopathic effect (CPE)	Virus
Rapid crenation and degeneration of the entire cell sheet	Enteroviruses
Syncytium or multinucleated giant cell formation	Measles, RSV, HSV
Diffuse roundening and ballooning of the cell line	HSV
Cytoplasmic vacuolations	SV 40
Large granular clumps resembling bunches of grapes	Adenovirus

Abbreviations: RSV, respiratory syncytial virus; HSV, herpes simplex virus; SV 40, Simian vacuolating virus-40.

- ❖ **Electron microscopy,** demonstrating the viruses in infected cell lines.

Shell Vial Technique

For viruses, such as CMV which take several weeks for cytopathic effect to develop, shell vial technique can be followed for early growth detection (1–2 days).

- ❖ It involves centrifugation of cell culture (mixed with the specimen) to enhance the cell contact and viral replication, followed by
- ❖ Detection of early viral antigen in the infected cells by direct fluorescence technique.

Problem Solving Exercise

Case Scenario 1: A patient with history of dog bite presents to emergency with hydrophobia, increased salivation and hyperexcitability. After the death of the patient, the brain biopsy was sent for histopathological examination (Fig. 4.4A). What is the etiological diagnosis?

Case Scenario 2: Serum specimen of a 23-year old man presented with fever, joint pain and myalgia is sent for dengue PCR (Fig. 4.6). Interpret the result. Discuss its principle?

Explanation

Case Scenario 1: Patient with history of dog bite, and presented with hydrophobia, increased salivation and hyperexcitability is suggestive of provisional diagnosis as rabies. Fig. 4.4A depicts intra-cytoplasmic inclusion body, described a Negri bodies which is characteristic of rabies.

Case Scenario 2: Fig. 4.6 depicts PCR for dengue virus from serum sample. Band of 290 bp appeared for the test and positive control indicates presence of dengue virus serotype-3 in the test serum.

CHAPTER 5

Laboratory Diagnosis of Parasitic Diseases

Laboratory diagnosis plays an important role in establishing the specific diagnosis of various parasitic infections. Following are the techniques used in the diagnosis of parasitic infections.

■ EXAMINATION OF FECES

As many parasites inhabit in the intestinal tract, stool examination is the most common diagnostic technique used for the diagnosis of parasitic infections.

Specimen Collection

Stool specimens should be collected in a wide-mouthed, clean, leak-proof, screw capped containers and should be handled carefully to avoid acquiring infection from organisms present in the stool (Fig. 5.1).
- ❖ **Timing:** Specimen should be collected before starting anti-parasitic drugs and closer to the onset of symptoms
- ❖ **Frequency:** At least three stool specimens collected on alternate days (within 10 days) are adequate to make the diagnosis of intestinal parasitic diseases (except for intestinal amoebiasis, for which six specimens may be recommended)

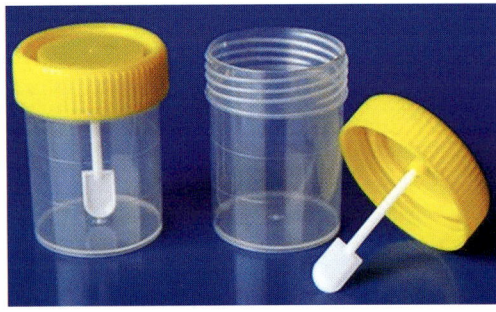

Fig. 5.1: Sample container for stool.

- ❖ **When to examine:** Liquid stool specimens should be examined within 30 minutes, semisolid stools within 1 hr (as on storage, trophozoites may disintegrate or become non-motile) and formed stools up to 24 hours after collection
- ❖ **For monitoring response to therapy:** Repeat stool examination can be done 3–4 weeks after the therapy for intestinal protozoan infection, and 5–6 weeks for *Taenia* infection
- ❖ **If delay in transport:** Fecal specimens should be kept at room temperature; pre-servatives (e.g., 10% formalin) can be used to maintain the morphology of the parasitic cysts and eggs
- ❖ **Specimens other than stool:**
  - *Perianal swabs* (cellophane tape or NIH swab): Useful for detecting eggs of *Enterobius vermicularis* deposited on the surface of perianal skin. It is also used for eggs of *Schistosoma mansoni* and *Taenia* species
  - *Duodenal contents:* It is very useful for the detection of small intestine parasites like, *Giardia intestinalis* and larva of *Strongyloides stercoralis*. Duodenal fluid can be collected by endoscopy or by Entero-test.

Macroscopic Examination

Macroscopic examination of stool may provide clue about various parasitic infections.
- ❖ **Mucoid bloody stool:** Found in acute amoebic dysentery, intestinal schistosomiasis, and invasive balantidiasis
- ❖ **Color:** Dark red stool indicates upper gastrointestinal tract (GIT) bleeding and a bright red stool is suggestive of bleeding from lower GIT

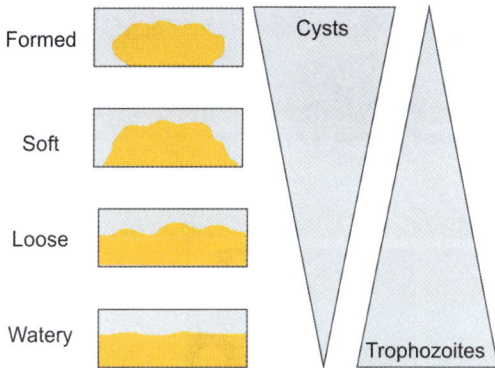

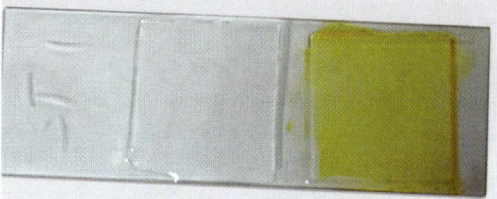

Fig. 5.3: Saline and iodine wet mount.
Source: Department of Microbiology, JIPMER, Puducherry *(with permission).*

Fig. 5.2: Relative frequency of trophozoites and cysts in stool specimens with various consistencies.

❖ **Frothy pale offensive stool** (containing fat) is usually found in giardiasis.

Stool Consistency

In liquid stool, trophozoites are usually found; whereas in semi-formed stool both trophozoites and cysts are found and the cysts are mainly found in formed specimens (Fig. 5.2). Exceptions to this general statement include:
❖ Coccidian oocysts, helminths eggs can be found in any type of fecal specimen
❖ In cryptosporidiosis, oocysts load is higher in liquid stool
❖ Tapeworm proglottids and adult worms of *Enterobius* and *Ascaris* are occasionally found in the stool.

Microscopic Examination

Microscopic examination includes direct wet mount examination and permanent staining methods.

Direct Wet Mount (Saline and Iodine Mount)

Drops of saline and Lugol's iodine are placed on left and right halves of the slide respectively (Fig. 5.3).
❖ A small amount of feces (~2 mg) is mixed with a stick to form a uniform smooth suspension. If more or less fecal material has been taken for the stool wet mount, the chance of finding stool parasites decreases
❖ **Cover slip** is placed on the mount and examined under low power objective (10X) for detection of helminths eggs and larvae;

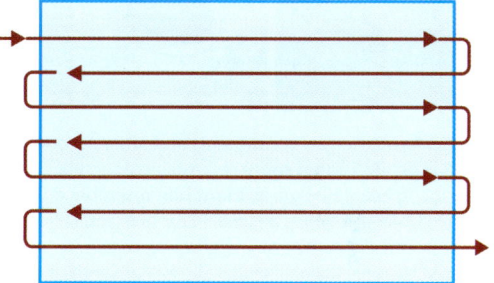

Fig. 5.4: Method of screening of slide during wet mount examination of stool.

followed by high power objective (40X) for protozoan cysts and trophozoites
❖ **Screening area:** The entire coverslip preparation should be examined in a zigzag fashion, first under low power and then under high power objective, before reporting a negative result (Fig. 5.4)
❖ **Motility:** If a finding is suspected to be a trophozoite, then examination for at least 15 seconds should be allowed to detect motility. Motility can be stimulated by—application of heat by placing a hot penny on the edge of a slide or tapping on the coverslip or increasing the intensity of the light source.

The following are the structures that can be visualized by microscopic examination of stool specimen, which may be confused with various protozoan trophozoites, cysts or helminthic eggs and larvae (Figs 5.5A to J).
❖ **Normal constituents:** These include plant fiber, starch cells (stains blue-black with iodine), muscle fibers, animal hair, pollen grains, yeast cells, bacteria, epithelial cells, fat globules, and air bubbles, etc.
❖ **Cellular elements:** Like pus cells (in inflammatory diarrhea), red blood cells (RBC) (in dysentery) may be present

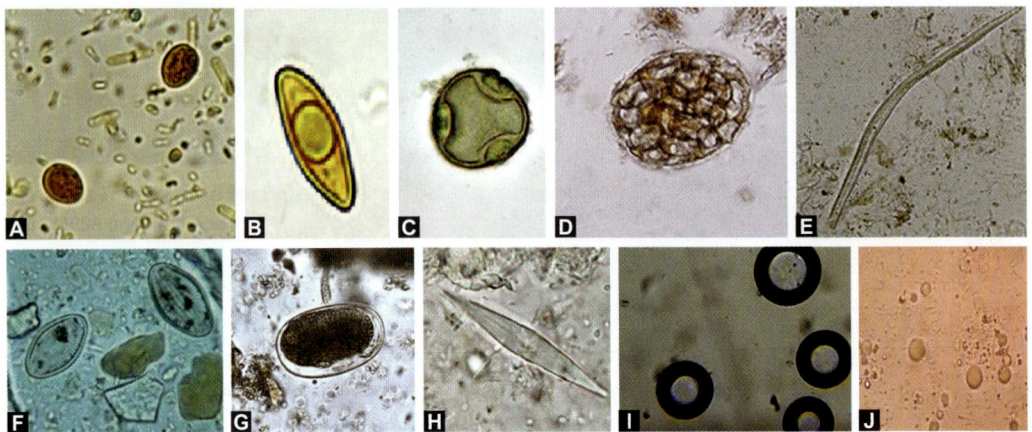

Figs 5.5A to J: Normal constituents and artifacts found in the stool in wet mount examination: (A) **Yeast cell** resembling *Giardia* cyst; (B) **Fungal spore** resembling oocyst of *Cystoisospora*; (C) **Pollen grain** resembling *Blastocystis*; (D) **Plant cell** resembling helminth egg; (E) **Plant hair** resembling *Strongyloides* larva; (F) Diatoms; (G) **Mite egg** resembling hookworm egg; (H) Charcot-Leyden crystals; (I) Air bubbles; (J) Fat globules.
Source: (A, B, D, E, F, G, H) DPDx Image Library, Centers for Disease Control and Prevention (CDC), Atlanta; (C) W Swierczynski G, Milanesi B. Atlas of Human Intestinal Protozoa Microscopic Diagnosis; (I and J) Department of Microbiology, JIPMER, Puducherry (*with permission*).

- **Charcot–Leyden crystals** (diamond-shaped): They are the breakdown products of eosinophils and may be seen in the stool or sputum of patients with parasitic diseases, such as amoebic dysentery, ascariasis, and allergic diseases, such as bronchial asthma (sputum).

Saline Mount

Saline mount is useful in the detection of trophozoites and cysts of protozoan parasites, and eggs and larvae of helminths. It has the following advantages than iodine mount.
- Motility of trophozoites and larvae in acute infection can be demonstrated
- Bile staining property can be appreciated—bile stained eggs appear golden brown and non-bile stained eggs appear colorless
- In stool specimen with preservatives, directly the wet mount can be prepared without using saline.

Iodine Mount

- **Advantages:** Nuclear details of protozoan cysts, helminthic eggs and larvae are better visualized, compared to saline mount
- **Disadvantages:** (i) Iodine immobilizes and kills the parasites, hence motility of the trophozoites and helminthic larvae cannot be appreciated, (ii) Bile staining property cannot be appreciated.

Non-bile Stained Eggs
Eggs of most of the intestinal parasites when they pass through intestine are stained by bile. The exceptions being *Enterobius*, hookworm and *Hymenolepis nana*; these eggs are non-bile stained.

Permanent Stained Smear

Permanent stained smears are required for accurate detection of protozoan cysts and trophozoites by staining their internal structures. Commonly used methods are:
- Iron-hematoxylin stain
- Trichrome stain
- Modified acid-fast stain—this is useful for coccidian parasites, such as *Cryptosporidium*, *Cyclospora* and *Cystoisospora*.

Concentration Techniques

If the parasite output is low in feces (egg, cysts, trophozoites and larvae) and direct examination may not be able to detect the parasites, then the stool specimens need to be concentrated. These methods are also useful in epidemiological analysis and for assessing the treatment response. The eggs, cysts and larvae are recovered after concentration procedures; however, the trophozoites get destroyed.

Commonly used concentration techniques are:

- ❖ **Sedimentation techniques:** The eggs and cysts settle down at the bottom following centrifugation. Example include formalin-ether concentration technique and formalin-ethyl acetate concentration technique
- ❖ **Flotation techniques:** It involves suspending the specimen in a medium (e.g., **saturated salt solution**) of greater density, so that the helminthic eggs and protozoan cysts float on the surface of the solution

Other flotation methods are:

- Zinc sulphate flotation concentration technique
- Sheather's sugar flotation technique (useful for *Cryptosporidium*, *Cystoisospora* and *Cyclospora*).

Sedimentation (Formol-ether) Technique

Principle: It involves concentration of stool specimen by centrifugation. The protozoan cysts and helminthic eggs are concentrated at the bottom of the tube because they have *greater density than the suspending medium.*

Procedure: About half teaspoonful of feces is mixed thoroughly 10 mL of 10% formalin, kept standing for 30 minutes and the filtered out with a gauge piece.

- ❖ The filtrate is mixed 5% with formalin and centrifuged. After discarding the supernatant, the sediment is again mixed with 5% formalin and centrifuged
- ❖ Finally 4–5 mL of ether is added to the sediment and the tube is closed with a stopper and shaken vigorously to mix well. The stopper is removed and the tube is centrifuged
- ❖ Four layers are formed—top layer consists of ether, second is a plug of debris, third is a clear layer of formalin and the fourth is the sediment (Figs 5.6A and B)
- ❖ The debris is removed from the side of the tube with the help of a glass rod and supernatant is discarded
- ❖ With a pipette, the sediment is removed and the saline or iodine mount is prepared and examined under the microscope.

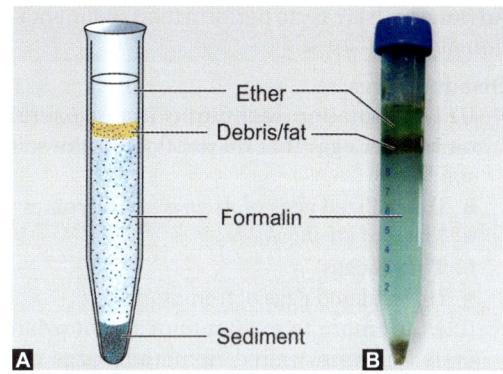

Figs 5.6A and B: Sedimentation (*Formol-ether*) technique.
Source: (B) Dr Anand Janagond, S Nijalingappa Medical College, Bagalkot, Karnataka, India (*with permission*).

Advantages:

- ❖ The sensitivity of detecting the ova or cysts increases by 8–10 folds
- ❖ The size and shape of the parasitic structures are maintained
- ❖ Inexpensive, easy to perform
- ❖ Fecal odor is removed
- ❖ As formalin kills the fecal parasites, no risk of acquiring laboratory-acquired infection.

Disadvantage: Trophozoite forms are killed and hence not detected in this method.

Flotation (Saturated Salt Solution) Technique

Principle: Flotation involves suspending the stool specimen in a medium of greater density than that of the helminthic eggs and protozoan cysts; e.g., saturated salt solution. After 15 minutes waiting period, the eggs and cysts float to the top and are collected by placing a glass slide on the surface of the meniscus at the top of the tube (Fig. 5.7).

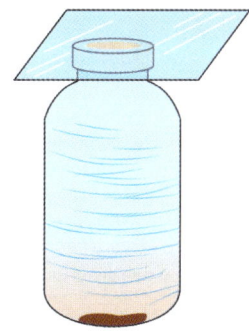

Fig. 5.7: Flotation (saturated salt solution) technique.

Advantage: It is easy to perform than sedimentation method.

Disadvantages:
- **ULTO:** Flotation technique is not useful for heavier eggs that do not float in the salt solution
  - **U**nfertilized eggs of *Ascaris lumbricoides*
  - **L**arva of *Strongyloides*
  - **T**aenia eggs
  - **O**perculated eggs of trematodes.
- If left for more than 20 minutes, protozoan cysts and thin-walled nematode eggs get collapsed and become distorted due to high specific gravity of the solution.

Various morphological forms of parasites seen in stool specimens are enlisted in Table 5.1.

EXAMINATION OF BLOOD

Blood examination is useful in the diagnosis of infection caused by blood parasites, such as *Plasmodium*, *Trypanosoma*, *Leishmania*, *Babesia*, *Wuchereria bancrofti*, *Brugia malayi*, *Loa loa* and *Mansonella*.

Various methods of examination of blood include:

1. **Direct wet mount examination:** It is useful for detection of malaria parasites and microfilariae in lymphatic filariasis
2. **Examination of blood smears:** Thin smear and thick smears are examined after staining with various Romanowsky stains, such as Leishman's stain, Giemsa stain, Field's stain and Jaswant Singh and Bhattacharjee (JSB) stain. This is the most common method of microscopic examination of peripheral blood, useful for most of the blood parasites
3. **Quantitative buffy coat (QBC):** This involves collection of the blood in a capillary tube coated internally with acridine orange stain, centrifugation and then examination of the buffy coat region under fluorescence microscopy. This is extremely useful for the detection of the malaria parasites and microfilariae
4. **Concentration of blood:** This is useful for detection of microfilariae from the blood specimen. Various concentration methods are:
   - Sedimentation technique
   - Cytocentrifugation (cytospin)
   - Knott concentration
   - Gradient centrifugation
   - Membrane filtration.

MICROSCOPIC EXAMINATION OF OTHER SPECIMENS

Microscopic examination of various specimens (other than stool) can also be performed to demonstrate different morphological forms of the parasites (Table 5.2).

Table 5.1: Morphological forms of parasites seen in stool specimens.

Morphological form	Parasites
Trophozoite and cyst	*Entamoeba histolytica* *Giardia lamblia*
Adult worm	*Ascaris lumbricoides* *Enterobius vermicularis*
Adult worm segments	*Taenia* species *Diphyllobothrium latum*
Egg	*Diphyllobothrium latum* *Taenia* species *Hymenolepis nana* *Schistosoma* species *Fasciola hepatica* *Fasciolopsis buski* *Ascaris lumbricoides* Hookworm *Enterobius vermicularis* *Trichuris trichiura*
Larva	*Strongyloides stercoralis*

Table 5.2: Various morphological forms of parasites seen in different specimens other than stool.

Specimen	Morphological form	Parasite
Peripheral blood smear	Ring form, schizont, gametocyte	*Plasmodium* spp.
	Amastigote	*Leishmania* spp.
	Trypomastigote	*Trypanosoma* spp.
	Microfilaria	Filarial nematodes*
Bone marrow, liver, lymph node, splenic aspirate	Tachyzoite	*Toxoplasma gondii*
	Amastigote	*Leishmania donovani*
Liver aspirate	Trophozoite	*Entamoeba histolytica*
Lymph node aspirate	Trypomastigote	*Trypanosoma* spp.

Contd...

CHAPTER 5 ◆ Laboratory Diagnosis of Parasitic Diseases

Contd...

Specimen	Morphological form	Parasite
Lymph node biopsy	Adult worm	Wuchereria bancrofti, Brugia malayi
Cerebrospinal fluid	Trophozoite	Naegleria fowleri, Acanthamoeba spp.
	Trypomastigote	Trypanosoma spp.
Urine	Trophozoite	Trichomonas vaginalis
	Microfilaria	Wuchereria bancrofti
	Egg	Schistosoma haematobium
Sputum	Adult worm	Paragonimus spp.
	Egg	Paragonimus spp.
	Larva (migrating)	Ascaris lumbricoides, Strongyloides spp. Hookworm
	Trophozoite	Entamoeba histolytica

Contd...

Contd...

Specimen	Morphological form	Parasite
Duodenal aspirate	Trophozoite	Giardia lamblia
	Larva	Strongyloides stercoralis
Corneal scrapings	Trophozoite	Acanthamoeba spp.
Skin	Amastigote	Leishmania spp.
	Microfilaria	Onchocerca volvulus
	Larva in skin ulcer fluid	Dracunculus medinensis
Muscle tissue	Encysted larva	Trichinella spiralis
	Cysticercus cellulosae	Taenia solium
Perianal area	Egg	Enterobius spp.

*Filarial nematodes found in the peripheral blood smears are Wuchereria bancrofti, Brugia malayi, Loa loa, Mansonella spp.

IMMUNODIAGNOSTIC METHODS

Immunodiagnostic methods involve detection of parasite specific antibodies in serum, and detection of circulating parasitic antigen in the serum.

Antibody Detection Tests

Antibodies are detected in various parasitic infections; mainly from serum (amoebic liver abscess, visceral leishmaniasis and toxoplasmosis); sometime from other specimens, such as CSF (neurocysticercosis) or pleural fluid (paragonimiasis).

Antigen Detection Tests

The antigen detection methods are available for various parasitic diseases, such as amoebiasis, malaria and lymphatic filariasis.

MOLECULAR METHODS

Molecular methods most frequently used in diagnostic parasitology include polymerase chain reaction (PCR), real time PCR and BioFire FilmArray.

Problem Solving Exercise

1. A laboratory technician is examining a stool specimen that has come as a screening test done under master health checkup. What are the structures that can be visualized by microscopic examination of stool specimen, which may be confused with various parasitic forms?
2. What are the various methods of wet mount examination of stool? Discuss their advantages and disadvantages.
3. What are the various stool concentration methods? Discuss their advantages and disadvantages.

Explanation

Refer text for detail.

Laboratory Diagnosis of Fungal Diseases

CHAPTER 6

■ CLASSIFICATION

Morphological Classification

Based on the morphology, there are four groups of fungi (Figs 6.1A to E).
1. **Yeast:** They grow as round to oval cells that reproduce by an asexual process called budding. Examples include *Cryptococcus neoformans* (Fig. 6.1A)
2. **Yeast-like:** They are oval budding cells with pseudohyphae (elongated budding cells remain attached to the mother cell to form long chain of daughter cells). They can be differentiated from true hyphae as they have constrictions at the septa. Examples include *Candida* (Fig. 6.1B)
3. **Molds:** They grow as long branching filaments of 2–10 μm wide called *hyphae* (mycelium) (Fig. 6.1E). Hyphae are either septate (i.e., form transverse walls) (Fig. 6.1D) or nonseptate (Fig. 6.1C). Examples of molds include dermatophytes, *Aspergillus, Penicillium, Rhizopus, Mucor,* etc.
4. **Dimorphic fungi:** They exist as molds at 25°C and as yeasts in human tissues at body temperature (37°C). Examples include *Histoplasma, Blastomyces, Coccidioides, Paracoccidioides, Penicillium marneffei* and *Sporothrix schenckii*.

Systemic Classification

Based on diseases, fungi are classified as follows:
- **Superficial mycoses:** Caused by *Malassezia furfur* and dermatophytes
- **Subcutaneous mycoses:** Caused by *Madurella* and others, *Sporothrix schenckii*, and *Rhinosporidium*
- **Systemic mycoses:** Agents are *Histoplasma, Blastomyces, Coccidioides,* and *Paracoccidioides*
- **Opportunistic mycoses:** Caused by *Candida* species, *Cryptococcus, Rhizopus, Mucor, Aspergillus* species and *Penicillium* species, and *Pneumocystis jirovecii*.

■ LABORATORY DIAGNOSIS

Specimen Collection

It depends on the site of infection. For example:
- For systemic mycoses—blood
- For cryptococcal meningitis—cerebrospinal fluid.

Details on specimen collection are described in the respective systems, where they cause the infections.

Microscopy

Following direct microscopic examination methods can be done:
- **Potassium hydroxide (KOH)** preparation (10%): Used for keratinized tissue specimens (skin scrapings, plucked hair samples), which digests the keratin material so that fungal hyphae will be clearly visualized (Fig. 6.2A)

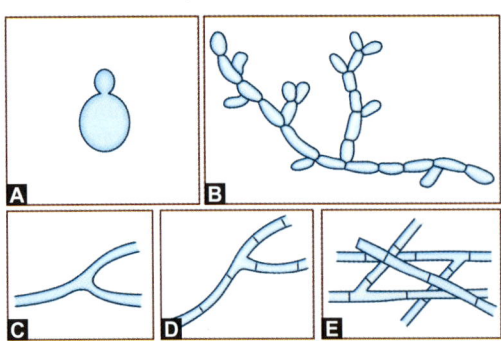

Figs 6.1A to E: Morphological forms of fungi: (A) Budding; (B) Budding yeast with pseudohyphae; (C) Aseptate hyphae; (D) Septate hyphae; (E) Mycelium.

CHAPTER 6 ◆ Laboratory Diagnosis of Fungal Diseases

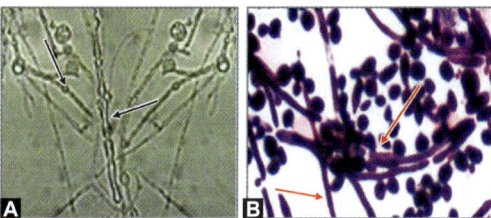
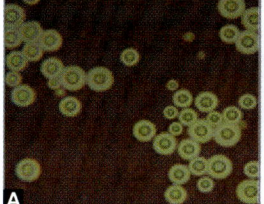
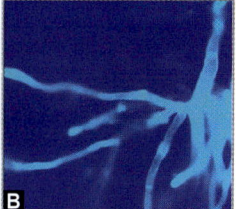

Figs 6.2A and B: (A) KOH mount showing fungal elements; (B) Gram staining showing gram-positive oval budding yeast cells with pseudohyphae.

Source: Department of Microbiology, Pondicherry Institute of Medical Sciences, Puducherry (*with permission*).

Figs 6.3A and B: (A) India ink staining shows clear refractile capsules surrounding round budding yeast cells *(Cryptococcus)*; (B) Calcofluor-white mount showing fungal elements.

Source: A. Public Health Image Library/A. Dr Leanor Haley, ID#:3771/ Centers for Disease Control and Prevention (CDC), Atlanta (*with permission*); B. Department of Microbiology, JIPMER, Puducherry (*with permission*).

- About 20–40% KOH is used for nail clipping (as takes longer time to dissolve)
- Biopsy specimens are usually dissolved in 10% KOH in a test tube and examined after overnight incubation (as they take longer time to dissolve).
❖ **Gram stain** is useful in identifying the yeast (e.g., *Cryptococcus*) and yeast-like fungi (e.g., *Candida*). They appear as gram-positive budding yeast cells (Fig. 6.2B)
❖ **India ink and nigrosin** stains are used as negative stains for demonstration of capsule of *Cryptococcus neoformans* (Fig. 6.3A)
❖ **Calcofluor-white stain:** This binds to cellulose and chitin of fungal cell wall and fluoresces under ultraviolet light (Fig. 6.3B)
❖ **Histopathological stains** are useful for demonstrating fungal elements (causing deep mycoses) from biopsy tissues
   - *Periodic acid-Schiff (PAS)* stain is the recommend stain for detecting fungi. PAS-positive fungi appear magenta/deep pink whereas the nuclei stain blue (Fig. 6.4A)
   - *Gomori methenamine silver (GMS) stain:* Fungi appear black whereas the background tissue takes pale green color (Fig. 6.4B)
   - *Mucicarmine stain* is used for *Cryptococcus* and *Rhinosporidium*
   - *Hematoxylin and eosin (H&E)* stain.
❖ **Lactophenol cotton blue (LPCB)** is used to study the microscopic appearance of the fungal isolates grown in culture (Fig. 6.4C).

Culture

Fungal culture is frequently performed for isolation and correct identification of the fungi.
❖ **Sabouraud's dextrose agar** (SDA) is the most commonly used media in diagnostic mycology. It contains peptone (1%) and dextrose (4%) and has a final pH of 5.6 (Figs 6.5A and B)

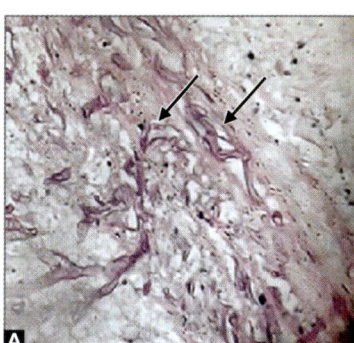
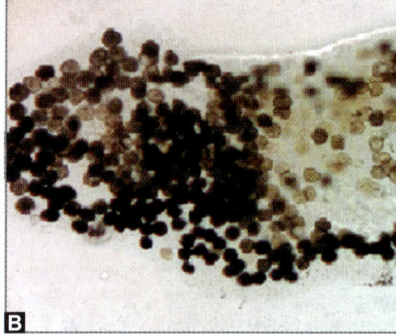
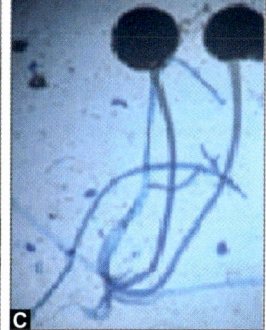

Figs 6.4A to C: (A) PAS stain showing fungal hyphae; (B) Gomori methenamine silver stain (fungi appear black, against pale green background); (C) Lactophenol cotton blue mount fungal isolate grown in culture.
Source: (A and B) Department of Pathology, and (C) Department of Microbiology, Pondicherry Institute of Medical Sciences, Puducherry (*with permission*).

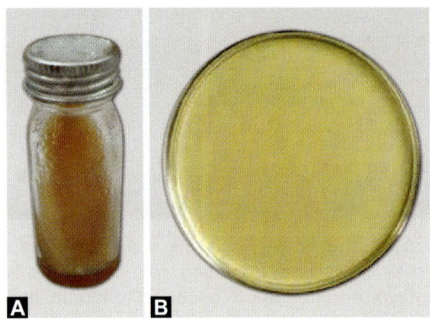

Figs 6.5A and B: (A) Sabouraud's dextrose agar slope in bottle; (B) Sabouraud's dextrose agar plate.
Source: Department of Microbiology, Pondicherry Institute of Medical Sciences, Puducherry (*with permission*).

- Specimen inoculated SDA plates are incubated at 25–30°C (except the dimorphic fungi that grow at both 25°C and 37°C) in biochemical oxygen demand (BOD) incubators for 2–3 weeks
- **Antibiotics**, such as cycloheximide, chloramphenicol and gentamicin can be added to the culture media to inhibit growth of bacteria and saprophytic fungi
- **Macroscopy:** Following macroscopic appearance of the colony are noted, such as (i) Rate of growth (yeasts and agents of opportunistic mycoses grow within 5 days; whereas dermatophytes take 1–4 weeks), (ii) Pigmentation (iii) Texture of the colony (waxy/leathery, velvety, cottony or granular/powdery), (iv) Colony topography (colony surface)
- **Microscopic appearance of fungi:** A bit of fungal colony is teased out (tease mount) from the culture tube and LPCB mount is made on a slide and viewed under microscope. Identification is based on the:
  - Nature of hyphae (septate or aseptate, hyaline or phaeoid, narrow or wide) and
  - Type of sporulation (conidia or sporangiospores).
- **Slide culture**: It gives the most accurate in situ (undisturbed) microscopic appearance of the fungal colony. Procedure—sterile slide is placed on a bent glass rod in a sterile petri dish. Two square agar blocks measuring around 1 cm^2 (smaller than the coverslip) are placed on the slide. Bit of the fungal colony is inoculated onto the margins (at the center) of the agar block. Then the coverslip is placed on the agar block and the petri dish is incubated at 25°C. After sufficient growth occurs, LPCB mounts are made both from the coverslip and the underneath slide (Fig. 6.6)
- **Cellophane tape mount:** Impressions are taken by placing the cellophane tape on the colonies present on the surface of SDA plate, and then LPCB mount is made from the cellophane tape. This is easy to perform and the in-situ fungal morphology is also maintained.

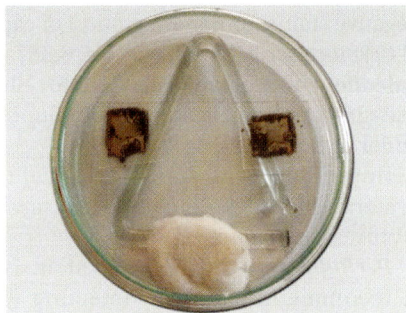

Fig. 6.6: Slide culture technique.
Source: Department of Microbiology, Pondicherry Institute of Medical Sciences, Puducherry (*with permission*).

Problem Solving Exercise

Case Scenario 1: CSF specimen is collected from a 32-year HIV positive patient with fever and neck rigidity. What is the stain recommended for direct microscopy and what is medium to be used for fungal culture.

Case Scenario 2: A young male presented with ring like annular skin lesions over the groin area. Which is the recommended direct microscopy technique to demonstrate the fungal elements and how will you perform fungal culture.

Explanation

Case Scenario 1: Patient with fever and neck rigidity is suggestive of a case of meningitis. India ink is recommended to demonstrate capsule of *Cryptococcus*. The recommended medium is Sabouraud's dextrose agar.

Case Scenario 2: Patient with ring like annular skin lesions over the groin area is suggestive of ring worm (Dermatophyte) infection. 10% KOH mount of the skin scraping is the recommended direct microscopy technique to demonstrate the fungal hyphae. The recommended culture medium is Sabouraud's dextrose agar.

Precipitation and Agglutination

CHAPTER 7

■ INTRODUCTION

The antigen–antibody reactions are specific and observable. Therefore, they are extensively used in the laboratories for the diagnosis of infectious diseases. The diagnostic tests based on Ag-Ab reactions are called as immunoassays. Most immunoassays are also called serological tests as they are performed using serum samples. However, other samples can also be used, such as urine, CSF, etc. Immunoassays can be broadly categorized into two types:
1. **Antigen detection assays:** Detect antigens in patient's sample by employing specific antibody
2. **Antibody detection assays:** Detect antibodies in patient's sample by employing specific antigen.

Immunoassays can be performed by both qualitative and quantitative methods.
- ❖ **Qualitative assays:** Here, the undiluted specimen containing the antibody is directly mixed with the suspension of antigen or vice versa. The exact amount of antigen or antibody present in the specimen cannot be estimated
- ❖ **Quantitative assays:** Here, the exact amount of antibody in serum can be estimated by serial dilution of the patient's serum and mixing it with a known quantity of antigen. The measurement of antibody is expressed as **titer** (defined as the highest dilution of serum that shows an observable reaction with the antigen).

Marrack's Lattice Hypothesis
When the sera containing antibody is serially diluted (in normal saline), gradually the antibody level decreases. When a fixed quantity of antigen is added to such a set of test tubes containing serially diluted sera, then it is observed that the Ag-Ab reaction

Contd...

Contd...

occurs at its best only in the middle test tubes where the amount of antigen and antibody are equivalent to each other (*zone of equivalence*). The Ag-Ab reaction is weak or fails to occur when the number of antigen and antibodies are not proportionate to each other (Figs 7.1A to C).
- ❑ In the earlier test tubes, *antibodies are excess*, hence the Ag-Ab reaction does not occur: This is called as **prozone phenomenon**
- ❑ In the later test tubes, *antigen is excess*, hence the Ag-Ab reaction fails to occur: This is called as **postzone phenomenon**.

Marrack (1934) proposed the **lattice hypothesis** to explain this mechanism. According to this concept the multivalent antigens combine with bivalent antibodies in varying proportions, depending on the antigen antibody ratio in the reacting mixture (Figs 7.1A to C).
- ❑ Ag-Ab reaction optimally occurs when a large lattice is formed consisting of alternating antigen and antibody molecules. This is possible only in the zone of equivalence
- ❑ In the zones of antibody or antigen excess (prozone/post zone), the lattice does not enlarge, due to inhibition of lattice formation by the excess antibody or antigen respectively.

Lattice hypothesis was described first for precipitation reaction, but it also holds true for agglutination and other techniques of Ag-Ab reactions.

The prozone phenomenon is of great importance in clinical serology, as sera rich in high titer of antibody may sometimes give a false-negative result, unless serial dilutions of sera are tested.

The antigen–antibody reactions used in diagnostic laboratories are based on various techniques which are broadly classified as conventional techniques and newer techniques (Table 7.1).

■ PRECIPITATION REACTION

Definition
When a **soluble antigen** reacts with its antibody in the presence of optimal temperature, pH and

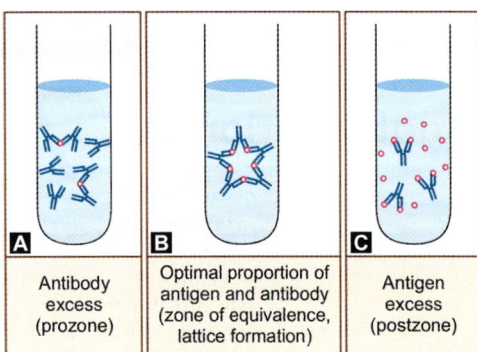

Figs 7.1A to C: (A) Prozone; (B) Zone of equivalence; (C) Postzone.

Table 7.1: Types of antigen–antibody reactions.

Conventional techniques	
• Precipitation reaction	• Agglutination reaction
Newer techniques	
• Enzyme-linked immunosorbent assay (ELISA)	
• Enzyme-linked fluorescent assay (ELFA)	
• Immunofluorescence assay (IFA)	
• Chemiluminescence-linked immunoassay (CLIA)	

• Rapid tests
  ➤ Lateral flow assay (immunochromatographic test)
  ➤ Flow through assay	

• Western blot	

electrolytes (NaCl), it leads to formation of the antigen–antibody complex in the form of:

❖ **Insoluble precipitation band** when gel or agar containing medium is used (called immunodiffusion) or

❖ **Insoluble floccules** when liquid medium is used (called flocculation test).

Clinical Applications

Earlier, precipitation reactions were one of the widely used serological tests. However, with the advent of simple and rapid newer techniques their application is greatly reduced. There are only limited situations where precipitation reaction is still in use; discussed below.

Slide Flocculation Test (for Syphilis)

It is used for serodiagnosis of syphilis, a sexually transmitted disease caused by *Treponema pallidum*.

❖ **Procedure:** When a drop of antigen is mixed with a drop of patient's serum (containing antibody) on a slide, then the precipitates formed remain suspended as floccules

❖ **Examples** include VDRL (Venereal Disease Research Laboratory) and RPR (Rapid Plasma Reagin) tests. Refer Chapter 43 for detail.

Elek's Gel Precipitation Test (Detecting Diphtheria Toxin)

The *Corynebacterium diphtheriae* strain isolated is streaked on to a medium containing a filter paper soaked with diphtheria antitoxin.

❖ If the strain is toxigenic, it produces the toxin, which diffuses in the agar, meets with the antitoxin and produces arrow-shaped precipitation band

❖ The precipitate bands of outbreak isolates (streaked adjacent) when meet with each other, three patterns may be observed based on relatedness between the strains (Fig. 7.3, Problem Solving Exercise 2).

Problem Solving Exercise 1

Venereal Disease Research Laboratory

A commercial sex worker with painless indurated genital lesions, presented to outpatient department for screening for sexually transmitted infections. One of the test done is demonstrated below (Figs 7.2A and B).
1. Identify the test and in which condition is it used?
2. Interpret the result.
3. What type of antigen is used in this test?
4. What is the principle of the test?

Explanation

History of commercial sex worker with painless indurated genital lesions is suggestive of syphilis. The test shown in the picture is Venereal Disease Research Laboratory (VDRL) test. It is the most widely used,

CHAPTER 7 ◆ Precipitation and Agglutination

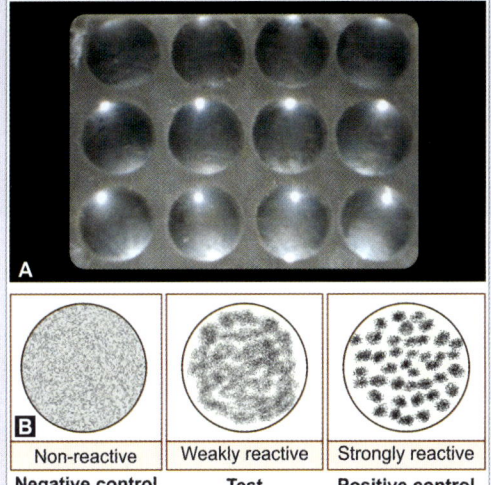

Figs 7.2A and B: VDRL slide and VDRL test results.
Source: Department of Microbiology, JIPMER, Puducherry *(with permission).*

simple, nonspecific and rapid serological test used for diagnosis of syphilis.

Procedure
50 µL of inactivated serum is mixed with a drop of VDRL antigen (cardiolipin antigen) in a *VDRL slide* containing 12 concave rings (Fig. 7.2A). Then the slide is rotated at 180 revolutions per minute for 4 minutes in a VDRL rotator and examined under microscope (10X). The results are read as follows:

- **Nonreactive:** Uniformly distributed fusiform crystals represent the presence of VDRL antigen only, which indicates a negative result.
- **Reactive:** It is indicated by formation of medium to large clumps of antigen–antibody complexes; visualized by focusing the slide under microscope (10x) (Fig. 7.2B).
- **Weakly reactive:** Slight roughness denotes weakly reactive test result (as in this case). In such cases, the test results should be confirmed by performing specific treponemal tests (Refer Chapter 43).

Problem Solving Exercise 2

Elek's Gel Precipitation Test
A cluster of diphtheria cases occurred affecting children in a remote village. The strains of *Corynebacterium diphtheriae* isolated from the clinical specimens were subjected for toxigenicity testing and the result is displayed in the Figure 7.3.
- Identify the test performed and interpret the result.
- Determine whether the relatedness between the strains isolated.

Explanation
The test performed in above case scenario is Elek's gel precipitation test. This is a type of immunodiffusion in gel described by Elek (1949)
- **Isolates 1 to 4** are toxigenic strains (as precipitation bands are formed due to binding of toxin produced by the strains with antitoxin released by the filter paper)
- **Isolates 1 and 2:** The precipitation bands crossed over, indicates the toxins are **not identical** and therefore strains are unrelated
- **Isolate 2 and 3:** There is partial fusion of precipitation bands, indicates the toxins are **partially identical** and therefore strains are partially related to each other
- **Isolates 3 and 4:** The precipitation bands fused with each other, indicates the toxins are **identical** to each other and therefore strains are completely related
- **Isolate 5** is non-toxigenic strain (no precipitation band is formed).

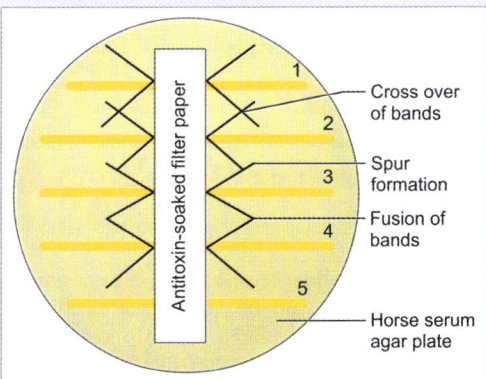

Fig. 7.3: Elek's gel precipitation test.

AGGLUTINATION REACTION

Definition

When a *particulate* or *insoluble* antigen is mixed with its antibody in the presence of electrolytes at a suitable temperature and pH, the particles are clumped or agglutinated.

Advantage

Agglutination is more sensitive than precipitation test as the clumps are better visualized and interpreted than bands or floccules. Hence, agglutination tests are widely used even in today's modern era of diagnosis.

Applications

Agglutination reactions are classified as direct, indirect (passive) and reverse passive agglutination reactions. All these agglutination tests are performed either on a slide, or in tube or in card or sometime in microtiter plates.

Direct Agglutination Test

Here, the antigen directly agglutinates with the antibody.

Slide Agglutination

It is usually performed to confirm the identification and serotyping of bacterial colonies grown in culture. It is also the method used for blood grouping and cross matching. The process follows:

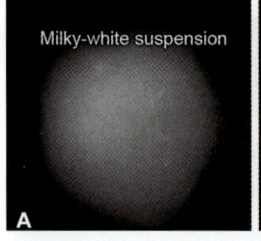 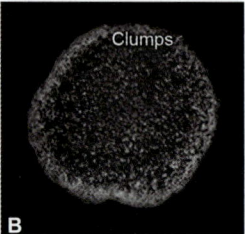

Figs 7.4A and B: Slide agglutination test: (A) Negative result; (B) Positive result (clumps).
Source: Department of Microbiology, JIPMER, Puducherry *(with permission)*.

Bacterial colony is mixed with a drop of saline on a slide to form a uniform, smooth, milky-white suspension
↓
To this, a drop of the antiserum (serum containing appropriate antibody) is added and the slide is shaken thoroughly (manually or by rotator) for few seconds
↓
A positive result is indicated by visible clumping with clearing of the suspension (Fig. 7.4B)
or
If the milky-white suspension remains unchanged, indicates a negative result (Fig. 7.4A).

Tube Agglutination

This is a standard quantitative test for estimating antibody in serum. Several tests are there that are done in various clinical conditions.

❖ **Widal test** in typhoid or enteric fever (Refer the Problem Solving Exercise 3) (Refer Chapter 18 for detail).

Problem Solving Exercise 3

Widal Test

A young adult male admitted to the hospital with fever of 10 days duration with step ladder pattern. A provisional clinical diagnosis of enteric fever was made. The following serological test was performed.
1. Identify the test performed and in which clinical condition this test is used?
2. What type of antigen–antibody reaction occurs in this test?
3. How will you interpret the positive and negative results and report the titer?
4. Name two other tests based on the same principle (Fig. 7.5).

Explanation

History of stepladder fever is suggestive of enteric fever. This is caused by *Salmonella* Typhi and *Salmonella* Paratyphi A and B. The test shown here is Widal test; titer of TO 1:160 and TH 1:320.

Widal test is an example of tube agglutination test used for quantitative estimation of antibody titer against *S.* Typhi and *Salmonella* Paratyphi A and B.

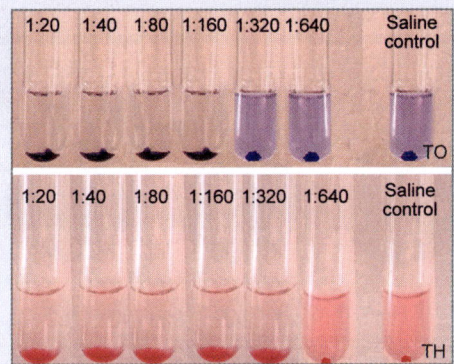

Fig. 7.5: Widal test
Abbreviations: TO and TH: Antibody titers of *S.*Typhi O and H in patient's serum.
Source: Department of Microbiology, Pondicherry Institute of Medical Sciences (*with permission*).

The *antibody titer* can be estimated as the highest dilution of the serum which produces a visible agglutination.

Procedure of Tube Agglutination Test

A fixed volume of antigen suspension is added to an equal volume of serial dilutions of a serum sample (containing appropriate antibody) in test tubes and overnight incubated at 37°C in water bath.
- Positive test indicates agglutination (matt formation at the bottom of the tube with clearing of the supernatant)
- Negative test indicates agglutination did not occur (antigen suspension forms button at the bottom of the tube with no clearing of supernatant).

- Standard agglutination test in acute brucellosis
- **Coombs antiglobulin test:** It is performed to diagnose Rh incompatibility by detecting Rh antibody from mother's and baby's serum.
- **Heterophile agglutination tests:**
  - Weil–Felix reaction in typhus fever
  - Paul–Bunnell test in infectious mononucleosis
  - Cold agglutination test in *Mycoplasma pneumoniae.*

Microscopic Agglutination

Here, the agglutination test is performed on a microtiter plate and the result is read under a microscope. Example is microscopic agglutination test (MAT), done for leptospirosis.

In Widal test: Antibodies against both H (flagellar) and O (somatic) antigens of *Salmonella* Typhi are detected.
- O antigen–antibody clumps appear as chalky-white granular dense deposits.
- H antigen–antibody clumps appear as loose fluffy clumps (Fig. 7.6).

Indirect or Passive Agglutination Test (for Antibody Detection)

As agglutination test is more sensitive and better interpreted than precipitation test, hence attempt has been made to convert a precipitation reaction into an agglutination reaction. This is possible by coating the soluble antigen on the surface of a carrier molecule (e.g., red blood cells, latex or bentonite), so that the antibody binds to the coated antigen and agglutination takes place on the surface of the carrier molecule.
- **Indirect hemagglutination test (IHA):** It is a passive agglutination test where RBCs are used as carrier molecules. IHA was used widely in the past, but is less popular at present
- **Latex agglutination test (LAT) for antibody detection:** Here, latex particles are used as carrier molecules which are capable of adsorbing several types of antigens. It is used for detection of antistreptolysin O antibody (ASO) titer (Refer the Problem Solving Exercise 4).

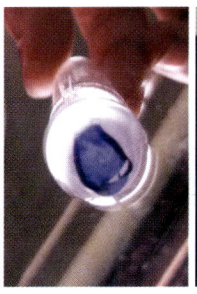 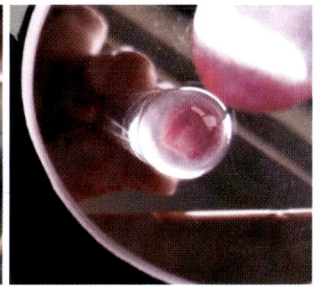

Fig. 7.6: O and H agglutination in Widal test (reading taken in a mirror).
Source: Department of Microbiology, Pondicherry Institute of Medical Sciences (*with permission*).

Problem Solving Exercise 4

Latex Agglutination Test for Antistreptolysin O (ASO) Antibody

A young child with history of recurrent sore throat was admitted to the hospital. His serum was sent to the laboratory and the test was performed. The test result is displayed in the Fig. 7.7.
1. Identify the test and interpret the result?
2. What is the principle of the test?
3. What is the nature of the antigen used in the test (Fig. 7.7)?

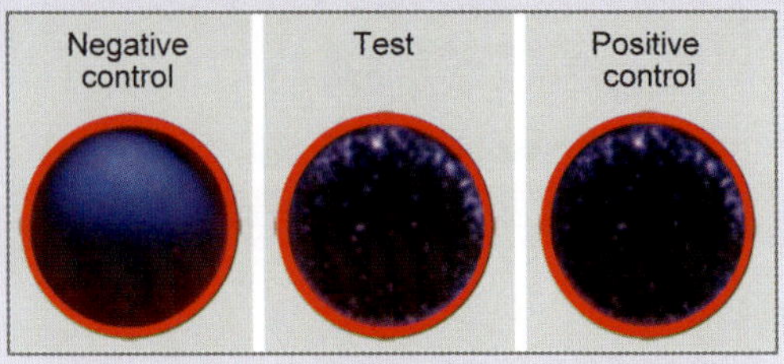

Fig. 7.7: ASO test by latex agglutination.
Source: Department of Microbiology, JIPMER, Puducherry (with permission).

Explanation

History of recurrent sore throat in a child raises the suspicion of streptococcal pharyngitis. The test shown here is a latex agglutination test, done for detection of ASO.

Principle

Here, polystyrene latex particles are used as carrier molecules which are capable of adsorbing several types of antigens. For better interpretation of result, the test is performed on a black color card.
- Drop of patient's serum (containing ASO antibody) is added to a drop of latex solution coated with the antigen and the card is rocked.
- **Positive result** appears as formation of visible clumps; is indicative of presence of ASO antibody.
- **Negative result** remains as milky-white suspension with no clumps; is indicative of absence of ASO antibody.
- **Quantitative test:** Once the test is positive, the test is repeated with serial dilution of serum. Highest dilution showing a positive result is indicative of titer of the test. ASO titer of >200 IU/mL is considered as the significant titre.
- Latex agglutination test is widely used as its simple and rapid test.

Reverse Passive Agglutination Test (for Antigen Detection)

In this test, the antibody is coated on a carrier molecule which detects antigen in patient's serum.
- **Reverse passive hemagglutination assay (RPHA):** Here, the RBCs are used as carrier molecules. RPHA was used in the past for detection of hepatitis B surface antigen (HBsAg); now obsolete
- **Latex agglutination test for antigen detection:** It is used widely for detection of CRP (C-reactive protein), RA (rheumatoid arthritis factor), capsular antigen detection in CSF (for pneumococcus, meningococcus and *Cryptococcus*) and streptococcal grouping
- **Coagglutination test:** Here, *Staphylococcus aureus* (protein A) acts as carrier molecule. This test was used in the past to detect antigen from clinical specimens now obsolete.

CHAPTER 8

ELISA, ELFA and Immunofluorescence

NEWER TECHNIQUES

The newer techniques use a detector molecule to label antibody or antigen which in turn detects the corresponding antigen or the antibody in the sample by producing a visible effect. Most of the newer techniques use this common principle, but they differ from each other by the type of labeled molecule used and the type of visible effect produced (Table 8.1).

Problem Solving Exercise

ELISA Test

A screening test for hepatitis B was performed on a group of hemophiliac patients attending outpatient department. The test done is demonstrated below.
1. Identify the test and interpret the result.
2. Name various types and their principles available for the test given below.
3. What are the advantages and disadvantages of this test format?
4. What are the applications of this test format (Fig. 8.1)?

Explanation

The test done here is ELISA for detection of hepatitis B surface antigen (HBsAg).

Interpretation

Sample 2, 4 and 5 are tested positive. Sample number 1, 3 and 6 are tested negative.

Answers to all other questions are explained below.

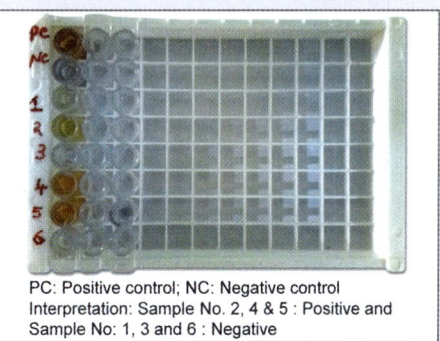

PC: Positive control; NC: Negative control
Interpretation: Sample No. 2, 4 & 5 : Positive and Sample No: 1, 3 and 6 : Negative

Fig. 8.1: ELISA for HBsAg.
Source: Department of Microbiology, Pondicherry Institute of Medical Sciences, Puducherry (*with permission*).

Table 8.1: Immunoassays and the types of molecules used for labeling.

Abbreviation	Immunoassay method	Molecules used for labeling	Type of visible effect
ELISA	Enzyme-linked immunosorbent assay	Enzyme-substrate-chromogen complex	Color change is detected by spectrophotometer
ELFA	Enzyme-linked fluorescent assay	Enzyme-substrate	Fluorometric detection
IFA	Immunofluorescence assay	Fluorescent dye	Emits light, detected by fluorescence microscope
CLIA	Chemiluminescence-linked immunoassay	Chemiluminescent compounds	Emits light, detected by luminometer
WB	Western blot	Enzyme	Color band (naked eye)
Rapid tests	Immunochromatographic test	Colloidal gold or silver	Color band (naked eye)
	Flow-through assay	Protein A conjugate	Color band (naked eye)

ELISA

Enzyme-linked immunosorbent assay (ELISA) is an immunoassay that detects either antigen or antibodies in the specimen, by using enzyme–substrate–chromogen system for detection.

Principle of ELISA

ELISA is so named because of its two components:
- **Immunosorbent:** Here, an absorbing material is used (e.g., polystyrene, polyvinyl) that specifically absorbs the antigen or antibody present in serum
- **Enzyme** is used to label one of the components of immunoassay (i.e., antigen or antibody).

Substrate-chromogen system: A substrate-chromogen system is added at the final step of ELISA.
- The enzyme reacts with the substrate, which in turn activates the chromogen to produce a color
- The classical example is, horseradish peroxidase used as enzyme which reacts with its substrate (hydrogen peroxide), that in turn activates the chromogen (tetramethyl benzidine) to produce a color
- The color change is detected by spectrophotometry in an ELISA reader. Intensity of the color is directly proportional to the amount of the detection molecule (Ag or Ab) present in test serum.

(Ag-Ab complex)-enzyme + substrate → activates the chromogen → color change → detected by spectrophotometry (ELISA reader, Fig. 8.2A)

Procedure of ELISA

ELISA is performed on a microtiter plate containing 96 wells (Fig. 8.1), made up of polystyrene, polyvinyl or polycarbonate material.

- ELISA kits are commercially available; contain all necessary reagents (such as enzyme conjugate, dilution buffer, substrate/chromogen, etc.)
- The procedure involves a series of steps done sequentially. At each step, a reagent is being added, and then incubated, followed by washing of the wells [manually or by an automated ELISA washer (Fig. 8.2B)].

Types of ELISA

There are several types of ELISA, which differ from each other in their principles.

Direct ELISA

It is used for detection of antigen in test serum. Here, the primary antibody (targeted against the serum antigen) is labeled with the enzyme.

Well + Ag (test serum) + primary Ab-enzyme + substrate-chromogen → color change (Fig. 8.3A)

Indirect ELISA

It is used for detection of antibody or less commonly antigen in serum. It differs from the direct ELISA in that the secondary antibody is labeled with enzyme instead of primary antibody. The secondary antibody is an anti-species antibody, e.g., anti-human Ig (an antibody targeted to Fc region of any human Ig). Indirect ELISA for antibody detection is described below (Fig. 8.3B).
- **Step 1:** The solid phase of the wells of microtiter plates are precoated with the Ag
- **Step 2:** Test serum (containing primary Ab specific to the Ag) is added to the wells. Ab gets attached to the Ag coated on the well

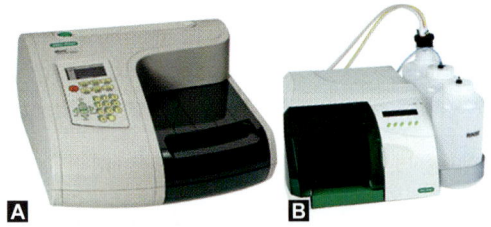

Figs 8.2A and B: (A) ELISA reader (Biorad); (B) ELISA washer.
Source: Biorad Pvt. Ltd (with permission).

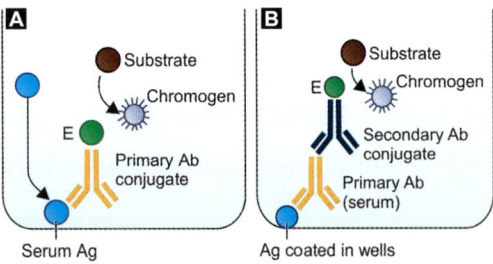

Figs 8.3A and B: (A) Direct ELISA (for antigen detection); (B) Indirect ELISA (for antibody detection).

- **Step 3:** After washing, enzyme-labeled secondary Ab (anti-human immunoglobulin) is added
- **Step 4:** After washing, a substrate-chromogen system is added and color is developed.

Wells are coated with Ag + primary Ab (test serum) + secondary Ab-enzyme + substrate-chromogen → development of color (Fig. 8.3B)

Sandwich ELISA

It detects the antigen in test serum. It is so named because the antigen gets sandwiched between a capture antibody and a detector antibody (Fig. 8.4A).
- **Step 1:** The microtiter well is precoated with the capture antibody (monoclonal Ab raised in rabbit) targeted against the test antigen
- **Step 2:** The test serum (containing antigen) is added to the wells. Ag gets attached to the capture antibody coated on the well
- **Step 3:** After washing, an enzyme labeled primary 'detector antibody' specific for the antigen is added. The detector antibody can be same as the capture antibody
- **Step 4:** After washing, a substrate–chromogen system is added and color is developed.

Wells coated with capture Ab + Ag (test serum) + primary Ab-enzyme + substrate-chromogen → color (Fig. 8.4A)

IgM Antibody Capture (MAC) ELISA

This is an enzymatically amplified sandwich-type immunoassay. This format of ELISA is widely used for dengue, Japanese encephalitis and West Nile virus, scrub typhus, leptospirosis, toxoplasmosis, etc. (Fig. 8.4B).
- It is based on capturing primary IgM Ab (in test serum) on a microtiter plate pre-coated with anti-human-IgM Ab, followed by addition of recombinant antigen (e.g., dengue antigen)
- Subsequently, enzyme labelled secondary antibody specific for the antigen is added, followed by addition of substrate-chromogen system
- The use of avidin-biotin system helps in amplifying the signal generated between enzyme-antibody complex, thus increases the sensitivity of the assay.

Wells coated with capture anti-IgM Ab + IgM Ab (test serum) + recombinant antigen + secondary Ab-biotin + avidin-enzyme + substrate-chromogen → color (Fig. 8.4B)

Competitive ELISA

Competitive ELISA is so named because, antigen in test serum competes with another antigen of the same type coated on well to bind to the primary antibody.
- **Step 1:** Primary antibody is first incubated in a solution with a serum sample containing the test antigen
- **Step 2:** This antigen–antibody mixture is then added to the microtiter well precoated with the same type of antigen
- **Step 3:** The free antibodies bind to the antigen coated on the well. More the test antigens present in the sample, lesser free antibodies will be available to bind to the antigens coated onto well
- **Step 4:** After washing (to remove free antibodies and antigens), enzyme-conjugated secondary antibody is added
- **Step 5:** After washing, a substrate–chromogen system is added and color is developed. Intensity of the color is inversely proportional to the amount of antigen present in the test serum (Fig. 8.5).

The competitive ELISA can also be used for the detection of antibody in serum. More so, different formats of competitive ELISA are available, such as direct, indirect and sandwich formats. The example given above is an indirect

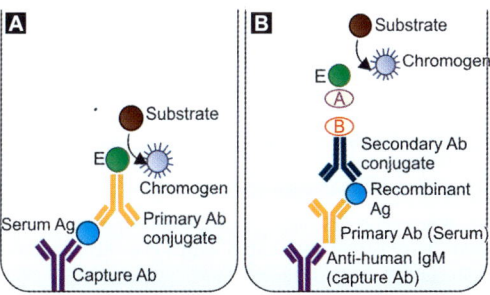

Figs 8.4A and B: (A) Sandwich ELISA (for antigen detection); (B) IgM antibody capture (MAC) ELISA.

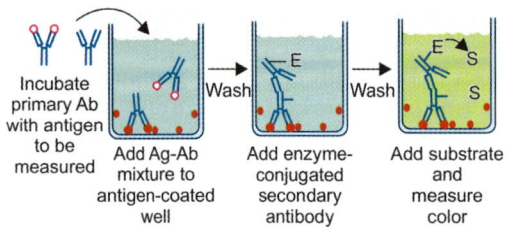

Fig. 8.5: Competitive ELISA for antigen detection.

competitive ELISA format used for antigen detection (Fig. 8.5).

Advantages of ELISA

ELISA is the method of choice for detection of antigens/antibodies in serum in modern days, especially in big laboratories as large number of samples can be tested together using the 96 well microtiter plate.
- It is economical, takes 2–3 hours for performing the assay
- ELISA has a high sensitivity; that is why, it is commonly used for performing screening test at blood banks and tertiary care sites
- Its specificity used to be low. But now, with use of more purified recombinant and synthetic antigens, and monoclonal antibodies, ELISA has become more specific.

Disadvantages of ELISA

- In small laboratories having less sample load, ELISA is less preferred than rapid tests as the latter can be performed on individual samples
- It takes more time (2–3 hours) compared to rapid tests which take 10–20 minutes
- It needs expensive equipment, such as ELISA washer and reader.

Applications of ELISA

ELISA can be used both for antigen and antibody detection.
- ELISA used for antigen detection: Hepatitis B [hepatitis B surface antigen (HBsAg) and precore antigen (HBeAg)], NS1 antigen for dengue, etc.
- ELISA can also be used for antibody detection against hepatitis B, hepatitis C, HIV, dengue, EBV, HSV, toxoplasmosis, leishmaniasis, etc.

ENZYME-LINKED FLUORESCENT ASSAY (ELFA)

ELFA is a modification of ELISA, differs from ELISA in two ways: (i) automated system, all steps are performed by the instrument itself, (ii) Ag-Ab-enzyme complex is detected by fluorometric method. VIDAS and miniVIDAS (bioMérieux) are commercially available systems based on ELFA technology (Fig. 8.6).

- **Procedure:** The solid phase receptacle (Fig. 8.6) present in reagent strip (equivalent to wells in microtiter plate in ELISA) serves as the solid phase; which is either coated with capture antigen (for antibody detection) or antibody (for antigen detection). Alkaline phosphatase is used as an enzyme and and the substrate used is a fluorescent molecule (4-methyl-umbelliferyl phosphate)
- **Advantages:** It has many advantages over ELISA: (i) an automated system, (ii) easy to perform and user friendly, (iii) less contamination chance, (iv) gives quantitative results and (v) more sensitive and specific
- **Disadvantages:** (i) Expensive, (ii) can run only 12–24 number of tests at a time (VIDAS), (iii) can run 2–4 types of tests at a time (mini-VIDAS)
- **Use:** It can be used to detect numerous parameters
    - *Infectious diseases:* Markers of hepatitis viruses and HIV (Ag and Ab), antibody to TORCH infection, measles, mumps, varicella, *H. pylori* and antigen to *C. difficile*, rotavirus, etc.
    - *Other uses:* Biomarkers (e.g., procalcitonin), hormones (e.g., thyroid), tumor

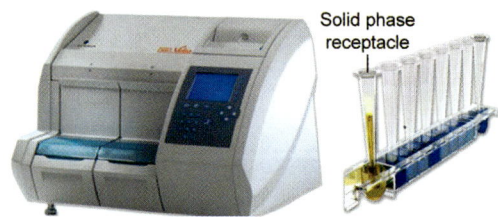

Fig. 8.6: miniVIDAS system and reagent strip (first well is solid phase receptacle coated with Ag or Ab and other wells contain various reagents).

Source: Department of Microbiology, JIPMER, Puducherry (*with permission*).

markers, cardiac markers and screening for allergy.

IMMUNOFLUORESCENCE ASSAY (IFA)

It is a technique similar to ELISA, but differs by some important features:
- Fluorescent dye is used instead of enzyme for labeling of antibody
- It detects cell surface antigens. It is also used to detect antibodies bound to cell surface antigens, unlike ELISA which detects free antigen or antibody.

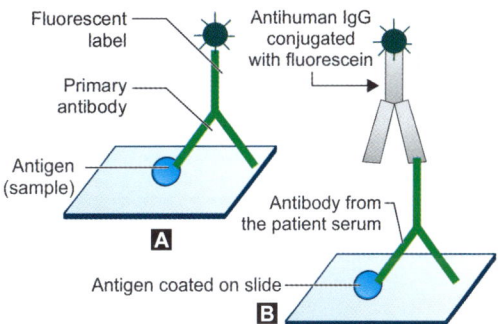

Figs 8.7A and B: Immunofluorescence assay: (A) Direct; (B) Indirect.

Principle

Fluorescence refers to absorbing high energy-shorter wavelength ultraviolet light rays by the fluorescent compounds and in turn emitting visible light rays with a low energy-longer wavelength.
- The fluorescent dye is used to conjugate the antibody and such labeled antibody can be used to detect the antigens or antigen–antibody complexes on the cell surface
- The fluorescent compounds commonly used is fluorescein isothiocyanate (FITC).

Types

Direct Immunofluorescence Assay
- **Step 1:** Sample containing cells carrying surface antigens is smeared on a slide
- **Step 2:** Primary antibody specific to the antigen, tagged with fluorescent dye is added
- **Step 3:** Slide is washed to remove the unbound antibodies and then viewed under a fluorescence microscope (Fig. 8.7A).

Indirect Immunofluorescence Assay
This detects antibodies in sample. Slides smeared with cells carrying known antigens are commercially available.
- **Step 1:** Test serum containing primary antibody is added to the slide

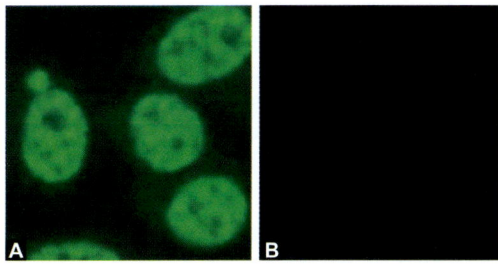

Figs 8.8A and B: Immunofluorescence assay for detection of antinuclear antibodies: (A) Positive result; (B) Negative result.
Source: EUROIMMUN AG Pvt Ltd. (with permission).

- **Step 2:** Slide is washed to remove the unbound antibodies. A secondary antibody (antihuman antibody conjugated with fluorescent dye) is added
- **Step 3:** Slide is washed and then viewed under a fluorescence microscope (Fig. 8.7B).

Applications: Immunofluorescence assay has various applications, such as:
- Detection of autoantibodies (e.g., antinuclear antibody) in autoimmune diseases (Figs 8.8A and B)
- Detecting microbial antigens, e.g., rabies antigen in corneal smear
- Detection of viral antigens in cell lines inoculated with the specimens.

CHAPTER 9

Western Blot, Rapid Tests and CLIA

■ WESTERN BLOT

Western blot detects specific proteins (antibodies) in a sample containing mixture of antibodies each targeted against different antigens of same microbe.
- ❖ It is so named for its similarity to Southern blot (detects DNA fragments) and Northern blot (detects mRNAs)

- ❖ The *Eastern blot* is the latest addition to the list; it is a modification of Western blot, which detects the carbohydrate epitopes present on proteins or lipids.

Procedure

Western blot comprises of three basic components as follows (Fig. 9.2):

Problem Solving Exercise 1

Western Blot

A commercial sex worker is presented with diarrhea for 1 month. Screening test [enzyme-linked immunosorbent assay (ELISA)] performed for human immunodeficiency virus (HIV) showed inconclusive (equivocal) result. For confirmation, the following test given below was performed.
1. Identify the test and interpret the result.
2. What is the principle of the test?
3. What are the other applications of the test (Fig. 9.1)?

Explanation

The test given in the picture is Western blot, done for detection of HIV antibodies.
  For HIV diagnosis, if the screening test (ELISA/rapid diagnostic test) shows inconclusive (equivocal) result, then it has to be confirmed by supplemental test.

Interpretation

Bands are positive for three antibodies against HIV antigens gp120, gp41, p24 and p55/51.

Final Report

Reactive for HIV-1 antibodies.
  Answers to the other questions are explained below.

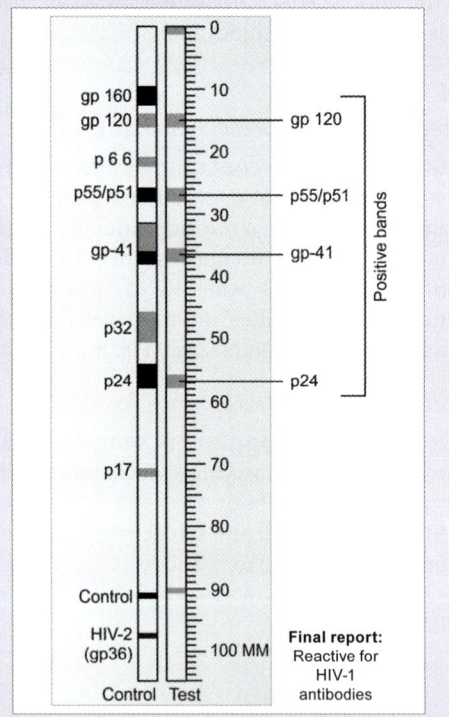

Fig. 9.1: Western blot for HIV.

2. Nitrocellulose Membrane Blotting

The gel is removed from the electrophoresis apparatus and placed over a protein-binding sheet, such as nitrocellulose or nylon and the antigen fragments in the gel are transferred (blotted) to the nitrocellulose membrane (NCM) sheet by the passage of an electric current.

3. Enzyme Immunoassay (to Detect the Antibodies)

- ❖ Nitrocellulose membrane strips containing protein antigen fragments are treated with patient's sample containing antibodies. Individual serum antibodies would bind to the respective antigen fragments, thus making Western blot highly specific
- ❖ Addition of enzyme-linked anti-human immunoglobulin (Ig), detects the individual serum antibodies bound to antigen fragments. Substrate/chromogen is added for development of colored bands.

Applications

Western blot has an excellent specificity. Hence, it is often used as a supplementary test to confirm the result of ELISA or other immunoassays having higher sensitivity. Western blot formats are available to detect antibody (Ab) in various diseases, such as human immunodeficiency virus (HIV) infection (discussed in Chapter 19), Lyme's disease, herpes simplex virus infection, cysticercosis, hydatid disease and toxoplasmosis.

■ RAPID TEST

Rapid tests are revolutionary in the diagnosis of infectious diseases.
- ❖ They are very simple to perform, rapid (result obtained in 10–20 minutes), require minimal training, and do not need any sophisticated instruments
- ❖ These tests are also called *point-of-care* (POC) tests, because unlike ELISA and other immunoassays, the POC tests can be performed independent of laboratory equipment and deliver instant results
- ❖ Two principles of rapid tests are available—lateral-flow assay and flow-through assay

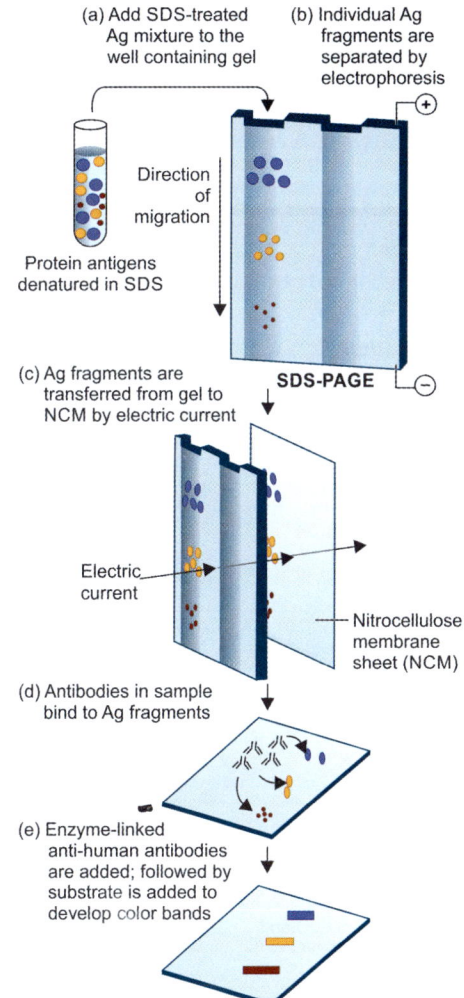

Fig. 9.2: Western blot (principle).
Abbreviations: SDS-PAGE, sodium dodecyl sulfate polyacrylamide gel electrophoresis; Ag, antigen.

1. Separation of Complex Protein Antigen Mixture by SDS PAGE

- ❖ **SDS:** The complex protein (antigen) mixture is treated with a strong denaturing detergent called SDS (sodium dodecyl sulfate)
- ❖ **PAGE:** Then the mixture is subjected to polyacrylamide gel electrophoresis (PAGE) which separates the antigenic components according to their molecular weight; lower molecular weight components migrate farther than higher molecular weight ones.

❖ Both the formats are available for the diagnosis of various diseases, such as malaria, viral hepatitis by hepatitis B and hepatitis C virus, HIV infection, leptospirosis, *Helicobacter pylori* infection, syphilis, etc.

Immunochromatographic Test (Lateral-flow Assay)

Problem Solving Exercise 2

Immunochromatographic Test
The following test was performed for a patient suffering from jaundice for 2 months for the diagnosis of hepatitis B virus infection.
1. Identify the test and interpret the result.
2. What is the principle of the test?
3. What are the other applications of the test (Fig. 9.3)?

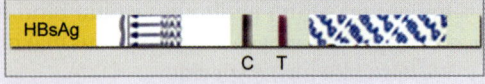

Fig. 9.3: ICT for HBsAg.

Explanation
The test performed here is immunochromatographic test.

Interpretation
The positive bands are formed at test line [hepatitis B surface antigen (HBsAg)] as well as control line.

Report
Positive for HBsAg.
Answers to the other questions are explained below.

Immunochromatographic test (ICT) is based on lateral-flow technique. It is widely used in diagnostic laboratories because of its simplicity, economy and rapidity. It can be used for both antigen and antibody detection in sample. Principle of antigen detection method is described below.

Principle (Antigen Detection)

The test system consists of NCM and an absorbent pad. Two formats are available—cassette or strip (Figs 9.4A and B). The NCM is coated at two places in the form of lines—a test line, coated with monoclonal Ab targeted against the test antigen, and a control line, coated with anti-human Ig. Specific Ab against the target Ag labeled with chromogenic marker (specific Ab tagged with *colloidal gold or silver*, a visually detectable marker) is infiltrated in the sample pad lining the sample window.

❖ The sample (serum) containing the test antigen is added to sample well, it reacts with Ab labeled with chromogenic marker (*colloidal gold* or *silver*, a visually detectable marker)
❖ Both "Ag-specific Ab-colloidal gold complex" as well as the "free colloidal gold-labeled Ab" in buffer moves *laterally* along the NCM
❖ **Test band:** At the test line, the Ag-labeled Ab complex is immobilized by binding to

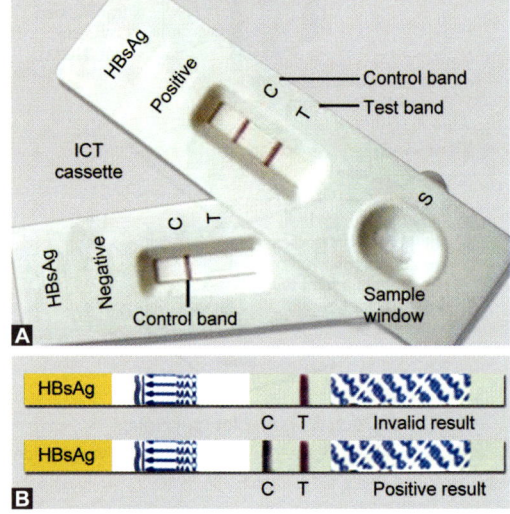

Figs 9.4A and B: Immunochromatographic test (ICT) for hepatitis B surface antigen (HBsAg) detection. (A) Cassette format; (B) Strip format.
Abbreviation: HBsAg, hepatitis B surface antigen.
Source: Department of Microbiology, Pondicherry Institute of Medical sciences, Puducherry (*with permission*).

the monoclonal Ab in the test line to form a colored band (Figs 9.4A and B)
❖ **Control band:** The free colloidal gold-labeled Ab can move further and binds to the anti-human Ig to form a colored control band. If the control band is not formed, then the test is considered invalid irrespective of whether the test band is formed or not (Figs 9.4A and B).

Flow-through Assay

Flow-through tests are another type of rapid diagnostic assays which differ from ICT in two aspects—(1) protein A is used for labeling Ab instead of gold conjugate, and (2) the sample flows *vertically* through the NCM as compared to lateral flow in ICT.

Flow-through tests can be used for both antigen and Ab detection. HIV TRI-DOT test is a classical example (described below, Fig. 9.5A). It detects antibodies to HIV-1 and 2 separately in patient's serum.

* The test system is in a cassette format, consisting of NCM and an absorbent pad. The NCM is coated at three regions—two test regions coated with HIV-1 and 2 antigens and the third control region coated with anti-human Ig
* Sample and buffer reagents are added sequentially from the top following which they pass through the membrane and excess fluid is absorbed into the underlying absorbent pad
* As the patient's sample passes through the membrane, HIV antibodies, if present, bind to the immobilized antigens (Fig. 9.5B)
* **Test dots:** Protein A conjugate (present in buffer) binds to the Fc portion of the HIV antibodies to give distinct pinkish purple DOT(s), separately for HIV-1 and 2 antibodies
* **Control dot:** Irrespective of whether the HIV antibodies are present or not, protein A can bind to any IgG present in serum and the IgG-protein A complex can further bind to the anti-human Ig at the control dot to give a pinkish purple DOT.

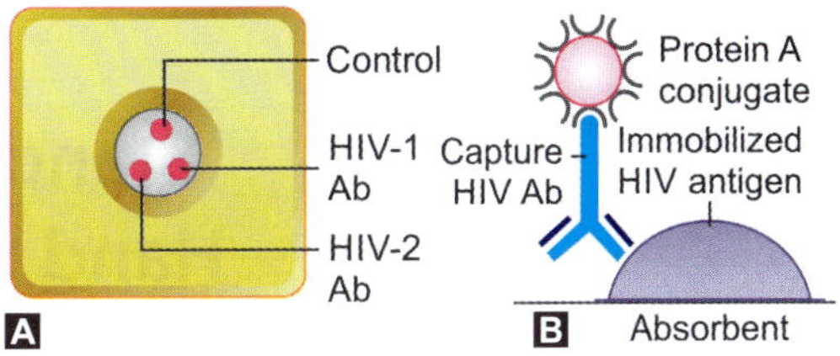

Figs 9.5A and B: Flow-through assays: (A) HIV TRI-DOT assay for HIV 1 and 2 antibodies detection; (B) Principle.
Source: Department of Microbiology, Pondicherry Institute of Medical sciences, Puducherry (*with permission*).

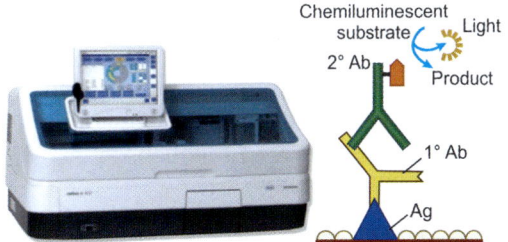

Fig. 9.6: Chemiluminescence system (CLIA) and its principle.
Source: Department of Microbiology, JIPMER, Puducherry (*with permission*).

CHEMILUMINESCENCE-LINKED IMMUNOASSAY (CLIA)

Chemiluminescence refers to the emission of light (luminescence), as a result of a chemical reaction. The principle of CLIA is similar to that of ELISA; however, the chromogenic substance is replaced by chemiluminescent compounds (e.g., luminol and acridinium ester) that generate light during a chemical reaction (luxogenic). The light (photons) can be detected by a photomultiplier, also called as luminometer (Fig. 9.6).

(Ag-Ab complex)-enzyme (e.g., HRP) + chemiluminescent substrate (e.g., luminol and acridinium ester) →

Contd...

product + light (photons) → detected by luminometer or photomultiplier.

Advantages of CLIA

CLIA claims to be 10 times more sensitive than ELISA.
* CLIA can be further modified by using an enhancer that potentiates the chemical reaction. This gives CLIA an overall improvement of 200 folds over ELISA
* Most samples have no 'background' signal, i.e., luminol compounds do not themselves emit light
* Measurement of chemiluminescence is not a ratio unlike the measurement of fluorescence (IFA) and or color (ELISA)
* Individual specimens can be tested in CLIA in contrast to ELISA which is preferred for testing multiple samples at a time.

Applications

Currently, CLIA is available for detection of antigens or antibodies against various infections, such as hepatitis viruses, HIV, TORCH infections (common congenital infection causing agents) and biomarkers, such as procalcitonin.

CHAPTER 10

Standard Precautions: Hand Hygiene and PPE

Healthcare-associated infections (HAIs) refer to (i) the infections acquired in the hospital by a patient admitted for a reason other than the infection in context, (ii) the infection should not be present or incubating at the time of admission, and (iii) the symptoms should appear at least after 48 hours of admission.

PREVENTION OF HAIs

The preventive measures for HAIs can be broadly categorized into (i) standard precautions and (ii) transmission-based or specific precautions (discussed in Chapter 11).

STANDARD PRECAUTIONS

Standard precautions are a set of infection control practices (see highlight box below) used to prevent transmission of diseases that can be acquired by contact with blood, body fluids, non-intact skin (including rashes), and mucous membranes. These measures should be followed when providing care to or handling:
- ❖ All individuals, whether they appear infectious/symptomatic or not
- ❖ All specimens (blood or body fluids) whether they appear infectious or not
- ❖ All needles and sharps whether they appear infectious or not.

Note: **Universal precautions** was a term used in the past to refer to the infection control practices to avoid contact with patients' body fluids, by means of wearing the nonporous articles, such as medical gloves, goggles, and face shields. Now it is replaced by the word "**standard precaution**" which in addition includes contact with all body fluids regardless of whether blood is present.

Standard Precautions
They are indicated while handling all patients, specimens and sharps. Components of standard precautions include:
- ❏ **Hand hygiene** (details explained later):
  - ➢ Wash hands promptly after contact with infective material
  - ➢ Use no touch technique wherever possible.
- ❏ **Personal protective equipment (PPE):** Described later
- ❏ **Biomedical waste:** All biomedical waste including sharp should be segregated and disposed appropriately (Refer Chapter 13)
- ❏ **Spillage cleaning:** Clean up spills of infective material promptly
- ❏ **Disinfection of patient care items:** Ensure that all patient-care items, such as instruments, devices and linens are disinfected before reuse
- ❏ **Environmental cleaning** of surface and floor (Refer Chapter 12)
- ❏ **Sharp:** Safe use and disposal of sharp (Refer Chapters 13 and 14)
- ❏ **Respiratory hygiene and cough etiquette** (Refer Chapter 11).

Hand Hygiene

Hands of the HCWs are the main source of transmission of infections in healthcare facilities. Hand hygiene is therefore the most important measure to avoid the transmission of harmful microbes and prevent healthcare-associated infections.

Types of Hand Hygiene Methods

Hand Rub

Alcohol based (70–80% ethyl alcohol) and chlorhexidine (0.5–4%) based hand rubs are available. The duration of contact has to be at least for 20–30 seconds (10.2).
- ❖ **Advantage:** After a period of contact, it gets evaporated of its own, hence drying of hands is not required separately

CHAPTER 10 ◆ Standard Precautions: Hand Hygiene and PPE

Problem Solving Exercise 1

Hand Hygiene
A nurse in an ICU records the pulse of a patient, records it in the case sheet and then goes back to nursing station. Then she draws blood of another patient. While transporting the specimen, a drop of blood fell on her palm. Then she enters the operation theater to assist for a surgery.
1. How many times she has to perform hand hygiene?
2. What are the hand hygiene methods she has to perform and for how much duration?
3. What are the hand hygiene products to be used?

Explanation
Nurse has to perform totally seven times hand hygiene: Five times hand rub, once hand wash and hand scrub each (Figs 10.1 to 10.3).

Hand rub: Nurse has to perform hand rub five times, 20–30 seconds in each time with 70–80% alcohol hand rub.
- Before recording pulse (WHO Moment 1)
- After recording pulse (WHO Moment 4)
- Before drawing blood (WHO Moment 2)
- After drawing blood (WHO Moment 3)
- After recording in the case sheet (WHO Moment 5).

Handwash: She has to perform handwash once (after blood drop fell on her palm), with 2–4% chlorhexidine hand wash for 40–60 seconds.

Hand scrub: She has to perform hand scrub once (before assisting for surgery), with 4% chlorhexidine hand wash for 3–5 minutes.
(Refer the text below for further details.)

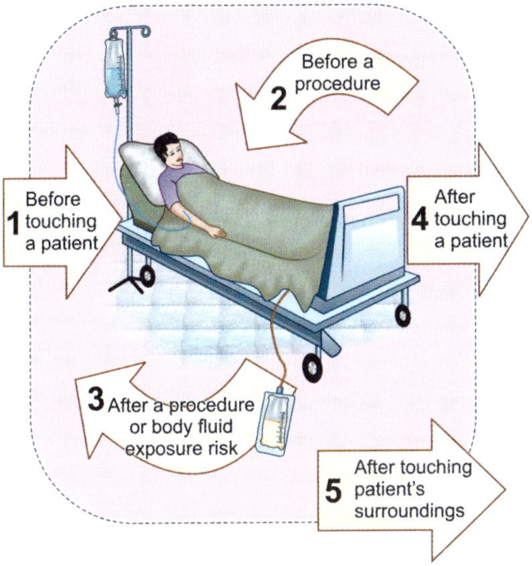

Fig. 10.1: My five moments for hand hygiene.
Source: World Health Organization (WHO) (with permission).

- **Indications:** Hand rub is indicated during routine patient care activities or taking rounds in the wards or ICUs—whenever opportunity for hand hygiene arises, except when the hands are visibly soiled with blood or other specimens.

Handwash
Antimicrobial soaps (liquid, gel or bars) are available containing 4% chlorhexidine. If facilities are not available, then even ordinary soap and water can also be used. The duration of contact has to be at least for 40–60 seconds (10.2). Handwashing is indicated in the following situations:
- When the hands are visibly soiled with blood, excreta, pus, etc.
- Before and after eating
- After going to toilet
- Before and after shift of the duty
- When giving care to a patient with diarrhea.

Surgical hand scrub (3–5 min): This is indicated prior to any surgical procedure and also in between the cases; using 4% chlorhexidine hand wash (Fig. 10.3).

My Five Moments for Hand Hygiene
Indications: The WHO has published standard guidelines describing the situations or opportunities when hand hygiene is indicated in healthcare sectors (Fig. 10.1)—known as 'My Five Moments for Hand Hygiene'; which include:
1. Before touching a patient
2. Before clean/aseptic procedures
3. After body fluid exposure/risk
4. After touching a patient
5. After touching patient's surroundings.

Steps of Hand Rubbing and Hand Washing
WHO has also laid down the guidelines describing the appropriate steps involved for an effective hand rubbing and hand washing (Fig. 10.2). The method of performing surgical hand scrub in depcited in Figure 10.3.

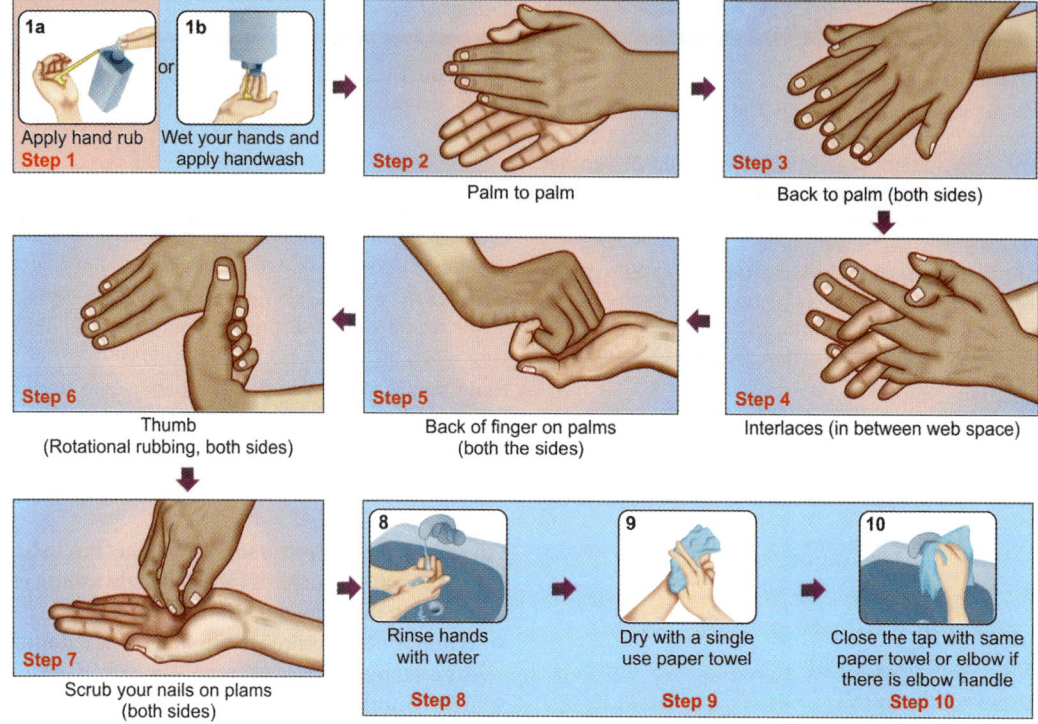

Fig. 10.2: Steps of hand rubbing and handwashing (WHO): Hand rub step 1 to 7 (20–30 seconds); Handwash step 1 to 10 (40–60 seconds).

Problem Solving Exercise 2

Personal Protective Equipment (PPE)

A 65-year-old patient was admitted to a hospital with complaints of dry cough, sore throat and fever. He was kept in an isolation room. His throat swab was sent for COVID-19 testing which came positive. A nurse is posted to give care to the patient.
1. What are the personal protective equipment (PPE), the nurse should wear while giving care to the patient?
2. Demonstrate the donning and doffing technique of each of the PPE.
3. What is the correct sequence of donning and doffing of PPE?
4. What are the precautions need to be followed while doffing of the PPE?

Explanation

PPE: The PPE needed for giving care to the COVID-19 patient are a pair of gloves, 3-ply mask, gown and goggles/face shield. If aerosol generating procedure are to be performed, N95 respirator need to be worn in place of 3-ply mask.

Technique and the correct sequence of donning and doffing of each of the PPE is explained subsequently in the text.

Precautions: Doffing should be performed with utmost precautions as even a minor breach in the doffing procedure would subject the HCW to a huge risk of acquiring the infection.
- Do not touch the exposed/contaminated area of PPE, such as front part of the mask or goggles and outer surface of gloves or gown.
- All PPE need to be doffed in the designated doffing area of the isolation room except the mask, which need to be doffed after coming out of the isolation room.
- Discard PPE into appropriate BMW bins:
  - Yellow bag: Gown/coverall, mask/respirator, shoe cover and cap
  - Red bag: Plastic apron, goggles/face shield, gloves
- Perform hand hygiene after removal of PPE

CHAPTER 10 ◆ Standard Precautions: Hand Hygiene and PPE

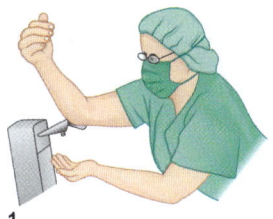

1
Put approximately 5 mL (3 doses) of alcohol-based handrub in the palm of your left hand, using the elbow of your other arm to operate the dispenser

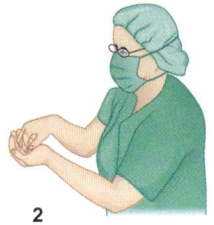

2
Dip the fingertips of your right hand in the handrub to decontaminate under the nails (5 seconds)

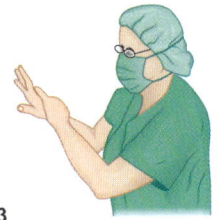

3
Images 3–7: Smear the handrub on the right forearm up to the elbow. Ensure that the whole skin area is covered by using circular movements around the forearm until the handrub has fully evaporated (10–15 seconds)

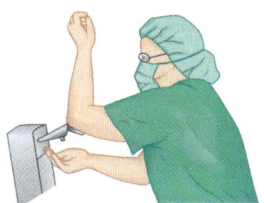

4
Put approximately 5 mL (3 doses) of alcohol-based handrub in the palm of your right hand, using the elbow of your other arm to operate the dispenser

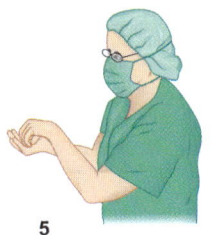

5
Dip the fingertips of your left hand in the handrub to decontaminate under the nails (5 seconds)

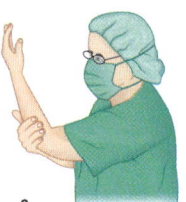

6
Smear the handrub on the left forearm up to the elbow. Ensure that the whole skin area is covered by using circular movements around the forearm until the handrub has fully evaporated (10–15 seconds)

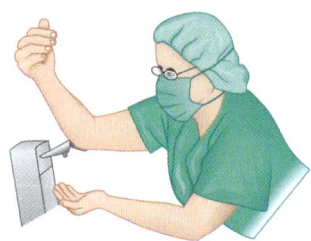

7
Put approximately 5 mL (3 doses) of alcohol-based handrub in the palm of your left hand, using the elbow of your other arm to operate the dispenser. Rub both hands at the same time up to the wrists, and ensure that all the steps represented in images 2–6 are followed (20–30 seconds)

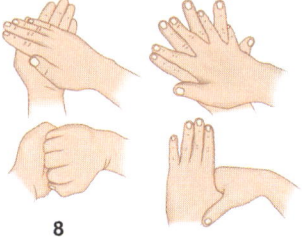

8
Perform hand rub steps as described in Fig. 10.2

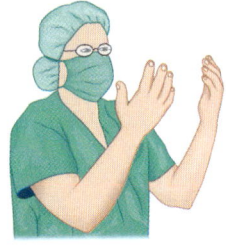

9
When the hands are dry, sterile surgical clothing and gloves can be donned

Fig. 10.3: Method of performing surgical hand scrub.

Personal Protective Equipment (PPE)

Personal protective equipment are used to protect the skin and mucous membranes of HCWs from exposure to blood and/or body fluids and from the HCW to the patient during sterile and invasive procedures.

❖ The various PPE used in healthcare settings are gloves, mask/respirator, gown/plastic apron/coverall, goggles or face shield, shoe cover and head cover (Figs 10.4A to N)

❖ Selection of appropriate PPE is based on:
  ■ The level of risk associated with contamination of skin, mucous membranes, and clothing by blood and body fluids during a specific patient care activity or intervention (as a part of standard precaution)

Table 10.1: Indications for appropriate use of glove use.

Indications for glove use
• As a part of standard precautions 　➤ Before a sterile procedure 　➤ Anticipation of contact with blood or body fluid, regardless of the existence of sterile conditions and including contact with non-intact skin and mucous membrane • As a part of contact precautions: Contact with a patient (and his/her immediate surroundings) • Heavy duty gloves: To protect from sharp injuries, mainly used by biomedical waste handlers (Fig. 10.4B)
Indications for glove removal
• As soon as gloves are damaged • Gloves are meant for single-use, must be changed in-between patients or patient care activities • When there is an indication for hand hygiene
Clinical situations where use of gloves is not recommended
• For routine patient care activities if there is no anticipated risk to blood/body fluid or no indication for contact precautions • Examples: Measuring blood pressure, temperature, and pulse, while administering medications (oral or injections), during maintenance of IV cannula, during dressing and transporting patient, writing in the patient's case sheet, etc.

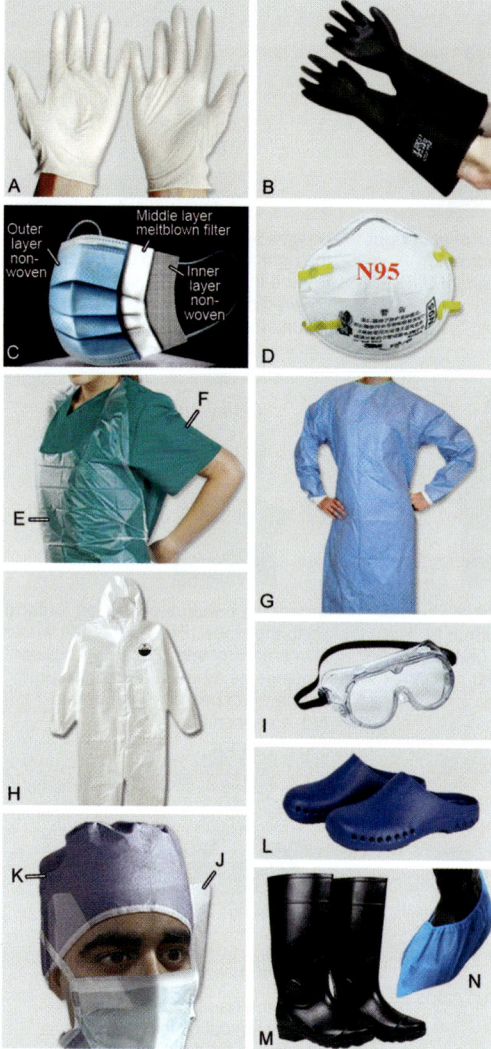

Figs 10.4A to N: Personal protective equipment (PPE): (A) Gloves; (B) Heavy duty gloves; (C) Surgical mask; (D) N95 respirator; (E) Plastic apron; (F) Linen gown; (G) Disposable gown; (H) Coverall; (I) Goggles; (J) Face shield; (K) Cap; (L) Shoes; (M) Gum boot; (N) Shoe cover.

colonized their hands. It is used as part of standard, contact and droplet precautions.

Gloves should be worn only when there is an indication (Table 10.1 and Fig. 10.4A). The use of gloves in situations when their use is not indicated represents a waste of resources and gives a false sense of security. Therefore, gloves should not be used when not clinically indicated (Table 10.1).

Hand Hygiene and Glove Use

Glove is not a substitute for hand hygiene. In no way does the glove use modify hand hygiene indications or replace hand hygiene. The following measures should be adapted during gloves use.

❖ **Hand hygiene before gloves use:** This is to prevent possible cross-contamination of gloves with HCW's flora
❖ **Handwash after glove use:** To prevent cross-contamination, perform hand wash immediately after the removal of gloves as it creates a moist, warm, and occlusive environment between the skin and the glove

- Route of transmission of suspected organisms—contact, droplet and inhalation (as a part of transmission-based precaution).
❖ The PPE must be removed immediately following the indication for which it was used.

Gloves

Gloves can protect both patients and HCWs from exposure to microorganisms that have

which is 'safe haven' for microorganisms. Furthermore, microtears can occur in gloves which may lead to transmission of organism if the HCW has had contact with blood or body fluid
- **Change:** Gloves should be worn for a single patient care activity and not beyond. Gloves must be changed between patient contacts and between separate procedures on the same patient
- **No hand hygiene over the gloved hand:** Gloved hands should neither be wiped with any form of handrub nor washed with soap and water.

The technique for donning and doffing of gloves has been depicted in Figures 10.5 and 10.6.

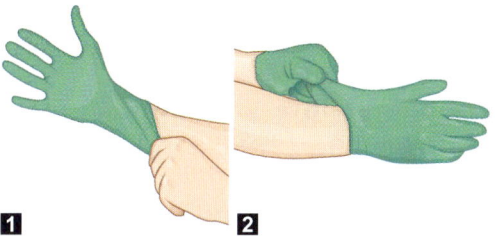

Fig. 10.5: Steps of gloves donning (wearing).
1. Donning of the first glove: Wear by touching and pulling only the edge of the cuff.
2. Donning of the second glove: Avoid touching the forearm skin by pulling external surface of second glove by the finger of gloved hand.

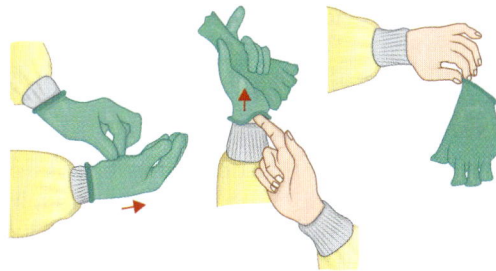

Fig. 10.6: Steps of gloves removal (doffing).
Do not touch the outside of the gloves (contaminated)
- Using a gloved hand, grasp the palm area of the other gloved hand peel off first glove.
- Hold removed glove in gloved hand slide fingers of ungloved hand under the other glove at wrist and peel off second glove over first glove.
- First glove will remain inside the pouch of the second glove.
- Perform hand hygiene after removal.

Surgical (3-ply) Mask and Respirators

Respiratory protection is essential when there is a risk of transmission of droplets and aerosols. There are two type of PPE available for respiratory protection; surgical mask and respirators.

Surgical Mask (3-ply Mask)

Surgical masks (also called as medical mask or 3-ply mask) are loose fitting, single-use item that cover the nose and mouth.
- They are used as part of standard precautions to prevent splashes or sprays from reaching the mouth and nose of the person wearing them
- They also provide some protection from respiratory secretions and are worn when caring for patients on droplet precautions.

Composition
It has three layers (Fig. 10.4C):
1. **Outer fluid repellent layer**: Hydrophobic layer that can repel water, blood and body fluids
2. **Middle filter layer:** It is made up of melt-blown material; filters bacteria/viruses and also filters out the water droplets. In contrast to N95 respirator, the filter pore size of a surgical mask is not standardized
3. **Inner hydrophilic layer**: Absorbs water, sweat and spit; made up of non-woven fabric.

Note: 2-ply masks may look similar to 3-ply mask in appearance. However, they have only two layers (outer and inner), but no middle filter layer. They should be used for hygienic and sanitation purposes—in restaurants, spa centers, food industry; but not in the hospitals.

Instructions
When using a surgical mask, the following measures should be considered:
- **Shelf-life:** Disposable (single-use); should be discarded or changed after 4-6 hours of use or earlier if it becomes soiled or wet
- **Donning:** Place the mask carefully, ensuring it covers the mouth and nose, adjust to the nose bridge, and tie it securely to minimize any gaps between the face and the mask
- **Hanging mask syndrome:** Masks should not be left dangling around the neck, a common practice observed among doctors, doing so may contaminate the inner side of mask

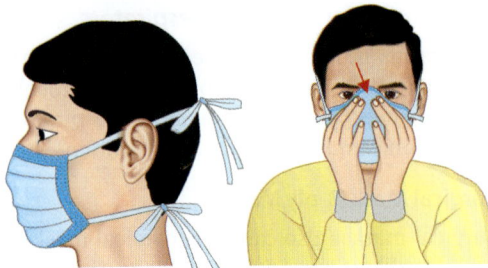

Fig. 10.7: Steps of mask donning (wearing).
- Pull the straps tight and pull the mask to below chin and then apply knots.
- Press on the nasal bridge part of the mask to seal tightly and for N95 respirator, perform fit check.

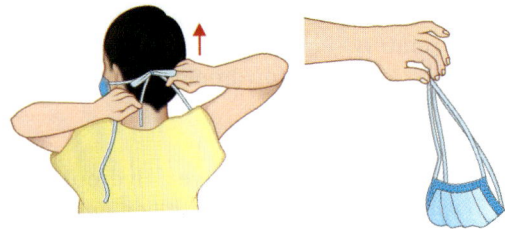

Fig. 10.8: Steps of mask removal (doffing).
- Do not touch front part of the mask.
- Untie the lower knot first, then the upper knot and remove the mask by holding its straps, without touching the front; handwash after removal.

❖ Touching the **front of the mask** while wearing should be avoided
❖ Mask should not be worn with beard or unshaven face
❖ Hand hygiene should be performed before donning the mask, upon touching or discarding a used mask.

The technique of donning and doffing of surgical mask has been depicted in Figures 10.7 and 10.8.

Respirator (N95 Respirator)

A respirator is a device designed to protect the wearer from airborne microorganisms (e.g., *M. tuberculosis*). There are many types of respirators. The most common respirator used in hospital settings is N95 respirator.
❖ N95 refers to 'not resistance to oil and ability to filter off 95% of airborne particles'
❖ **Composition:** The N95 respirator is comprised of four layers of material: an outer and inner layers of spun-bond polypropylene and middle two layers of cellulose/polyester, melt-blown polypropylene filter

❖ **Negative-pressure:** N95 respirators are described as "negative-pressure" because the pressure inside the facepiece is negative during inhalation compared to the pressure outside the respirator
❖ **Removal:** N95 respirator should be removed or changed once in 8 hours or earlier if it gets clogged, wet or dirty on the inside, or deformed, or torn
❖ **Single-use:** N95 respirator is for single-use only, should not be reused as it cannot be cleaned or disinfected
❖ **Fit checking:** After wearing the N95 respirator, the HCW must perform a fit check to ensure if it is properly fitted. No clinical activity should be undertaken until a satisfactory fit check has been achieved. It includes the following steps:
  ▪ **Sealing:** The respirator is compressed to ensure a seal across the face, cheeks and the nasal bridge
  ▪ **The positive pressure seal** of the respirator is checked by gently exhaling. If air escapes, the respirator needs to be adjusted
  ▪ **The negative pressure seal** of the respirator is checked by gently inhaling. If the respirator is not drawn in towards the face, or air leaks around the face seal, the respirator is readjusted.
❖ **Fit testing:** Fit testing is done to identify which size and style of N95 respirator is suitable for an individual and to train the HCW on how to don and doff N95 respirator. It should be done at the time of joining and thereafter annually.

Protective Body Clothing

Laboratory coats, plastic aprons, disposable gowns and coverall (full body cover) are examples of protective body wears used in hospitals. They are worn when there is a risk that clothing may become exposed to blood or body fluids
❖ **Laboratory coats:** They are used as a part of a standard precaution by all laboratory staff which protect their clothing and skin from the splash of blood or body fluid; however, they are not fluid resistant
❖ **Plastic aprons:** Worn when there is a low risk of contamination of blood/body fluid. They are fluid-resistant and for single-use only, i.e.,

used for one procedure or one patient care activity (Fig. 10.4E)
- ❖ **Disposable gowns:** They are long-sleeved, fluid resistant; indicated when there is a moderate risk of contamination with blood/body fluid (Fig. 10.4G)
- ❖ **Coverall:** It comprises of a gown with pant and hood, which covers the whole body including the head. Coverall should be used in the following situations
  - Anticipated risk of splashing with a **large volume** blood/body fluid (e.g., cardiac surgeries)
  - Anticipated risk of extensive skin to skin contact with a patient known to harbor organisms of contact transmission (e.g., lifting a patient with uncontrolled diarrhea)
  - Handling patients infected with pathogens of high mortality (e.g., Nipah or Ebola) or in the laboratory while handling their specimens (Fig. 10.4H).
- ❖ **Donning:** Gown should be fully covered, torso from neck to knees, arms to end of the wrist and then wrapped around the neck. It should be fastened in the back of neck and waist (Fig. 10.9)
- ❖ **Doffing:** Once the task is performed, the gown must be removed immediately after use by unfastening the gown ties taking care that sleeves should not contact the body while reaching for the ties (Fig. 10.10).

Protective Eye/Face Wear

Protective eyewear (goggles, or face-shields) are used to protect the mucous membranes of the eyes, nose, and mouth

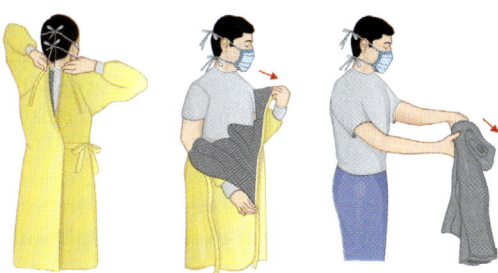

Fig. 10.10: Steps of gown removal (doffing).
Do not touch front part of the gown
- Unfasten gown ties, taking care that sleeves do not touch the body when reaching for ties.
- Pull the gown away from neck and shoulders, touching inside of gown only.
- Turn gown inside out and roll into a bundle and discard.
- Perform hand hygiene after removal.

- ❖ Prevents exposure to blood and/or body fluids that may be splashed, sprayed, or splattered into the face during clinical procedures
- ❖ Eyewear must be worn during procedures that are likely to generate droplets or aerosols of blood and/or high-risk body fluids (Figs 10.4I and J).

Head Cover and Shoe Cover

- ❖ **Head cover or cap** (Fig. 10.4K) is used when spillage of blood is suspected, e.g., during major cardiac surgeries, etc.
- ❖ **Shoe covers** include: (1) Surgical shoes (slippers) and shoe covers (Figs 10.4L and N): Used mainly in ICUs and operation theaters to protect HCWs from organisms present in floor and (2) Gumboots: Used for anticipated risk of sharp injuries (e.g., for biomedical waste handlers, laundry staff and housekeeping staff) (Fig. 10.4M).

Donning and Doffing

In order to minimize the risk of transmission of infection, donning (wearing) and doffing (removing) of PPE must be performed in a particular sequence.

Donning (wearing): Gown first → Mask or respirator → Goggles or face shield → Gloves
Doffing (removing): Gloves first → Face shield or goggles → Gown → Mask or respirator.

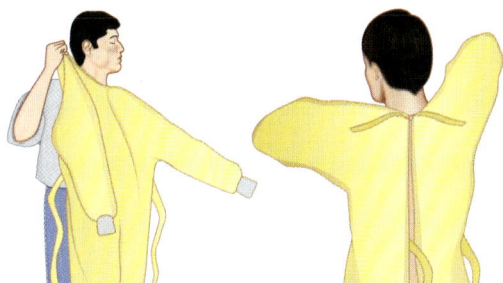

Fig. 10.9: Steps of gown donning (wearing).
Fully cover torso from neck to knees, arms to end of wrists, and wrap around the back. Fasten it in the back of neck and waist.

Doffing is extremely important as even a minor breach in the doffing procedure would subject the HCW to a huge risk of acquiring the infection. This could be a potential reason why many HCWs got infected during COVID-19 pandemic.

- All PPE should be removed just before exiting the patient room **except a respirator**, which should be removed after leaving the patient room and closing the door
- Discard into appropriate BMW bins:
  - Yellow bag: Gown/coverall, mask/respirator, shoe cover and cap
  - Red bag: Plastic apron, goggles/face shield, gloves.

Blood Spill Management

Spillage of blood and body fluid poses a substantial risk for the transmission of blood-borne viruses, such as hepatitis B, C and HIV. Therefore, any spillage (small, few drops to large, few mL) should be considered infectious, and need to be cleaned at the earliest.

Steps of Spill Management (CDC)

The following steps need to be sequentially followed for the management of blood or body fluid spillage.
1. Any spillage, should be attended immediately
2. Mark the spill area, place the wet floor signage
3. Wear appropriate PPE (gloves and gown) as mentioned in the spill kit
4. Confine the spill and wipe immediately with an absorbent towel or cloth, which is spread over the spill to solidify the blood or body fluid. Then it is disposed as infectious waste
5. Clean with hypochlorite (freshly prepared)
   - For large spills (>10 cm size): Use 1:10 dilution of 5% hypochlorite (5000 ppm), i.e., 0.5%
   - For small spills (<10 cm size): Use 1:100 dilution of 5% hypochlorite (500 ppm), i.e., 0.05%
6. Allow the disinfectant to remain wet on the surface for at least a contact time of 10 min
7. Rinse the area with clean water to remove the disinfectant residue.

CHAPTER 11

Transmission-based Precautions

▮DEFINITION

Transmission-based precautions (TBPs), also called as specific precautions are set of infection control practices which should be followed over and above the standard precautions.
- ❖ TBPs should be practiced when giving care for the patients who are infected with infectious agents having specific mode of transmissions, such as contact, droplet and airborne
- ❖ Accordingly, there are three types of TBPs—contact precautions, droplet precautions and airborne precautions
- ❖ TBPs should be followed even when the specific infections are suspected and may be discontinued later when the diagnosis is ruled out.

▮CONTACT PRECAUTIONS

Contact precaution should be followed when there is a definitive or suspected evidence of certain infectious agents that are transmitted by direct or indirect contact during patient care.
- ❖ **Direct transmission** occurs when infectious agents are transferred from one person to another person without a contaminated intermediate object or person. For example, direct contact through contaminated hands (most common mode of transmission of organism in healthcare settings)

Problem Solving Exercise 1

Contact Precautions

A 70-year-old woman after surgery for total knee replacement, is transferred to the postoperative ward. Four days later, patient develops erythema and pus discharge at the wound site. Wound swab sent for culture shows growth of MRSA (methicillin-resistant *S. aureus*); sensitive only to vancomycin and linezolid. Total of 10 patients are housed in the same ward and only two nurses are posted. Hand rub is available only at the entrance and at the nursing station. There is only one stethoscope, blood pressure (BP) apparatus and thermometer in the ward. It is a practice in the ward to use same gloves continuously, due to shortage of supply. After 2 days, another patient following appendectomy develops discharge from the wound site and MRSA grows on culture with same antimicrobial sensitivity pattern.

Identify the risks for transmission and the type of transmission-based precaution applicable?

Explanation

A cluster of cases of surgical site infection occurred with MRSA infection which resulted from lack of standard and contact precautions of the index case.
- ❑ **Inadequate staffing:** Ten patients are there in the ward and only two sisters are posted there for their care
- ❑ **Inaccessibility to handrub:** Handrub are available only at the entrance and nursing station but not at the bedside
- ❑ **No patient dedicated equipment:** There was only one stethoscope, BP apparatus and thermometer, etc., in the ward
- ❑ **Inappropriate use of gloves:** HCWs are using the same gloves in multiple occasions, without changing them when indicated
- ❑ **Patient placement is not followed:** Patient isolation or cohorting are not followed.

❖ **Indirect transmission** involves the transfer of an infectious agent through a contaminated intermediate object (clothes, patient-care devices, environmental surfaces, fomite) or person.

> **Agents Transmitted Through Contact**
> ☐ MRSA (methicillin resistant *S. aureus*)
> ☐ CRE (carbapenem resistant Enterobacteriaceae)
> ☐ VRE (vancomycin resistant enterococci)
> ☐ MDR (multi-drug resistant) nonfermenting gram-negative bacilli, such as *Acinetobacter, Pseudomonas*, etc.
> ☐ Agents of conjunctivitis (e.g., adenovirus, gonococcus, *Chlamydia*)
> ☐ Any highly contagious skin lesions (abscess, impetigo, infected ulcers) infected with Group A *Streptococcus, Staphylococcus*, HSV lesions
> ☐ Skin infestations (e.g., scabies)
> ☐ Agents of diarrhea, such as rotavirus, *Vibrio, C. difficile*
> ☐ Enterically transmitted hepatitis viruses (HAV and HEV).

Infection Control Measures

The following infection control measures should be applied in addition to other standard precaution measures.
- ❖ **Hand hygiene:** Strict adherence to hand hygiene is an absolute requirement of contact precaution as transmission via contaminated hands accounts for majority of contact transmission
- ❖ **PPE:** Gloves and gown are the essential personal protective equipment (PPE) that the healthcare worker (HCW) should wear upon entry to the patient-care area and must be removed before leaving the patient-care area. Surgical mask and protective eyewear are optional PPEs, needed if there is a risk of exposure to splashes or spray of blood and body substances into the face and eyes
- ❖ **Equipment**: Single-use patient-dedicated equipment (e.g., blood pressure cuffs, stethoscopes, thermometers) must be used. If not possible, then the equipment should be cleaned and allowed to dry before use on another patient
- ❖ **Patient placement: Single isolation room** with a bathroom facility is preferred. If not available, then cohorting is recommended. **Cohorting** may be carried out in various ways
  - Patients with similar infections requiring contact precautions can be placed together either in the same isolation room, or in the same cubicle or corner of a ward or
  - Spatial separation of minimum of **3 feet distance** between the beds with privacy curtains.
- ❖ **Transfer of patients:** Patient movement should be limited only to medically-necessary purposes. When transport is necessary, the HCW must wear PPE before transport and the infected areas of the patient's body should be covered to contain the infection
- ❖ **Disinfection of the rooms:** Patient rooms must be frequently cleaned and disinfected adequately (e.g., at least daily and before use by another patient) focusing on frequently-touched surfaces and equipment in the immediate vicinity of the patient.

▌DROPLET PRECAUTIONS

Droplet precautions when used in addition to standard precautions are intended to prevent the spread of infectious agents that are transmitted through respiratory droplet via close respiratory or mucous membrane contact with respiratory secretions.
- ❖ Respiratory droplets are large-particles (>5 μm in size) that are generated by a patient who is coughing, sneezing or talking
- ❖ Transmission via large droplets requires close contact (<3 feet) as droplets do not remain suspended in the air and generally, only travel shorter distances
- ❖ Some infectious agents transmitted by droplet route can also be significantly transmitted by contact mode. This is because the larger droplets settle on the surfaces and inanimate objects within 1-meter distance, which subsequently spread to other individuals when they touch the contaminated surfaces and then touch their eyes, nose or mouth.

> **Agents Transmitted Through Droplets**
> ☐ Diphtheria (pharyngeal)
> ☐ *Haemophilus influenzae* type b
> ☐ *Neisseria meningitidis*
> ☐ Pertussis (whooping cough)
> ☐ Pneumonic plague

Contd...

CHAPTER 11 ◈ Transmission-based Precautions

Problem Solving Exercise 2

Droplet Precautions

A cluster of cases of upper respiratory tract infection (URTI) occurred in a long-term care facility, following a group activity held in a common food area of the hospital. All cases who attended the group activity had food, sitting close to each other at the dining table. One of the individual who attended the group activity was already suffering from URTI since four days. Due to the lack of waste bins in the dining room, used tissues were placed on the dining room tables. The shared bathrooms were far from the dining area, therefore hand hygiene was not performed during the event. Eight individuals reported symptoms consistent with COVID-19, which was later confirmed by molecular test. Discuss the infection control breach occurred. What type of transmission based precautions needed for these cases when they are admitted in ward?

Explanation

A cluster of COVID-19 (URTI) cases occurred in a long-term care facility following a group activity where one of the attendants was already suffering from URTI. The factor which promoted the spread of infection include:

- **Overcrowding:** Group activity held in a common food area and individuals had food, sitting close to each other at the dining tables
- **Lack of droplet precaution by the index case:** The index case did not follow any measures of droplet precaution, such as wearing surgical mask, hand hygiene, etc. He should not have attended any group activity when suffering from URTI
- **Inappropriate respiratory hygiene:** Due to the lack of waste bins in the dining room, used tissues were placed on the dining room tables
- **Inadequate hand hygiene due to** hand hygiene facility was far away from the dining area.

Contd...

- *Mycoplasma* pneumonia
- Streptococcal (group A) pharyngitis
- Influenza viruses, seasonal
- SARS-CoV2 (COVID-19)
- Viral hemorrhagic fevers due to Lassa, Ebola, Marburg, Crimean Congo Fever viruses
- Other viruses: Mumps, Parvovirus B19, Rhinovirus, Rubella, Adenovirus

Infection Control Measures

The following infection control measures should be applied in addition to standard precautions.

1. Hand Hygiene

Droplet transmission is also associated with contact transmission (as discussed earlier). Therefore, hand hygiene is an important component of droplet precautions.

2. Personal Protective Equipment

Healthcare workers (HCWs) should wear a **surgical mask** when close contact (<3 feet) with the patient is anticipated and also upon room entry.
- Patients should wear a surgical mask (all the time)
- HCWs should wear protective eyewear if there is a risk of splashes or spray to eye/face. Gown and gloves should also be worn to prevent contact transmission

- ❖ The primary function of surgical mask is for '**source control**'; which prevents the transmission of droplets from the wearer to the environment. N95 respirator does not provide additional environmental protection and therefore, should not be used for this purpose
- ❖ Secondary function of the surgical mask is to protect the person wearing it from larger droplets in the environment
- ❖ **AGPs:** For certain diseases like seasonal influenza, viral hemorrhagic fever or COVID-19, the HCWs should wear N95 respirator during aerosol generating procedures (AGPs), described subsequently in this chapter.

3. Respiratory Hygiene/Cough Etiquette

The following measures are recommended for all individuals with respiratory symptoms (Fig. 11.1).

- ❖ Directly coughing or sneezing on hands or rubbing of the nose should be strictly avoided
- ❖ Mouth and nose should be covered with a tissue when coughing or sneezing. Tissues should be disposed into the yellow waste bins after use
- ❖ If no tissues are available, coughing or sneezing can be done into the inner elbow (sleeves), turning away from other patients

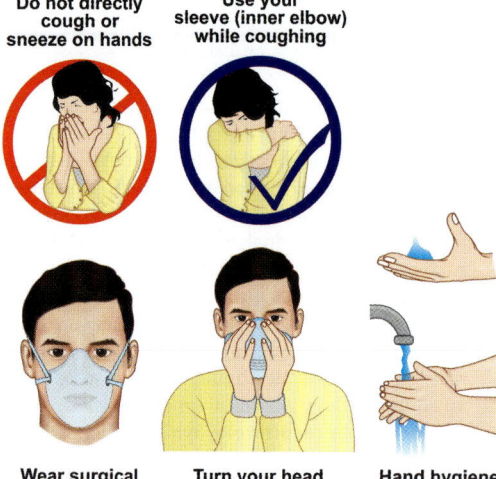

Fig. 11.1: Respiratory hygiene/cough etiquette.

- Hand hygiene should be performed after having contact with respiratory secretions
- Contaminated hands should be kept away from the mucous membranes of the eyes
- In outpatient settings, patients with respiratory symptoms should be segregated separately, provided with mask and attending the cases must be fast-tracked

❖ **Social distancing:** Individuals with respiratory symptoms should always maintain a distance of least 1 meter from others.

4. Patient Placement

A single room is preferred for patients who require droplet precautions. If not available, alternative placement options can be looked for similar to contact precaution, such as cohorting, spatial separation of >3 feet and drawing the curtain between patient beds.

5. Transfer of Patients

Transfer of patients on droplet precautions should be limited as there is a high-risk of transmission. If unavoidable, then the following precautions should be undertaken.
- ❖ The patient should wear a surgical mask while they are being transferred
- ❖ Patients should follow respiratory hygiene and cough etiquette
- ❖ HCW transporting the patient should wear surgical mask, gloves, gown and protective eyewear.

6. Disinfection of the Rooms

Patient-care items, bedside equipment, frequently touched surfaces area and environmental surfaces should be cleaned daily with appropriate disinfectants according to the hospital policy.

AIRBORNE PRECAUTIONS

Problem Solving Exercise 3

Airborne Precautions

An intern is posted in tuberculosis isolation ward, which comprises of individual isolation rooms. His nature of job is to draw blood specimen, giving injections, measuring blood pressure, changing the dress of the patient etc.
1. What type of transmission-based precaution is needed in tuberculosis isolation ward? Discuss its components.
2. What are the recommended personal protective equipment (PPE) to be worn before he enters into an isolation room?
3. Demonstrate the method of donning and doffing of each PPE with correct sequence.
4. What are the precautions need to be followed while donning and doffing of each PPE?

Explanation

M. tuberculosis is transmitted through aerosol. Therefore, aerosol precaution is needed. The recommended PPE to be worn before entering into an isolation room are gloves, gown, N95 respirator and goggles/face shield.
For the answers to the other questions, refer text below and also Chapter 10.

Airborne precautions when used in addition to standard precautions are intended to prevent the spread of infectious agents that are transmitted through respiratory aerosols.

Aerosols are small-particles (<5 μm) generated by an infectious person during coughing, sneezing, talking or performing certain aerosol-generating procedures (e.g., intubation). These smaller droplets remain suspended in air for long periods and may disperse to a distant place along with the air current.

Agents Transmitted Through Aerosols
- *Mycobacterium tuberculosis*
- Measles virus
- Varicella (chickenpox and zoster)
- Smallpox (variola) and monkeypox virus
- Aerosolizable spore-containing powders, such as *Bacillus anthracis*
- *Aspergillus* (pulmonary aspergillosis)

Aerosol-generating Procedures (AGPs)

AGPs are procedures that can generate much higher concentrations of aerosols as compared to coughing, sneezing, or speaking and are associated with higher risk of pathogen transmission.
❖ Therefore, it is recommended to follow airborne precautions, such as isolating the patient in negative pressure room and wearing appropriate PPE like N95 respirator
❖ Examples of AGPs include: Endotracheal intubation, open respiratory and airway suctioning, tracheostomy care, cardiopulmonary resuscitation, sputum induction and bronchoscopy.

Infection Control Measures

A prudent approach is to implement infection control measures at the earliest based on clinical suspicion, and discontinue it later if the patient is subsequently diagnosed with a disease that does not require airborne precautions.

1. PPE

While giving care to a patient with airborne precaution, the HCWs must wear N95 or higher level respirator. The HCW must perform *fit checking* every time before donning the N95 respirator to ensure it is properly applied. Gloves, gown and protective eyewear may be needed if the exposure risk is likely to be present.

2. Patient Placement

Patients should be placed in an airborne infection isolation room (AIIR). The components of AIIR include: adequate ventilation, ultraviolet germicidal irradiation (UVGI) and filtration.

3. Ventilation

Ventilation can reduce the risk of infection through dilution and removal of room air containing infectious aerosols by introduction of clean or fresh air into the room, either by natural or mechanical ventilation.

Natural Ventilation

Natural ventilation refers to the fresh air that enters and leaves a room through openings, such as windows or doors.
❖ The effect of natural ventilation is maximized when the door and windows are placed at opposite to each other and are kept open to maintain airflow at all times
❖ In a consultation room with natural ventilation, the seating arrangement for patient and doctor should be made in such that doctor should sit away from the direction of natural airflow, thus has a lesser risk of exposure (Figs 11.2A and B)

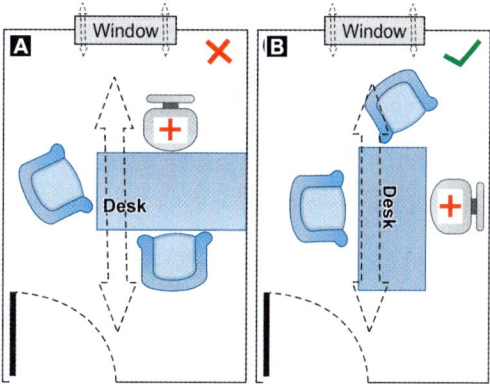

Figs 11.2A and B: Schematic diagram showing seating directions of patient and doctor in a consultation room.
- In room (A), the seating arrangement is along with direct of natural ventilation of air flow, so that the doctor has a higher risk of exposure to the potentially infected air.
- In room (B), doctor is sitting away from the direction of natural airflow, thus has a lesser risk of exposure.

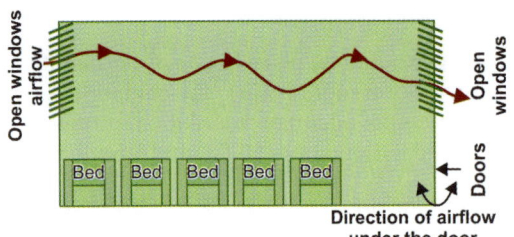

Fig. 11.3: Schematic diagram of a room with natural ventilation.

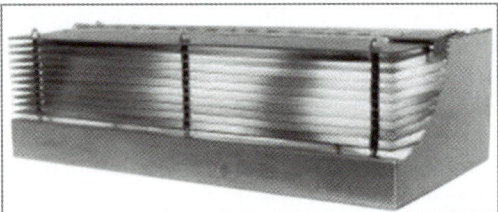

Fig. 11.4: Wall mounted ultraviolet germicidal irradiation.

- In ward set-up, the beds should be placed away from air flow (door-window direction) (Fig. 11.3).

Mechanical Ventilation (Negative-pressure Room)

Negative-pressure room includes a mechanical ventilation system which maintains the pressure of the room slightly lesser than the pressure of the entry area (i.e., creating a "negative pressure"), so that it allows air to flow into the isolation room but not escape from the room, as air naturally flows from areas with higher pressure to the areas with lower pressure, thereby preventing contaminated air from escaping the room.

4. Ultraviolet Germicidal Irradiation

If adequate ventilation is not possible, wall mounted ultraviolet germicidal irradiation (UVGI) devices can be used as in addition to negative pressure ventilation (Fig. 11.4).

5. Filtration

The room air directly exhausted to the outside through an exhaust fan or through HEPA (high efficiency particulate air) filtration. Exhaust fans must be properly installed closely fitting to the window (Figs 11.5A and B).

6. Transfer of Patients

The patient on airborne precaution should be transferred outside the negative pressure

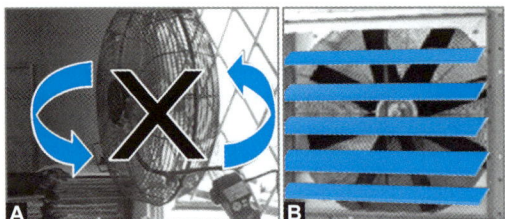

Figs 11.5A and B: Exhaust fan: (A) Poorly-installed in an open window space; (B) well-installed, closely fitted.

room only when it is absolutely necessary. In such a case, the following measures should be undertaken.

- The patient should wear a surgical mask and follow respiratory hygiene and cough etiquette
- Any skin lesions associated with the condition (e.g., chickenpox) should be covered
- The HCW must wear N95 respirator and other PPE as indicated.

7. Respiratory Hygiene

Patients must be explained in detail about cough hygiene as described under droplet precautions and Figure 11.1.

8. Visitors and Staff

Entry of the visitors and staff should be absolutely restricted or they should wear PPE before entry into the room.

The infection control measures need to be taken for various standard and transmission-based precautions have been summarized in Table 11.1.

Table 11.1: Measures be followed during standard and transmission-based precautions.

Type	Isolation room or cohorting	Hand hygiene	Gloves	Apron or gown	Mask	Eye protection	Handling of equipment	Visitors
Standard	Not required	Yes	As required*	If soiling likely#	As required$	As required$	Single use or reprocessed	No additional precautions
Contact	Essential	Yes	Essential	Essential	As required$	As required$	Same as standard	Same precautions as for HCWs
Droplet	Essential	Yes	As required*	If soiling likely#	Surgical mask is essential	As required$	Same as standard	Restricted. Precautions, same as for HCWs
Airborne	Essential (negative pressure)	Yes	As required*	If soiling likely#	N95 respirator is essential	As required$	Same as contact	Same as for droplet

*Gloves are used when there is likely exposure to blood, body fluids and contaminated items.
$Mask or eye protection is required during procedures likely to generate droplets or anticipated splash of specimens on face respectively.
#Soiling is likely to occur during procedures that are expected to generate contamination from blood and body fluids.
Environmental cleaning with an appropriate disinfectant is required for all type of precautions.

Sterilization and Disinfection

CHAPTER 12

■ INTRODUCTION

The sterilization and disinfection practices in a hospital is of paramount importance in preventing transmission of healthcare-associated infections.

Definitions

Sterilization, disinfection and cleaning—aim at removing or destroying the microorganisms from materials or from body surfaces. However, they vary in their efficacy of destroying the microorganisms (Table 12.1).

Sterilization

Sterilization is a process by which all living microorganisms including viable spores, are either destroyed or removed from an article, surface or medium.

Table 12.1: Level of sterilant/disinfectants according to their microbicidal action.

Level of disinfectant/sterilant	Bacterial spores	Tubercle bacilli	Non-enveloped viruses	Fungi	Vegetative bacteria	Enveloped viruses
Sterilant	Yes	Yes	Yes	Yes	Yes	Yes
Disinfectant						
High level	+/–	Yes	Yes	Yes	Yes	Yes
Intermediate level	No	Yes	Yes	Yes	Yes	Yes
Low level	No	No	+/–	+/–	Yes	Yes

❖ Results in reduction of ≥10^6 log colony forming units (CFU) of microorganisms and their spores
❖ The agents which achieve sterilization are called as sterilants (Table 12.2).

Table 12.2: Agents used in the hospital for achieving sterilization, disinfection and cleaning.

Agents	Physical methods	Chemical methods
Sterilants		
Agents of sterilization	• Steam sterilizer (autoclave) • Dry heat sterilizer (hot air oven) • Filtration • Radiation: Ionizing and non-ionizing (infrared)	• Ethylene oxide (ETO) sterilizer • Plasma sterilizer
Disinfectants		
High-level disinfectants	No physical methods in this category	• Aldehydes—glutaraldehyde, orthophthaldehyde • Peracetic acid • Hydrogen peroxide
Intermediate-level disinfectants	• Heat-based methods: Boiling • Ultraviolet (non-ionizing) radiation	• Alcohols—ethyl alcohol and isopropyl alcohol • Phenolics—phenol, cresol, lysol • Halogens—iodine and chlorine
Low-level disinfectants	No physical methods in this category	• Quaternary ammonium compound (QAC) • Chlorhexidine
Cleaning		
Agents of cleaning	Automated washers, such as ultrasonic washers, washer-disinfector and automated cart washers	• Enzymatic solution • Detergent • Soap (antimicrobial or plain soap)

Disinfection

It refers to a process that destroys or removes most if not all pathogenic organisms but may or may not destroy bacterial spores.
- ❖ Results in reduction of ≥10^3 log CFU of most microorganism but not spores
- ❖ Achieved by a physical agent or a chemical agent and are normally used only on inanimate objects, not on body surfaces
- ❖ The agents which achieve disinfection are called as disinfectants (Table 12.2)
- ❖ Depending upon their efficacy, the disinfectants are further classified into three categories (Table 12.1)—high, intermediate and low level disinfectants.

Note: **Antiseptics** are a type of disinfectants which are safe to apply on body surfaces (skin and mucosa) resulting in the destruction of organisms present on the body surfaces. This type of disinfection is termed as **asepsis**.

Cleaning (Decontamination)

Cleaning refers to the reduction in the pathogenic microbial population to a level at which items are considered as safe without protective attire
- ❖ Results in reduction of at least ≥1 log CFU of most of the microorganism but not spores
- ❖ Achieved by manual or mechanical cleaning by soap and detergents to eliminate debris or organic matter from the medical devices or surfaces.

In a healthcare facility, most of the sterilization practices for surgical instrument and other critical care items are carried out in Central Sterile Supply Department (CSSD). Therefore, it is important to understand the workflow of CSSD.

Central Sterile Supply Department (CSSD)

CSSD is an integrated place in hospitals that performs sterilization of medical devices, equipment and consumables; that are used in the operating theater (OT) of the hospital and also for other aseptic procedures.
The processing area of CSSD consists of four unidirectional zones starting from an unsterile area to a sterile area separated by a physical barrier (Fig. 12.1).
Decontamination area → Packaging area → Sterilization area → Sterile storage area

Contd...

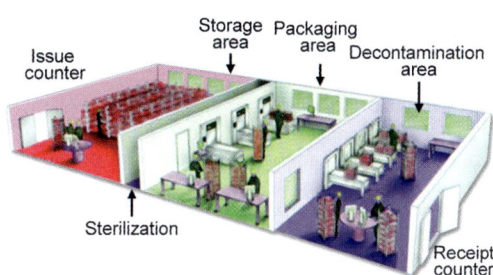

Fig. 12.1: Central Sterile Services Department (CSSD).

Contd...

1. **Decontamination area:** The items are collected and then decontaminated/cleaned by either manual wash or by automated machines (ultrasonic washer and washer-disinfector)
2. **Packaging area:** Here, the items (medical devices) are enclosed in materials or a container designed to allow the penetration and removal of the sterilant during sterilization and then to protect the device from contamination and other damage following sterilization and until the time of use
3. **Sterilization area:** The packed medical devices received from the packaging area are subjected to sterilization process by steam sterilizer, ethylene oxide sterilizer (ETO) or plasma sterilizer
4. **Sterile storage area:** After sterilization the sterilized items are stored in this area. It has an issue counter to supply the items to OTs and various other areas of the hospital.

■ STERILANTS

Steam Sterilizer (Autoclave)

Steam sterilizer functions similar to a pressure cooker; by providing moist heat of >100°C. It is a pressure chamber; consists of a cylinder, a lid and an electrical heater.
- ❖ **Pressure chamber:** It consists of:
  - A large **cylinder** (vertical or horizontal) made up of gunmetal or stainless steel, in which the materials to be sterilized are placed
  - A **steam jacket** (water compartment).
- ❖ **Lid:** It bears the following:
  - A discharge tap for the passage of air and steam
  - A pressure gauge (sets the pressure at a particular level)
  - A safety valve (to remove the excess steam).

❖ **Electrical heater**: It is attached to the jacket; that heats the water to produce steam.

> **Sterilization Conditions**
> The steam sterilizer can be set to provide higher temperatures by adjusting the pressure provided to the vessel. The most commonly used sterilization condition is 121°C for 15 min at a pressure of 15 pounds per square inch (psi).

Uses of Steam Sterilizer (Autoclave)

Steam sterilizer is the most commonly used sterilization method in the hospital. It is used for:
❖ All critical and semi-critical items that are heat and moisture resistant: surgical instruments, anesthetic equipment, dental instruments, implanted medical devices and surgical drapes and linens
❖ Culture media preparation
❖ Biomedical waste treatment of waste and sharps.

Types of Steam Sterilizer

Steam sterilizers are available in various sizes and dimensions.
❖ **Horizontal type** (large volume capacity) (Figs 12.2A and B): It is used in CSSD, large-size laboratories and for biomedical waste treatment
❖ **Vertical type** (small volume capacity) (Fig. 12.2C): It is used for small-size laboratories.

Sterilization Control

The effectiveness of the sterilization achieved by steam sterilizer can be monitored by biological indicator, such as spores of *Geobacillus stearothermophilus*:

Ethylene Oxide (ETO) Sterilizer

Ethylene oxide (ETO) is one of the widely used gaseous chemical sterilants in CSSD.
❖ **Sterilization cycle:** It is carried out in a special equipment called ethylene oxide sterilizer (Fig. 12.3)
❖ **Uses:** ETO is used by CSSD to sterilize critical items (and sometimes semicritical items) that are moisture or heat sensitive and cannot be sterilized by steam sterilization. Examples include:
  ▪ Heart-lung machine components
  ▪ Sutures, catheters and stents

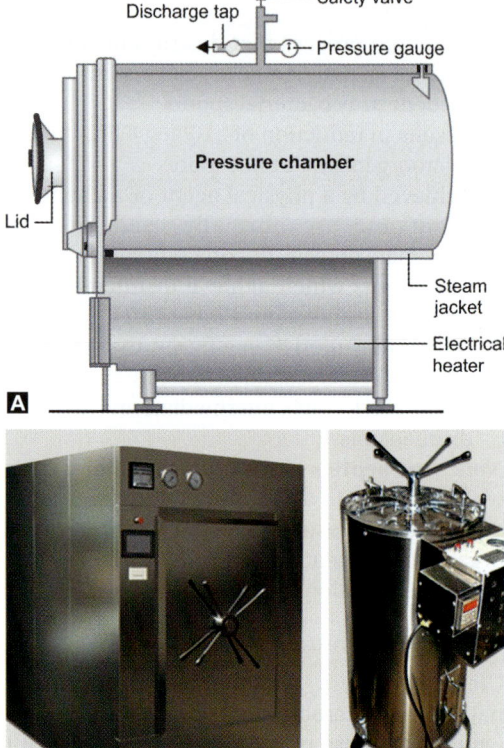

Figs 12.2A to C: Steam sterilizer (autoclave): (A) Schematic diagram; (B) Horizontal autoclave; (C) Vertical autoclave.

  ▪ Respirators and dental equipment
  ▪ Devices with electronic components
  ▪ Multi-lumen tubings, etc.
❖ **Advantages of ETO:** (i) Large chamber capacity, (ii) low temperature (55°C) is maintained, therefore suitable for heat sensitive items, (iii) high penetration power- ETO is highly diffusible, penetrates areas that cannot be reached by steam, (iv) non-corrosive to plastic, metal and rubber materials
❖ **Disadvantages:** (i) ETO is highly inflammable, irritant, explosive and carcinogenic, (ii) long duration of cycle (12–14 hours), (iv) high cost of instrument and consumables
❖ **Sterilization control:** By using spores of *Bacillus atrophaeus*.

Plasma Sterilization

Plasma sterilizer is a special device used to create the plasma state (commercial brands, such as Sterrad, Fig. 12.4).

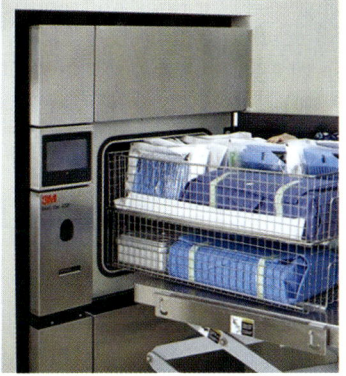
Fig. 12.3: Ethylene oxide sterilizer.
Source: 3M India Pvt. Ltd.

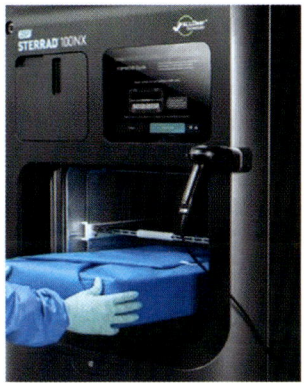
Fig. 12.4: Plasma sterilizer (Sterrad).
Source: Johnson & Johnson Pvt. Ltd.

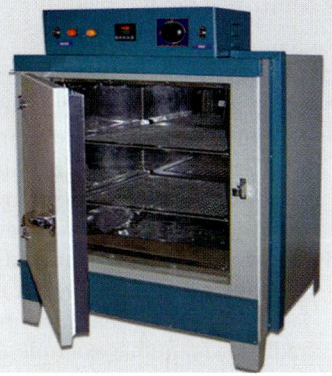
Fig. 12.5: Dry heat sterilizer (hot air oven).

- It uses hydrogen peroxide as chemical sterilant
- The cycle is run for 24–75 min, at low temperature (37–44°C)
- **Sterilization control:** Spores of *Bacillus stearothermophilus* is used as a biological indicator
- **Uses:** It is used by CSSD for sterilization of materials and devices that cannot tolerate high temperature and humidity of steam sterilizer, such as some plastics, electrical devices, and corrosion-susceptible metals, such as arthroscope, micro and vascular instruments, spine sets and laparoscope.

Dry Heat Sterilizer (Hot Air Oven)

This method is used for materials that might be damaged by moist heat or that are impenetrable to the moist heat (e.g., glass wares, powders, petroleum products, sharp instruments) (Fig. 12.5).

- The most common cycle used is 160°C for 120 minutes
- **Sterilization control:** Spores of *Bacillus atrophaeus*.

Filtration

Filtration acts by removing microorganisms, not by killing. Membrane filters are the most widely used filters in hospitals. They retain all the particles on the surface that are larger than their pore size (Fig. 12.6). Membrane filtration has two wider applications in hospital settings—filtration of air and water.

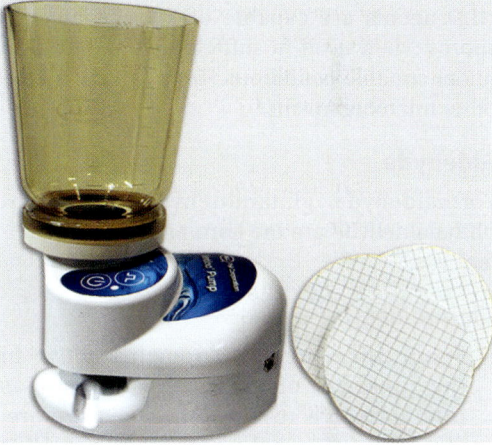
Fig. 12.6: Filter apparatus with membrane filter.
Source: Department of Microbiology, JIPMER, Puducherry.

- **Filtration of air:** (1) HEPA filters (High-efficiency particulate air filters) in hospitals are used in biological safety cabinets, airflow system, operation theatre, and isolation rooms. (2) Filters are also used in surgical (3-ply) mask and N95 respirators
- **Filtration of liquid:** (1) Used for bacteriological examination of water in hospital settings, especially dialysis water. (2) It is also used to remove bacteria from heat labile liquids, such as sera, sugar, toxin, vaccine and antibiotic solutions.

The sterilization control of membrane filters includes *Brevundimonas diminuta* and *Serratia marcescens*.

Radiation

Radiations are of two types:
- **Ionizing radiation** (e.g., cobalt 60 gamma rays): It is a low-temperature sterilization method (called as **cold sterilization**) that has been used for a number of medical products (e.g., tissue for transplantation, pharmaceuticals, medical devices)
- **Non-ionizing radiation:** Infrared radiation technology can be used for sterilization for selected heat-resistant instruments. Ultraviolet radiation is another example, described under intermediate level disinfectant.

HIGH-LEVEL DISINFECTANTS (HLD)

HLD agents are capable of killing bacterial spores when used in sufficient concentration under suitable conditions. They can kill all the other microorganisms.

Aldehyde

Formaldehyde, glutaraldehyde and ortho-phthalaldehyde are the commonly used disinfectants.

Glutaraldehyde

- **Semicritical items:** It remains active in the presence of organic matter and is non-corrosive to equipment. Therefore, glutaraldehyde is the most common HLD used for semicritical equipment, such as endoscopes and cystoscopes
  - It is used at 2% or 2.4% concentration (e.g., Cidex). It disinfects objects within 20 minutes but may require longer time to kill spores (10–14 hours)
  - It is available in inactive form; has to be activated by alkalinization before use. Once activated, it remains active only for 14 days.
- **Aerial disinfection and cleaning:** It is also used for fogging and cleaning of floor and surfaces of critical areas, such as operation theater (e.g., Bacilocid Extra).

Ortho-phthalaldehyde (0.55%)

This can also be used for disinfection of semicritical items, has many advantages over glutaraldehyde—(1) it does not require activation, (2) better odor, (3) less eye irritation, (4) acts faster (5–10 min). However, it does not kill spores effectively and stains skin gray.

Peracetic Acid

Peracetic acid is used in automated machines. It is also available for manual immersion; 0.1–0.2%, used for 5–15 min.

Use: It can be used to sterilize medical (e.g., endoscopes, arthroscopes), surgical, and dental instruments. Peracetic acid in combination with hydrogen peroxide has been used for disinfecting hemodialyzers

Hydrogen Peroxide (H_2O_2)

H_2O_2 works by producing destructive hydroxyl free radicals that can attack various cell components.

Uses: H_2O_2 has several usages at various concentrations. It is sporicidal only at >4–5%
- 3% H_2O_2 is used for environmental surface disinfection, fogging and for wound cleaning
- 3–6% H_2O_2 is used to disinfect soft contact lens, tonometer biprisms, ventilators, fabrics, and endoscopes, etc.
- 6–7.5% H_2O_2 is used as chemical sterilant in plasma sterilization
- Vaporized H_2O_2 is used for industrial sterilization of medical devices and for decontamination of large and small area.

INTERMEDIATE-LEVEL DISINFECTANTS

Alcohol

Ethyl alcohol and isopropyl alcohol are the most popular alcohols used in hospitals.
- **Uses:** Alcohol (60–80%) is used for various purposes
  - **Alcohol-based handrub** (ABHR), e.g., Sterillium, a popular commercial product
  - Disinfecting **smaller non-critical instruments,** such as thermometers, which are immersed in alcohol for 10–15 minutes
  - Disinfection of **small medical items/ surfaces,** such as rubber stoppers of

multiple-dose medication vials or vaccine bottles and hubs of the central line
- Disinfection of **external surfaces of equipment,** such as stethoscopes, ventilators, manual ventilation bags, ultrasound machines, etc.
- Disinfection of **non-critical surfaces,** such as laboratory bench, medication preparation areas
- **Spirit** (70% alcohol): Used a skin antiseptic.
❖ **Disadvantages:** (i) Flammable and must be stored in a cool, well-ventilated area, (ii) Evaporate rapidly.

Phenolics

Phenol (carbolic acid) was the first widely used antiseptic and disinfectant.
❖ **Used as disinfectants:** Cresol, and lysol are the common phenolics used for disinfecting environmental surfaces (e.g., bedside tables, bedrails, and laboratory surfaces) and noncritical medical devices. They are toxic to skin, hence not used as antiseptics. **5% phenol** is mycobactericidal, used for disinfection of sputum specimen
❖ **Used as antiseptics:** Certain phenolics are compatible with skin and are widely used as antiseptics. The classical example is chloroxylenol (the active ingredient of the commercial brand, Dettol)
❖ Phenolics are the only ILD that retain activity in the presence of organic materials.

Halogens

Among the halogens, iodine and chlorine have antimicrobial activity. They exist in free state, and form salt with sodium and other metals.

Iodine

Two preparations are available.
❖ **Tincture of iodine:** It used as antiseptic for wound cleaning. It can stain the skin
❖ **Povidone iodine** (e.g., Betadine): It is prepared by complexing iodine with carrier (povidone) which helps in sustained-release of iodine. It is nonstaining and free of skin toxicity. It is used as antiseptics at different concentrations

❖ 5% topical solution and ointment is used for wound cleaning
❖ 10% is used for surgical skin preparation.

Chlorine and Hypochlorite

Chlorine is one of the most commonly available disinfectant in hospital.
❖ **Preparations:** Chlorine occurs as—(1) free chlorine, (2) hypochlorite—it is available in two preparations
- Liquid form (sodium hypochlorite or household bleach), or
- Powder form (calcium hypochlorite or bleaching powder)
- Other forms: Include sodium dichloroisocyanurate (NaDCC) available as tablets and chlorine dioxide.
❖ **Uses (free chlorine):** Chlorine is used for disinfection of municipal water supplies and swimming pool water. It is also employed in the dairy and food industries
❖ **Uses (sodium hypochlorite):** It is available at 5.25–6.15%, which is equivalent to 50,000 ppm of available chlorine. It should be used in appropriate dilutions (by adding with water) for disinfection of various hospital supplies. The contact time is about 10–20 minutes
- Large blood spill: 0.5% (1:10 dilution or 5,000 ppm) is used
- Small blood spill: 0.05% (1:100 dilution, or 500 ppm) is used
- Pre-treatment of liquid waste before disposal: 1% (1:5 dilution, 10,000 ppm) is used
- Laundry items: 0.1% (1 in 50 dilution 1,000 ppm) is used
- Surface disinfectant: 0.5% (1:10 dilution or 5,000 ppm) is used
- *C. difficile* (diarrheal stool): Hypocholrite is sporicidal only >0.5% (5000 ppm).
❖ **Advantages:** Hypochlorites are broad spectrum, rapid in its action, non-flammable, low cost and are widely available
❖ **Disadvantages:** (1) Inactivated by organic matter, (2) Toxic to skin and mucosa, and carcinogenic, (3) Daily preparation is required (4) Corrosive to fabrics and carpets.

Ultraviolet (UV) Radiation

UV radiation has been employed for disinfection of air and/or surfaces as in operating rooms, isolation rooms, and biologic safety cabinets. It can also be used for disinfection of drinking water, titanium implants and contact lenses. Its effectiveness is influenced by the presence of organic matter.

■ LOW-LEVEL DISINFECTANTS

Low-level disinfectants (LLD) destroy vegetative bacteria and enveloped viruses, variable action on nonenveloped viruses, and fungi, but no action on tubercle bacilli and spores.

Quaternary Ammonium Compound (QAC)

QAC are commonly used in environmental sanitation of noncritical surfaces, such as floors, furniture, and walls. Some products are also used for disinfecting non-critical medical equipment that contacts intact skin (e.g., blood pressure cuffs). QAC are also good cleaning agents as they have surfactant like action. Benzyl ammonium chloride is the classical example of QAC.

Chlorhexidine Gluconate (CHG)

CHG is widely used in antiseptic products, at various concentrations
- ❖ **Hand hygiene product:** Hand rub (0.5%), handwash (4%) (e.g., Microshield, a commercial product)
- ❖ **Mouthwash** (0.1–0.2%)
- ❖ **Body wash** solutions (used before surgery)
- ❖ **Skin disinfectant** before surgery (2%)
- ❖ **Antiseptic** for wound cleaning: Commercially available as **Savlon** which is a combination of CHG 0.3%, cetrimide and isopropyl alcohol.

■ CLEANING AGENTS

Most disinfectants act well only when the instrument or the surface is free from organic matter, such as dirt, blood, or other specimens. Therefore, cleaning is a very important step which needs to be performed before the disinfectants are applied. Broadly two types of cleaning agents are available.
1. **Enzymatic (proteolytic) cleaners:** They contain enzymes, such as amylase, lipase, cellulase, protease which breakdown proteinaceous matter present on equipment. Enzymatic cleaners are not disinfectants; they only remove protein from surfaces
2. **Cleaning chemicals (detergents):** These agents act by reducing surface tension and dissolving fat and organic matter.

■ ENVIRONMENTAL CLEANING

Environmental cleaning of the floor and surface of hospitals play a vital role in controlling the spread of infections. The general principles of environmental cleaning are as follows.
- ❖ **Cleaning followed by disinfections:**
  - ■ **Cleaning:** Always cleaning with a detergent is performed first, before applying disinfectant
  - ■ **Disinfection:** CDC recommends to use low- to intermediate-level disinfectants for environmental cleaning, such as QAC, hypochlorite and improved hydrogen peroxide.
- ❖ **Cleaning sequence:** Cleaning should be performed in correct sequence to prevent recontamination
  - ■ **Cleaner to dirtier:** The cleaner areas are cleaned first, followed by the dirtier areas; e.g., low-touch surfaces should be cleaned first followed by high-touch surfaces
  - ■ **High to low:** Top area should be cleaned first, then proceed towards bottom (e.g., bedrails → bed legs and table surfaces → floors)
  - ■ **Inward to outwards:** Clean the farthest point from the door first and then proceed towards the door.
- ❖ **Frequency of cleaning for common situations:**
  - ■ Non-critical surfaces and floors can be cleaned 2–3 times a day
  - ■ Mattress used for patients should be cleaned weekly and after discharge
  - ■ Doors, windows, walls and ceiling should be cleaned once a month and spot-cleaning when soiled
  - ■ **High touch areas**, such as doorknobs, elevator buttons, telephones, bedrails, light switches, computer keyboards,

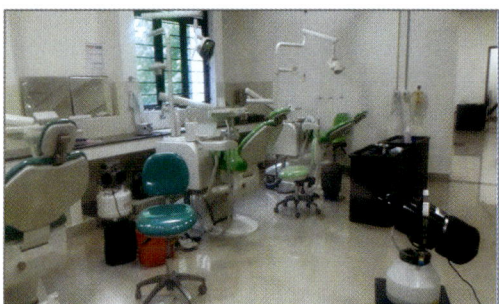

Fig. 12.7: Fogging of dental unit following construction.
Source: Sanitary Department, JIPMER, Puducherry.

monitoring equipment should be cleaned more frequently, every 3–4 hours.

Disinfection of Operation Theater

Environmental cleaning in operation theater (OT) minimizes patients' and HCWs' exposure to potentially infectious microorganisms.

- ❖ **Surface disinfection:** Cleaning should be performed first with a cleansing agent, followed by disinfection by using an aldehyde-based disinfectant. Disinfection of OT is carried out in the following situations
  1. First cleaning of the day (before cases begin)
  2. In between cases (cleaning 3 to 4 feet perimeter around the OT table)
  3. Terminal cleaning of OT after the last case
  4. Detailed wash-down of the OT complex once a week
  5. During renovation or construction of OT or nearby places.
- ❖ **Fogging:** Also called aerial disinfection, involves spraying of a disinfectant (e.g., glutaraldehyde, H_2O_2 or QAC based product) with the help of a fogger machine (Fig. 12.7)
  - The procedure takes around 1-2 hours, during which OT should be closed down and personnel need to be vacated
  - **Indication:** Routine periodic fogging is not recommended, but is indicated only when any outbreak of infection is suspected or any change in infection control practice implemented or during renovation or construction of OT or nearby places.

METHODS TO TEST EFFICACY OF STERILIZERS

The efficacy of sterilizers can be assessed by using physical, chemical and biological indicators.

Physical Indicator

These are the digital displays of the sterilizer equipment showing parameters, such as temperature, time and pressure, etc.

Chemical Indicator

They use heat or chemical sensitive materials which undergo a color change if the sterilization parameter (e.g., time, steam quality and temperature) for which it is issued is achieved. Common types used are:

- ❖ **Class I:** Also called as exposure indicator or external pack control. They are used on the external surface of each pack, to indicate that the pack has been directly exposed to the sterilant. However, it does not assure sterility (Fig. 12.8A)
- ❖ **Class II:** It is called as Bowie–Dick test or as equipment control; i.e., it checks the efficacy of air removal, air leaks and steam penetration and ensures that the steam sterilizer is functioning well
- ❖ **Class IV and V:** Also called as internal pack control indicator. It is placed inside the packs and therefore it verifies whether the critical parameters, such as time, steam quality and temperature are attained inside the pack or not (Fig. 12.8B).

Biological Indicator

It is the most reliable indicator as it uses bacterial spores to check the effectiveness of sterilization.

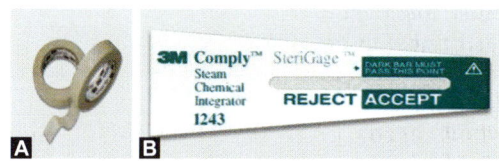

Figs 12.8A and B: Chemical indicator: (A) Type I (autoclave tape); (B) Type V (internal pack control indicator).
Source: Department of CSSD, JIPMER, Puducherry.

The spores are highly resistant and will be destroyed only when the effective condition is achieved.
- *Geobacillus stearothermophilus* for steam sterilizer and gas plasma (hydrogen peroxide) and liquid acetic acid sterilizer
- *Bacillus atrophaeus* for ethylene oxide sterilizer and dry heat sterilizer (hot air oven)
- Spore containing vials are incubated. Depending upon the incubators used, the result is obtained in 24 minutes to 48 hours time (Figs 12.9A and B).

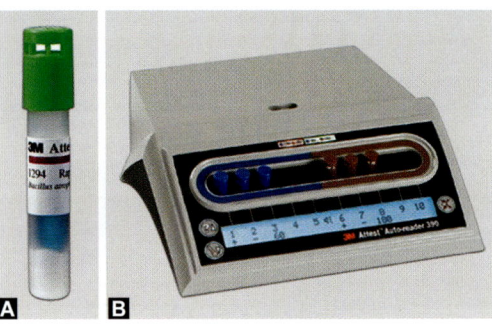

Figs 12.9A and B: Biological indicator: (A) Vial; (B) Incubator.
Source: Department of CSSD, JIPMER, Puducherry.

Problem Solving Exercise

What are the recommended methods for sterilization/disinfection of following items in a healthcare facility—endoscope, culture media, handrub, ventilator tubes, operation theatre disinfection, cleaning of surgical instrument, stethoscope, wound disinfection?

Explanation

The recommended methods for sterilization/disinfection of following items in a healthcare facility are:
- **Endoscope:** 2% Glutaraldehyde or 0.55% ortho-phthalaldehyde
- **Culture media:** Should be sterilized by autoclave (121°C for 15 min)
- **Handrub:** Hands should be disinfected with either alcohol-based hand rub (60–80%) or chlorhexidine alcohol hand rub after contact with patient or its surrounding
- **Ventilator tubes:** Can be sterilized at CSSD by ethylene oxide sterilizer, plasma sterilizer
- **Operation theatre disinfection:** Cleaning with a detergent, followed by disinfection with a high level disinfectant, such as glutaraldehyde or hydrogen peroxide
- **Cleaning of surgical instruments:** The surgical instruments should be cleaned first with enzymatic (proteolytic) cleaners before sending to CSSD for sterilization
- **Stethoscope:** The external surfaces of stethoscope should be disinfected with alcohol 60–80% (isopropyl alcohol) after each use
- **Wound disinfection:** Povidone iodine (5% topical solution and ointment) is recommended for wound disinfection.

Biomedical Waste Management

CHAPTER 13

Problem Solving Exercise

Biomedical Waste Segregation Audit

While examining the biomedical waste receptacles at the common collection point in a hospital, the following items were found. Find out how many items are segregated appropriately according to biomedical waste rule 2016.

Yellow bag	Red bag	White box	Blue box
1. N95 Mask 2. Cyclophosphamide vial 3. Nitrile gloves 4. Central venous catheter 5. Coverall	1. Syringe 2. IV set 3. Blood bag 4. Nasogastric tube 5. Syringe with fixed needle	1. Microscopy slide 2. Metallic implant 3. Needle 4. Scalpel 5. Broken glass ampoule	1. Cytotoxic drug bottle 2. Glass ampoule (amikacin) 3. Stained cloth 4. Stained cotton 5. BacT/ALERT bottle

Explanation: The following are the correct items segregated in the biomedical waste receptacles

Yellow bag	Red bag	White box	Blue box
Correctly segregated 1. N95 Mask 2. Cyclophosphamide vial 3. Coverall **Not segregated correctly** 1. Nitrile gloves (red) 2. Central venous catheter (red)	**Correctly segregated** 1. Syringe 2. IV set 3. Nasogastric tube **Not segregated correctly** 1. Blood bag (yellow) 2. Syringe with fixed needle (white)	**Correctly segregated** 1. Needle 2. Scalpel **Not segregated correctly** 1. Microscopy slide (blue) 2. Metallic implant (blue) 3. Broken glass ampoule (blue)	**Correctly segregated** 1. Glass ampoule (amikacin) **Not segregated correctly** 1. Cytotoxic drug bottle (yellow) 2. Stained cloth (yellow) 3. Stained cotton (yellow) 4. BacT/ALERT bottle (red)

■ INTRODUCTION

Biomedical wastes (BMW) are defined as wastes that are generated during the laboratory diagnosis, treatment or immunization of human beings or animals, or in research activities pertaining thereto, or in the production of biologicals.

Waste Generated in Hospitals

It is estimated that the quantity of solid waste generated in hospitals varies from 1/2 to 2 kg/bed; which can be divided into two categories:
1. **General (non-hazardous solid waste, 80%):** A large amount of waste falls in the general waste category, which may be disposed of with the usual domestic and urban waste management system. They do not cause any harm to humans. They are not considered as BMW. They should not be mixed with BMW.
2. **Biomedical waste:** BMW accounts for a minor proportion of the total waste generated in the hospitals; which includes infectious waste (10%) and chemical/radioactive waste (5%).

Hazards Associated with BMW

Inappropriate and inefficient disposal of BMW can lead to infectious hazards, malignancies, malformations, and environmental (air, land

and water) pollution not only to the current generation but also for future generations. The various hazards are:
- **Hazards from infectious sharps:** They may lead to transmission of blood borne viruses (hepatitis B, C and HIV)
- **Hazards from chemical wastes:** They are toxic, corrosive, explosive and flammable; can cause chemical burns
- **Pharmaceutical waste:** Exposure to these agents may cause several adverse effects
- **Hazards from cytotoxic waste:** They can be mutagenic, teratogenic, or carcinogenic
- **Hazards from radioactive waste:** They are genotoxic, in higher doses can cause tissue destruction.

BIOMEDICAL WASTE RULE, INDIA

The Ministry of Environment and Forests (MoEF) has formulated biomedical waste rule in 2016 with an amendment added in 2018 and 2019 (Table 13.1).
- It was implemented with a vision of simplifying categorization of BMWs, while improving the ease of segregation, transportation and disposal methods to decrease environmental pollution
- According to this new rule, there are four categories of BMWs, each is segregated by a single color-coded container.

Steps of BMW Management

The management of BMW can overall be summarized into five simple steps:
1. Waste segregation (at the point of generation) into color-coded containers
2. Pre-treatment for laboratory liquid waste
3. Transport of waste from generation site to central storage area of the hospital
4. Transport of waste from central storage area to common biomedical waste treatment facility (CBMWTF)
5. Treatment and/or disposal (within 48 hours of generation).

Waste Segregation in Hospitals

Waste segregation refers to the basic separation of different categories of waste generated at source in the hospital and thereby reducing the risks as well as the cost of handling and disposal. According to BMW Rule (2016), segregation of waste should be done by using containers of four different colors—each is designated for segregation of a particular waste category (Table 13.1).
- Yellow bag—for infectious non-plastic waste
- Red bag—for infectious plastic waste
- White or translucent sharp container (puncture-proof box)—for metal sharps
- Blue container (puncture-proof box)—for broken glass items and metal implants.

The following general principles need to be followed during segregation, transport and storage of BMW:
- **Waste receptacles:** The waste receptacles should have the following properties
  - **Plastic bags** must be labeled with biohazard logos (Fig. 13.1) and should be non-inflammable, autoclave stable and non-chlorinated
  - **Containers** should have well-fitting lids, either removable by hand or preferably operated by a foot pedal
  - **Sharp box** should be puncture-proof, leak-proof and tamper-proof impermeable container.
- **Importance of segregation:** Segregation is the most crucial step in BMW management. Wrong segregation may lead to serious consequences, such as:
  - Needle stick injury transmitting hepatitis B or HIV (if sharp items are segregated in to yellow or red bags)
  - Production of carcinogens (if plastic items are wrongly segregated into yellow bag

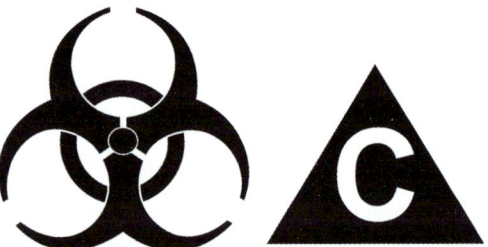

Biohazard symbol   Cytotoxic hazard symbol

Fig. 13.1: Logos used for segregation of biomedical waste.

Table 13.1: Biomedical Waste Management Rule, India, 2016 (including the amendment added in 2018 and 2019).

Category	Type of waste	Type of bag/container	Treatment/disposal options
Yellow	A. Human anatomical waste	Yellow-colored non-chlorinated plastic bags	Incineration/plasma pyrolysis/deep burial
	B. Animal anatomical waste		
	C. Soiled waste		Incineration/plasma pyrolysis/ deep burial/ autoclaving or hydroclaving + shredding/mutilation
	D. Expired/discarded medicines—pharmaceutical waste, cytotoxic drugs	Yellow-colored containers/non-chlorinated plastic bags with cytotoxic label	Sent back to manufacturer/CBMWTF for incineration (cytotoxic drugs at temperature >1200°C)
	E. Chemical solid waste	Yellow-colored containers/nonchlorinated plastic bags	Incineration or plasma pyrolysis or encapsulation
	F. Chemical liquid waste, such as discarded disinfectants, infected body fluids and secretions, liquid from housekeeping-related activities	To be discharged into separate collection system, which leads to effluent treatment system. Not to be discarded into yellow bag	Pre-treated[1] before mixing with other wastewater
	G. Discarded linen waste contaminated with blood/body fluids, mask, cap, gown and shoe cover	Non-chlorinated yellow plastic bags/suitable packing material	Non-chlorinated chemical disinfection[2] followed by incineration/plasma pyrolysis
	H. Microbiology, other clinical laboratory waste, blood bags, live attenuated vaccines	Autoclave safe plastic bag/container	Pre-treat to sterilize with non-chlorinated chemicals[2] on-site as per NACO/ WHO guidelines (Blue book 2014) + incineration
Red	**Infectious plastic waste** Disposable items, such as tubing, bottles, intravenous tubes and sets, catheters, urine bags, syringes (without needles and fixed needle syringes) and vacutainer with their needles cut), gloves, plastic apron and goggles	Red-colored non-chlorinated plastic bags or containers	• Autoclaving/microwaving/hydroclaving + shredding • Mutilation/sterilization+ shredding Treated waste sent to authorized recyclers or for energy recovery
White (Translucent)	**Waste sharps including metal sharps** Needles, syringes with fixed needles, needles from needle tip cutter or burner, scalpels, blades, or any other contaminated sharp (used or discarded)	Puncture-proof, leak-proof, tamper-proof containers	Autoclaving/dry heat sterilization followed by: • Shredding or mutilation or encapsulation in metal container or cement concrete or • Sanitary landfill or • Designated concrete waste sharp pit

Contd...

Contd...

Category	Type of waste	Type of bag/container	Treatment/disposal options
Blue	a. **Glasswares:** Broken or discarded and contaminated glass including medicine vials and ampoules except those contaminated with cytotoxic wastes, microscope slides b. **Metallic body implants** Dental implants, other body implants and plates	Puncture-proof and leak-proof container	Disinfection can be carried out by: • Soaking the washed glass waste after cleaning with detergent and sodium hypochlorite treatment (1–2%) or • Autoclaving/microwaving/hydroclaving and then it is sent for recycling

Note:
- Biomedical waste rule does not specify any specific color coded bag for general waste segregation in hospital. Depending upon the local policy, hospitals choose any color-coded bag for general waste (for e.g., JIPMER uses black bag for general waste).
- [1]**Chemical treatment:** Hypochlorite should be used at 1–2% concentration having 30% residual chlorine with contact time of 20 minutes.
- [2]**Non-chlorinated chemicals** include 5% phenol, 5% cresol or 5% lysol.
- The chlorinated plastic bags (except blood bags) and gloves should be phased out and replaced with non-chlorinated bags and gloves.
- Every healthcare facility should have their own STP (sewage treatment plant).
- Barcoding system should be introduced to monitor the segregation compliance.

Abbreviations: NACO, National AIDS Control Organization; WHO, World Health Organization; CBMWTF, common biomedical waste treatment facility.

and subjected to incineration, leads to production of carcinogenic furans).
- ❖ **Securement:** All the bags used for waste collection need to be sealed once they are filled to 3/4th of their capacity
- ❖ **Labeling:** Bags and containers should be labeled properly with the date and place
- ❖ **Pre-treatment:** The laboratory liquid waste should always be pre-treated either with chemical (1–2% hypochlorite) or autoclave before segregating into appropriate containers
- ❖ **Transport:** The waste should be transported within 24 hours by **dedicated trolley** to the central BMW storage facility of the hospital. Separate routes should be used for transport to prevent exposure to staff and patients and to minimize the passage of loaded carts through patient care and other clean areas. Interim storage of the waste at ward is strongly discouraged
- ❖ **Central storage area:** This is a temporary storage facility present within a hospital where different types of waste should be brought for safe retention until it is treated or collected for transport to CBMWTF
- ❖ **PPE:** HCWs handling BMW during transport or in the storage area should wear appropriate personal protective equipment (PPE), such as heavy duty gloves, 3-ply mask, gowns and gumboots (Fig. 10.4, Chapter 10).

Treatment and Disposal Methods

As per the mandate of the BMWM rules, 2016, the final disposal and recycling must be performed at common biomedical waste treatment facility (CBMWTF). Only when there is no CBMWTF within 75 km, the hospital can create its own the disposal facility. The various methods used for treatment/disposal of BMW are—incineration, autoclave, chemical disinfection (hypochlorite), microwave, effluent treatment plant, hydroclaving, shredder, deep burial and sharp pit.

Needle Stick Injury

CHAPTER 14

Problem Solving Exercise 1

A 32-year-old staff working in biomedical waste department reported to HICC with complaints of needle stick injury while segregating a yellow bag. The incident happened 18 hours back. He did not perform any first aid measures at the time of injury. He has not received any hepatitis B vaccination before. Discuss the post-exposure prophylaxis measures that should be undertaken.

Explanation

The source is unknown as the prick happened while segregating a yellow bag. Therefore, the following post-exposure prophylaxis measures need to be taken.
- **For HIV:** First dose of ART has to be given immediately (within 2hr of exposure); followed by full course of ART for 28 days (Refer the text for the drugs given in ART and the dosage)
- **For hepatitis B:** He should receive hepatitis B immunoglobulin plus hepatitis B vaccine series (three doses); 1st dose to be taken now, followed by 2nd and 3rd dose after 1 month and six month respectively.

Problem Solving Exercise 2

A 28-year-old medicine resident reported to HICC with complaints of needle stick injury on his left thumb while recapping the needle. The incident happened 1 hr back. On enquiry, he mentioned that he had immediately washed his finger with running tap water for 2 minutes. The source sample was tested and was found to be positive for hepatitis B surface antigen and reactive for HIV antibodies. The resident had received a complete course (one series) of hepatitis B vaccine 10 years back, following which he had an anti-HBs titer of 550 mIU/mL. Discuss the post-exposure prophylaxis measures that should be undertaken.

Explanation

The source sample was found to be positive for hepatitis B surface antigen and reactive for HIV antibodies. Therefore, the following post-exposure prophylaxis measures need to be taken.
- **For HIV:** First dose of ART has to be given immediately (within 2hr of exposure); followed by full course of ART for 28 days (Refer the text for the drugs given in ART and the dosage)
- **For hepatitis B:** As he was vaccinated and protected with anti-HBs titer of 550 mIU/mL; therefore no further action (post-exposure prophylaxis) is necessary.

Problem Solving Exercise 3

A 41-year-old surgeon reported to HICC with complaints of surgical blade injury on his left thumb, 3 hr back. The source sample was tested positive for hepatitis B surface antigen, but negative for HIV antibodies and HCV antibodies. The surgeon had received two doses of hepatitis B vaccine 2 years back. Discuss the post-exposure prophylaxis measures that should be undertaken.

Explanation

The source sample was found to be positive for hepatitis B surface antigen but non-reactive for HIV. Therefore, the following post-exposure prophylaxis measures need to be taken.
- **For HIV:** No further action (post-exposure prophylaxis) is necessary

- **For hepatitis B:** He was partially vaccinated for hepatitis B, therefore, he should be given hepatitis B immunoglobulin plus the third dose hepatitis B vaccine.

INTRODUCTION

An occupational exposure is defined as:
- Percutaneous injury, e.g., needle stick injury (NSI) or other sharp injury
- Splash injury:
  - Contact with the mucous membrane (e.g., eye or mouth)
  - Contact with non-intact skin (abraded skin or afflicted with dermatitis)
  - Contact with the intact skin when the duration is prolonged (e.g., several minutes or more).

An occupational injury is often loosely termed as needle stick injury though it includes injury through needle or other sharps and splashes.

Agents transmitted: Hepatitis B virus (HBV), hepatitis C virus (HCV) and HIV are three major blood-borne viruses (BBVs) that are transmitted through NSI. The risk of transmission is highest for HBV (30%) followed by HCV (3%) and HIV (0.3%).

POST-EXPOSURE MANAGEMENT

Steps of Post-exposure Management

The following are the sequential steps to be followed following an occupational exposure (Table 14.1):
1. **First aid:** First aid has to be started as early as possible (Table 14.2)
2. **Report to the designated nodal center:** Every hospital must have a nodal center for the management of NSI. In most hospitals, HICC office acts as a nodal center, other hospitals may designate staff clinic or casualty for the purpose. Nodal centers perform the following functions as mentioned below (steps 3–9)
3. **Take first dose of PEP for HIV:**
   - The first dose of PEP for HIV should be taken as early as possible. Effect is maximum if taken <2 hours and effect is nil if taken after 72 hours of exposure
   - **NACO recommendation:** The first dose regimen comprises of a fixed-dose combination of five tablets; given on the first day of exposure
     - Tenofovir 300 mg + Lamivudine 300 mg, one tablet once daily and
     - Lopinavir (200 mg) + Ritonavir (50 mg) two tablets twice daily.
   - If the HIV negative status of the source is documented in patient's case record or in the hospital information system, then the first dose of PEP is not required
   - If test report is not available, then administer the first dose regimen immediately without waiting for the laboratory result.
4. **Testing for BBVs:** The following tests are done for both source and HCW. The test format should be a rapid method (immunochromatographic test or flow

Table 14.1: Steps of post-exposure management.

1. First aid
2. Report to designated nodal center
3. Take first dose of PEP for HIV
4. Testing for BBVs
5. Decision on PEP for HIV and HBV
6. Documentation and recording of exposure
7. Informed consent and counseling
8. Follow-up testing of HCWs
9. Precautions during the follow-up period

Abbreviations: PEP, post-exposure prophylaxis; HCW, healthcare worker; BBV, blood-borne virus.

Table 14.2: First Aid: Management of exposed site.

Do's	Don'ts
Earlier the first aid, lesser is the chance of transmission of BBVs	• Do not panic
• For splash injury: Irrigate thoroughly the site (e.g., eyes or mouth or other exposed area) vigorously with water at least for 5 minutes	• Do not place the pricked finger into the mouth reflexively
• Spit fluid out immediately if gone into mouth and rinse the mouth several times	• Do not squeeze blood from wound
• If wearing contact lenses, leave them in place while irrigating. Once the eye is cleaned, remove the contact lens and clean them in a normal manner	• Do not use antiseptics and detergents

through assay) and result should be available within 1–2 hours
- Anti-HIV antibody detection
- HBsAg detection
- Anti-HCV antibody detection
- Anti-HBs antibody (done for HCW if previously vaccinated for HBV and titer not tested).

HCW's baseline status is determined because later it may be difficult to attribute whether the infection was acquired due to this occupational exposure or any other prior exposure. This may guide while taking a decision, when the HCW claims for compensation from the health authorities.

5. **Decision on post-exposure prophylaxis** (PEP) for HIV and HBV is taken based on standard guidelines (NACO for HIV and CDC for HBV) as described in Tables 14.3 and 14.4 respectively
6. **Informed consent and counseling:** Almost every person feels anxious after exposure. They should be counseled and provided with psychological support
   - They should be informed about the risks and benefits of PEP medications
   - PEP is not mandatory. If the exposed person refuses to take the PEP, it should be documented. However, he should be made to understand about the risk

Table 14.3: Revised NACO Guidelines for post-exposure prophylaxis (PEP), 2018.

Exposure code (EC)	Source HIV status code (SC)	PEP Recommendation
1, 2 or 3	Negative	Not warranted
1	1	Not warranted
1	2	PEP is recommended
2	1	Duration of PEP: 28 days
2	2	**Primary TL+LR regimen*:** Regimen comprises of fixed dose combination of five tablets to be taken every day.
3	1 or 2	• Tenofovir (300 mg) + Lamivudine (300 mg), one tablet once daily and
2 or 3	Unknown (in area with high prevalence)	• Lopinavir (200 mg) + Ritonavir (50 mg) two tablets twice daily
		Alternative TLE regimen: Fixed dose combination of tenofovir (300 mg)+ Lamivudine (300 mg) + Efavirenz (600 mg), one tablet once daily

Exposure code:
1. **EC-1 (Mild exposure):** Mucous membrane/non-intact skin exposure with small volumes, or less duration
2. **EC-2 (Moderate exposure):**
   - Mucous membrane/non-intact skin with large volumes/splashes for several minutes or more duration OR
   - Percutaneous superficial exposure with solid needle or superficial scratch
3. **EC-3 (Severe exposure):** Percutaneous exposure with:
   - Large volume transfer
   - By hollow needle, wide bore needle or deep puncture
   - Visible blood on device
   - Needle used in patient's artery or vein

Source HIV Status Code (SC):
1. **SC-1:** HIV positive, asymptomatic or low viral load (<400 copies/mL)
2. **SC-2:** HIV positive, symptomatic (advanced AIDS or primary HIV infection), high viral load
3. **SC Unknown:** Status of the patient is unknown and neither the patient nor his/her blood is available for testing
4. **HIV negative:** Tested negative according to NACO strategy

The first dose of PEP
Should be started within 2 hours (for greater impact) and definitely within 72 hours.

Side effects and compliance to PEP:
- Common side effects are: Nausea, diarrhea, myalgia, headache or fatigue, anemia and leukopenia
- **PEP should never be discontinued** as compliance of >95% to the PEP schedule is required to maximize the efficacy of PEP.

*Regimen for exposure in pregnant women is essentially same as that of non-pregnant persons.
Abbreviations: NACO, National AIDS Control Organization; ART, antiretroviral therapy.

Table 14.4: Post-exposure prophylaxis (PEP) for hepatitis B.

HCW status	If source is positive or unknown for HBsAg	If source is negative for HBsAg
If the exposed person is completely vaccinated and the antibody titer is protective (≥10 mIU/mL)	No further treatment is required: • Regardless of the HBV status of the source* • Regardless if the titer falls down later*	
If the exposed person is completely vaccinated and the titer is not protective (<10 mIU/mL)	HBIG-1 dose should be started immediately; maximum within 7 days Vaccine: Start the second series (3 doses)	Vaccine: Start the second series (3 doses)
If the exposed person is not vaccinated or partially vaccinated	HBIG-1 dose should be started immediately; maximum within 7 days Vaccine: Complete the vaccine series from the last dose given (do not restart)	Vaccine: Complete the vaccine series from the last dose given (do not restart)
Nonresponders (If the exposed person is vaccinated for 2 series, i.e., 6 doses and the titer is not protective)	HBIG-2 doses at 1 month apart (0.06 mL/kg or 10–12 IU/kg)	Nothing is required

Note:
- HCW is said to be protected when titer rises (anti-HBs ≥10 mIU/mL), after three or more doses of vaccination. Rise of titer after one or two doses of vaccine should not be considered as protective.
- HCWs who are not protected must be checked for their HBsAg status at baseline and follow-up testing 6 months later, regardless of their vaccination status.
- Anti-HBs antibody titer should be checked only after 2 months of last dose of vaccine and 6 months after HBIG administration; otherwise, it will give erratic results.
- HBIG and HBV vaccine can be administered simultaneously but at different sites.
- HBIG provides a temporary protection for 3–6 months.
- Previous report of Anti-HBs titer is acceptable only if it is documented. Verbal reports should not be considered.

* In a previously protected person, the memory B cells will start producing antibodies soon after the antigenic challenge, hence revaccination by booster doses is not recommended even if the titer falls down later.
Adapted from CDC guideline, 2013.
Abbreviations: HBIG, hepatitis B immunoglobulin; HCW, healthcare worker; HBsAg, hepatitis B surface antigen.

of acquiring infection if PEP is not taken.
7. **Documentation and recording of exposure:**
   - A *structured proforma* should be used to collect the detail information related to exposure, such as date, time, and place of exposure, type of procedure done, type of exposure, duration of exposure, source status, volume and type of specimen involved
   - *Consent form:* For prophylactic treatment, the exposed person must sign a consent form. If the individual refuses to initiate PEP, it should be documented. The designated officer for PEP should keep this document.
8. **Follow-up testing** of HCWs for BBVs should be done if the source status is positive/unknown
   - *HIV testing follow-up is done:* At 6 weeks, 3 months and 6 months after exposure
   - HBV and HCV follow-up testing is done at 6 months after exposure.
9. **Precautions during the follow-up period:** If the source status is positive/unknown, then the following precautions should be adopted by the HCW during the follow-up period, especially the first 6–12 weeks
   - Refraining from blood, semen, organ donation
   - Abstinence from sexual intercourse or use of latex condom till both baseline and 3 months HIV tests are found negative
   - Women should not breastfeed their infants
   - The exposed person is advised to seek medical evaluation for any febrile illness that occurs within 12 weeks of exposure.

CHAPTER 15

Environmental Surveillance

The various environmental sources from which microorganisms can be transmitted to patients and healthcare workers include water, air and environmental surfaces. Therefore, monitoring of microbiological quality of water, air and surfaces are of paramount importance for safe hospital environment.

■ WATER SURVEILLANCE

Problem Solving Exercise

Water Surveillance
Water surveillance was performed in a newly constructed ICU of a tertiary care hospital and the result is shown in Figure 15.2. Interpret the result using McCrady statistical Table (Table 15.3). Discuss the procedure of this test. What is the further test advised to perform.

Explanation
❏ The test performed in Fig. 15.2 is a **multiple tube method**, performed on an unpolluted water sample. It shows positive result for one 50 mL tube and two numbers of 10 mL tubes.

When matched with McCrady statistical Table (Table 15.3), the **presumptive coliform count** (MPN) is estimated as 6 coliforms per 100 mL water sample. The quality of water supply is of 'Intermediate quality' (Table 15.4).
❏ **Differential Coliform Count (Eijkman Test)** needs to be performed to find out whether the organism is thermotolerant *E. coli*. If tested positive, the quality of water supply is reported as 'unsatisfactory'.

Microbial contamination of water in healthcare settings is broadly of two types.
1. **Enteric pathogens:** This results from fecal contamination of drinking water supplies. Most of them cause diarrheal outbreaks. These include **bacteria** (*Salmonella, Shigella, Vibrio cholerae*), **viruses** (rotavirus, and others), **parasites** (*Entamoeba histolytica, Giardia* and others)
2. **Common hospital pathogens:** These include multidrug resistant gram-negative bacilli, legionellae, etc., commonly present in hospital environment; can contaminate various hospital water supplies and can lead to waterborne outbreaks in healthcare settings.

The methods employed for detection of microbial contamination of water must have capability to detect both the category of pathogens (Table 15.1).

Test of Drinking Water Contaminated with Enteric Pathogens

Hospital drinking water should be regularly tested to confirm that they are free from contamination with enteric pathogens. As enteric pathogens (*Salmonella, Shigella*)

Table 15.1: Microbiological testing methods for water analysis.

Bacteriological examination	Indications
Multiple-tube method	• Extensively used for drinking water analysis • For highly turbid samples
Membrane filtration method	• For testing dialysis water • For testing clean water, where the bacterial count in water is expected to be low • For testing large volume of water

Table 15.2: Indicator organisms of fecal pollution of water.

Indicator organisms	Interpretation
	Presence in water indicates:
Coliform (other than *Escherichia coli*)	Remote contamination—either by fecal (presumptive) or soil and vegetation
Fecal (thermotolerant) *Escherichia coli*	Confirms recent fecal contamination of water; most sensitive indicator
Other indicators	Less reliable, such as Fecal streptococci, *Clostridium perfringens*, *Pseudomonas aeruginosa*

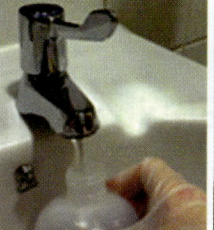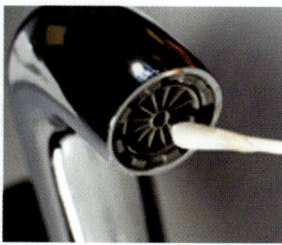

Fig. 15.1: Water sampling methods.

are usually present in small quantity, it is impracticable to detect the presence of all types. Instead, the water supplies are tested for those microorganisms which indicate that fecal contamination has taken place (**indicator organisms**) (Table 15.2).

Indicator Organisms

Indicator organisms are usually the commensal bacteria of intestine which satisfy two properties:
1. They should be present in excess number than any pathogen so that they can be detected easily; at the same time, they should not be able to proliferate in water to any extent
2. They should be more resistant than the pathogens to the stresses of aquatic environment and disinfection processes.

Mere presence of these indicator organisms does not assure the presence of water borne pathogens; but their presence in water supplies indicates that there is a contamination of sewage and the water supplies needs to be disinfected.

There are a number of intestinal commensals, used as indicator organisms as enlisted in Table 15.2.

Collection and Transport of Water Sample

Water specimen should be collected in a screw-capped wide sterile container.
- **Volume:** At least 150–200 mL of water should be collected
- **Neutralizer:** Sodium thiosulfate is added to neutralize the bactericidal effect of residual chlorine present in water if any
- **Sampling points** in hospitals must represent different sources from which water is obtained, such as portable water from pipelines, endoscopy rinse water, dialysis water, dental chair unit waterline, etc.
- **Sampling method from the tap:** Care should be taken while collecting water to minimize extraneous contamination. Hand washing should be performed and gloves should be worn before collection (Fig. 15.1)
- **Tap swabs:** Sterile swab is inserted into the nozzle of the tap carefully, without touching the outer tap surface. The swab is then rubbed around, i.e., moved backwards and forwards and up and down, as much as possible, on the inside surface of the tap outlet or flow straightener (Fig. 15.1).

Multiple-tube Method

It is the most common method used for water surveillance. It is so named as it involves mixing of specific volume of water samples to multiple tubes containing a special culture medium—MacConkey purple broth.
- **Procedure:** Most of the hospital water supplies are non-turbid and unpolluted. As per WHO guideline, for testing of unpolluted water samples the following method should be followed (Fig. 15.2)
  - 50 mL of water is added to one tube having 50 mL of culture medium
  - 10 mL of water is added to each of five tubes containing 10 mL of culture medium.
- **Positive result:** After incubated for 24–48 hours, the medium turns to yellow from purple (due to lactose fermentation), along with turbidity of the medium and gas collected in the Durham's tube
- **Determination of MPN:** The number of tubes giving positive reaction is compared

CHAPTER 15 ❖ Environmental Surveillance

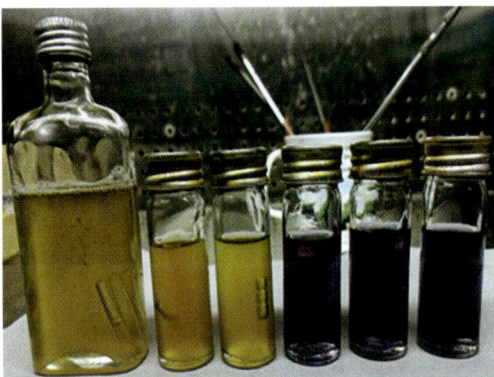

Fig. 15.2: MacConkey purple broth for multiple tube method (one 50 mL and five 10 mL tubes are needed for testing unpolluted water); if negative, media appears purple; if positive, media turn yellow.
Source: Department of Microbiology, JIPMER, Puducherry (*with permission*).

with McCrady statistical table (Table 15.3) to determine the most probable number (MPN) of coliform count present per 100 mL of water. This is called as presumptive coliform count.

For example: As shown in Figure 15.2, multiple tube method performed on an unpolluted water sample gives positive result for one 50 mL tube and two numbers of 10 mL tubes. When matched with Table 15.3, the presumptive coliform count (MPN) is estimated as 6 coliforms per 100 mL water sample

❖ **Quality of water supply:** Depending upon the MPN/100 mL, the quality of the water specimen can be interpreted as excellent, satisfactory, intermediate or unsatisfactory (Table 15.4).

Differential Coliform Count (Eijkman Test)

Detection of coliform bacteria does not always indicate fecal contamination as some of them may be found in environment. Hence, it is further tested by differential coliform count to detect the fecal *E. coli*. This is done by sub-culturing the positive tubes (from the multiple tube method) on lactose containing medium, such as brilliant green bile broth for:
❖ Detection of lactose fermentation with the production of acid and gas at 44°C and
❖ Demonstrating a positive indole test at 44°C.

Table 15.3: MPN values per 100 mL of sample for non-polluted/treated water samples (McCrady statistical table).

No. of tubes giving a positive reaction out of		MPN per 100 mL of water
1 of 50 mL	5 of 10 mL	
0	0	<1
0	1	1
0	2	2
0	3	4
0	4	5
0	5	7
1	0	2
1	1	3
1	2	6
1	3	9
1	4	16
1	5	>18

Table 15.4: Classification of quality of drinking water supply.

Quality of drinking water supply	Most probable number (MPN)/100 mL of water	
	Coliform count/ 100 mL	Thermotolerant *E. coli* count/ 100 mL
Excellent	0	0
Satisfactory	1–3	0
Intermediate	4–9	0
Unsatisfactory	≥10	≥1

Membrane Filtration Method

This method is based on the filtration of a known volume (e.g., 100 mL) of water through a cellulose membrane of pore size 0.2 or 0.45 μm. It is the recommended method for—(1) testing dialysis water, (2) for testing clean water, where the bacterial count in water is expected to be low and (3) for testing a large volume of water. However, It is not suitable for turbid water.

Test of Water Contaminated with Healthcare Associated Pathogens

Most of the healthcare associated pathogens are recovered by membrane filtration method, followed by plating on to a suitable culture medium, e.g., *Legionella,* on to buffer charcoal yeast extract (BCYE) medium.

Endotoxin Detection

Dialysis water, devices, etc. contaminated with endotoxin can cause serious toxic effects.

Therefore, the dialysis water used for hemodialysis is tested for presence of endotoxin.
- **Method:** Gel clot assay (Limulus amebocyte lysate assay)
- **Permissive level:** Water used to prepare dialysate and to reprocess hemodialyzers should contain endotoxin unit <0.25 EU/mL.

AIR SURVEILLANCE

Air is an important vehicle of transmission of many pathogenic organisms. Therefore, the examination of air to detect the number of bacteria carrying particles is important particularly in critical areas, such as operation theaters (OTs), bone marrow transplant units, etc.

Indication (CDC Recommendations)

Routine air sampling (i.e., random or periodic sampling) is not recommended. CDC recommends targeted air surveillance, which should be carried out for the following indications:
- Investigation of an outbreak
- For research purpose
- After reconstruction or newly constructed buildings
- After fogging (to monitor the quality)
- For short-term evaluation of a change in infection control practice.

Evaluation of the Quality of Air in OT

Evaluation of the quality of air includes both microbiological and non-microbiological (physical) parameters.

Microbiological Parameters

There are two principle means of monitoring the microbiological parameters present in the air, passive monitoring and active sampling.

Passive Monitoring (Settle Plate) Method

Standard Petri dishes containing culture media (e.g., blood agar) are exposed to the air for a given time and then the plates are incubated at 37°C for 24 hours aerobically.

1,1, 1 method: Here, the plates are placed at different locations in the OT one meter away from the side walls, one meter above the floor and for a duration of one hour.

Active Monitoring (Slit Sampler Method)

In active monitoring, a microbiological air sampler (e.g., sieve impactor) is used. It has a vacuum pump, and a perforated lid (Fig. 15.3B), in which an agar plate can be placed.
- The vacuum pump physically draws a known volume of air through the perforated lid and allows it to impact on the agar plate (e.g., blood agar)
- Following incubation, the quantity of microorganisms present in the culture plate is measured in terms of CFU/m^3 of air (Fig. 15.3A)
- Active monitoring is applicable when the concentration of microorganisms is not very high, such as in an operating theater, bone marrow transplant unit, etc.

Air Particle Counters

Air particle counters have been developed recently, that are capable of detecting airborne particles containing microorganisms in real time.

Non-microbiological Parameters

The number of bacteria in air at any given point of time depends upon various non-microbiological parameters, such as air changes per hour,

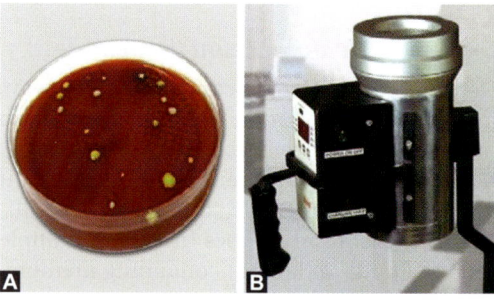

Figs 15.3A and B: (A) Air sampler method showing blood agar with bacterial colonies; (B) Air sampler (HiMedia).
Source: Department of Microbiology, JIPMER, Puducherry *(with permission).*

air velocity, positive pressure environment, temperature and relative humidity inside OT, etc. Therefore, there should be periodic monitoring of these parameters.

SURFACE SURVEILLANCE

Environmental surface sampling has been used to determine (a) reservoirs of potential environmental pathogens, and (b) the sources of the environmental contamination.

- **Locations:** It is required for high-risk locations, such as operation theaters and ICU settings
- **Sites for sampling (high touch areas):** Surface sampling is taken from sites where there is high-risk of contaminations
- **Indications (CDC recommendation):**
  - Surface sampling is currently indicated for research, as a part of an epidemiologic investigation, or during an outbreak investigation
  - Routine periodic surface surveillance is not recommended.
- **Method:** Moistened sterile swabs (soaked in sterile saline) are used to collect the samples from high-risk areas and then inoculated on to blood agar for the recovery of aerobic bacteria
- **Reporting:** Only pathogenic organisms isolated are reported. A semi-quantitative report (as heavy, moderate or light growth) should be provided. Contaminants, such as aerobic spore bearers are not reported.

SECTION 2

Systemic Microbiology (Infectious Diseases)

SECTION OUTLINE

16. Cardiovascular System Infections: Infective Endocarditis and Acute Rheumatic Fever
17. Bloodstream Infections
18. Bacterial Infections of Bloodstream: Enteric Fever, Scrub Typhus, Brucellosis, and Leptospirosis
19. Viral Infections of Bloodstream: HIV/AIDS and Dengue
20. Parasitic Infections of Bloodstream: Malaria, Visceral Leishmaniasis and Lymphatic Filariasis
21. Fungal Infections of Bloodstream: Systemic Candidiasis and Systemic Mycoses
22. Bacterial Diarrhea: Shigellosis, Cholera and Others
23. Viral Gastroenteritis: Rotaviruses and Others
24. Intestinal Protozoan Infections: Intestinal Amoebiasis, Giardiasis and Coccidian Parasitic Infections
25. Intestinal Helminthic Infections
    - Intestinal Cestode Infections: Intestinal Taeniasis, Hymenolepiasis and Others
    - Intestinal Trematode Infections: *Fasciolopsis buski*, *Schistosoma mansoni* and Others
    - Intestinal Nematode Infections: Trichuriasis, Enterobiasis, Ascariasis, Hookworm Infection, Strongyloidiasis

26. Viral Hepatitis
27. Parasitic Infections of Hepatobiliary System: Amoebic Liver Abscess, Hydatid Disease and Others
28. Staphylococcal Infections
29. Beta-hemolytic Streptococcal Infections
30. Miscellaneous Bacterial Infections of Skin and Soft Tissues: Anaerobic Infections including Gas Gangrene, Leprosy and Anthrax
31. Viral Exanthems and Other Cutaneous Viral Infections: Herpes Simplex, Measles, Rubella and Others
32. Superficial and Subcutaneous Fungal Infections
33. Bacterial Pharyngitis: *Streptococcus pyogenes* Pharyngitis and Diphtheria
34. Bacterial Pneumonia: Pneumococcal Pneumonia, *Haemophilus influenzae* Pneumonia, *Klebsiella pneumoniae* Pneumonia and Others
35. Tuberculosis
36. *Pseudomonas* and *Acinetobacter* Infections
37. Viral Infections of Respiratory Tract: Influenza, COVID-19, Infectious Mononucleosis, and Others
38. Parasitic and Fungal Infections of Respiratory Tract: Paragonimiasis, Zygomycosis, Aspergillosis, Pneumocystosis and Others
39. Bacterial Meningitis
40. Viral Meningitis and Viral Encephalitis (Enteroviruses including Polio, Rabies, Japanese Encephalitis and Others)
41. Parasitic and Fungal Infections of Central Nervous System: Neurocysticercosis, Free-living Amoebae Infections, Toxoplasmosis, Cryptococcal Meningitis and Others
42. Urinary Tract Infections
43. Infective Syndromes of Genital Tract (Sexually-transmitted Infections) : Syphilis, Gonorrhoea, Non-gonococcal Urethritis (*Chlamydia trachomatis*), Vulvovaginitis (Trichomoniasis, Vaginal Candidiasis) and Others
44. AETCOM in Microbiology
45. University Practical Examination

Cardiovascular System Infections: Infective Endocarditis and Acute Rheumatic Fever

CHAPTER 16

▮ INTRODUCTION

Cardiovascular system infections include infections of heart and blood vessels.
- ❖ **Infections of heart:** This includes infection of the three layers of the heart wall endocarditis, myocarditis and pericarditis
- ❖ **Infections of blood vessels**: Infections of blood vessels include mycotic aneurysm, and infective endarteritis
- ❖ **Device-related infections:** These include CRBSI (catheter-related bloodstream infection) and suppurative thrombophlebitis
- ❖ **Autoimmune-mediated:** Acute rheumatic fever.

▮ INFECTIVE ENDOCARDITIS

Infective endocarditis (IE) refers to microbial invasion of the heart valves or mural endocardium—characteristically results in formation of bulky friable *vegetations*, composed of mass of platelets, fibrin, microcolonies of organisms, and scanty inflammatory cells.

Problem Solving Exercise 1

Infective Endocarditis

A 75-year-old man was hospitalized with fever (101°F), severe back-pain and weakness in lower limbs. On examination, few non-tender, small erythematous nodular lesions on soles were seen. Echocardiogram showed valvular vegetations on mitral valve. He was diagnosed to have a cardiac valve vegetations 3 years back. Laboratory tests showed CRP 2.5 mg/dL, ESR 66 mm/h, leukocytes 15.6×10^9/L and creatinine 4.6 mg/dL. Two pairs of blood cultures were sent in BacT/ALERT bottles; both flagged positive. The smear made from BacT/ALERT broth and subculture done on blood agar have been depicted in the Figures 16.1A and B. The patient was immediately started on benzyl penicillin.
1. What is the probable clinical diagnosis?
2. What are the typical etiological agents of this clinical condition?
3. Describe the diagnostic criteria used for this condition.
4. How will you collect specimen for this clinical condition?

Explanation

This is a case of Infective endocarditis, caused by viridans streptococci

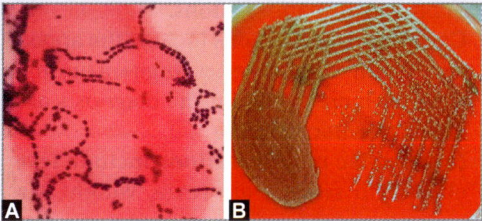

Figs 16.1A and B: Viridans streptococci: (A) Gram-positive cocci in long chains; (B) α-hemolytic colonies on blood agar.
Source: Department of Microbiology, Pondicherry Institute of Medical Sciences, Puducherry (*with permission*).

- ❑ The **typical agents of IE** include: Viridans streptococci, *Streptococcus gallolyticus*, HACEK group, *Staphylococcus aureus* or enterococci
- ❑ **Modified Duke criteria** is the diagnostic criteria applied in this clinical condition—two major criteria and two minor criteria are fulfilled here.
  - ➢ *Major criteria 1:* Blood culture criterion is fulfilled. The smear made from BacT/ALERT broth showed gram-positive cocci in chain (Fig. 16.1A) and subculture on blood agar grew minute, α-hemolytic colonies (Fig. 16.1B). This finding is suggestive of viridans streptococci.

Optochin susceptibility test can be performed to rule out pneumococcus. MALDI-TOF can be performed for species identification
- *Major criteria 2:* Echocardiogram showed valvular vegetations on mitral valve
- *Two minor criteria fulfilled are:* (1) Fever (101°F), (2) Vascular phenomena: few non-tender, small erythematous nodular lesions on soles, described as Janeway lesions

- **Collection specimen:** Blood cultures should be collected before starting antibiotic therapy
  - Two blood culture sets should be collected at an interval of >12 hr between 1st and 2nd set
  - Alternatively, three blood culture sets can be collected over one hour (e.g., 30 min gap between 1st and 2nd set and 30 min gap between 2nd and 3rd set)

Note: Blood culture set refers to 'pair of bottles'; collected from different venipuncture sites.

Classification

Infective endocarditis can be classified into acute and subacute forms based on rapidity of evolution, severity of infection and virulence of the implicated organism (Table 16.1).

Etiological Agents of IE

The causative organisms of IE differ depending on the underlying risk factors such as native or prosthetic valve IE, acute or subacute IE, other risk factors such as IV drug abuser (Table 16.2).

Clinical Manifestations

The clinical spectrum of IE includes both cardiac and noncardiac manifestations.
- ❖ **Cardiac manifestations** include the appearance of a new/worsened regurgitant murmur, which is more useful for the diagnosis of IE involving a normal valve
- ❖ **Noncardiac manifestations** include fever, chills and sweats, anorexia, weight loss, myalgia, arthralgia, arterial emboli, splenomegaly, clubbing, petechiae, neurologic manifestations and peripheral manifestations (Osler's nodes, subungual hemorrhages, Janeway lesions)
- ❖ **Laboratory manifestations** such as anemia, leukocytosis, microscopic hematuria, elevated erythrocyte sedimentation rate (ESR), C-reactive protein (CRP), or rheumatoid factor.

Table 16.1: Differences between acute and subacute endocarditis.

Acute endocarditis	Subacute endocarditis
Evolution is rapid	Evolution is slow
Involves normal cardiac valve	Involves previously damaged heart (scarred or deformed valve)
Implicated organism is of high virulence, e.g., *S. aureus*	Implicated organism is of low virulence, e.g., viridans streptococci
Causes substantial morbidity and mortality even with the appropriate antibiotic therapy and/or surgery	Follows a gradually progressive course of weeks to months; most patients recover after antibiotic therapy
Less common type, accounts for 10–20% of all cases	More common type, accounts for 50–60% of all cases

Table 16.2: Agents of infective endocarditis.

Etiological agents of infective endocarditis
• *Staphylococcus aureus:* Overall, the most common cause of IE
• Coagulase-negative staphylococci (e.g., *Staphylococcus epidermidis*): Associated with prosthetic valve endocarditis
• Streptococci (viridans streptococci and others): Most common cause of subacute bacterial endocarditis
• Enterococci: Associated with left-sided (mitral valve) endocarditis in IV drug abusers
• Pneumococci
• Fastidious gram-negative coccobacilli (HACEK* group), *Coxiella burnetii*, *Brucella* species, etc.)
• Enterobacteriaceae
• *Pseudomonas* spp. (usually in drug users)
• *Candida* species
• Diphtheroids

*HACEK, *Haemophilus* species, *Aggregatibacter* species, *Cardiobacterium hominis*, *Eikenella corrodens*, and *Kingella kingae*.

Diagnosis (Modified Duke Criteria)

The diagnosis of IE is established with the help of a highly sensitive and specific diagnostic schema—known as the **modified Duke criteria**; which is based on clinical, laboratory, and echocardiographic findings (Table 16.3).

Blood Cultures

Isolation of the causative microorganism from blood cultures is critical for diagnosis,

determination of antimicrobial susceptibility, and planning of treatment. Blood cultures should be collected before antibiotic therapy.
- Two blood culture sets should be collected at an interval of >12hr between 1st and 2nd set
- Alternatively, three blood culture sets can be collected over one hour (e.g., 30 min gap between 1st and 2nd set and 30 min gap between 2nd and 3rd set).

Note: Blood culture set refers to 'pair of bottles'; collected from different venipuncture sites.

A major criterion can be fulfilled (Table 16.3), if:
- A typical IE organism is isolated from two separate blood cultures, or
- Agent other than typical IE organisms is isolated persistently from blood cultures (Table 16.3) in the absence of an extracardiac focus of infection.

A minor criterion is considered to be fulfilled (Table 16.3) if blood cultures show positive but not meeting major criterion.

Blood culture collection technique and processing is discussed in detail in Chapter 17.

Non-blood-culture Tests

Various non-blood-culture tests that can be used for the diagnosis of IE include:
- Serologic tests can be used to implicate some organisms that are difficult to recover by blood culture: *Brucella, Bartonella, Legionella, Chlamydophila psittaci,* and *Coxiella burnetii*
- Isolation of the pathogens in vegetations by culture
- Direct fluorescence antibody techniques
- PCR to recover unique microbial DNA or 16S rRNA that, when sequenced, allows identification of the etiologic agent.

Echocardiography

Echocardiography allows anatomic confirmation of infective endocarditis, sizing of vegetations, detection of intracardiac complications, and assessment of cardiac function.

Treatment of Infective Endocarditis

1. **Regimen for *S. aureus* IE:**
   - For native valve IE: Cloxacillin or vancomycin is given for 6 weeks

Table 16.3: Modified Duke criteria for the clinical diagnosis of infective endocarditis.

Major Criteria

1. **Positive blood culture:** Any one of the following:
A. Typical IE organism isolated from two separate blood cultures (Viridans streptococci, *Streptococcus gallolyticus*, HACEK group, *S. aureus* or enterococci) or
B. Persistently positive blood culture with agents other than typical IE organisms:
  ➤ Blood culture sets drawn >12 h apart; or
  ➤ All of 3 sets or a majority of ≥4 separate blood cultures, with first and last drawn at least 1 h apart
C. Single positive blood culture for *Coxiella burnetii* or phase I IgG antibody titer of >1:800

2. **Evidence of endocardial involvement:** Any one
A. Positive echocardiogram
  ➤ Oscillating intracardiac mass on valve *or*
  ➤ Abscess, *or*
  ➤ New partial dehiscence of prosthetic valve
B. New valvular regurgitation

Minor Criteria
1. **Predisposition:** Predisposing heart conditions or IV drug use
2. **Fever** ≥ 38.0°C (≥100.4°F)
3. **Vascular phenomena:** Major arterial emboli, septic pulmonary infarcts, mycotic aneurysm, intracranial hemorrhage, conjunctival hemorrhages or Janeway lesions
4. **Immunologic phenomena:** Glomerulonephritis, Osler's nodes, Roth's spots or rheumatoid factor
5. **Microbiologic evidence:** Positive blood culture but not meeting major criterion as noted previously[a] or serologic evidence of active infection with organism consistent with infective endocarditis

Definite endocarditis if the followings are present:
- Two major criteria or
- One major criterion and three minor criteria or
- Five minor criteria

[a]Excluding single positive blood cultures for coagulase-negative staphylococci and diphtheroids, which are common culture contaminants, and organisms that do not cause endocarditis frequently, such as gram-negative bacilli.

Abbreviation: IE, infective endocarditis.

- For prosthetic valve IE: In addition to the above regimen, rifampin (for 6 weeks) and gentamicin (for 2 weeks) are added.

2. **Regimen for Viridans Streptococci and *S. gallolyticus* IE**
   - For native valve IE: Penicillin or ceftriaxone is given for 4 weeks
   - For prosthetic valve IE: Gentamicin is added for 6 weeks

ACUTE RHEUMATIC FEVER

Problem Solving Exercise 2

Acute Rheumatic Fever

A 8-year-old female child presented to the cardiology OPD with swollen, red, and/or tender joints, which migrates from one joint to another (knees, ankles, hips, and elbows) over a period of hours. The child was having an abnormal gait. She also complained of painless, small, mobile lumps beneath the skin overlying bony prominences, particularly of the hands, feet, and elbows. On auscultation of CVS, murmur was heard over the mitral valve area. ECG showed prolongation of P-R interval. On inquiry, it was found that the child had an episode of sore throat 3 weeks back.
1. What is the probable clinical diagnosis and its etiological agent?
2. Describe the diagnostic criteria used for this clinical condition.
3. How will you prevent recurrence of such episodes?

Explanation

This is a case of Acute Rheumatic Fever; which occurred as a sequel to streptococcal sore throat

Modified Jones criteria is the diagnostic criteria applied in this condition—four major criteria and one minor criteria are fulfilled here.
- *Major criteria fulfilled are:*
  - Migratory polyarthritis: Swollen, red, and/or tender joints, which migrates from one joint to another (knees, ankles, hips, and elbows) over a period of hours
  - Subcutaneous nodules: Painless, small, mobile lumps beneath the skin overlying bony prominences, particularly of the hands, feet, and elbows
  - Carditis: On auscultation, murmur was heard over the mitral valve area
  - Chorea: Child has abnormal gait
- Minor criterion fulfilled was: ECG showed prolongation of P-R interval.

Refer text for the explanation of other questions.

Acute rheumatic fever (ARF) is a multisystem disease that occurs in people previously affected with streptococcal (group A) sore throat, as a result of an autoimmune reaction.

- **Autoimmune mechanism:** Antibodies targeted against streptococcal antigens (M protein) during past episode of sore throat, cross react with human tissue antigens (e.g., heart and joint)
- Although ARF may involve many parts of the body, almost all the manifestations resolve completely; except the cardiac valvular damage, which is called as rheumatic heart disease (RHD).

Group A *Streptococcus* (*S. pyogenes*) principally causes infections of skin and soft tissues and pharyngitis (Chapter 29 and 33).

Clinical Manifestations

Primary ARF is mainly a disease of children, of 5–14 years age. The clinical manifestations usually appear after period of ~3 weeks following precipitating group A streptococcal infection. The prior streptococcal infection may be either subclinical (more common) or presents as sore throat.

Acute rheumatic fever affects heart, joints, skin and brain. The common manifestations in the order of frequency include:
- **Migrating polyarthritis:** It is the most common manifestation; affects the large joints—most commonly the knees, ankles, hips, and elbows
- **Pancarditis,** affecting endocardium, pericardium, or myocardium
- **Subcutaneous nodules:** Occur as painless, small, mobile lumps beneath the skin overlying bony prominences, particularly of the hands, feet, and elbows
- **Chorea (Sydenham's):** It is an abnormal involuntary movement disorder, mainly affecting head and limbs

Table 16.4: Diagnostic criteria for rheumatic fever—modified Jones criteria (2015).

Major criteria	
Low-risk population	**High-risk population**
Carditis (clinical or subclinical)	Carditis (clinical or subclinical)
Arthritis—only polyarthritis	Arthritis—monoarthritis or polyarthritis
	Polyarthralgia
Chorea	Chorea
Erythema marginatum	Erythema marginatum
Subcutaneous nodules	Subcutaneous nodules
Minor criteria	
Low-risk population	**High-risk population**
Polyarthralgia	Monoarthralgia
Hyperpyrexia (≥38.5ºC)	Hyperpyrexia (≥38.0ºC)
ESR ≥60 mm/h and/or CRP ≥3.0 mg/dL	ESR ≥30 mm/h and/or CRP ≥3.0 mg/dL
Prolonged PR interval	Prolonged PR interval
Diagnostic criteria	
Initial ARF	Two major or One major + two minor
Recurrent ARF (with a reliable past history of ARF/RHD)	Two major or One major + two minor or Three minor criteria

Abbreviations: ESR, erythrocyte sedimentation rate; CRP, C-reactive protein; ARF, acute rheumatic fever; RHD, rheumatic heart disease.

Note: The supporting evidence (of previous streptococcal infection), which was a part of previous version of Jones criteria (1992), has been removed from the new modified Jones criteria, 2015.

❖ **Erythema marginatum:** They are pink macular rashes that appear and disappear before the examiner's eyes.

Diagnosis of ARF (Jones Criteria)

The diagnosis of ARF is made based on diagnostic criteria known as revised Jones criteria (2015). It is based on the presence of a combination of typical clinical features together with ECG and laboratory (ESR, CRP) findings (Table 16.4).

Treatment

Penicillin is the drug of choice; can be given orally (as penicillin V for 10 days) or intramuscularly (as single dose of benzathine penicillin G).

Prevention

Primary Prevention

It includes timely and complete treatment of group A streptococcal sore throat with antibiotics (penicillin) within 9 days of sore throat onset, which will prevent almost all cases of ARF.

Secondary Prevention

The mainstay of controlling ARF and RHD is secondary prevention. Patients with ARF are at much higher risk of developing recurrent ARF. Therefore, long-term (5-10 yrs or even longer) penicillin prophylaxis is indicated to prevent recurrences.

CHAPTER 17

Bloodstream Infections

Problem Solving Exercise 1

Sepsis

A 42-year-old female presented with fever, chills and rigors, confusion, anxiety, difficulty in breathing, malaise and vomiting. On examination, the following signs were noticed: body temperature 102°F, heart rate 106 per minute and respiratory rate 24 per minute, blood pressure 90/60 mm of Hg. Urine output was significantly decreased.
1. What is the probable clinical diagnosis?
2. What scoring system is used to assess the severity of infection and extent of organ failure?
3. How will you collect the specimen?
4. Describe the laboratory diagnosis in detail.

Explanation

The provisional diagnosis in this case is sepsis; as it satisfies the bed side **qSOFA (Quick SOFA)** criteria— respiratory rate ≥22/min, altered mentation and systolic blood pressure ≤100 mm Hg

SOFA scoring system: Sepsis is clinically diagnosed by SOFA (sepsis-related organ failure assessment) score which in turn depends on six parameters:
1. Respiratory system (PaO2/FiO2)
2. Coagulation system (platelet count)
3. Liver (serum bilirubin)
4. Cardiovascular (mean arterial pressure)
5. CNS (Glasgow coma scale score)
6. Renal (serum creatinine and urine output).

Refer Table 17.1 for detail.
Collection of blood culture and laboratory diagnosis of sepsis is discussed in the text below.

▮ INTRODUCTION

Bloodstream infections (BSI) refer to the presence of microorganisms in blood, which constitute one of the most serious situations among infectious diseases; as they are a threat to every organ in the body.
- ❖ Microbial invasion of bloodstream can have serious immediate consequences such as shock, multiple organ failure, and DIC (disseminated intravascular coagulopathies)
- ❖ Therefore, timely detection of the causative agent is one of the most important goals of the microbiology laboratory.

Terminologies

The suffix 'emia' is derived from the Greek word meaning "blood" and refers to the presence of a substance in the blood.
- ❖ Bacteremia refers to the presence of bacteria in blood without any multiplication
- ❖ Septicemia is a condition in which bacteria circulate and actively multiply in the bloodstream and may produce their products (e.g., toxins) that cause harm to the host
- ❖ Similarly, the presence of viruses, parasites and fungi in blood can be described as 'viremia', 'parasitemia' and 'fungemia' respectively.

▮ CLINICAL MANIFESTATIONS

Bloodstream infections have a bacteremia stage followed by a septicemic stage. The clinical manifestations are evident only in the septicemic stage. In this stage, the bacteria multiply and release their products (e.g., toxins) which travel to various organs affecting their functions. Based on the severity and the extent of organ failure; bloodstream infection can be divided into two stages: sepsis and septic shock (Table 17.1).
- ❖ **Sepsis:** The common signs and symptoms include:

- Fever or hypothermia with/without chills and rigors
- Hyperventilation leads to excess loss of CO_2 and subsequent respiratory alkalosis
- Skin lesions, change of mental status and diarrhea.

❖ **Septic shock:** This is the gravest late stage complication of septicemia and is manifested as—hypotension, DIC and multiorgan failure (e.g., acute respiratory distress, renal failure, tissue destruction, etc.). The endotoxins of gram-negative bacteria have a direct effect on the pathogenesis of septic (or endotoxic) shock.

In sepsis, the severity and degree of organ failure can be determined by an assessment score called as SOFA (sepsis-related organ failure assessment) score Quick SOFA criteria (Table 17.1).

The common agents implicated in sepsis are gram-negative organisms such as *Escherichia coli, Klebsiella pneumoniae, Pseudomonas, Acinetobacter* and gram-positive cocci such as *Staphylococcus aureus* and *Enterococcus species*.

■ LABORATORY DIAGNOSIS

Diagnosis of bloodstream infection depends on the isolation of the causative agent from blood by performing blood culture.

Specimen Collection for Blood Culture

Extreme care should be taken while collection of blood for culture, as there is a high-risk of contamination with skin flora.

- ❖ **Site:** Blood for culture should always be collected in **pairs;** from two separate venipunctures and 2 separate skin decontamination processes. If a central line is present, then one sample from the central line and one from the venipuncture should be collected
- ❖ **Preparation of the site:** To avoid contamination with skin flora, blood should be collected under strict aseptic conditions using sterile disposable syringe (Fig. 17.1)
- ❖ **Skin decontamination:** Skin should be disinfected by two-step procedure—first, treated with 70% isopropyl alcohol and then a second antiseptic solution such as povidone iodine or chlorhexidine should be applied

Table 17.1: Definition of sepsis and the assessment of severity and organ failure.

Sepsis
Sepsis is defined as life-threatening organ dysfunction caused by a dysregulated host response to infection
SOFA score
Sepsis is diagnosed by SOFA (sepsis-related organ failure assessment) score which in turn depends on six parameters.   1. Respiratory system—PaO_2/FiO_2 2. Coagulation system—platelet count   3. Liver—serum bilirubin   4. Cardiovascular—mean arterial pressure (MAP)   5. Central nervous system—Glasgow coma scale score   6. Renal—serum creatinine and urine output   Organ dysfunction can be identified as an acute change in the total SOFA score ≥2 points following the infection
qSOFA (Quick SOFA) Criteria
Determination of SOFA score takes considerable time as it depends upon a number of laboratory parameters. However, before the result of SOFA score is available, sepsis can promptly be identified at the bedside with qSOFA score   • Respiratory rate ≥22/min   • Altered mentation   • Systolic blood pressure ≤100 mm Hg
Septic shock
It is a subset of sepsis in which underlying circulatory and cellular/metabolic abnormalities are profound. Patients with septic shock can be identified with a clinical construct of sepsis with: • Persisting hypotension requiring vasopressors to maintain MAP (mean arterial pressure) ≥65 mm Hg and   • Serum lactate level >2 mmol/L (18 mg/dL) despite adequate volume resuscitation   Patients with septic shock have a mortality of >40% in contrast to 10%, for sepsis cases

Note: PaO_2/FiO_2 is the ratio of arterial oxygen partial pressure to fractional inspired oxygen.

- The disinfectants should be applied in a circular motion (5 cm in diameter), starting from the center to the periphery
- The area should be allowed to air dry before venipuncture.

❖ **Timing of collection:** Blood should be collected before starting antimicrobial therapy. If the antimicrobial agent is already started, then the best time of collection is just before the next dose of the antimicrobial agent

❖ **Blood volume:** Blood specimen is drawn using a sterile syringe and needle. Higher

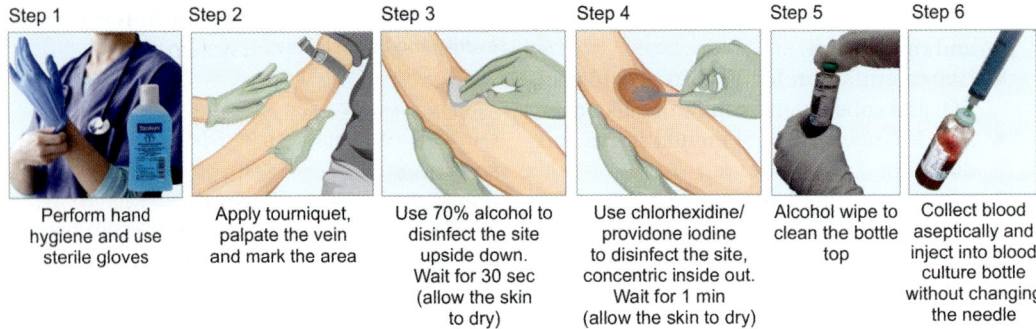

Fig. 17.1: Steps of collection of blood for culture.

the volume of blood, greater is the chance of isolation (yield increases by 3.2% per mL of blood cultured). At least **8–10 mL** of blood per bottle for an adult and **1–3 mL** per pediatric bottle is recommended

- **Number of blood cultures:** At least 2–3 blood culture sets (each set consists of two bottles: 1 aerobic and 1 anaerobic) are required to have good isolation rate (around 65%, 80% and 95% with one, two and three sets respectively). Multiple blood cultures should be collected for endocarditis cases
- **Dispensing:** Collected blood is then directly dispensed into either blood culture bottle at the bedside; either a conventional or automated blood culture. Change of needle between collection and dispensing, an old practice is no longer recommended
- **Transport of blood specimen:** The collected blood is gently mixed with the broth and then transported immediately to the Microbiology laboratory. In case of delay, blood culture bottle **should never be refrigerated**. It can be kept at 35°C in an incubator (if available) or left at room temperature.

- **Dilution:** The blood is inoculated in the medium at a dilution of 1:5 so that the antibacterial components in the blood, if any, will get diluted
- **SPS** (sodium polyanethol sulfonate) is added to the medium as an anticoagulant. It also counteracts the bactericidal action of blood
- **Incubation:** Upon receipt, the bottles should be directly incubated in the upright position at 37° C for up to 7 days
- **Repeat subcultures** are made from the BHI broth onto blood agar and MacConkey agar
  - **From monophasic medium:** Subcultures are made when the broth becomes turbid or periodically (blind subcultures) for one week. There is a risk of contamination due to opening of the cap of the bottle every time when subcultures are done

Conventional Culture Medium

The method used for the conventional blood culture is as follows (Refer Chapter 3.6).
- **Types of media:** There are two types of conventional blood culture media (Figs 17.2A and B)
  - Monophasic medium: It contains 50–100 mL of brain heart infusion (BHI) broth
  - Castaneda's biphasic medium: It consists of BHI agar slope and BHI broth (50 mL).

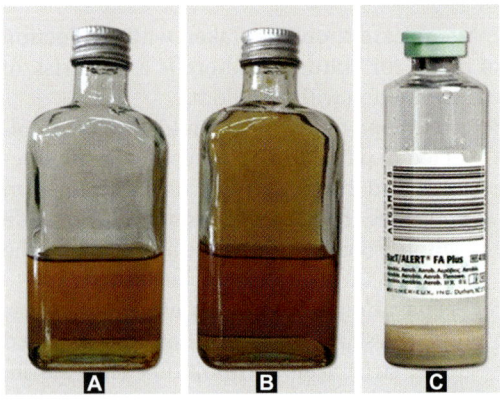

Figs 17.2A to C: Blood culture bottles: (A) Monophasic medium (BHI broth); (B) Biphasic medium (Castaneda's), containing BHI broth and BHI agar slant; (C) BacT/ALERT bottle.

Source: Department of Microbiology, JIPMER, Puducherry (*with permission*).

- **In biphasic medium,** the subcultures can be made just by tilting the bottles so that the broth runs over the agar slope. There is lower risk of contamination as it obviates the opening of the cap of the bottle. The colonies appear over the agar slant, which is further used for identification.

Automated Culture Media

BACTEC and BacT/ALERT are the automated blood culture systems. The most advanced system is Bact/ALERT Virtuo. In these systems, the growth is continuously monitored and reading is recorded every 15–20 min (Fig. 17.2C).

When the growth is detected, the system gives a positive signal. Then the bottle is removed and processed similarly as done for conventional bottles. Automated systems are much superior to conventional media in terms of faster isolation and increased sensitivity. More so, they also help in diagnosing catheter related bloodstream infection (CRBSI) by determining the differential time to positivity.

Identification

The isolated organism is identified by colony morphology, Gram staining, followed by either conventional biochemical reactions or automated identification system such as MALDI-TOF or VITEK.

Antimicrobial Susceptibility Test (AST)

Antimicrobial susceptibility test is carried out for guiding the institution of appropriate therapy. Minimum inhibitory concentration (MIC) based method (e.g., VITEK) is preferred over disk diffusion method when testing for blood isolates. It is ideal for endocarditis isolates, especially while reporting AST result of penicillin.

Treatment of Sepsis/Bloodstream Infection

Due to higher prevalence of multidrug resistant bacteria (MDROs) and higher mortality in sepsis, antibiotics should be instituted at the earliest, as soon as sepsis is clinically suspected. De-escalation approach is usually followed which means:

- ❖ Empirical treatment consists of higher class of antimicrobials with both gram-negative and gram-positive coverage; e.g., carbapenem such as meropenem plus vancomycin
- ❖ Definitive treatment can be tailored according to the culture sensitivity report.

Problem Solving Exercise 2

Catheter-related Bloodstream Infection (CRBSI)

A 42-year-old male on central line presented with fever (>103°F), altered mental status, heart rate of 102 per minute and respiratory rate of 24 breaths per minute. Blood was collected both from central line and venepuncture separately in BacT/ALERT bottles and sent for culture. Both central line and venepuncture bottles flagged positive for *Staphylococcus aureus* after 4 hours and 7 hours of incubation respectively. What is the clinical condition and how will you diagnose this condition?

Explanation

This is a case of CRBSI (catheter-related bloodstream infection) as the following criteria are met:
- ❑ Patient is on central line
- ❑ **Presence of signs of sepsis:** Fever with altered mental status, increased heart rate, respiratory rate.
- ❑ **Culture criteria** (differential time to positivity >2 hours): Culture of both central line and venepuncture blood specimens revealed the same pathogen (*Staphylococcus aureus*); with central line bottle flagged positive (at 4 hours of incubation) >2 hours earlier than the venepuncture bottle (flagged at 7 hours of incubation).

Bacterial Infections of Bloodstream: Enteric Fever, Scrub Typhus, Brucellosis, and Leptospirosis

CHAPTER 18

ENTERIC FEVER (TYPHOIDAL SALMONELLA)

Problem Solving Exercise 1

A 12-year-old boy was admitted with high-grade fever, abdominal pain, nausea, vomiting and anorexia for the past 5 days. On examination, tongue was coated and spleen was palpable. Blood specimen was collected for culture in automated culture bottle (Fig. 18.1C) and results of all the investigations done are shown in the Figures 18.2, 18.4 to 18.7 and Table 18.3.
- How will you collect the blood sample and send it to the laboratory for culture?
- Identify the test and interpret the result.
- Interpret the antimicrobial susceptibility test result and suggest the antibiotic to be used.
- Name two vaccines to prevent the infection.

Explanation

Clinical Diagnosis

Fever, abdominal discomfort for 5 days and palpable spleen in endemic area, such as India is suggestive of enteric fever.

In first week, blood culture is the investigation of choice. Blood specimen should be collected aseptically (Fig. 18.1C), preferably in automated blood culture bottle (if facilities are available).

Identification
- Positive blood culture bottles or conventional blood culture in biphasic media when subcultured on MacConkey agar reveals NLF colonies (Fig. 18.2).
- Biochemical reactions (Fig. 18.5) and agglutination with *Salmonella* polyvalent and O9 antisera suggests the identification as *Salmonella* Typhi (Fig. 18.6).

Antimicrobial Susceptibility Test

Antibiogram (Fig. 18.7 and Table 18.3) reveals the strain is sensitive to ceftriaxone, chloramphenicol, azithromycin, ampicillin and co-trimoxazole and intermediate to ciprofloxacin. Ceftriaxone being the drug of choice, should be the first line of treatment given.
(For answers to other questions, refer below.)

Clinical Manifestations of Enteric Fever

Enteric fever is a misnomer as the manifestations are more extraintestinal than intestinal. It is transmitted by ingestion of contaminated food or water. Various manifestations include:
- **Fever:** Described as step ladder pattern type of remittent fever
- **Other symptoms:** Headache, chills, cough, sweating, myalgia and arthralgia
- **Rashes** (called as *rose spots*)
- **Early intestinal manifestations,** such as abdominal pain, nausea, vomiting, anorexia, diarrhea or constipation and loss of appetite
- **Important signs** include hepatosplenomegaly, epistaxis and relative bradycardia
- **Complications:** Gastrointestinal bleeding and intestinal perforation can occur mostly in the third and fourth weeks of illness.
- **Neurologic manifestations** occur rarely which include meningitis, cerebellar ataxia and neuropsychiatric symptoms.

Laboratory Diagnosis

Specimen collection largely depends on the duration of illness (Table 18.1).

Culture

Blood Culture

Blood culture is the ideal method for diagnosis in the first week of fever, which becomes positive

Table 18.1: Tests used for diagnosis of enteric fever.

Duration of illness	Specimen used and test done

First week	• Culture of:
	  ➤ Blood
	  ➤ Bone marrow aspirate
	  ➤ Duodenal aspirate

Second week and Third week	• Serum:
	  ➤ For antibody detection by Widal test
	  ➤ For antigen detection
	• Stool and urine culture

Fourth week	Stool and urine culture
Carriers	• Stool and urine culture • Serum: For detection of antibodies to Vi antigen • Sewage culture—indirect way

in about 90% of cases. Thereafter, the positivity declines to 75% in the second week and 60% in the third week and 25% till the fever subsides.

❖ **Culture medium:** Blood culture bottles are the recommended media. There are two types of media:
1. Conventional blood culture media:
   ♦ Monophasic medium: Brain heart infusion (BHI) broth (Fig. 18.1A)
   ♦ Castaneda's biphasic medium: Consists of BHI agar slope and BHI broth (Fig. 18.1B)
2. Automated blood culture bottles: BACTEC or BacT/ALERT (Fig. 18.1C)

❖ **Procedure:** 10–20 mL of fresh blood is directly injected at the bedside through a hole present on the cap of the bottle rather than opening the bottle
❖ **Incubation:** Blood culture bottles are incubated at 37°C for 24 hours
❖ **Repeat subcultures:**
  ■ From monophasic medium: Repeat subcultures are made onto blood agar and MacConkey agar periodically for one week. There is a risk of contamination due to opening of the cap of the bottle every time when subcultures are made
  ■ Biphasic medium is preferred as the subcultures can be made just by tilting the bottles so that the broth runs over the agar slope. Bottle is incubated in the upright position. If colonies appear over the agar slant, it is used for further identification
  ■ From positive BacT/ALERT bottles subcultures are done.
❖ *Colony appearance*:
  ■ Blood agar: Nonhemolytic moist colonies
  ■ MacConkey agar: Colonies are round, translucent, pale and lactose nonfermenting (Fig. 18.2).

Stool and Urine Culture

This is useful for isolation of *Salmonella* in the third and fourth weeks of illness. They remain positive even after antibiotic treatment. Stool and urine culture are also done for detection of carriers.

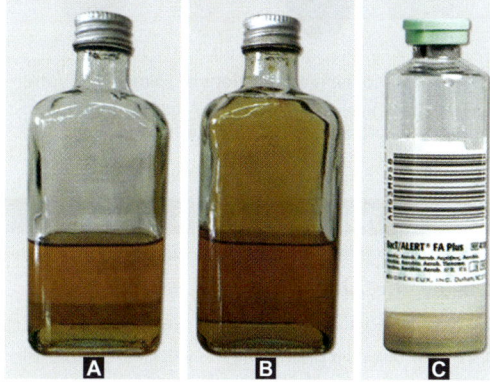

Figs 18.1A to C: Blood culture bottles: (A) Monophasic medium (BHI broth); (B) Biphasic medium (Castaneda's), containing BHI broth and BHI agar slant; (C) BacT/ALERT bottle.

Source: (A to C) Department of Microbiology, JIPMER, Puducherry (*with permission*).

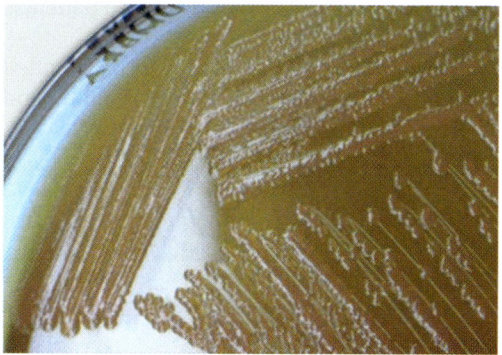

Fig. 18.2: MacConkey agar showing nonlactose fermenter colonies of *Salmonella.*

Source: Department of Microbiology, Pondicherry Institute of Medical Sciences, Puducherry (*with permission*).

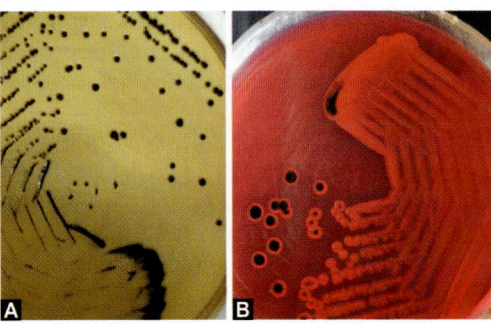

Figs 18.3A and B: Colonies of *S.* Typhi: (A) DCA (Deoxycholate citrate agar) showing pale colonies with black center; (B) XLD agar (Xylose lysine deoxycholate) showing red colonies with black center.
Source: Department of Microbiology, JIPMER, Puducherry (*with permission*).

- ❖ **Urine culture:** Urine is centrifuged and the deposit is inoculated onto MacConkey agar.
- ❖ **Stool culture** is done similar to that is followed for *Shigella*.
  - ■ **Enrichment broth,** such as Selenite F broth, tetrathionate broth and gram-negative broth are used
  - ■ **Selective media,** such as MacConkey agar and DCA or XLD are used.
    - ♦ DCA: It produces non-lactose-fermenting pale colonies with black center (Fig. 18.3A)
    - ♦ XLD agar: It produces red colonies with black center (Fig. 18.3B).

Other Specimens Include

- ❖ **Bone marrow** culture is useful during the first week of illness (55–90% sensitive); when blood culture is negative, especially when patient is on antibiotics
- ❖ **Duodenal aspirate** culture is recommended during first week of illness if both blood and bone marrow cultures turn negative.

Identification

In culture smear, *Salmonella* appear gram-negative bacilli (Fig. 18.4). Motility testing by hanging drop reveals that they are motile with peritrichous flagella.

Biochemical Identification (Fig. 18.5)

Two common enteric fever isolates (*S.* Typhi and *S.* Paratyphi A) show the following biochemical properties (Table 18.2).

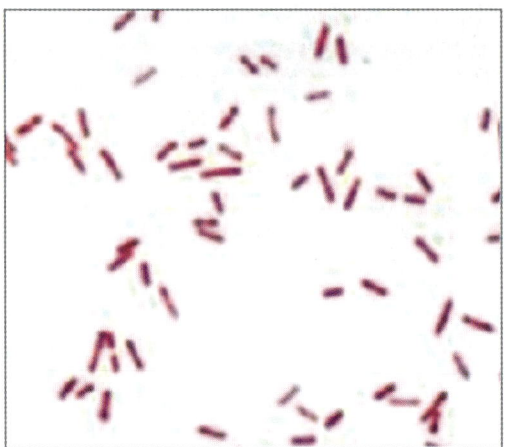

Fig. 18.4: Gram-stained smear showing gram-negative bacilli (*Salmonella*).
Source: Department of Microbiology, Pondicherry Institute of Medical Sciences, Puducherry (*with permission*).

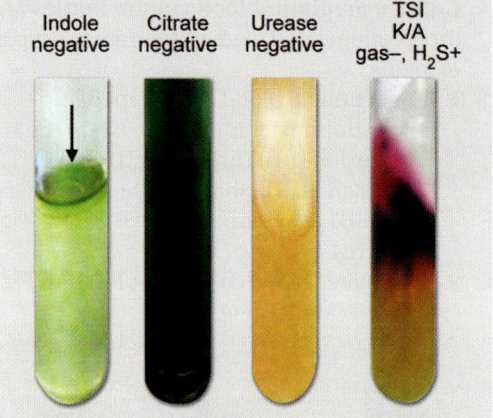

Fig. 18.5: Biochemical reactions of *Salmonella* Typhi.
Source: Department of Microbiology, Pondicherry Institute of Medical Sciences, Puducherry (*with permission*).

Table 18.2: ICUT reaction for *Salmonella*.

	S. Typhi	*S.* Paratyphi A
Indole	Negative	Negative
Citrate	Negative	Negative
Urease	Negative	Negative
TSI	Alkaline slant/acidic butt, gas absent, speck of H_2S present	Alkaline slant/acidic butt, gas present, H_2S absent

Slide Agglutination Test

Identification of *Salmonella* at genus level can be confirmed by slide agglutination using

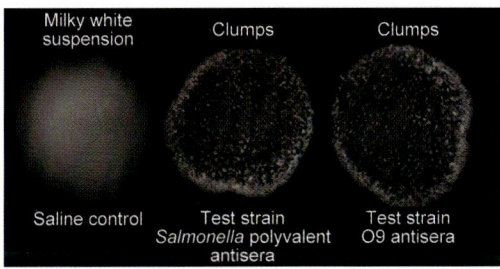

Fig. 18.6: Bacterial agglutination with antisera: Test strain is tested with *Salmonella* polyvalent antisera and then with O9 antisera. (Presence of clumps indicates test is positive and the stain is identified as *Salmonella* Typhi).
Source: Department of Microbiology, Pondicherry Institute of Medical Sciences, Puducherry (*with permission*).

polyvalent O antisera. Then, the serotypes can be identified by using type specific O antisera.
- *S.* Typhi: Agglutinates with O9 antisera (Fig. 18.6)
- *S.* Paratyphi A: Agglutinates with O2 antisera.

Antimicrobial susceptibility testing (Fig. 18.7): This is done on Mueller-Hinton agar by disk diffusion method (Table 18.3).

Widal Test (Detection of Antibodies)

Widal test is widely used serological tests for diagnosis of enteric fever. Also refer Problem Solving Exercise 3 of Chapter 7.
- **Principle:** It is an agglutination test where H and O antibodies against *S.* Typhi and *S.* Paratyphi A and B are detected.
- **Antigens used:** Four antigens are used.
  1. O antigen of *S.* Typhi (TO)
  2. H antigen of *S.* Typhi (TH)
  3. H antigen of *S.* Paratyphi A (AH)
  4. H antigen of *S.* Paratyphi B (BH).

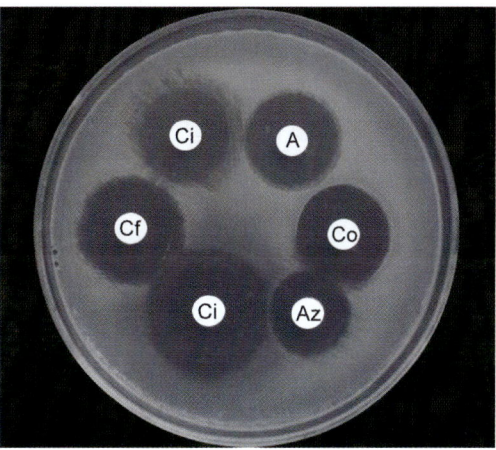

Fig. 18.7: Antimicrobial susceptibility testing on Mueller-Hinton Agar for *Salmonella* Typhi (Refer Table 18.3 for CLSI zone interpretation).
Abbreviations: Cf, ciprofloxacin; Ci, ceftriaxone; C, chloramphenicol; Az, azithromycin; A, ampicillin; Co, cotrimoxazole; CLSI, Clinical and Laboratory Standards Institute.
Source: Department of Microbiology, Pondicherry Institute of Medical Sciences, Puducherry (*with permission*).

(As the paratyphoid O antigens cross react with the typhoid O antigen due to their sharing of factor 12, hence, they are not used in the test.)
- **Procedure of Widal test:**
  - Patient's serum is serially diluted in normal saline in test tubes from 1 in 10 to 1 in 640 dilutions. Four such sets are made
  - To each set of diluted sera, respective four antigen suspensions are added
  - Control tubes containing the antigens and normal saline should be kept to check for auto-agglutination

Table 18.3: Interpretative categories (CLSI) and observed zone size diameter (mm) to various antimicrobial agents tested for *Salmonella* Typhi.

Antimicrobial agents	Disk strength (µg)	CLSI interpretative criteria for *Salmonella* Typhi (in mm)			Observed zone size (Fig.18.7) (in mm)	Interpretation
		Resistant	Intermediate	Sensitive		
Ciprofloxacin (Cf)	5	≤20	21–30	≥31	21	Intermediate
Ceftriaxone (Ci)	30	≤19	20–22	≥23	28	Sensitive
Chloramphenicol (C)	30	≤12	13–17	≥18	19	Sensitive
Azithromycin (Az)	15	≤12	-	≥13	16	Sensitive
Ampicillin (A)	10	≤13	14–16	≥17	19	Sensitive
Cotrimoxazole (Co)	1.25/23.75	≤10	11–15	≥16	20	Sensitive

Abbreviation: CLSI, Clinical and Laboratory Standards Institute.

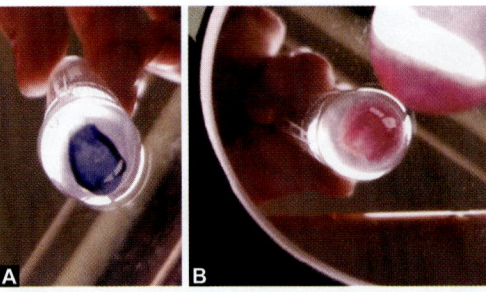

Figs 18.8A and B: O and H agglutination in Widal test reading taken in a mirror.
Source: Department of Microbiology, Pondicherry Institute of Medical Sciences, Puducherry (*with permission*).

- Test tubes are incubated in water bath at 37°C overnight.
- **Results:**
  - O agglutination appears as compact granular chalky clumps (disk-like pattern), with clear supernatant fluid (Fig. 18.8A)
  - H agglutination appears as large loose fluffy cotton-woolly clumps, with clear supernatant fluid (Fig. 18.8B)
  - If agglutination does not occur, *button* formation occurs due to deposition of antigens and the supernatant fluid remains hazy
  - *Titer*: The highest dilution of sera, at which agglutination occurs, is taken as the antibody titer.

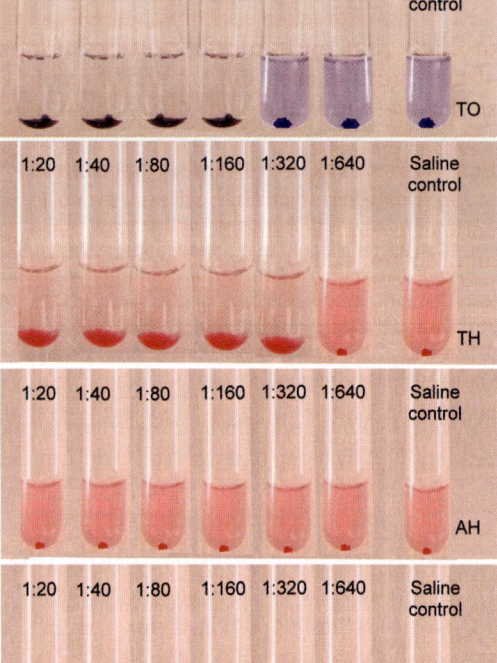

Fig. 18.9: Widal test (titer TO 1:160; TH 1: 320; AH <1:20; BH <1:20. Titer suggestive of enteric fever due to *S.* Typhi.
Source: Department of Microbiology, Pondicherry Institute of Medical Sciences, Puducherry (*with permission*).

Interpretation (Table 18.4 and Fig. 18.9):

- **Significant titer:** Higher titers are only significant. The cut-off varies from place to place depending on endemicity of the disease. Significant titer in most of the places in India is taken as:
  - H agglutinin titer >200 and
  - O agglutinin titer >100
- **False positive:** Widal test may occur due to:
  - **Anamnestic response:** It refers to a transient rise of titer due to unrelated infections (malaria, dengue) in persons who have had prior infection or immunization
  - Persons with inapparent infection or
  - Persons with prior immunization (with TAB vaccine).
- **Four-fold rise** in antibody titer demonstrated by testing paired sera at 1 week interval is more meaningful than a single high titer. Rise in titers in anamnestic responses are transient that usually fall down after 1 week whereas, in

Table 18.4: Interpretation of Widal test.

Widal test result	Suggestive of
Rise of TO and TH antibody (Fig. 18.9)	Enteric fever due to *S.* Typhi
Rise of TO and AH antibody	Enteric fever due to *S.* Paratyphi A
Rise of TO and BH antibody	Enteric fever due to *S.* Paratyphi B
Rise of only TO antibody	Recent infection—due to any serotype—*S.* Typhi or *S.* Paratyphi A or B
Rise of only TH antibody	? Convalescent stage/anamnestic response
Rise of all three TH, AH, BH antibodies	Post-TAB vaccination

true infection, the titer increases by four-fold after 1 week
- **False negative** Widal test may occur in:
  - Early stage (first week of illness)
  - Late stage (after fourth week)
  - Carriers
  - Patients on antibiotics
  - Due to prozone phenomena (antibody excess): This can be obviated by serial dilution of sera.
- **O agglutinins** appear early and disappear early and indicate recent infection. H agglutinins appear late and disappear late
- **O antibodies** are serotype nonspecific. They are raised in all infections, i.e., *S.* Typhi, *S.* Paratyphi A and B
- **H antibodies** are specific. TH, AH and BH antibodies are raised in *S.* Typhi, *S.* Paratyphi A and B infections, respectively.

Other Antibody Detection Tests

Various commercial methods available are:
- **Typhidot test:** OMP (outer membrane protein) antigen is used, detects both immunoglobulin (Ig) M and IgG antibodies
- **IDL Tubex test:** O9 antigen is used, detects only IgM antibodies against *S.* Typhi.

Demonstration of Serum Antigens

Antigens of typhoidal salmonellae are consistently present in the blood in the early course of the disease, and also in the urine of patients during the late phase. Several methods, such as ELISA are available for antigen detection.

Molecular Methods

Several polymerase chain reaction (PCR)-based methods (e.g., nested PCR) are available to detect and differentiate typhoidal salmonellae by targeting various genes, such as *flagellin* gene, *Iro B* and *FliC* gene.

Detection of Carriers

Typhoid carriers are detected by:
- **Culture:** Stool and bile culture (detects fecal carriers) and urine culture (detects urinary carriers)
- **Detection of Vi antibodies**
- **Isolation from sewage** is carried out to trace the carriers in the communities.

Treatment

Treatment of enteric fever depends on the susceptibility of the strains. The drugs usually given are:
- Third generation cephalosporins, e.g., ceftriaxone
- Azithromycin
- Ciprofloxacin (currently increasing resistance has been reported, hence not a preferred drug).

Vaccines for Typhoid Fever

The following are vaccines available for typhoid.
- **Parenteral Vi polysaccharide vaccine:** It is composed of purified Vi capsular polysaccharide antigen.
  - *Dosage*: Single dose containing 25 µg of Vi antigen is given intramuscularly or subcutaneously
  - Vaccine confers protection for 2 years
  - *Age*: It is given only after 2 years of age.
- **Typhoral:** Oral, live attenuated vaccine.
  - Typhoral is a stable live attenuated mutant of *S.* Typhi strain Ty2 1a
  - It is given orally before food, on alternate days 1, 3, 5 and/or 7 (total of three or four doses).
  - **Boosters** are recommended every 3 years for people residing in endemic areas.

SCRUB TYPHUS

Weil-Felix Test

It is heterophile agglutination test works on the principle of antigenic cross reactivity.
- **Antigen:** Group specific alkali stable lipopolysaccharide (LPS) antigen found in some rickettsiae is also shared by certain strains of *Proteus* (OX19, OX2 and OXK strains). Hence, rickettsial antibodies are detected by using *Proteus* antigens
- **Procedure:** It is a tube agglutination test; serial dilutions of patient's serum are treated with nonmotile strains of *Proteus vulgaris* OX19 and OX2 and *Proteus mirabilis* OXK
- **Results:**
  - *In epidemic and endemic typhus*: Sera agglutinate mainly with OX19 and sometimes with OX2
  - *In tickborne spotted fever*: Antibodies to both OX19 and OX2 are elevated

Problem Solving Exercise 2

A 49-year-old man from village area near Puducherry presented with vesicular rashes, lymphadenopathy and eschar on upper limb. There was history of high grade fever, myalgia and respiratory distress for the past 2 days. A serological test was performed as shown in the picture below (Fig. 18.10):
1. Identify the test and interpret the result. How will you confirm the diagnosis?
2. What is the clinical diagnosis and its causative organism and mode of transmission?
3. What are the clinical manifestations seen in this conditions?
4. What are the various modalities of laboratory diagnosis?
5. How will you treat this condition?

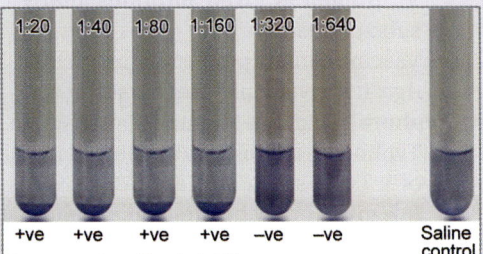

Interpretation: Titer is 1:160
Patient serum is serially diluted and *Proteus mirabilis* OX K antigen is added to all tubes. Clumps formation with clearing of supernatant fluid indicates positive test.

Fig. 18.10: Weil Felix test.

Explanation
Clinical Diagnosis
The history of triad of an eschar (at the site of bite), regional lymphadenopathy and maculopapular rash; however seen only in 40–50% of cases. Patient may also present with non-specific symptoms, such as fever, headache, myalgia, cough, and gastrointestinal symptoms.

Complication: Encephalitis and interstitial pneumonia may occur rarely in the late stage (due to vascular injury).

Etiological agent: *Orientia tsutsugamushi*

Vector: It is transmitted by trombiculid mite.

Serological test: The test shown here is Weil-Felix test (Fig. 18.10). Raised antibody titer against OX-K is suggestive of scrub typhus. As it is a heterophile agglutination test, it should be confirmed by serological test detecting specific antibody, such as IgM ELISA for scrub typhus (using 56-kDa recombinant major surface protein antigens) and indirect immunofluorescence test (IFA, gold standard test).

Molecular test: PCR detecting specific genes, such as major 56-kDa gene, 47-kDa gene and 16S rRNA gene.

Treatment: Doxycycline is the drug of choice. Azithromycin is given alternatively.

Details of the Weil-Felix test is explained below.

- *In scrub typhus:* Antibodies to OXK are raised (Fig. 18.10).
- The test is negative in rickettsial pox, Q fever, ehrlichiosis and bartonellosis.

❖ **False positive titer** may be seen in presence of underlying *Proteus* infection. Hence, four-fold rise of antibody titer in paired sera is more meaningful than a single high titer

❖ **False negative result** may occur due to excess antibodies in patient's sera (*prozone* phenomenon). This can be obviated by testing with serial dilutions of patient's sera.

BRUCELLOSIS

Clinical Manifestations

Brucella is a zoonotic pathogen; infect various animals.
❖ *B. melitensis* is the most pathogenic species to man. It infects sheep, goat and camel
❖ *B. abortus* infects cattle and buffalo
❖ *B. suis* infects pigs.

Transmission: Man usually gets infection (1) most commonly by direct contact from infected animals tissue, urine, etc.; (2) ingestion of infected raw milk; and (3) inhalation of dust or aerosols.

Manifestations are of following types:
❖ **Classic triad:** Though the manifestations vary (40–50%), the classic triad of fever with profuse night sweats; arthralgia/arthritis and hepatosplenomegaly are present in most patients
❖ **Typhoid-like illness:** Overall, brucellosis resembles typhoid-like illness except that it is less acute, less severe with undulating pattern of fever (remittent course) and more musculoskeletal symptoms (vertebral osteomyelitis and septic arthritis).

Problem Solving Exercise 3

A 52-year-old slaughterhouse worker presented with on and off fever with profuse night sweats and joint pain. On examination, hepatosplenomegaly was found. A serological test performed is displayed in Figure 18.11.
1. Identify the serological test and interpret the result.
2. What is the clinical diagnosis?

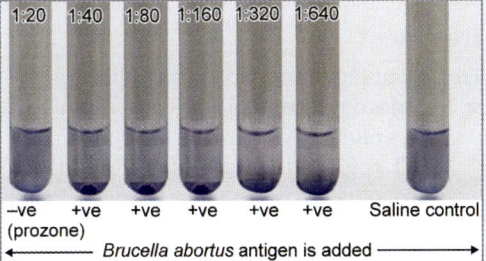

Fig. 18.11: Serological test.
Source: Department of Microbiology, Pondicherry Institute of Medical Sciences, Puducherry (*with permission*).

3. How the disease is transmitted?
4. What are the various modalities of laboratory diagnosis?
5. How will you treat this condition?

Explanation
Clinical Diagnosis

The history is suggestive of brucellosis. Points in favor are:
- Slaughterhouse worker (occupational exposure).
- Triad of fever (on and off) with profuse night sweats, joint pain and hepatosplenomegaly.

Standard Agglutination Test

This is the serological test shown in Figure 18.11.
- First tube do not show agglutination (button formed) due to prozone phenomena.
- All other tubes show agglutination; clump formation with clearing of supernatant.
- Saline control is satisfactory (no agglutination).
- *Interpretation*: The test is found be positive with a titer of ≥1:640 (significant).

(For answers to other questions, refer text below).

Laboratory Diagnosis

Culture and Identification

Blood and bone marrow, CSF, joint fluid or other tissues are the useful specimens. Blood and body fluids are inoculated and processed in blood culture bottles (monophasic or Castaneda's biphasic media) or automated systems, such as BACTEC and BacT/ALERT as discussed earlier.
- **Subcultures** are made from positively flagged blood culture bottles onto blood agar and then incubated in candle jar at 37°C overnight
- **Identification** is done by—Culture Smear (small, gram-negative coccobacilli), automated identification systems (MALDI-TOF or VITEK) or conventional biochemical tests (catalase and oxidase positive, rapid urease positive).

Serological Tests (Antibody Detection)
Standard Agglutination Test (SAT)
- **Procedure:** It is a tube agglutination test. Equal volumes of serial dilutions of patient's sera are mixed with the killed smooth suspension of a standard strain of *B. abortus* and incubated at 37°C for 48 hours

- **Result:**
  - Positive reaction—characterized by clumps formation with clearing of supernatant
  - Negative reaction—characterized by button formation.
- **Significant titer:**
  - Titer of >1:160 is considered as significant in nonendemic areas
  - In endemic area or following occupational exposure: Titer of ≥1:320 or rising titer by repeating the test after 2–4 weeks is considered diagnostic.
- **Interpretation:** A positive SAT result indicates either acute or chronic brucellosis. As SAT detects total antibodies (IgM + IgG); it cannot differentiate between acute and chronic infection
- **2-mercaptoethanol (2ME) SAT test:** 2ME destroys IgM antibodies. Therefore, SAT performed with 2ME treated serum detects only IgG and confirms chronic brucellosis
  - SAT positive and 2ME SAT negative—indicates acute brucellosis (IgM)
  - SAT positive and 2ME SAT positive—indicates chronic brucellosis (IgG).

- **False negative SAT** may occur due to:
  - Prozone phenomenon (due to excess of antibodies in patient's sera)
  - Presence of blocking or non-agglutinating antibodies.
- **False positive SAT** may occur due to antigenic cross-reactions with some other gram-negative bacteria having similar O chains.

Other Antibody Detection Tests

- **ELISA** is a highly sensitive test; uses either cytoplasmic proteins or LPS antigens to detect IgM, IgG, and IgA antibodies individually. Therefore, it is useful for diagnosis chronic brucellosis. However, the result has to be confirmed by SAT. ELISA is also useful in diagnosis neurobrucellosis
- **Dipstick assays** for anti-*Brucella* IgM are available for diagnosis of acute infection, but is less sensitive.

Molecular Method

Polymerase chain reaction is rapid, sensitive and specific and can also differentiate between the species and biovars.

Diagnosis of Brucellosis in Animals

- Isolation from milk and dairy products
- **Antibody detection in milk,** such as milk ring test, Rose Bengal card test and whey agglutination test.

Treatment

Treatment regimen used for brucellosis are:
- **Standard regimen in adults:** Gentamicin for 7 days plus doxycycline for 6 weeks.
- **WHO regimen in adults:** Rifampin for 6 weeks plus doxycycline for 6 weeks. Relapse or treatment failure occurs in 5–10% of cases
- **For CNS involvement:** Ceftriaxone is added and treatment is prolonged for 3–6 months.

LEPTOSPIROSIS

Problem Solving Exercise 4

A young farmer presented with fever, headache, and myalgia and yellow discoloration of skin and sclera. On examination, he had conjunctival inflammation and hepatosplenomegaly. His blood count showed a neutrophilia with thrombocytopenia.

Liver function tests showed an elevated conjugated bilirubin with mild elevation of transaminases. He was also found to be oliguric and uremic. A rapid serological test was performed as shown in the picture below (Fig. 18.12):
1. What is the clinical diagnosis and how this disease is transmitted?
2. What are the clinical manifestations seen in this disease?
3. What are the various modalities of laboratory diagnosis?
4. How will you treat this condition?

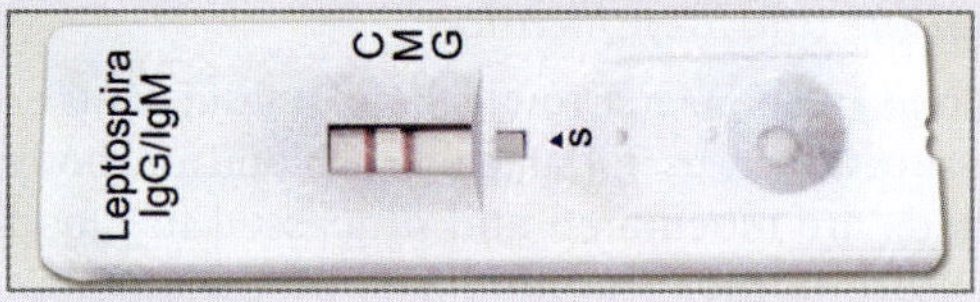

Fig. 18.12: ICT for *Leptospira* antibody.
Source: Department of Microbiology, Pondicherry Institute of Medical Sciences, Puducherry (*with permission*).

Explanation

This is a case of leptospirosis. The points in favor are:
- The history of fever, conjunctival inflammation and hepatosplenomegaly
- Jaundice with ↑ bilirubin and liver enzymes
- The rapid serological test detected anti-*Leptospira* IgM antibodies (Fig. 18.12).

(For answers to other questions, refer below).

Clinical Manifestations (Leptospirosis)

Leptospirosis is zoonotic disease caused by *Leptospira interrogans*. It is transmitted by contact with water, moist soil and wet surfaces contaminated with rodent urine. Direct human-to-human transmission does not occur. Disease is presented in two forms:

Mild Anicteric Febrile Illness

It occurs in 90% of patients. It is biphasic:
- Septicemic phase occurs first, presented with fever, headache, conjunctival suffusion, abdominal pain
- Followed by immune phase, presented with meningitis, uveitis and rash.

Weil's Disease

It is also called as hepatorenal-hemorrhagic syndrome. It is a severe form of icteric illness with renal dysfunction, occurs in 10% patients.

Laboratory Diagnosis

Cerebrospinal fluid and blood (in first 10 days of infection) and urine (between 10–30 days of infection) are useful specimens.

Microscopy

- **Under dark-ground microscope (Fig. 18.13):** They are tightly and regularly coiled, with characteristic hooked ends, such as umbrella handle
- **Staining:** They do not stain by ordinary stain, but can be stained by *sliver impregnation stains*, such as Fontana stain and modified Steiner technique
- **Appearance:** *L. interrogans* is 6–12 μm long; tightly and regularly coiled, with characteristic hooked ends, such as umbrella handle (hence the species name *interrogans*—resembling interrogation or question mark)
- **Disadvantage:** Microscopy is less sensitive and requires technical expertise.

Isolation

Leptospira is obligate aerobe, fastidious and grows slowly. Cultures should be incubated at 30°C for 4–6 weeks in media, such as:

- EMJH (Ellinghausen, McCullough, Johnson, Harris) medium
- Korthof's media with rabbit blood
- Fletcher's semisolid media.

Serology for Antibody Detection

- IgM antibodies appear early within one week of illness, reach peak levels in third or fourth week and then decline slowly and become undetectable within six months
- IgG antibodies appear later than IgM; reach peak level after few weeks of illness and may persist at low level for years (Fig. 18.14).

Antibody detection tests can be broadly classified into:

- **Genus specific tests:** They use broadly reactive genus-specific antigen prepared from nonpathogenic *Leptospira biflexa* Patoc 1 strain. They cannot detect the infecting serovar. Various tests available are:
  - Macroscopic slide agglutination test
  - Microcapsule agglutination test
  - Latex agglutination test
  - Enzyme-linked immunosorbent assay (ELISA)
  - Immunochromatographic test (ICT): It detects IgM and IgG antibodies separately (Fig. 18.14).

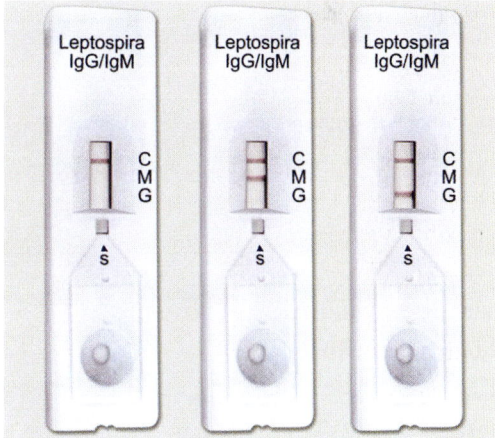

Fig. 18.14: Genus-specific rapid diagnostic test for leptospirosis.
Source: Department of Microbiology, Pondicherry Institute of Medical Sciences, Puducherry (*with permission*).

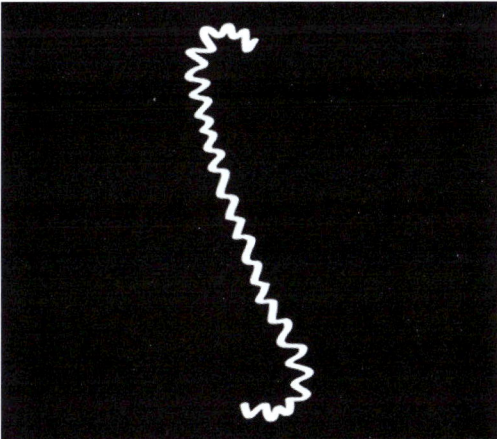

Fig. 18.13: Dark-ground microscopy demonstrating *Leptospira interrogans* (schematic diagram).

- **Serovar-specific test:** *Microscopic agglutination test* detects antibodies against specific serovars of *L. interrogans*. It is the *gold standard* method and *reference test* for the diagnosis of leptospirosis
- **Cross agglutination and absorption test (CAAT):** It is done to detect the relatedness between the strains.

Molecular Methods

Polymerase chain reaction (PCR) has been found particularly useful in severe disease, before seroconversion occurs.

- Various genes, such as *16S* or *23S* rRNA or *IS1533* insertion sequence are targeted
- However, PCR is not serovar specific.

Treatment

- **Mild leptospirosis** should be treated with oral doxycycline (100 mg twice a day for 7 days)
- **Severe leptospirosis:** Penicillin is the drug of choice.

CHAPTER 19

Viral Infections of Bloodstream: HIV/AIDS and Dengue

■ HIV/AIDS

Problem Solving Exercise 1

In a blood bank, samples received from six donors were subjected to a serological test as shown in Figure 19.1 (for HIV infection screening).
1. Interpret the test result.
2. Which test you will do further to establish the diagnosis according to National AIDS Control Organization (NACO) strategy?
3. Mention the various modes of transmission of HIV infection.
4. What are the various generations of HIV enzyme-linked immunosorbent assay (ELISA)?

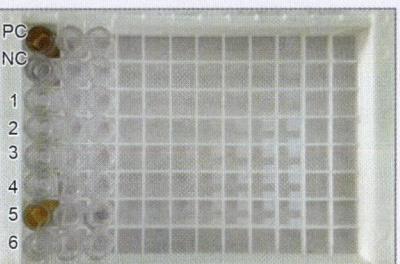

Fig. 19.1: Screening test of six blood donors for HIV.
Abbreviations: PC, positive control; NC, negative control.
Source: Department of Microbiology, Pondicherry Institute of Medical Sciences, Puducherry (*with permission*).

Explanation
The test shown here is HIV ELISA. Out of six samples, sample no. 5 is reactive for HIV and samples 1, 2, 3, 4 and 6 are not reactive for HIV. The positive (PC) and negative controls (NC) are satisfactory.

National AIDS Control Organization (NACO) Strategy I
- Testing for HIV infection in blood bank belongs to NACO strategy I.
- Here, if first test comes positive, no further test is required to carry out. The blood sample is discarded.
- Result is not reported to the donor. However, the donor is advised to attend the Integrated Counseling and Testing Centre (ICTC) clinic for further evaluation.

HIV Transmission
The various modes of transmission of HIV include:
- **Sexual intercourse** (anal >vaginal; male to female > female to male). It is the most common mode of transmission (75% of total cases in the world)
- **Parenteral:** Blood transfusion, injection drug abuse, needle stick exposure
- **Vertical:** Mother to fetus.
  Answer to all the others questions are explained in the text of this chapter.

HIV ELISA: There are four generations of HIV ELISA. (Details have been explained below under laboratory diagnosis).

Problem Solving Exercise 2

The Government of a newly formed state was interested to determine the prevalence of HIV infection in the state. Specimens (serum) were collected from various general populations and subjected to the following serological screening test (Fig. 19.2).
1. Interpret the test results and what is the most probable diagnosis?
2. Which test you will do further to establish the diagnosis according to NACO strategy?

Explanation
The test shown here (Fig. 19.2), is rapid test which works on immunocomb principle. Out of 12 samples tested:
- Sample no. 9, 10 are reactive for HIV

- Samples no. 1, 2, 3, 4, 5, 6, 7, 8, 12 are nonreactive for HIV
- Test for sample 11 is not valid as internal control is not satisfactory
- The internal control is satisfactory for the remaining samples.

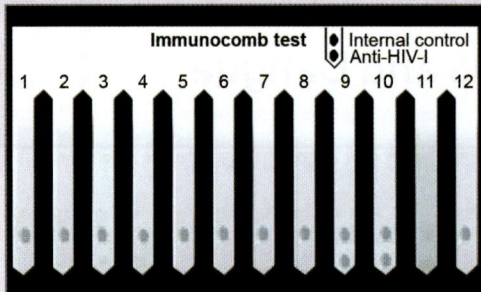

Fig. 19.2: Serological screening test.
Source: Department of Microbiology, Pondicherry Institute of Medical Sciences, Puducherry (*with permission*).

NACO Strategy IIA

For seroprevalence or epidemiological purpose, NACO strategy IIA is done.
- Here confirmation of HIV-1 diagnosis is done by a second screening test which works on either different principle or uses different antigens than the first screening test.
- If both the tests are reactive; it is reported as "REACTIVE".
- In case if second test is nonreactive, then the result is taken as negative for sentinel surveillance purposes.

Problem Solving Exercise 3

A 25-year-old male with history of multiple sex partners is admitted with complaints of unexplained fever, progressive loss of weight, persistent diarrhea and generalized lymphadenopathy for the past 6 months.
1. Interpret the test result and what is the most probable diagnosis?
2. What further test you will do to establish the diagnosis according to NACO strategy?

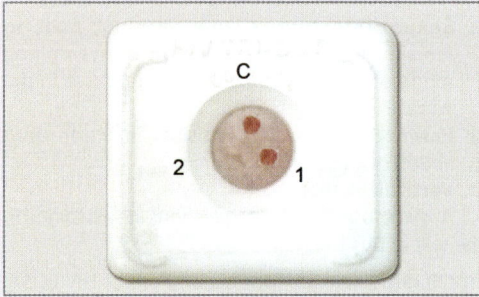

Fig. 19.3: HIV TRI-DOT test.
Source: Department of Microbiology, Pondicherry Institute of Medical Sciences, Puducherry (*with permission*).

Explanation

Clinical Diagnosis

History of unexplained fever, progressive loss of weight, persistent diarrhea and generalized lymphadenopathy for the past 6 months in a male having multiple sex partner—most likely diagnosis is HIV infection.

Microbiological Diagnosis

Test shown here is HIV TRI-DOT test (Fig. 19.3), a rapid test for HIV which works on flow through assay principle. Both control dot and test dot at HIV-1 region have shown reactive, hence the test is reactive for HIV-1 antibodies.

NACO Strategy IIB

- Diagnosis of HIV in symptomatic individual belongs to *NACO strategy IIB*.
- Here, positive result of first test should be confirmed by a second screening test which works on either different principle or uses different antigens than the first screening test.
- In case sample is positive by first test, and positive by second test, then sample is reported as reactive and post-test counseling should be given.
- In case sample is positive by first and negative by second test, then third test is done.
- If third test is reactive then sample is reported as indeterminate and repeat testing is done after 2–4 weeks. In case if third test is negative, sample is reported as negative.
- In case of indeterminate result, sample should be sent to reference laboratory for confirmation by western blot or reverse transcriptase polymerase chain reaction (RT-PCR).
- **3Cs: C**ounseling, informed **C**onsent and **C**onfidentiality are must in these cases.

Problem Solving Exercise 4

A patient was waiting for appendectomy surgery. The surgeon wanted to rule out HIV status preoperatively. A serological test was performed as shown in Figure 19.4.
1. Interpret the test result and diagnosis.
2. What further test you will do to establish the diagnosis according to NACO strategy?

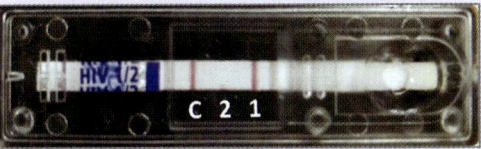

Fig. 19.4: Serological test.
Source: Department of Microbiology, Pondicherry Institute of Medical Sciences, Puducherry (*with permission*).

Explanation
NACO Strategy III
It is a case of diagnosis of HIV in asymptomatic individual which belongs to NACO strategy III. Test show here is HIV rapid test, which works on lateral flow or immunochromatographic assay principle. Both control band and also test band at HIV-1 region had shown reactive.
- Here, the confirmation of HIV-1 diagnosis is done by performing second and third screening tests which work on either different principle or uses different antigens.
- If all three tests are positive, then reported as "REACTIVE".
- If first and second tests are positive, still third test should be done to report as HIV reactive. If third test is negative then sample is reported as indeterminate and repeat testing is done after 2–4 weeks.
- In case sample is positive by first test and negative by 2nd and 3rd tests, then:
  - If patient belongs to high-risk category, reported as intermediate or
  - If belongs to low-risk category then reported as non-reactive.
- In case of indeterminate result, sample should be sent to reference laboratory for confirmation by western blot or RT-PCR.
- **3Cs: C**ounseling, informed **C**onsent and **C**onfidentiality are must in these cases.

LABORATORY DIAGNOSIS OF HIV/AIDS

The various modalities available for the laboratory diagnosis of HIV/AIDS are enlisted in Table 19.1.

Diagnosis of HIV/AIDS is not like other infectious diseases. A number of moral, ethical, legal and psychosocial issues are associated with a positive HIV status. The following care should be taken **(3Cs)** while performing the test for HIV.
- ❖ **Consent** in written format should be taken before the test is done. The patient should be explained about the nature of the test being performed
- ❖ **Confidentiality** of a positive test result is a must. Patient name or the word "HIV positive" should not be written on the report form
- ❖ **Counseling** should be provided to motivate the individual to tell the spouse/family and induce behavioral change.

Antibody Detection

Detection of anti-HIV antibodies is the mainstay of diagnosis of HIV. Tests to detect specific HIV antibodies can be classified into:

Table 19.1: Laboratory diagnosis of HIV/AIDS.

Specific Tests for HIV Infection
• **Screening tests** (antibody detection):   ➢ ELISA (takes 2–3 hours)   ➢ Rapid/Simple test (takes <30 minutes)
• **Supplemental tests** (antibody detection):   ➢ Western blot assay   ➢ Line immunoassay (LIA)

• **Confirmatory tests**
 ➢ p24 antigen detection (after 12–26 days of infection)
 ➢ Viral culture—by Co-cultivation technique
 ➢ HIV RNA (best confirmatory method)—can be detected 10–14 days after infection
   ♦ Reverse transcriptase PCR (RT-PCR)
   ♦ Branched DNA assay
   ♦ NASBA (nucleic acid sequence-based amplification)
   ♦ Real time RT-PCR for estimating viral load
 ➢ HIV DNA detection: Useful for diagnosis of pediatric HIV

Non–specific Immunological Methods
• Low CD4 T cell count   • Hypergammaglobulinemia: ➢ Neopterin   ➢ β2-macroglobulin   • Altered CD4: CD8 T cell ratio

Screening Assays

Screening assays usually take less time (2–3 hours for ELISA, less than 30 minutes for rapid/simple tests):

- ❖ **High sensitivity and specificity:** NACO recommends the use of ELISA and rapid kits which have a sensitivity of ≥99.5% and a specificity of ≥98%
- ❖ **Should be confirmed:** Results of a single screening test should never be used as the final interpretation of HIV status. It is always subjected to confirmatory tests
- ❖ Antigens used in most of the screening tests are:
  - HIV-1 specific (p24, gp 120, gp160, gp41)
  - HIV-2 specific gp36.
- ❖ They detect HIV-1 and 2 either separately or together.

ELISA (Enzyme-linked Immunosorbant Assay)

ELISA is the most commonly performed screening test at blood banks and tertiary care sites. It is easy to perform, adaptable to large number of samples. It is sensitive, specific, and cost effective.

ELISA kits: Most of the currently available ELISA kits are of two types:
1. *3rd generation ELISA* that uses recombinant and/or synthetic peptides as antigen to detect HIV antibodies
2. *4th generation ELISA* that detects both HIV antibodies and p24 antigen by using combination of recombinant/synthetic peptides as well as monoclonal antibodies respectively. It reduces the window period considerably.

Types of ELISA: Various ELISA formats are in use depending on different principles, such as: (i) indirect ELISA, (ii) competitive ELISA, (iii) sandwich ELISA.

Rapid/Simple Test

These assays have been developed for ease of performance and quick results. They generally require less than 30 minutes to perform and do not require special equipment. They are the most commonly used tests in India. They work on various principles, such as:

- ❖ Dot blot assays (or Immunoconcentration or flow through method, e.g., Tridot test, Fig. 19.3)
- ❖ Immunochromatography (or ICT, lateral flow assay, Fig. 19.4)
- ❖ Particle agglutination assays (using latex, gelatin, RBCs)
- ❖ Dip stick/Comb tests (Enzyme immune assay-based tests, Fig. 19.2).

Supplemental Tests

These assays are highly specific antibody detection methods; hence used for validation of positive results of screening tests. They are expensive, labor intensive, need expertise to interpret, and may also give equivocal/indeterminate results.

Western Blot

It is the most commonly used supplemental test available and is also recommended by NACO.

- ❖ It works on the principle of immunoblot technique (described in Chapter 9)
- ❖ It detects individual antibodies in serum separately against various antigenic fragments of HIV (Fig. 19.5)
  - Antibody to *gag* gene products (p55, p40, p24, p18)
  - Antibody to *pol* gene products (p65/66, p55/51, p31)
  - Antibody to *env* gene products (gp 120, gp160, gp41).
- ❖ The antigen antibody complexes appear as distinct bands on nitrocellulose strip
- ❖ Reactive results are interpreted as per:
  - *WHO criteria:* presence of at least two envelope bands (out of gp120, gp160 or gp41) with or without gag or pol bands
  - *CDC criteria:* presence of any two; out of p24, gp120, gp160 and gp41 bands.

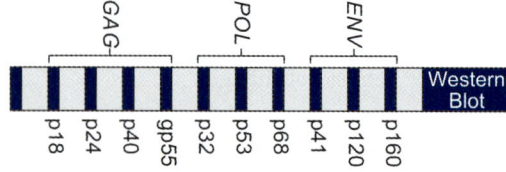

Fig. 19.5: Western blot test strip.

Problem Solving Exercise 5

A commercial sex worker presented with diarrhea and loss of weight for 2 months. Screening tests performed for HIV showed equivocal results (Fig. 19.6). For confirmation, the following test given below was performed.
1. Identify the test and interpret the result.
2. What is the principle of the test?
3. What are the other tests can be used for confirmation?

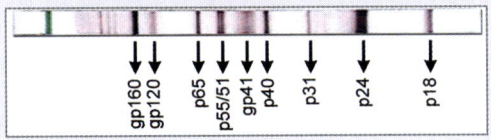

Fig. 19.6: HIV Western blot test strip.
Source: Department of Microbiology, JIPMER, Puducherry (with permission).

Explanation
The test given in the picture is Western blot, done for detection of HIV antibodies.

For HIV diagnosis, if the screening tests show inconclusive (equivocal) result, then it has to be confirmed by supplemental test.

Interpretation
Colored bands are present for antibodies against HIV antigens gp160, gp120, gp41 (*env* gene products), p65, p55/51, p31 (*pol* gene products), p40, p24, p18 (*gag* gene products).

Final Report
Reactive for HIV-1 antibodies; as antibodies to p24, gp120, gp160, gp41 antigens are specific to HIV-1.

Detection of p24 Core Antigen

The p24 antigen becomes detectable after 12–26 days of infection and lasts for 3–4 weeks thereafter. Again, it is elevated during the late advanced stage of AIDS. p24 Ag is detected by 4th generation ELISA (described earlier).
- **It is less sensitive** (~30%) because once the antibody is formed, it binds to the p24 protein and the antigen-antibody complex gets eliminated from the blood
- Recently, **antigen dissociation assay** has been developed that involves pretreatment of serum to an agent, that liberates p24 antigen from the immunocomplexes. This has shown better sensitivity
- **Uses of p24 antigen detection test:**
  - For confirmation of diagnosis of HIV/AIDS
  - Diagnosis of HIV during the window period
  - To diagnose the late stage of HIV/AIDS (immune collapse) or CNS disease
  - Diagnosis of HIV in infants (not reliable)
  - Monitoring the progress of HIV infection
  - To resolve equivocal western blot results.

Viral RNA Detection

Detection of viral RNA is the **"gold standard"** method for confirmation of HIV diagnosis. Various formats are available targeting *pol* and *env* genes.

- Reverse transcriptase polymerase chain reaction (RT-PCR)
- Branched DNA assay
- NASBA: Nucleic acid sequence-based amplification
- Real time RT-PCR: For estimating viral load.

Apart from the routine diagnosis of HIV, RNA detection has several other uses, such as:
- It is the **most sensitive** and **specific** method, detects even few copies of viral RNA and is the best method **for confirmation** of HIV
- It is the best tool for diagnosis of HIV during **window period**, detects HIV earlier than all available methods (10–14 days post-exposure)
- **Viral load monitoring:** Real time RT-PCR can quantify the viral load and is the most appropriate tool for monitoring the response to antiretroviral therapy
- **Typing:** RT-PCR can successfully differentiate between HIV-1 and HIV-2 infections and can detect the specific genotype or subtype
- Detection of **drug resistance** genes.

DNA PCR

PCR detecting proviral DNA is extremely useful for diagnosis of pediatric HIV and to differentiate latent HIV infection from active viral transcription. It is also useful during the window period, viral load estimation (real time PCR) and detection of genotypes.

Isolation of the Virus

Isolation is time consuming, expensive, takes longer time (6 weeks or more) and not sensitive. It is used only for research and not for routine diagnostics.

Co-cultivation is the method used for virus isolation. Here, the peripheral blood mononuclear cells (PBMCs) obtained from the patient are co-cultured along with the PBMCs from healthy donor; followed by detection of viral RNA or antigen in culture suspension.

Non-specific/Immunological Tests

- ❖ **CD4 T cell count:** Measurement of CD4 T cell count is carried out by flow cytometry method. It is useful for:
    - Assessing the risk of opportunistic infections
    - Initiation of antiretroviral therapy—previously used. Current guideline says treatment should be started in all patients regardless of CD4 T cell count
    - Monitoring the response to antiretroviral therapy.
- ❖ **Abnormal proteins,** such as neopterin and beta 2-microglobulin are elevated.

NACO Strategy for HIV Diagnosis

For the resource poor countries, it is impracticable to confirm the result of HIV screening tests by PCR or western blot as these assays are expensive and available only at limited centers.

NACO (National AIDS Control Organization, India) has formulated a strategic plan (Fig. 19.7) for HIV diagnosis. The guidelines are as follows:
- ❖ Depending on the situation/condition, for which the test is done, the positive result of the first screening test should be either considered as such or confirmed by another one or two screening tests

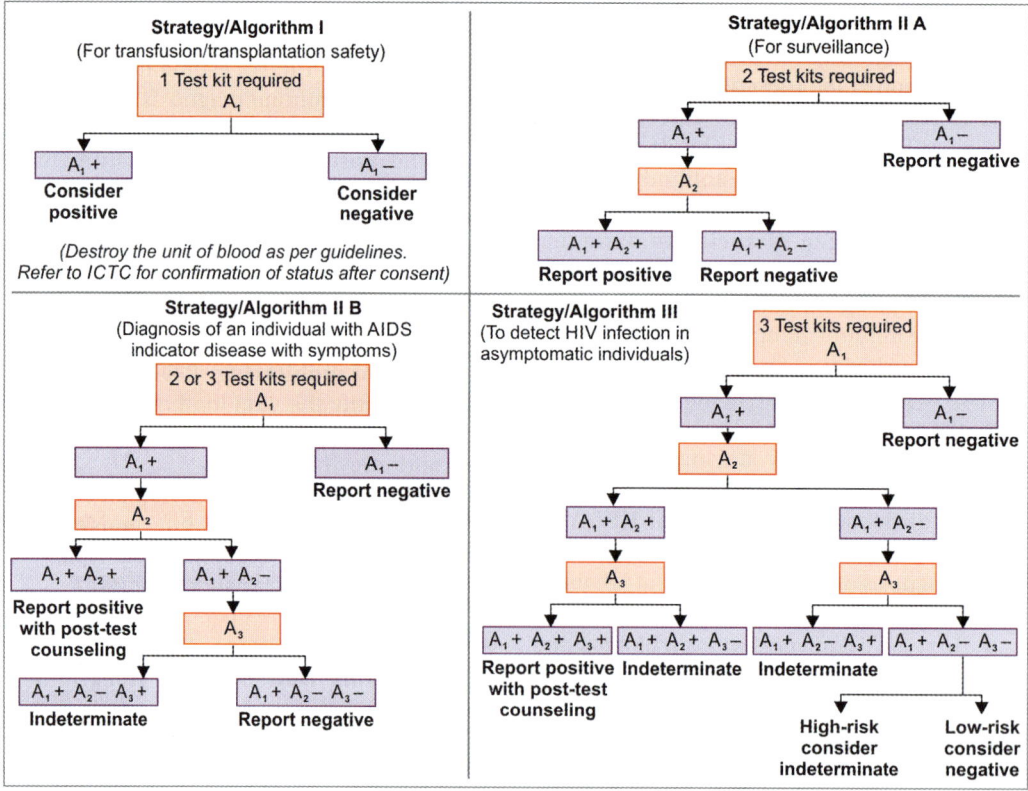

Fig. 19.7: NACO strategies/algorithms for diagnosing HIV infection.
Abbreviations: NACO, National AIDS Control Organization; ICTC, Integrated Counselling and Testing Centre.

- The first screening test should be highly sensitive, whereas the second and third screening tests should have high specificity
- The three screening tests should use different principles or different antigens. The same kit should not be used again
- Supplemental or confirmatory tests should be used only when the screening test(s) results are equivocal/intermediate.

Prognosis/Monitoring of HIV

Various tools available for monitoring the response to antiretroviral therapy include:
- **CD4 T cell count:** Most commonly used
- **HIV RNA load:** Most consistent and best tool at present
- p24 antigen detection
- Neopterin and β2 macroglobulin level.

Note: Viral antibody levels are inconsistent and variable during late stage due to immune collapse; hence not reliable for prognosis.

Diagnosis of Pediatric HIV Infection

The routine screening methods (ELISA or rapid/simple tests) detect IgG antibodies.
- They cannot differentiate between baby's IgG or maternally transferred IgG, hence cannot be used for the diagnosis of pediatric HIV
- As all maternal antibodies would disappear by 18 months; therefore IgG assays can be performed after 18 months of birth.

Various methods used for diagnosis of pediatric HIV include:
- **HIV DNA PCR:** This is the most recommended method for diagnosis of pediatric HIV. Baby is tested for HIV DNA PCR at 6 weeks by DBS (Dry Blood Spot) collection. If found positive, then is reconfirmed by a repeat HIV DNA PCR. Then it is reported as positive and the baby is then initiated on lifelong ART
- HIV RNA detection
- p24 antigen detection
- IgG ELISA only after 18 months of age.

Diagnosis of HIV in Window Period

Window period refers to the initial time interval between the exposure and appearance of detectable levels of antibodies in the serum.
- The antibodies appear in blood within 2–8 weeks after infection, but usually become detectable after 3 weeks to 12 weeks with the assays available presently. It can be as low as 22 days; when third generation antibody detection kits with high sensitivity are used
- p24 antigen detection (30% sensitive; by 4th generation ELISA): It can be detected by 12–26 days after infection
- HIV RNA detection (by RT-PCR) is the best method—it detects HIV RNA around 10–14 days after infection.

Treatment of HIV infection (ART Guideline, NACO 2018)

Indication to start ART: TREAT ALL; i.e., antiretroviral therapy (ART) has to be started in all patients irrespective of CD4 count, clinical stage, age, population or associated opportunistic infections (OIs).
- **HAART:** Highly active antiretroviral therapy (HAART) is use of combination of at least three antiretroviral drugs to maximally suppress the HIV and stop the progression of the disease
- **TLE regimen:** Tenofovir + Lamivudine + Efavirenz is used to treat HIV-1 infection in adults
- **TL + LR regimen:** Tenofovir-Lamivudine + Lopinavir-Ritonavir is indicated for HIV-2 infection, for HIV-1/2 co-infection and for post-exposure prophylaxis for healthcare workers (Chapter 14).

DENGUE

Problem Solving Exercise 6

A 29-year-old female came to casualty with complaints of high-grade fever, severe joint pain, back pain and myalgia for last 2 days. Gradually, she developed petechial rashes over the body. On examination, she was found to have jaundice, hepatomegaly and a low platelet count (20,000/mm³). A tourniquet test done over the cubital fossa demonstrated 25 petechial spots/square inch area. On inquiry, she told that she stays in area, where mosquitoes are prevalent. Her blood sample was sent for a dengue NS1 antigen enzyme-linked immunosorbent assay (ELISA). Test result is displayed in Figure 19.8.

1. Interpret the test result.
2. What is your clinical diagnosis?
3. What is the pathogenesis of this disease?
4. What are the different modalities of laboratory diagnosis?
5. List the viruses that cause hemorrhagic fever.

Explanation

Clinical Diagnosis

The history is suggestive of dengue hemorrhagic fever. Points in favor are:
- High-grade fever, severe joint pain, back pain and myalgia
- Petechial rashes all over the body with positive tourniquet test
- Low platelet count.

Confirmation

Positive dengue NS1 ELISA along with other clues as already described above the etiological agent can be identified as dengue virus.

Viral hemorrhagic fevers (VHF)

VHF are as a group of illnesses caused by different families of viruses that cause vascular damage that results in symptomatic bleeding (hemorrhage). VHFs are caused by viruses of three distinct groups:
1. **Arboviruses:** Transmitted by arthropod vectors. Examples include dengue, yellow fever viruses
2. **Filoviruses** such as Ebola and Marburg viruses
3. **Rodent borne** viruses such as Hantaviruses and Arenaviruses.

(For answers to other questions, refer below.)

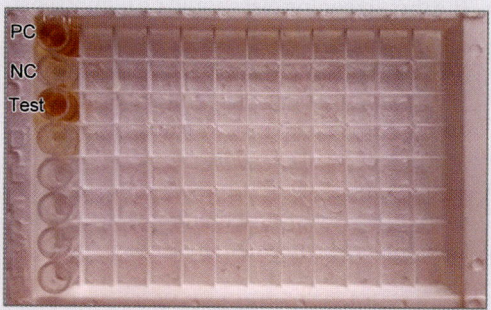

Fig. 19.8: ELISA for detection of NS1 antigen of Dengue.

Pathogenesis of Dengue

Primary dengue infection occurs when a person is infected with dengue virus for the first time with any one serotype.

Secondary dengue infection: It is more severe form of dengue illness; appear months to years later. It occurs due to infection with another second serotype which is different from the first serotype causing primary infection.
- ❖ **ADE:** During secondary dengue infection, there occurs an immunolgical phenomenon called antibody dependent enhancement (ADE)
- ❖ This in-turn leads to development of complications, such as dengue hemorrhagic fever (DHF) and dengue shock syndrome (DSS).

Clinical Classifications of Dengue

The Traditional (1997) WHO Classification

This classification divides dengue into three clinical stages:
1. **Dengue fever (DF):** It is characterized by:
   - Abrupt onset of high fever (also called biphasic fever, break bone fever or saddle back fever)
   - Maculopapular rashes over the chest and upper limbs
   - Severe frontal headache
   - Muscle and joint pains
   - Lymphadenopathy
   - Retro-orbital pain
   - Loss of appetite, nausea and vomiting.
2. **Dengue hemorrhagic fever (DHF):** It is characterized by:
   - High-grade continuous fever
   - Hepatomegaly
   - Thrombocytopenia (platelet count <1 Lakh/mm^3)
   - Raised hematocrit (packed cell volume) by 20%
   - Evidence of hemorrhages which can be detected by:
     - ♦ Positive tourniquet test (>20 petechial spots per square inch area in cubital fossa
     - ♦ Spontaneous bleeding from skin, nose, mouth and gums.
3. **Dengue shock syndrome (DSS):** Here, all the above criteria of DHF are present, and in addition manifestations of shock are present, such as:
   - Rapid and weak pulse

- Narrow pulse pressure (<20 mm Hg) or hypotension
- Presence of cold and clammy skin
- Restlessness.

2009 WHO Classification

This is the most recently described classification by WHO which grades dengue into two stages based on the severity of infection:
1. **Dengue with/without warning signs,** such as abdominal pain, persistent vomiting, mucosal bleed, lethargy, liver enlargement, Increase in hematocrit and rapid decrease in platelet count
2. **Severe dengue:** Criteria included are severe plasma leakage leading to shock and fluid accumulation with respiratory distress, severe bleeding and severe organ involvement (elevated liver enzymes, impaired consciousness, etc.).

Laboratory Diagnosis of Dengue

The outline of laboratory diagnosis of dengue is mainly dependent on serological tests.

NS1 Antigen Detection

ELISA and ICT formats are available for detecting NS1 antigen in serum. They gained recent popularity because of the early detection of the infection.
- NS1 antigen becomes detectable from day 1 of fever and remains positive up to 18 days
- **Highly specific:** It differentiates between flaviviruses. It can also be specific to different dengue serotypes.

Antibody Detection

- **In primary infection:** Antibody response is slow and of low titer. IgM appears first after 5 days of fever and disappears within 90 days. IgG is detectable at low titer in 14–21 days of illness, and then it slowly increases
- **In secondary infection:** IgG antibody titers rise rapidly. IgG is often cross reactive with many flaviviruses and may give false positive result after recent infection or vaccination with yellow fever virus or JE. In contrast, IgM titer is significantly low and may be undetectable
- **In past infection:** Low levels of IgG remain detectable for over 60 years and in the absence of symptoms, is a useful indicator of past infection
- **MAC-ELISA** (IgM antibody capture ELISA): This is the recommended serological testing in India. Kits are supplied by NIV, Pune
  - **Principle** (Fig. 8.4B, Chapter 8): It is a double sandwich ELISA; which captures human IgM antibodies on a microtiter plate using anti-human-IgM antibody followed by the addition of dengue virus four serotypes specific envelope protein antigens (this step makes the test specific). There is a signal enhancement due to use of avidin-biotin complex (ABC) which makes the test more sensitive
  - Cross-reactivity with other flaviviruses is a limitation of this test.

Molecular Method

Detection of specific genes of viral RNA (3'-UTR region) by real time RT-PCR: It is the most sensitive (80–90%) and specific assay (95%), can be used for detection of serotypes and quantification of viral load in blood (within –1 to +5 days of onset of symptoms).

Treatment

There is no specific antiviral therapy for dengue. Treatment is symptomatic and supportive such as:
- Replacement of plasma losses
- Correction of electrolyte and metabolic disturbances
- Platelet transfusion if needed.

Parasitic Infections of Bloodstream: Malaria, Visceral Leishmaniasis and Lymphatic Filariasis

CHAPTER 20

■ MALARIA

Problem Solving Exercise 1

Plasmodium falciparum

A 36-year-old female from Odisha presented with fever, chills and rigor for 5 days with anemia. The patient developed seizures prior to admission. She was started on ceftriaxone by a private medical practitioner and she did not improve. On physical examination, splenomegaly was present and signs of meningeal irritation were absent. Her blood sample was collected and sent to laboratory for peripheral blood smear examination and for other laboratory investigations (Figs 20.4A and B).
1. What is the etiological agent based on test performed?
2. What is the host, infective form, pathogenic form, diagnostic form, habitat and mode of transmission of the parasite?
3. What are the various complications seen?
4. What are the various diagnostic modalities?
5. How will you treat this clinical condition?

Explanation

This is a case of cerebral malaria due to *Plasmodium falciparum*.

Clinical Diagnosis—Points in Favor
- From Odisha (endemic for falciparum malaria)
- Presented with splenomegaly, anemia, and fever with chills and rigor
- Central nervous system involvement such as history of seizure and absence of meningeal irritations-classical feature of cerebral malaria.

Identification

Peripheral thin blood smear examination: Figure 20.4A shows red blood cells (RBCs) containing multiple ring forms, accole forms and double dot ring forms and Fig. 20.4B shows banana-shaped gametocyte; hence the diagnosis is cerebral malaria due to *P. falciparum*. For answers to the other questions, refer text below and Table 20.1.

Problem Solving Exercise 2

Plasmodium vivax

A 13-year-old boy from Mangaluru, presented with high grade fever rises every third day with chills and rigor. His serum sample was subjected to a rapid diagnostic test (RDT) (Fig. 20.1).
1. What is the etiological agent based on interpretation of the test?
2. What is the principle of this test?
3. How will you treat this condition?

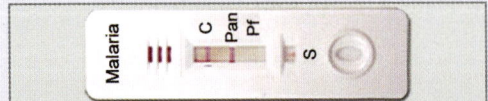

Fig. 20.1: Rapid diagnostic test for malaria.

Explanation

This is a case of vivax malaria.

Clinical Diagnosis
- From Mangaluru (endemic for vivax malaria).
- Presented with high grade fever rises every third day with chills and rigor.

Identification

Rapid diagnostic test for malaria, works on immunochromatographic test.

In Figure 20.1, bands present at panmalarial (genus specific) region, but absent at *P. falciparum* (Pf) region—indicates infection is caused by one of the non-falciparum *Plasmodium* species. The most common non-falciparum *Plasmodium* species (in India) is *Plasmodium vivax*.

Treatment

For answers to the other questions, refer text below and Table 20.1.

Table 20.1: Features of malaria parasites.

Features or characteristics of malaria parasites	
Host	• Definitive host (vector): Female *Anopheles* mosquito • Intermediate host: Man
Infective form and modes of transmission	*For human:* • Sporozoites when transmitted by mosquito bite • Trophozoites and merozoites when transmitted by blood transfusion *For mosquito*—gametocytes
Habitat in man	Hepatocytes and red blood cells (RBCs)
Manifestations (benign malaria)	• Paroxysms of fever with chills and rigor • Anemia • Splenomegaly
Complications (malignant malaria)	Seen in only *Plasmodium falciparum* (due to sequestration of parasites in the blood vessels of deep viscera and cytoadherence of infected RBCs to endothelial cells) • Cerebral malaria • Blackwater fever • Algid malaria (shock) • Pulmonary edema • Hypoglycemia • Renal failure
Treatment	Vivax malaria—chloroquine Falciparum malaria—quinine and artemisinin

Laboratory Diagnosis of Malaria

The diagnostic tests for malaria can be divided into microscopic and nonmicroscopic tests.

Peripheral Blood Smear

Peripheral smear study still remains the simple and gold standard confirmatory test for detection of malarial parasites.

Specimen

Peripheral blood is the specimen of choice, collected from earlobe or by finger prick in older children and adults and from the great toe in infants.
- Blood films should be prepared directly from the capillary blood. In case of anticoagulated blood, smears should be made within an hour of collection of blood
- **Time for taking blood:** Blood should be collected few hours after the height of the paroxysm of fever and before taking antimalarial drugs. Parasite density is maximum during this period
- **Frequency:** Smears should be examined at least twice daily until parasites are detected.

Types of Peripheral Blood Smear

It is of two types—(1) thin, and (2) thick smears. Both the smears are made at the same time from capillary blood either on the same or different slides (Fig. 20.2). At least two thick and two thin smears should be made.
- **For thick smear**, a big drop of blood is spread over 1–2 cm square area on a clean glass slide. The thickness of the film should be such that it allows newsprint to be read
- **For thin smear**, a small drop of blood is taken on a corner of a slide. It is spread by another spreader slide at an angle of 45° and then is lowered to an angle of 30° and is pushed gently to the left, till the blood is exhausted
- The **surface of a good thin** film is: (i) even and uniform, (ii) consists of a single layer of RBCs, (iii) forms a "feathery tail end" near the center of the slide, and (iv) margins of the film do not touch the sides of the slide
- **Stains:** They are stained with one of the Romanowsky's stains such as Leishman's, Giemsa and Field's, Wright's or JSB (Jaswant Singh and Bhattacharya) stain
- **Examination:** Both the smears are examined. The thin smear is screened near the feathery tail end. At least 200–300 oil immersion fields should be examined before the smears are considered as negative

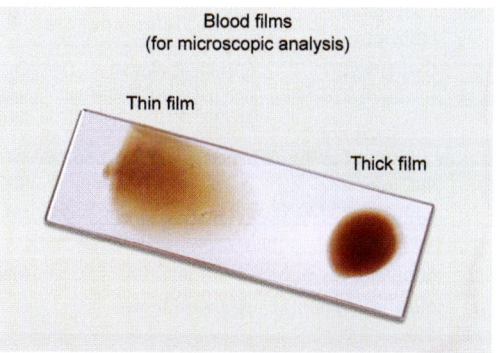

Fig. 20.2: Glass slide showing thin and thick blood smears.

- ❖ **Advantages:** Peripheral smear is simple, rapid and cheap
  - Thick smear is useful in—(1) **Detecting the parasites:** It is 40 times more sensitive than thin smear, can detect as low as 5–10 parasites per µL of blood; (2) Quantification of parasitemia; (3) Demonstrating the malaria pigments
  - Thin smear is useful in speciation of malaria parasites (Table 20.2).
- ❖ **Disadvantages:** (1) It is labor intensive and requires experienced microscopist; (2) Low sensitivity—the detection limit of thin smear is >200 parasites per µL of blood.

The *speciation* by thin smear is based on the detection of the various parasitic morphological forms. In falciparum malaria, only gametocytes and ring forms are demonstrated (but not schizonts and late trophozoites) (Table 20.2 and Figs 20.3 to 20.6).

Quantitative Buffy Coat Examination

The quantitative buffy coat (QBC) is an advanced microscopic technique for malaria diagnosis. It consists of three basic steps:

Table 20.2: Differences between the four malarial parasites (Figs 20.3 to 20.6).

	Parasitic changes	*Plasmodium vivax*	*Plasmodium falciparum*	*Plasmodium malariae*	*Plasmodium ovale*
1.	Forms seen in peripheral blood smear	Trophozoites (early/ring forms and late), gametocytes, schizonts	Ring forms (early trophozoites), gametocytes	Similar to that of *P. vivax*	Similar to that of *P. vivax*
2.	Ring forms (early trophozoites): Vacuole in the center, peripheral thin rim of blue cytoplasm, surrounding the red nucleus	Ring occupies 1/3rd of the size of red blood cell (RBC), cytoplasm opposite to the nucleus is thicker (Fig. 20.5A)	Rings are smaller than in *P. vivax* occupying 1/6th of RBC (Fig. 20.4A). Variants of ring forms are: • Multiple rings • Accole forms • Double dot ring forms	Similar to that of *P. vivax* but thicker	Similar to that of *P. vivax*, more compact (Fig. 20.6B)
3.	Late trophozoites	Large, amoeboid, prominent vacuole	Small, compact, rounded, slightly amoeboid, vacuole inconspicuous, not seen in smear	Small, compact, band forms seen, vacuole inconspicuous (Fig. 20.6A)	Small, compact, rounded, coarse pigment, vacuole inconspicuous
4.	Schizont	Large, 9–10 µm, completely fills the enlarged RBC (Fig. 20.5B)	Small, 4.5–5 µm size, Fills 2/3rd of normal sized RBC	Small, 6.5–7 µm size, almost fills a normal sized RBC	Small, 6.2 µm size, Fills 3/4th of enlarged oval RBC
5.	Merozoites/schizonts	12–24 no.	18–24 no.	6–12 no.	8–12 no.
6.	Gametocyte	Spherical, almost occupies the RBC (Fig. 20.5B)	Crescent/banana shaped, larger than RBC size (Fig. 20.4B)	Similar to that of *P. vivax*	Similar to that of *P. vivax*
Changes in RBCs					
1.	RBC infected	Young RBC	RBC of all age	Old RBC	Young RBC
2.	RBC size	Enlarged, round	Normal in size	Normal in size	Enlarged, oval, fimbriated margin
3.	Stippling	Schuffner's dots	Maurer's cleft	Ziemann's dots	James's dots
4.	Malarial pigments	Yellowish brown	Dark brown	Dark brown	Dark yellowish brown

Note: In falciparum malaria, only the gametocytes and ring forms are demonstrated in peripheral blood but not schizonts and late trophozoites (as the later stages of erythrocytic cycle occurs in deep vessels, not in peripheral blood).

CHAPTER 20 ◆ Parasitic Infections of Bloodstream

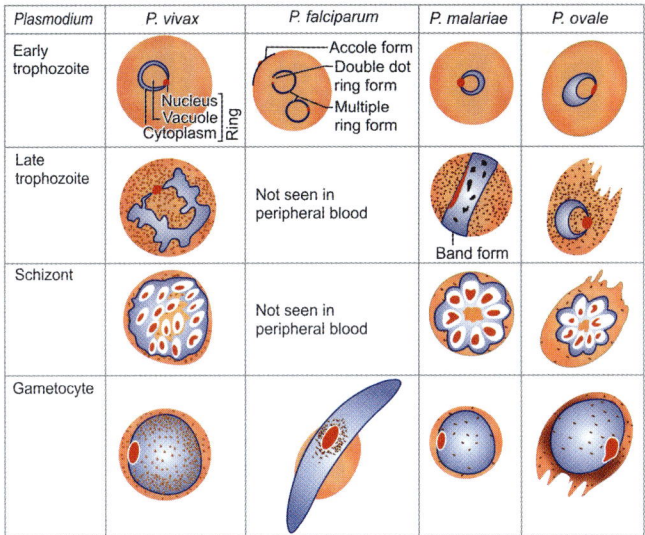

Fig. 20.3: Morphological forms of malaria parasites seen in the peripheral smear.

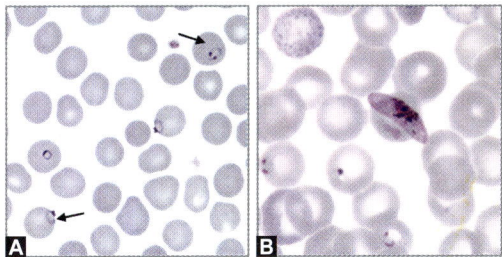

Figs 20.4A and B: Thin smear showing *Plasmodium falciparum*. (A) Accole form and double dot (headphone shaped) ring forms; (B) Gametocyte (banana shaped).
Source: DPDx Image Library, Centers for Disease Control and Prevention (CDC), Atlanta (*with permission*).

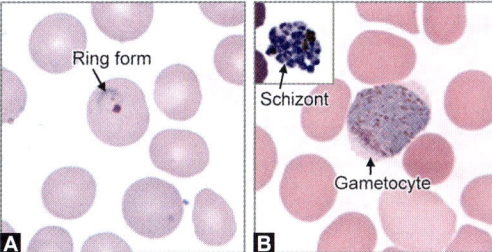

Figs 20.5A and B: Thin smear showing *Plasmodium vivax*. (A) Ring form; (B) Schizont and gametocyte.
Source: DPDx Image Library, Centers for Disease Control and Prevention (CDC), Atlanta (*with permission*).

1. Blood (60 μL) is collected in a capillary tube coated internally with acridine orange (Fig. 20.7A)
2. Capillary tube is centrifuged, which causes separation of components of blood according to their densities, forming discrete layers as RBCs, WBCs, lymphocytes and platelets (Fig. 20.7B)
3. Examination of capillary tube at the buffy coat region under ultraviolet (UV) light source (Figs 20.7C and D).

Interpretation

Acridine orange has a property of staining the nuclear DNA fluorescent brilliant green. Normal

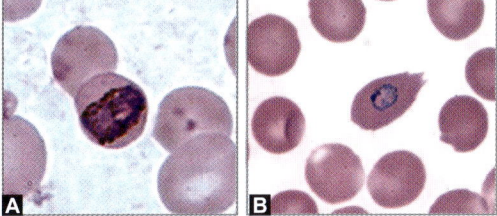

Figs 20.6A and B: Thin smear showing ring form of: (A) *Plasmodium malariae* (band form); (B) *Plasmodium ovale*.
Source: DPDx Image Library, Centers for Disease Control and Prevention (CDC), Atlanta (*with permission*).

RBCs do not take up the stain (as they are a nucleated). However, parasitized RBCs appear as brilliant green dots. WBCs also take up the stain (Figs 20.7C and D).

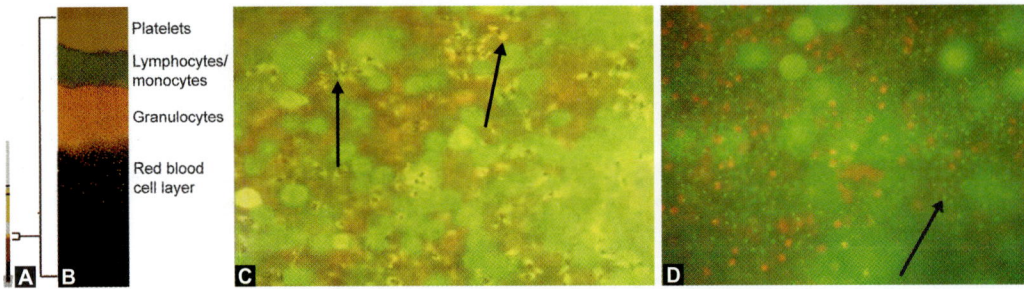

Figs 20.7A to D: (A) QBC capillary tube; (B) Magnified view of QBC capillary tube after centrifugation; (C) Crescent-shaped gametocyte of *Plasmodium falciparum*; (D) Ring forms of *Plasmodium falciparum* seen as fluorescent dots.
Source: (C and D) Department of Microbiology, Sri Siddhartha Medical College, Tumkur, Karnataka (*with permission*).

Advantages

QBC is faster (the entire tube can be screened within minutes), more sensitive (at least as good as a thick film), and quantification is possible.

Disadvantages

It is expensive, less specific and speciation is difficult.

Antigen Detection (Rapid Diagnostic Tests)

Rapid diagnostic tests (RDTs) have revolutionized the diagnosis of malaria.
- ❖ **Antigens:** Several malarial antigens can be detected:
  - **pLDH (Parasite lactate dehydrogenase):** It is produced by all *Plasmodium* species. Currently available test kits can differentiate pan-LDH common to all species and Pf-LDH specific to *P. falciparum*
  - **Parasite aldolase:** Produced by all four *Plasmodium* species
  - **Histidine rich protein-2 (HRP-II):** It is produced only by *P. falciparum*.
- ❖ **Principle:** Test kits currently available use a nitrocellulose membrane (NCM) strip with two parasite detection lines and a control line (Fig. 20.8A):
  - Test line-1: Coated with capture antibodies specific for *P. falciparum* (e.g., HRP-II or Pf-LDH)
  - Test line-2: Coated with capture antibodies common to all *Plasmodium* spp. (e.g., pan-LDH or aldolase).
- ❖ **Procedure:** Drop of blood specimen is added along with a buffer solution to sample window. Malarial antigens combine with polyclonal malarial antibody labeled with colloidal gold present in buffer and move along with NCM to meet its corresponding antibodies at different test lines (Fig. 20.8A)
- ❖ **Interpretation** is based on immobilization of malarial antigens at test lines 1 and/or 2 forming colored bands (Figs 20.8A and B)
  - If band is formed at only test line 1: Indicates *P. falciparum* infection
  - If band is formed at only test line 2: Indicates *Plasmodium* species other than *P. falciparum* infection

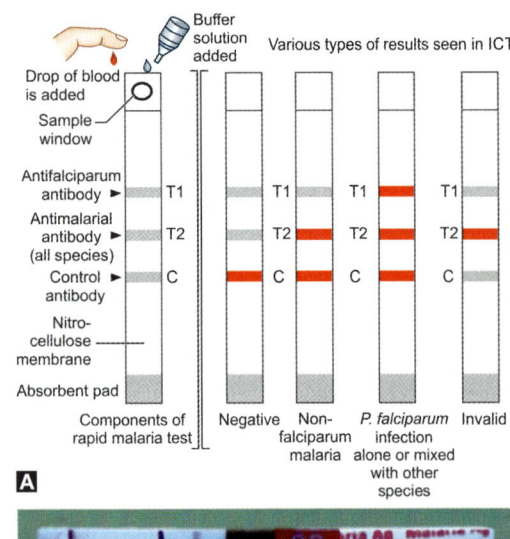

Figs 20.8A and B: (A) Schematic diagram of rapid diagnostic test kit showing negative, non-falciparum, pure or mixed infection with *Plasmodium falciparum* and invalid result of malaria; (B) Real image of rapid diagnostic test kit.
Source: (B) Department of Microbiology, Sri Siddhartha Medical College, Tumakuru, Karnataka (*with permission*).

- If bands are formed at both test lines 1 and 2: Indicates infection with *P. falciparum* or mixed infection.

Note: The band at control line must come to validate the test; if it does not come, test is considered invalid. Control line is coated with antibody against polyclonal malarial antibody present in buffer.

Advantages of Rapid Diagnostic Tests

Rapid diagnostic tests are simple to perform, do not need extra equipment or trained microscopist.
- **Sensitivity:** Rapid diagnostic tests are more than 90% sensitive at >100 parasites/µL. But the sensitivity is markedly reduced at <100 parasites/µL
- **Prognosis:** pLDH is produced by the viable parasites, hence it is used to monitor the response for treatment (microscopy is the best to assess prognosis)
- **Pregnancy:** HRP-II is a reliable marker to diagnose malaria in pregnancy
- **Severity:** Intensity of the band is directly proportional to the parasitemia and severity of the disease.

Disadvantages of Rapid Diagnostic Tests

RDTs have several disadvantages.
- It cannot differentiate between the non-falciparum malaria species
- Expensive than peripheral smear
- Gametocytes cannot be detected
- Low sensitivity: The lower limit to detect HRP-II is 40 parasites/µL and pLDH is 100 parasites/µL
- RDT has not been developed for *P. knowlesi* yet. Comparison of peripheral smear, QBC and RDTs are described in Table 20.3.

Antibody Detection

Antibodies persist even after the clinical cure. Serology does not detect current infection, but only measures past exposure. Therefore, Government of India has banned the use of antibody detection tests for malaria diagnosis.

Other Nonspecific Tests

Other nonspecific tests include normocytic hemolytic anemia, leukopenia, metabolic acidosis, raised ESR, and hypoglycemia.

Treatment

For vivax malaria: The recommended regimen is chloroquine 25 mg/kg (divided over three days) and primaquine 0.25 mg/kg body weight (daily for 14 days; to prevent relapse)

For falciparum malaria:
- North-Eastern states: **ACT-AL regimen**—artemisinin combination therapy-artemether-lumefantrine for 3 days *plus* **Primaquine** single dose on second day (to kill gametocytes of *P. falciparum*)

Table 20.3: Comparison of peripheral smear, quantitative buffy coat and rapid diagnostic tests.

Features	Peripheral smear	Quantitative buffy coat	Rapid diagnostic tests
Method	Cumbersome	Easy	Easy
Time	Longer, 60–120 minutes	Faster, 15–30 minutes	Faster, 15–30 minutes
Sensitivity	Detection limit: • 5 parasites/µL in thick film • 200 parasites/µL in thin film	Claimed to be more sensitive, at least as good as a thick film	• >100 parasites/µL, sensitivity >90% • <100 parasites/µL, sensitivity falls
Specificity	Gold standard	False positives—artifacts may be reported as positive by nontrained technicians	False positive in RA factor (rheumatoid arthritis) positive cases
Speciation	Accurate, gold standard	Difficult	Detect *Plasmodium falciparum* but cannot differentiate non-falciparum species
Cost	Inexpensive	Costly equipment and consumables	Kits are costly but no extra equipment required. Good for field study
Experienced Microscopist	Required	Not required, minimal training is sufficient	Not required, minimal training is sufficient

- Other states: **ACT-SP regimen**—artesunate for 3 days *plus* sulfadoxine/pyrimethamine given on first day *plus* **Primaquine** single dose on second day.

VISCERAL LEISHMANIASIS

Problem Solving Exercise 3

A 31-year-old man from Bihar presented with splenomegaly, anemia and fever. The bone marrow aspirate collected was sent for Giemsa staining (Fig. 20.9B).
1. Identify the etiological agent and the clinical diagnosis based on the smear focused.
2. What is the host, infective form, pathogenic form, diagnostic form, habitat and mode of transmission of the parasite?
3. What are the various diagnostic modalities?
4. How will you treat this condition?

Explanation

This is a case of visceral leishmaniasis. Points in favor are:
- Residence from Bihar
- Presented with splenomegaly, anemia and fever
- Figure 20.9 B shows Leishman Donovan bodies (LD bodies, i.e., amastigotes filled within a macrophage)
- Treatment: Amphotericin B.

(For answer to the other questions, refer Tables 20.4 and 20.5).

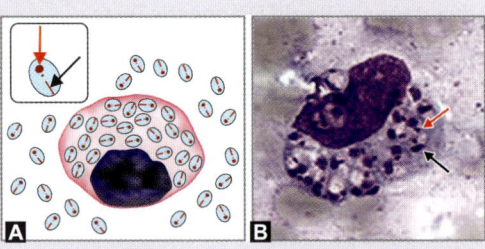

Figs 20.9A and B: *L. donovani* amastigotes: showing a macrophage containing multiple *Leishmania* amastigotes: (A) Schematic; (B) In bone marrow smear stained with Giemsa. Note that each amastigote has a nucleus (red arrow) and a rod-shaped kinetoplast (black arrow).
Source: (B) DPDx Image Library, Centers for Disease Control and Prevention (CDC), Atlanta (*with permission*).

Table 20.4: Features/characteristics of *Leishmania donovani*.

Features	*Leishmania donovani*
Host	Man Vector: Sandfly (*Phlebotomus*)
Morphological forms	• Amastigote in human • Promastigote in sandfly
Infective form	Promastigote
Transmission	Bite of sand fly
Habitat	Reticuloendothelial cells of spleen, bone marrow, lymph node, liver and peripheral blood
Pathogenic form	Amastigote form
Major manifestations of kala-azar	Due to Leishman Donovan bodies deposit in various organs: • Splenomegaly: most consistent sign • Bone marrow involvement leads to pancytopenia and hypergammaglobulinemia • Lymphadenopathy (African cases) • Hyperpigmentation (on face, hands, feet, and abdomen) and fever are the common presentations in Indian cases; hence the name kala-azar or black fever
Diagnostic form (Figs 20.9A and B)	Amastigote forms reside inside the macrophages, called as LD (Leishman Donovan) body
Treatment	Pentavalent antimonials—drug of choice Liposomal amphotericin B is the first-line drug in Bihar (due to resistance to antimonials)

Table 20.5: Laboratory diagnosis of *Leishmania donovani*.

Methods	Salient features
Specimen	• Splenic aspirate (most sensitive) • Bone marrow aspirate (most common) • Lymph node aspirate (in African cases) • Peripheral blood (in HIV-infected patients)
Direct microscopy	Leishman or Giemsa stain reveals LD bodies (macrophages filled with amastigote forms of 3–5 µm) (Fig. 20.9A and B).
Culture	• NNN (McNeal, Novy, Nicolle) media or Schneider's *Drosophila* media are used • Amastigotes transform into promastigote forms which are detected in culture fluid microscopy by staining with Giemsa stain (Figs 20.10A and B).
Antibody detection (nonspecific)	Hypergammaglobulinemia detection by: • Napier's aldehyde test • Chopra's antimony test
Antibody detection (specific)	Uses Leishmania specific antigen: • ELISA • ICT detecting antibody to recombinant kinesin antigen (rk-39). Recently, ICT based on another novel antigen rKE16 (from *L. donovani*) has been developed • Direct agglutination test (DAT)—100% sensitive and specific
PCR	Detecting kinetoplast DNA
Montenegro skin test	• It is hypersensitivity type IV reaction, characterized by induration following injection of *L. donovani* killed antigen • It is positive when CMI is good, i.e., positive in all stages of leishmaniasis; except active VL and diffuse CL
Animal inoculation	Chinese and golden hamsters

Abbreviations: LD, Leishman Donovan; ELISA, enzyme-linked immunosorbent assay; ICT, immunochromatographic test; CMI, cell-mediated immunity; VL, visceral leishmaniasis; CL, cutaneous leishmaniasis; PCR: polymerase chain reaction.

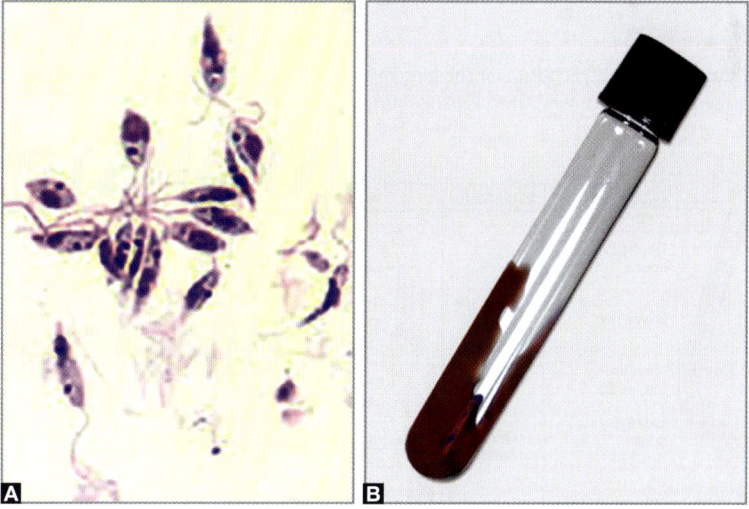

Figs 20.10A and B: (A) Smear made from culture fluid shows promastigote forms (Giemsa stain); (B) NNN medium.
Source: (A) DPDx Image Library, Centers for Disease Control and Prevention (CDC), Atlanta (*with permission*); (B) World Health Organization, "Manual on visceral leishmaniasis control" (Slide22/Alvar) (*with permission*).

LYMPHATIC FILARIASIS

Problem Solving Exercise 4

A 25-year-old male from a village in Puducherry came to this hospital with history of fever on and off for the past 1 year and recent unilateral swelling of the left lower limb. His blood sample was collected, and sent for peripheral blood smear examination (Fig. 20.11A).
1. Identify the parasite.
2. Draw a neat, labeled diagram of the etiological agent focused.
3. Which is the infective stage of the parasite for man?
4. How does man acquire this infection and what is the vector involved?
5. What are the different modalities of diagnosis of this clinical condition?

Explanation

It is a case of lymphatic filariasis due to *Wuchereria bancrofti*. Points in favor are:
- Fever with unilateral lower limb swelling
- Peripheral blood smear examination revealed microfilaria, 240 µm in length, tail tip pointed free of nuclei (Fig. 20.11A).
- Neat labeled diagram of microfilaria is shown in Figure 20.12.
- Microfilaria of *W. bancrofti* is often confused with that of *Brugiya malayi* (Fig. 20.11B); the differentiating features of both are depicted in (Fig. 20.13).

For answer to other questions, refer Table 20.6.

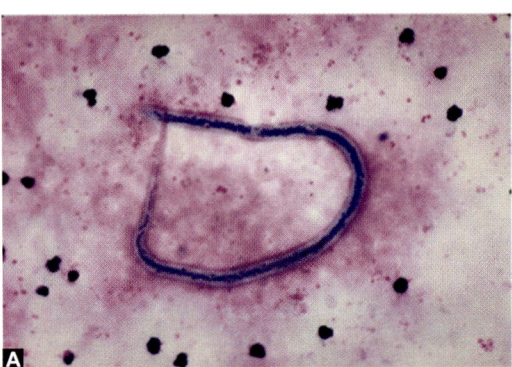
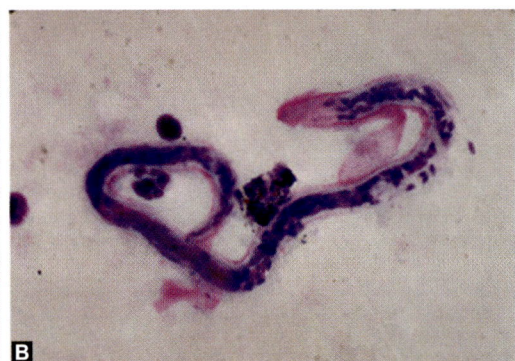

Figs 20.11A and B: Peripheral blood smear showing microfilaria of: (A) *Wuchereria bancrofti*; (B) *Brugiya malayi*.
Source: (A) ID# 3009/; (B) ID# 3003; Dr Mae Melvin, Public Health Image Library, Centers for Disease Control and Prevention (CDC), Atlanta (*with permission*).

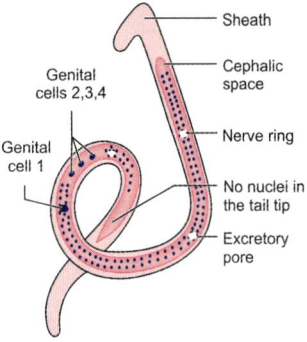

Fig. 20.12: Microfilaria of *Wuchereria bancrofti*.

Microfilaria	Head end	Tail end	Features*
Wuchereria bancrofti	Sheath Cephalic space (1:1) Coarse nuclei well-separated	No nuclei in the tail tip Pointed tail tip	A: 240–300 mm B: Nocturnal C: Sheathed D: Blood
Brugia malayi	Sheath Cephalic space (2:1) Darkly stained large coarse overlapping nuclei	Four to five nuclei in the tail region Two widely spaced nuclei in tail tip	A: 220 mm B: Nocturnal C: Sheathed D: Blood

Fig. 20.13: Differences between microfilaria of *Wuchereria bancrofti* and *Brugiya malayi*.
Key: *A: Size, B: Periodicity, C: Sheath, D: Habitat.

Table 20.6: Characteristics of lymphatic filarial worms.

Characteristics	Filarial worm

Host	- Definitive—humans
	- Intermediate—mosquito, for example:
	   › *Wuchereria*: *Culex fatigans, Aedes* and *Anopheles*
	   › *Brugiya*: *Mansonella* and *Anopheles*

Infective form	Filariform (L3) larva
Transmission	Mosquito bite
Habitat	Lymphatics
Pathogenic form	Adult worms in lymphatics
Manifestations of lymphatic filariasis	*Acute filariasis (acute adenolymphangitis)* - Fever - Transient local edema - Dermatolymphangitis: Plaque-like lesion
	Chronic filariasis: It develops 10–15 years after infection. - Hydrocele - Elephantiasis (swelling of lower limb or less commonly arm, vulva or breast) - Chyluria—excretion of chyle in urine
Occult filariasis	- This is a hypersensitivity reaction to microfilarial antigens mainly affecting lungs causing tropical pulmonary eosinophilia. - Microfilaria will be absent from peripheral blood
Diagnostic form (Fig. 20.11)	**Demonstration of microfilariae** by thin or thick smear stained with Giemsa or by QBC examination—blood collected during night hours (or day time after DEC provocation test) Detects microfilaria; based on which *Wuchereria* and *Brugia* can be differentiated
Other methods of laboratory diagnosis	- **Antigen detection** (ELISA, ICT)—detects Ag by using monoclonal antibodies to Og4C3 Ag and AD12 Ag - Antibody detection—IFA, ELISA ELISA detecting antibody to AD12 and Og4C3 antigen - Imaging methods—USG, X-ray - Molecular methods—real-time PCR detecting genes such as *SspI* repeat, *pWb12* repeat, *pWb-35* etc. - Eosinophilia and elevated IgE
Treatment	In India: DEC + albendazole African cases: DEC + Ivermectin

Abbreviations: ELISA, enzyme-linked immunosorbent assay; IFA, immunofluorescent antibody; ICT, immunochromatographic test; USG, ultrasonography; PCR, polymerase chain reaction; DEC, diethylcarbamazine

Fungal Infections of Bloodstream: Systemic Candidiasis and Systemic Mycoses

CHAPTER 21

▮ SYSTEMIC CANDIDIASIS

Problem Solving Exercise

A 29-year-old HIV-infected male presents to the clinic with history of high-grade fever and altered mental status. On examination, his blood pressure was found as 90/60 mm of Hg, and respiratory rate was increased to 28 per minute. Blood cultures were collected in BacT/ALERT bottles, which flagged positive after 22 hours of incubation. Gram stain of blood culture broth is shown in the Figure 21.1A.
a. What is the clinical diagnosis and the likely etiological agent?
b. Name the risk factors predisposing this clinical condition.
c. What are the other clinical manifestations caused by this organism?
d. Describe the laboratory diagnosis of this clinical condition in detail.

Explanation:
It is a case of sepsis due to systemic candidiasis
- Low blood pressure, increased respiratory rate and altered mental status is suggestive of clinical diagnosis of sepsis
- Blood culture broth smear (Fig. 21.1A) reveals gram-positive oval budding yeast cells with pseudohyphae—suggestive of *Candida* species.

The explanation for the remaining questions have been discussed subsequently in the text.

Introduction

Candidiasis is the most common fungal disease in humans, affecting the skin, mucosa, and various internal organs; caused by *Candida*, a yeast-like fungus that produces pseudohyphae. Pseudohypha is an important virulence factor, helps in invasion. Various species of *Candida* include:
- *Candida albicans:* It is the most pathogenic species of *Candida* infecting humans
- Other *Candida* species which can also cause infection are *C. tropicalis* (most common species), *C. glabrata*, *C. krusei*, *C. parapsilosis*, *C. dubliniensis*, *C. kefyr*, *C. guilliermondii*, *C. viswanathii* and *C. auris*.

Predisposing Factors

Predisposing factors that are associated with increased risk of infection with *Candida* include:
- **Physiological state:** Extremes of age (infancy, old age), pregnancy
- **Low immunity:** Patients on steroid or immunosuppressive drugs, post-transplantation, malignancy, HIV-infected people
- Patients on **broad spectrum antibiotics**—suppress the normal flora
- **Others:** Diabetes mellitus, febrile neutropenia and zinc or iron deficiency.

Clinical Manifestations

Candida species produce a spectrum of infections ranging from skin and mucosal infection to invasive and allergic infections.
- **Invasive candidiasis:** It results from hematogenous or local spread of the fungi. Various forms are:
  - Urinary tract infection
  - Pulmonary candidiasis
  - Septicemia (mainly by *C. albicans* and *C. glabrata*)
  - Arthritis and osteomyelitis
  - Meningitis

CHAPTER 21 ♦ Fungal Infections of Bloodstream: Systemic Candidiasis and Systemic Mycoses

- Ocular—keratoconjunctivitis and endophthalmitis
- Hepatosplenic candidiasis
- Disseminated candidiasis
- Nosocomial candidiasis (mainly by *C. glabrata*).

❖ **Mucosal candidiasis:** The various mucosal manifestations include oropharyngeal candidiasis (oral thrush), vulvovaginitis, etc.

❖ **Cutaneous candidiasis:** The cutaneous manifestations seen in candidiasis are intertrigo (pustules in the skin folds) and nail infections such as paronychia and onychomycosis

❖ **Allergic candidiasis,** such as candidid reaction

❖ *Candida auris* has recently emerged as a potentially multi-drug resistant species of *Candida* known to cause severe disease in healthcare setting.

Laboratory Diagnosis

Specimen Collection

Depending on the site of infection, various specimens can be collected, such as urine or blood.

Direct Microscopy

Gram staining reveals gram-positive oval budding yeast cells (4–6 μm size) with pseudohyphae (Fig. 21.1A). It has to be differentiated from true hyphae (Table 21.1).

Culture

Specimens can be inoculated onto SDA with antibiotic supplements and then incubated at 37°C. *Candida* can also grow in bacteriological culture media, such as blood agar. Blood for culture can be inoculated into blood culture bottles (conventional or automated blood culture bottles, such as BacT/ALERT).

❖ Colonies appear in 1–2 days and described as creamy white, smooth, and pasty with typical yeasty odor (Fig. 21.1B)

❖ Gram staining of the colonies shows gram-positive budding yeast cells with pseudohyphae except for *C. glabrata* which does not show pseudohyphae.

Tests for Species Identification

❖ **Germ tube test:** It is a specific test for *C. albicans*; also called Reynolds Braude phenomenon
  - Colonies are mixed with human or sheep serum and incubated for 2 hours. Wet mount preparation is examined under microscope
  - Germ tubes are formed, described as long tube-like projections extending from the yeast cells
  - It is differentiated from pseudohyphae as there is no constriction at the origin (Fig. 21.1D, Table 21.1)

Table 21.1: Differences between pseudohyphae and true hyphae.

Features	Pseudohyphae	True hyphae
Morphology	Elongated chains of budding yeast cells	Elongated branching filaments
Grows by	Budding	Apical elongation
Septa	Constricted	No constriction

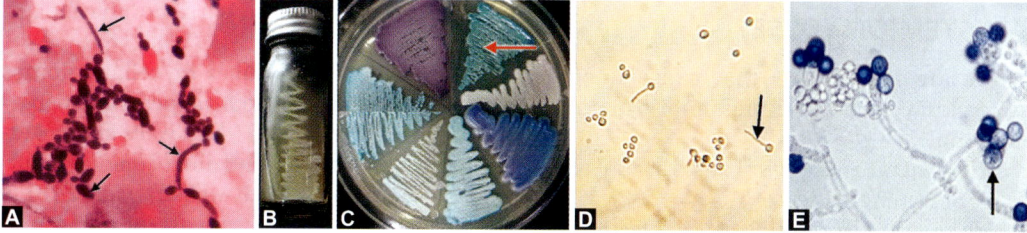

Figs 21.1A to E: (A) *Candida albicans*—gram-positive oval budding yeast cells with pseudohyphae; (B) *Candida albicans* on SDA shows creamy white colonies; (C) CHROMagar showing colonies of various *Candida* species producing different colors (e.g., light-green color by *C. albicans*, red arrow); (D) *Candida albicans* shows positive germ tube test (arrow showing); (E) *Candida albicans* shows thick walled chlamydospores (arrow showing).

Source: (A to D) Department of Microbiology, Pondicherry Institute of Medical Sciences, Puducherry; (E) ID#:2917/Centers for Disease Control and Prevention (CDC), Atlanta (*with permission*).

- Though the test is specific for *C. albicans*, it may also be positive for *C. dubliniensis*.
- **Dalmau plate culture:** Culture on cornmeal agar can provide clue for species identification. *C. albicans* produces thick walled chlamydospores (Fig. 21.1E)
- **CHROMagar:** Different *Candida* species produce different colored colonies on CHROMagar (Fig. 21.1C)
- **Automated systems**, such as MALDI-TOF and VITEK can also be used for speciation
- **Molecular methods**, such as PCR using species specific primers are useful for species identification.

Immunodiagnosis

- **Antibody detection:** Various formats, such as ELISA, latex agglutination tests are available detecting serum antibodies against cell wall mannan antigen
- **Antigen detection:** *Candida* specific antigen, such as cell wall mannan and cytoplasmic antigens can be detected by ELISA
- **β-d-Glucan assay:** It is a marker of invasive fungal infections, (including invasive candidiasis) and can also be used for monitoring response to treatment. It can be detected in blood by colorimetric enzyme immunoassay.

Treatment

- The antifungal drugs recommended for systemic candidiasis are liposomal amphotericin B or caspofungin or voriconazole/fluconazole
- *C. glabrata* and *C. krusei* exhibit resistance to azoles and are refractory to treatment with azoles.

SYSTEMIC MYCOSES

There are four agents that cause deep or systemic mycoses. These fungi are also thermally dimorphic.
- *Histoplasma capsulatum* causes histoplasmosis or Darling's disease
- *Blastomyces dermatitidis* causes blastomycosis
- *Coccidioides immitis* causes coccidioidomycosis
- *Paracoccidioides brasiliensis* causes paracoccidioidomycosis.

Histoplasmosis

Histoplasmosis is a systemic granulomatous disease caused by dimorphic fungus, *Histoplasma capsulatum*.

Pathogenesis

H. capsulatum is transmitted by inhalation of spores (i.e., microconidia) which usually circulate in the air after contaminated soil is disturbed.

Clinical Manifestations

Clinically, the classical histoplasmosis ranges from asymptomatic infection (in immunocompetent people) to life-threatening illness seen in people with low case mix index. The various clinical types include:
- **Pulmonary:** It is the most common form
- **Mucocutaneous:** Skin and oral mucosal lesions seen
- **Disseminated form:** most commonly involving the bone marrow, spleen, liver, eyes and adrenal glands, in immunocompromised host.

Laboratory Diagnosis

Histoplasmosis can be diagnosed by:
- **Specimens** helpful for establishing the diagnosis include sputum, aspirate from bone marrow and lymph node, blood and biopsies from skin and mucosa
- **Direct microscopy:** Histopathological staining (such as periodic acid–Schiff, Giemsa or Gomori methenamine silver) of the specimens reveal tiny oval yeast cells (2–4 μm size) with narrow based budding within the macrophages and underlying granulomatous response (Fig. 21.2A)
- **Culture:** *Histoplasma* is a dimorphic fungus, hence:
  - At 25°C: It produces mycelial colonies which on LPCB mount appears as tuberculate macroconidia (thick walls and finger-like projections) and microconidia (smaller, thin and smooth-walled) (Fig. 21.2B)
  - At 37°C: It produces yeast form (creamy-white colonies).

Treatment

Liposomal amphotericin B is the antifungal of choice in acute pulmonary and disseminated

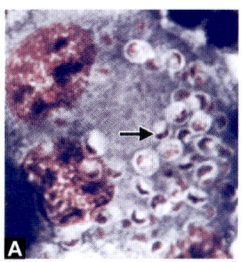 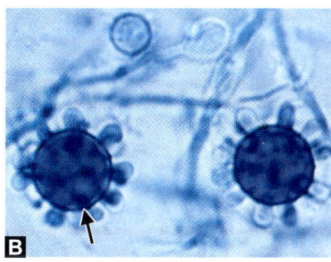 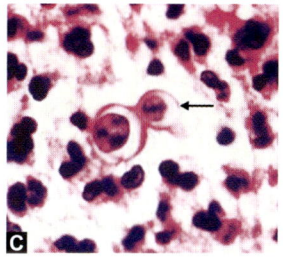

Figs 21.2A to C: (A) *H. capsulatum* [yeast cells with narrow-based budding (Giemsa stain)]; (B) Mold form of *H. capsulatum*, septate thin hyphae with tuberculate macroconidia (arrows showing); (C) *Blastomyces* [histopathological stain- shows broad-based budding yeast cells (figure of 8 appearance)].

Source: (A) Dr Lucille K. Georg/ID#:15365; (B) Dr Libero Ajello/ID#:15364; (C) ID#:493/Centers for Disease Control and Prevention (CDC), Atlanta *(with permission)*.

histoplasmosis. Itraconazole is recommended for chronic cavitary pulmonary histoplasmosis.

Blastomycosis

This disease is caused by *Blastomyces dermatitidis*; endemic in North America.

- ❖ **Clinical manifestations:** Acute pulmonary form is the most common. Extrapulmonary manifestations include verrucose skin lesions, osteomyelitis and rarely CNS involvement in AIDS patients
- ❖ **It is diagnosed by** histopathological staining of the tissue biopsy specimens which reveals thick-walled round yeast cells of 8–15 μm size with single broad-based budding (*figure of 8 appearance*) (Fig. 21.2C).

Coccidioidomycosis

Also called as desert rheumatism or Valley fever; caused by *Coccidioides immitis*.

- ❖ **Clinical manifestations:** Most patients are asymptomatic (60%). In remainders, pulmonary form is the most common followed by skin lesions and arthritis. Disseminated form occurs in AIDS patients with low CMI
- ❖ **Laboratory diagnosis:**
  - Histopathological staining of sputum or tissue biopsy specimens demonstrates spherules. **Spherules** are large sac, such as structures (20–80 μm size), have thick, doubly refractive wall, and are filled with endospores (Fig. 21.3A)
  - Cultures on SDA produces mycelial growth which on LPCB mount reveals fragmented hyphae consisting of barrel-shaped arthrospores with alternate cells distorted (empty cells) (Fig. 21.3B).

Paracoccidioidomycosis

This disease is caused by *Paracoccidioides brasiliensis*; endemic in South America.

- ❖ **Clinical manifestations:** It occurs in two forms
  - Acute form (or juvenile type): It is less common but more severe form, affects young adults; manifests as disseminated infection involving multiple viscera and is refractory to treatment
  - Chronic form (or adult form): It is more common, less severe form, affects older men, manifests as progressive pulmonary disease.
- ❖ **Laboratory diagnosis:** Histopathological staining of pus, tissue biopsies or sputum reveals round thick-walled yeasts, with multiple narrow-necked buds attached circumferentially giving rise to *Mickey Mouse or pilot wheel appearance* (Fig. 21.3C).

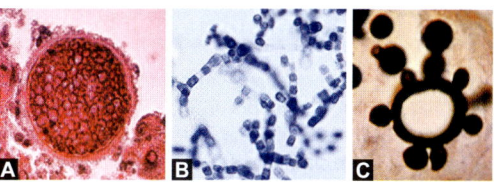

Figs 21.3A to C: *Coccidioides* (A) Spherule (PAS staining); (B) Hyphae with arthroconidia (LPCB mount)]; (C) Paracoccidioidomycosis [Methenamine silver staining shows yeast from (pilot wheel appearance)].

Source: Public Health Image Library/(A) ID#:14499; (B) ID#:12196; (C) Dr Lucille K Georg/ID#:527/Centers for Disease Control and Prevention (CDC) Atlanta *(with permission)*.

CHAPTER 22
Bacterial Diarrhea: Shigellosis, Cholera and Others

■ INTRODUCTION

The diarrheal diseases are one of the leading cause of illness globally; cause significant morbidity and mortality. Diarrhea and dysentery are the two important clinical types:
1. **Diarrhea** is defined as passage of three or more loose or liquid stools per day, in excess than the usual habit for that person. It may be watery type of diarrhea (non-inflammatory) or stool mixed with pus (inflammatory type)
2. **Dysentery** is characterized by diarrhea with increased blood and mucus, often associated with fever, abdominal pain, and tenesmus (feeling of constant need to pass stools, despite an empty colon).

Bacterial Etiology

Bacterial agents account for a significant proportion of diarrheal diseases.
- ❖ **Bacterial agents causing diarrhea:** Mostly enterotoxin mediated
  - ■ *Vibrio cholerae*
  - ■ *Diarrheagenic Escherichia coli*
    - ♦ Enteropathogenic *E. coli*
    - ♦ Enterotoxigenic *E. coli*
    - ♦ Enteroaggregative *E. coli*.
  - ■ *Clostridium perfringens*
  - ■ *Bacillus cereus*
  - ■ *Staphylococcus aureus*
  - ■ *Aeromonas hydrophila*
  - ■ *Plesiomonas shigelloides*.
- ❖ **Predominantly inflammatory diarrhea:**
  - ■ Non-typhoidal salmonellae
  - ■ *Yersinia enterocolitica*
  - ■ *Listeria monocytogenes*
  - ■ *Clostridioides difficile*
  - ■ *Plesiomonas shigelloides*.
- ❖ **Predominantly dysentery:**
  - ■ *Shigella* species
  - ■ *Campylobacter jejuni*
  - ■ Diarrheagenic *E. coli*
    - ♦ Enterohemorrhagic *E. coli*
    - ♦ Enteroinvasive *E. coli*.
  - ■ *Vibrio parahaemolyticus*.

Important bacterial pathogens of GIT are discussed here. The viral and parasitic agents are discussed in subsequent chapters.

■ SHIGELLOSIS

Problem Solving Exercise 1

A 6-year-old child presented with tenesmus, abdominal pain and passage of blood-tinged stool 10 times for one day. Stool specimen was subjected to culture (Fig. 22.1), Gram staining of culture smear (Fig. 22.2), biochemical reactions (Fig. 22.3) and agglutination test with specific antisera (Fig. 22.4). The antimicrobial susceptibility test (AST) is demonstrated in Figure 22.5 with zone interpretation chart in Table 22.1.
- ❏ What is the clinical diagnosis and its causative organism?
- ❏ What are the various modalities of laboratory diagnosis?
- ❏ How will you treat this condition?

Explanation

Clinical Diagnosis

The history of passage of blood-tinged stool, tenesmus and abdominal pain is suggestive of dysentery.

The common agents of dysentery include *Shigella*, enteroinvasive *Escherichia coli*, enterohemorrhagic *E. coli*, *Campylobacter jejuni*, *Vibrio parahemolyticus* and parasites, such as *Entamoeba histolytica* and *Balantidium coli*.

Identification
Based on the culture on MacConkey agar (Fig. 22.1A), Gram staining of culture smear (Fig. 22.2), biochemical reactions (Fig. 22.3), and positive agglutination with *Shigella* polyvalent antisera (Fig. 22.4), the causative organism can be identified as *Shigella*.

Antimicrobial Susceptibility Test and Treatment
Antimicrobial susceptibility test on Mueller-Hinton agar (Fig. 22.5) with zone interpretation chart (Table 22.1) shows that the pathogen is sensitive to ciprofloxacin, ampicillin and co-trimoxazole. As the patient is 6-year-old boy, preferred treatment option would be ampicillin or co-trimoxazole.
(For answers to other questions, refer text below).

Shigella is one of the important agent of bacillary dysentery; characterized by frequent passage of bloody mucopurulent stools with increased tenesmus and abdominal cramps. There are four species or serogroups which are further divided into serotypes:
1. Serogroup A: *S. dysenteriae* (15 serotypes)
2. Serogroup B: *S. flexneri* (8 serotypes)
3. Serogroup C: *S. boydii* (19 serotypes)
4. Serogroup D: *S. sonnei* (one serotype).

Pathogenesis
- **Mode of transmission:** Infection occurs by ingestion through contaminated fingers (most common), food, and water or rarely flies
- **Infective dose:** As low as 10–100 bacilli are capable of initiating the disease
- **Invasion:** Bacilli enter the mucosa via M cells (spread cell to cell) and are then engulfed by macrophages and induce recruitment of inflammatory cells releasing cytokines, which cause acute colitis—the hallmark of shigellosis
- **Exotoxin production:** *Shigella* produce exotoxins, such as enterotoxins and shiga toxin (causes local vascular damage of intestine, kidney and brain).

Clinical Manifestations
- **Incubation period:** It usually lasts for 1–4 days
- **Dysentery:** Frequent passage of bloody mucopurulent stools with increased tenesmus and abdominal cramps
- **Complications:** Theses are toxic megacolon, perforations and rectal prolapse.

Laboratory Diagnosis
- **Specimen collection:** Fresh stool sample is collected. Rectal swabs are not satisfactory
- **Transport media:** Specimens should be transported immediately. If delay is inevitable, specimens should be transported in a suitable medium, such as Sach's buffered glycerol saline
- **Wet mount preparation** of feces shows large number of pus cells, red blood cells and macrophages.

Culture
To inhibit the commensals, fecal specimen is inoculated simultaneously onto enrichment broth and selective media.
- **Enrichment broth,** such as *Selenite F broth, tetrathionate broth* and *Gram-negative broth* are used. Turbidity indicating growth appears in 18–24 hours, from which again subcultures are made onto selective media
- **Selective media,** such as:
  - *Mildly selective media*: On MacConkey agar, *Shigella* produces translucent non-lactose fermenting (NLF) colonies (Fig. 22.1A)
  - *Highly selective media:* They contain of bile salts as inhibitory agent
    - Deoxycholate citrate agar (DCA): It produces translucent NLF colonies (Fig. 22.1B)
    - Xylose lysine deoxycholate agar (XLD): Colonies of *Shigella* appear red without black center.

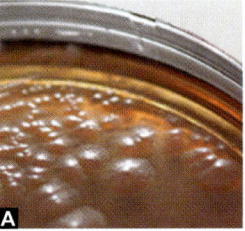 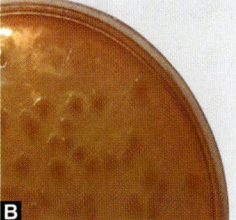

Figs 22.1A and B: *Shigella* producing translucent non-lactose fermenters colonies on (A) MacConkey agar; (B) Deoxycholate citrate agar.

Source: Department of Microbiology, Pondicherry Institute of Medical Sciences, Puducherry (*with permission*).

Identification

- **Culture smear and motility testing:** Gram stain of colonies reveal short, gram-negative bacilli (Fig. 22.2). They are nonmotile
- **Biochemical reactions:** Biochemically *Shigella* is an organism of exceptions. *Shigella* species and their serotypes can be differentiated by an array of biochemical tests
  - *Catalase*: All shigellae are catalase positive, except *S. dysenteriae* serotype-1
  - *Oxidase test* is negative for all species
- ICUT tests (Fig. 22.3): Indole test (negative), citrate test (negative), urease test (negative) and TSI (triple sugar iron agar) test shows alkaline/acid, gas absent, H_2S absent
- All *Shigella* species are mannitol fermenters; except *S. dysenteriae*.
- Identification of *Shigella* from colonies also can be made by automated identification systems such as VITEK
- **Serotyping:** Because of biochemical variations, identification of *Shigella* is always confirmed by slide agglutination with polyvalent antisera (genus specific). Then, the species identification can be done by using group specific antisera specific for serogroups. Serotypes under each species are further detected by using type specific antisera (Fig. 22.4)
- **Antimicrobial susceptibility testing** is done on Mueller-Hinton agar by disk diffusion test (Fig. 22.5 and Table 22.1).

Treatment

Because of the prompt transmissibility, current recommendation is that every case of shigellosis should be treated with antibiotics (for 3-5 days).
- Ciprofloxacin is the drug of choice
- Alternative drugs which are effective are— ceftriaxone or azithromycin.

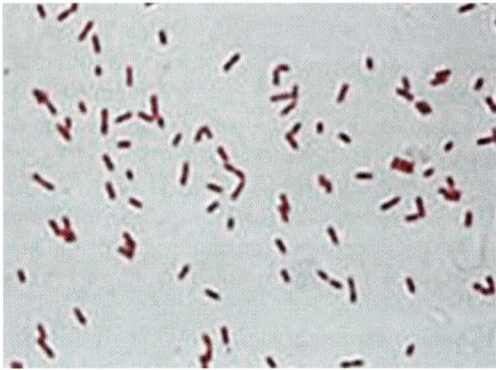

Fig. 22.2: Gram-stained smear showing short gram-negative bacilli (*Shigella*).
Source: Department of Microbiology, Pondicherry Institute of Medical Sciences, Puducherry (*with permission*).

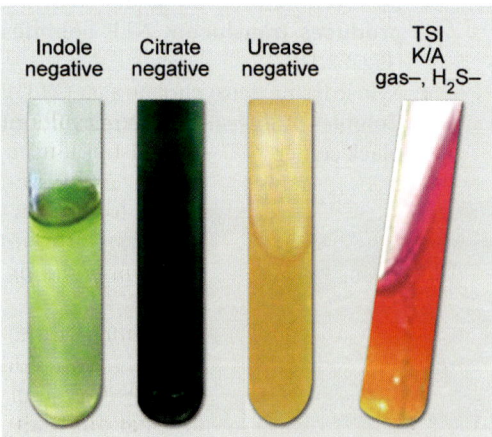

Fig. 22.3: Biochemical reactions of *Shigella*.
Source: Department of Microbiology, Pondicherry Institute of Medical Sciences, Puducherry (with permission).

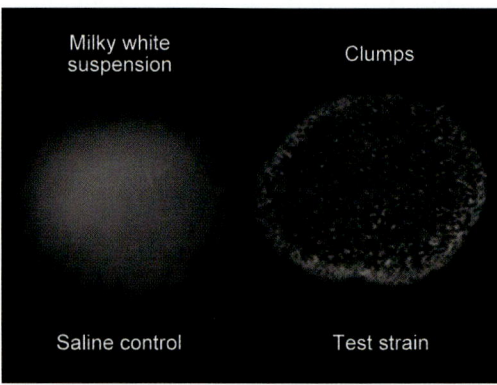

Fig. 22.4: Bacterial agglutination test: Test strain is tested with *Shigella* polyvalent antisera; presence of clumps indicates test is positive and the isolate can be identified as *Shigella*.
Source: Department of Microbiology, Pondicherry Institute of Medical Sciences, Puducherry (*with permission*).

Table 22.1: Interpretative categories (CLSI) and observed zone size diameter (mm) to various antimicrobial agents tested for *Shigella* species.

Antimicrobial agents	Disk strength (µg)	CLSI interpretative criteria for *Shigella* species (in mm)			Observed zone size (Fig. 22.5) (in mm)	Interpretation
		Resistant	Intermediate	Sensitive		
Ciprofloxacin (Cf)	5	≤21	22–25	≥26	27	Sensitive
Ampicillin (A)	10	≤13	14–16	≥17	21	Sensitive
Cotrimoxazole (Co)	1.25/23.75	≤10	11–15	≥16	19	Sensitive

Abbreviation: CLSI, Clinical and Laboratory Standards Institute.

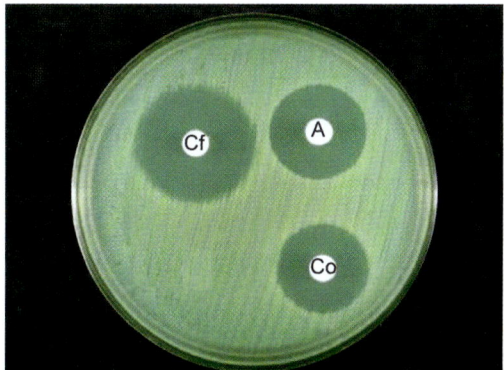

Fig. 22.5: Antimicrobial susceptibility testing on Mueller-Hinton Agar for *Shigella* species (Table 22.1 for CLSI zone interpretation).
Abbreviations: Cf, ciprofloxacin; A, ampicillin; Co, cotrimoxazole; CLSI, Clinical and Laboratory Standards Institute.
Source: Department of Microbiology, Pondicherry Institute of Medical Sciences, Puducherry (*with permission*).

DIARRHEAGENIC ESCHERICHIA COLI INFECTIONS

Although *E. coli* is a normal flora of GIT, certain types of *E. coli* (called diarrheagenic *E. coli*) are known to cause diarrhea. Diarrheagenic *E. coli* are of six pathotypes:

1. **Enteropathogenic E. coli (EPEC):** EPEC frequently causes infantile diarrhea (outbreaks) and occasionally cause sporadic diarrhea in adults. It acts by attachment and disruption of GI mucosa
2. **Enterotoxigenic E. coli (ETEC):** It is the most common agent of traveler's diarrhea; mediated by toxins, such as heat labile (LT) and heat stable (ST) toxins
3. **Enteroinvasive E. coli (EIEC):** It invades intestinal mucosa, causes dysentery
4. **Enterohemorrhagic E. coli (EHEC):** It also causes dysentery. The most common serotype of *E. coli* involved is O157:H7. It is mediated by verocytotoxin (or shiga-like toxin). It can cause complications, such as hemorrhagic uremic syndrome and hemorrhagic colitis
5. Enteroaggregative *E. coli* (EAEC)
6. Diffusely adherent *E. coli* (DAEC).

NON-TYPHOIDAL SALMONELLOSIS (NTS)

The *Salmonella* serotypes other than *S.* Typhi and *S.* Paratyphi can colonize the intestine of a broad range of animals, including mammals, reptiles, birds and insects. They also infect humans causing food-borne gastroenteritis and occasionally septicemia. Majority of infections due to NTS are caused by *S.* Typhimurium and *S.* Enteritidis and others.

Gastroenteritis

- Infection with NTS most often results in gastroenteritis—characterized by nausea, vomiting, watery diarrhea, fever and onset of abdominal cramps 6-48 hours after the ingestion of contaminated food (gastroenteritis is uncommon in typhoidal salmonellae)
- NTS is zoonotic, most commonly transmitted by consumption of contaminated animal food products, especially eggs, poultry, undercooked ground meat and dairy products
- Gastroenteritis caused by NTS is usually self-limited. Diarrhea resolves within 3-7 days.

CHOLERA

Problem Solving Exercise 2

A 8-year-old boy developed severe watery diarrhea (10–12 times) and vomiting for 2 days. Stool collected has a rice water type of appearance. The specimen was subjected to Gram staining (Fig. 22.6), culture (Fig. 22.7B) and biochemical reactions (Fig. 22.8), agglutination with antisera (Fig. 22.11). The antimicrobial susceptibility test (AST) is demonstrated in Figure 22.12 with zone of interpretation chart in Table 22.3.
- What is the clinical diagnosis and its causative organism?
- List the virulence factors and its mechanism of action.
- What are the various modalities of laboratory diagnosis?
- How will you treat this condition?

Explanation
Clinical Diagnosis
The history of severe watery diarrhea (rice water stool) and vomiting is suggestive of cholera.

Identification
- Based on the curved (comma shaped) gram-negative bacilli (Fig. 22.6), yellow-colored colonies on thiosulfate-citrate-bile salt-sucrose agar (TCBS agar; Fig. 22.7B), and biochemical reactions (Fig. 22.8), the identification is *Vibrio cholerae*
- Based on agglutination with specific antisera—the serotype is identified as "ogawa" (Fig. 22.11).

Antimicrobial Susceptibility Test
Antimicrobial susceptibility test on Mueller-Hinton agar (Fig. 22.12) with zone of interpretation (Table 22.3) shows that the isolate is sensitive to tetracycline, ampicillin, chloramphenicol and resistant to ciprofloxacin.
(For answers to other questions, refer text below).

Clinical Manifestations (Cholera)

Vibrio cholerae is the causative agent of cholera characterized by *painless* watery diarrhea.
- The stool is watery (rice water in appearance) with mucus flakes without blood or pus cells with a fishy, nonoffensive odor. Vomiting and muscle cramps are present but fever is usually absent
- **Complications:** Occurs late, include increased thirst, postural hypotension, tachycardia, decreased skin turgor and renal failure.

Virulence Factor

The following are the important virulence factors of *V. cholerae*:
- **Toxin coregulated pilus:** It helps in adhesion of *Vibrio* to intestinal mucosa
- **Cholera toxin:** It has two fragments. Fragment A is active, causes ADP-ribosylation of G protein, which in turn up regulates the activity of adenylate cyclase results in intracellular accumulation of cyclic adenosine monophosphate (cAMP), leads to accumulation of sodium chloride in the intestinal lumen, further leads to severe diarrhea.

Laboratory Diagnosis

Specimens
- Freshly collected watery stool is the specimen of choice; collected before starting the antibiotics
- Rectal swab is preferred for carriers.

Transport/Holding Media
Specimens should be transported immediately. If delay is expected, transport media are used, such as:
- Venkatraman-Ramakrishnan (VR) medium
- Cary-Blair medium
- Autoclaved sea water.

Direct Microscopy
- **Gram staining** of fecal smear (mucus flakes) reveals short curved *comma-shaped* gram-negative rods, typically arranged in parallel rows, described by Koch as *"fish in stream"* appearance (Fig. 22.6)
- **Motility testing by hanging drop method:** They are actively motile, described as *darting motility*. *V. cholerae* becomes nonmotile after stool specimen treated with flagellar (H) antiserum.

CHAPTER 22 ◆ Bacterial Diarrhea: Shigellosis, Cholera and Others

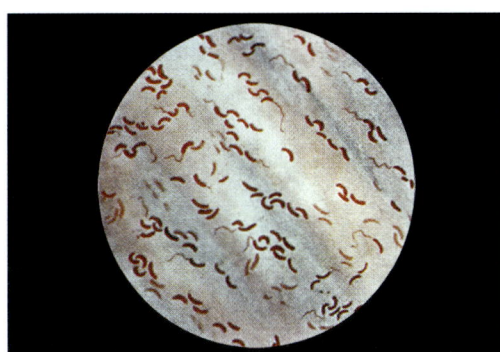

Fig. 22.6: *Vibrio cholerae* (Gram stain): Curved comma-shaped gram-negative rods (fish in stream appearance).
Source: Public Health Image Library, ID#:5324/Centers for Disease Control and Prevention (CDC) (*with permission*).

Culture

Vibrio cholerae is nonfastidious, strongly aerobic. Stool specimen is inoculated onto enrichment broth and selective media.

Enrichment Broth
- Alkaline peptone water (APW)
- Monsur's taurocholate tellurite peptone water.

Selective Media
- Alkaline bile salt agar (BSA)
- Monsur's gelatin taurocholate trypticase tellurite agar (GTTT)
- **TCBS agar:** This medium is widely in use at present (Fig. 22.7B). *V. cholerae* produces yellow-colored colonies due to sucrose fermentation
- **MacConkey agar:** *V. cholerae* produces translucent non-lactose fermenting (NLF) colonies.

Culture smear and Motility Testing
- Culture smear of the colonies reveals short curved gram-negative bacilli
- Hanging drop shows typical darting motility.

Bacterial Identification

Identification is made either by automated systems, such as MALDI-TOF or VITEK; or by conventional biochemical tests. The key biochemical properties include:
- Catalase and oxidase positive
- **ICUT test**—shows the following reactions (Fig. 22.8):
  - Indole test—positive
  - Citrate test—variable
  - Urease test—negative
  - TSI (triple sugar iron agar test)—Being sucrose fermenter, it shows acid/acid, gas absent, H_2S absent.
- **Hemodigestion:** On blood agar, it causes nonspecific lysis of blood cells, seen as greenish clearing around the main inoculum (Fig. 22.7A)
- **String test:** When a colony of *Vibrio* is mixed with a drop of 0.5% sodium deoxycholate on a slide, the suspension loses its turbidity, and becomes mucoid. When tried lifting the suspension with a loop, it forms a string (Fig. 22.9).

Typing of Vibrio cholerae (Fig. 22.10)
Serogrouping

Specific serogroups can be identified by using group-specific antisera. First the colony is tested

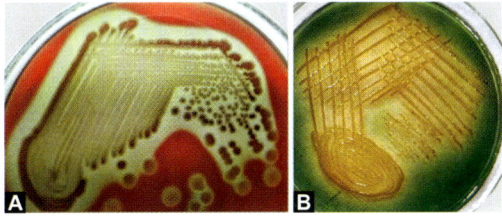

Figs 22.7A and B: (A) *Vibrio cholerae* on blood agar (hemodigestion); (B) TCBS agar with yellow-colored colonies of *Vibrio cholerae*.
Source: Department of Microbiology, Pondicherry Institute of Medical Sciences, Puducherry (*with permission*).

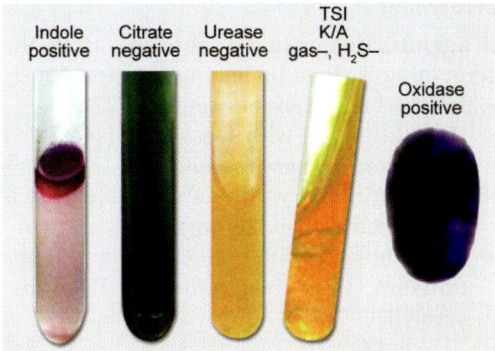

Fig. 22.8: Biochemical reactions of *V. cholerae*.
Source: Department of Microbiology, Pondicherry Institute of Medical Sciences, Puducherry (*with permission*).

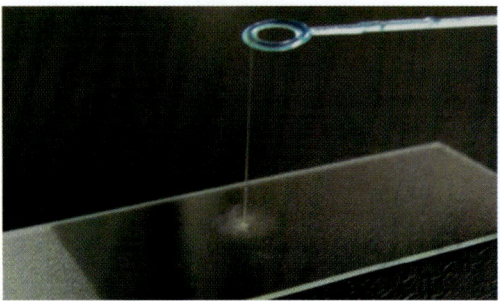

Fig. 22.9: String test (positive).
Source: Department of Microbiology, Pondicherry Institute of Medical Sciences, Puducherry (*with permission*).

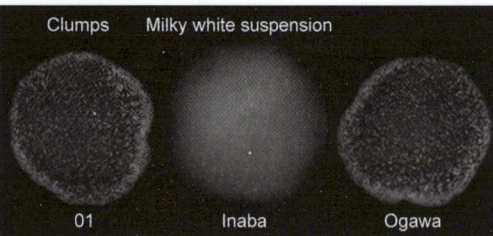

Fig. 22.11: Agglutination positive with O1 antisera and Ogawa antisera.
Source: Department of Microbiology, Pondicherry Institute of Medical Sciences, Puducherry (*with permission*).

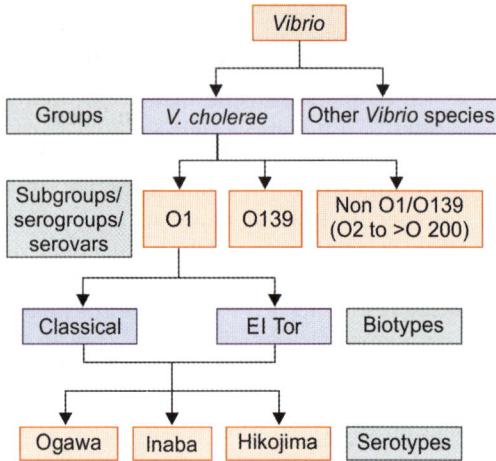

Fig. 22.10: Typing of *V. cholerae* (Gardner and Venkatraman classification).

with O1 antisera→ If found negative, then tested with O139 antisera (Fig. 22.11).

Serotyping

If agglutinated with O1 antisera, then the serotyping is done by testing simultaneously with Ogawa and Inaba antisera (Fig. 22.11).
- If agglutinated with Ogawa antisera, it is designated as Ogawa serotype
- If agglutinated with Inaba antisera, it is designated as Inaba serotype
- If agglutinated with both Ogawa and Inaba antisera, it is designated as Hikojima serotype.

Biotyping

Vibrio cholerae serogroup O1 can be further differentiated to biotypes classical and El Tor by various tests (Table 22.2). However, most of the strains are hybrid variety showing mixed results of both classical and El Tor biotypes.

Antimicrobial Susceptibility Testing

It is done on Mueller-Hinton agar by disk diffusion test. Interpretation is based on Clinical and Laboratory Standards Institute (CLSI) guideline (Fig. 22.12 and Table 22.3).

Table 22.2: Differences between classical and El Tor *Vibrio cholerae*.

Biotypes of *V. cholerae* O1	Classical	El Tor
Hemolysis on sheep blood agar	Negative	Positive
Polymyxin B (50 IU)	Susceptible	Resistant
VP test	Negative	Positive
Cholera toxin gene	CTX-1	CTX-2

Abbreviation: VP, Voges-Proskauer test.

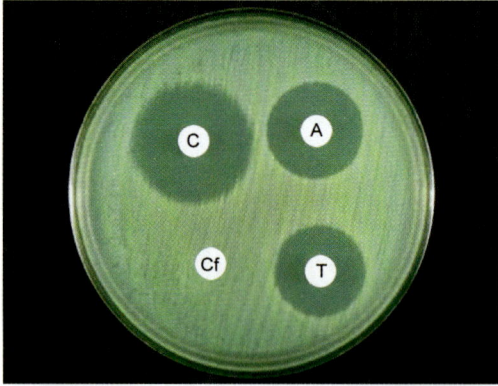

Fig. 22.12: Antimicrobial susceptibility testing on Mueller-Hinton Agar for *Vibrio cholerae* (Table 22.3 for CLSI zone interpretation).
Abbreviations: C, chloramphenicol; A, ampicillin; Cf, ciprofloxacin; T, Tetracycline; CLSI, Clinical and Laboratory Standards Institute.
Source: Department of Microbiology, Pondicherry Institute of Medical Sciences, Puducherry (*with permission*).

Table 22.3: Interpretative categories (CLSI) and observed zone size diameter (mm) to various antimicrobial agents tested for *Vibrio cholerae*.

Antimicrobial agents	Disk strength (µg)	CLSI interpretative criteria for *Vibrio cholerae* species (in mm)			Observed zone size (Fig. 22.12) (in mm)	Interpretation
		Resistant	Intermediate	Sensitive		
Ciprofloxacin (Cf)	5	≤15	16–20	≥21	6	Resistant
Ampicillin (A)	10	≤13	14–16	≥17	21	Sensitive
Tetracycline (T)	30	≤11	12–14	≥15	19	Sensitive
Chloramphenicol (C)	30	≤12	13–17	≥18	26	Sensitive

Abbreviation: CLSI, Clinical and Laboratory Standards Institute.
Note: Doxycycline should be tested by a MIC based method only (as there is no disk diffusion break point).

Treatment

- **Fluid replacement** is crucial. Oral rehydration solution is given in mild cases. In severe cases, intravenous fluid replacement with Ringer's lactate (or normal saline) is advised
- **Antibiotics** have a minor role as the pathogenesis is toxin mediated; recommended only in severe cases. Azithromycin or erythromycin are the drugs of choice. Alternatively doxycycline or tetracycline can be given.

Vaccine Prophylaxis

Oral cholera vaccines are currently in practice.
- **Killed whole-cell** vaccine and whole-cell recombinant B subunit cholera vaccine (WC/rBS) (Dukoral); given two oral doses
- **Oral live attenuated vaccines:** They use mutant strains that lack the gene encoding for cholera toxin, e.g., CVD 103-HgR vaccine (*Orochol*).

CLOSTRIDIOIDES DIFFICILE DIARRHEA

Problem Solving Exercise 3

A seriously-ill patient on ventilator in ICU developed diarrhea after 10 days of hospitalization. He was on ceftriaxone and clindamycin for 10 days. Stool sample was subjected to the following test shown in Figure 22.13C.
1. What is the clinical diagnosis and its causative organism?
2. Write the principle of the test.
3. How will you treat this condition?

Explanation
- **Clinical Diagnosis:** The history of severe diarrhea in a hospitalized patient after prolonged intake of antibiotics raises the suspicion of *C. difficile* diarrhea.
- **Identification:** The detection of toxin and glutamate dehydrogenase (GDH) antigen by the immunological test done on fecal specimen confirms the diagnosis (Fig. 22.13C)
- **Test Principle:** C. DIFF QUIK CHEK test: It is a rapid cassette assay that simultaneously detects both organism specific glutamate dehydrogenase (GDH) antigen and toxins of *C. difficile* in fecal specimens (Figs 22.13A to C).
- **Treatment:** Oral vancomycin and/or oral metronidazole are the recommended antibiotics for treatment.

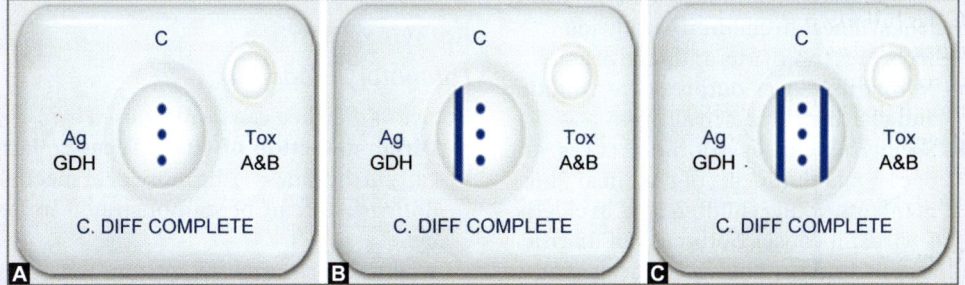

Figs 22.13A to C: *C. DIFF* QUIK CHEK test: (A) Only control band positive indicate test is negative; (B) Control band and glutamate dehydrogenase (GDH) band positive indicates nontoxigenic *Clostridioides difficile* present in stool (commensal); (C) Control band and GDH band positive indicates toxigenic *C. difficile* present in stool.

CHAPTER 23
Viral Gastroenteritis: Rotaviruses and Others

Problem Solving Exercise

A 4-year-old child was admitted to the pediatrics' ward with abdominal distress, diarrhea and mild dehydration, fever and vomiting for 2 days. Stool sample was for rotavirus antigen detection by ELISA (Fig. 23.1).
- Interpret the test result.
- What are the other viral agents that may cause similar illness?
- Name the mode of transmission of this infection.
- What are the different modalities of laboratory diagnosis?
- How will you prevent such disease in future?

Explanation

A 4-year-old child with symptoms of acute gastroenteritis, most common etiological agents would be gastroenteritis causing viruses. ELISA positive for rotavirus antigen in stool confirms the diagnosis as rotavirus gastroenteritis.
(For answers to other questions, refer below).

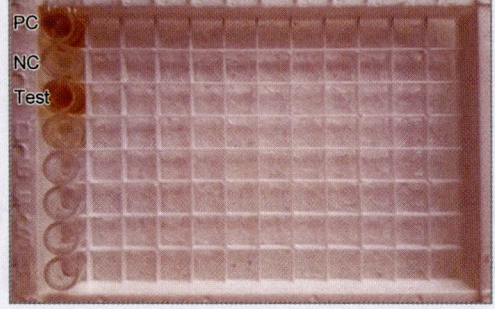

Fig. 23.1: Rotavirus antigen detection by ELISA.
Source: Department of Microbiology, Pondicherry Institute of Medical Sciences, Puducherry (*with permission*).

■ VIRAL GASTROENTERITIS

Viral etiology accounts for the most of the acute infectious gastroenteritis worldwide. The mode of transmission of infection is by consumption of contaminated food and water. The viral agents are:

- *Rotavirus*: Most common cause of severe diarrheal illness in children worldwide
- Caliciviruses (norovirus and sapovirus)
    - *Norovirus* causes outbreaks of vomiting and diarrheal illness in all ages
    - *Sapovirus* causes sporadic cases and occasional outbreaks of diarrheal illness in infants, young children, and in elderly.
- Astrovirus: It causes outbreaks of diarrheal illness in infants, young children, and in elderly
- Adenovirus (type 40 and 41): Second most common viral agent of endemic diarrheal illness of infants and young children worldwide.

Rotaviruses are transmitted by fecal–oral route, then they progress further to destroy enterocytes of small intestine to cause diarrhea.

Rotavirus Diarrhea

Laboratory Diagnosis

Rotavirus diarrhea can be diagnosed by:
- **Direct detection of virus:** Feces collected early in the illness is the most ideal specimen. Rotaviruses can be demonstrated in stool by:
    - *Immunoelectron microscopy*: Rotaviruses have sharp-edged, triple-shelled capsids;

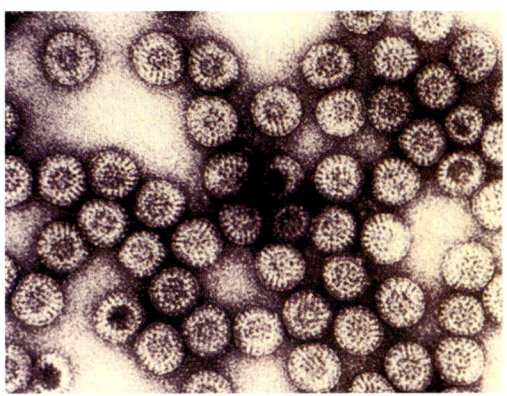

Fig. 23.2: Rotavirus (electron micrograph).
Source: Public Health Image Library, ID# 15194; Centers for Disease Control and Prevention (*with permission*).

look-like spokes grouped around the hub of a wheel (Fig. 23.2)
- *Isolation* of rotavirus is difficult. Rolling of tissue cultures may be attempted to enhance viral replication.
❖ **Detection of viral antigen** in stool—by ELISA and latex agglutination based methods
❖ **RT-PCR** is the most sensitive detection method for detection of rotavirus from stool
❖ **Serologic tests (ELISA)** can be used to detect the rise in antibody titer. This may be useful for seroprevalence purpose.

Treatment

Treatment is mainly supportive, to correct the loss of water and electrolytes, such as oral or parenteral fluid replacement.

Vaccine

Two brands of rotavirus vaccine are available:

Rotavac

It contains live attenuated rotavirus 116E (G9P[10] strain). It provides cross protection against many types including G1P[8] type.
❖ It is manufactured by Bharat Biotech, India
❖ It is introduced under national immunization schedule of India (2020), in selected states—Andhra Pradesh, Assam, Haryana, Himachal Pradesh, Jharkhand, Madhya Pradesh, Odisha, Rajasthan, Tamil Nadu, Tripura and Uttar Pradesh
❖ Three doses (5 drops/dose): Administered orally at 6, 10 and 14 weeks along with DPT and OPV
❖ Overall efficacy in first 2 years of life is about 55%
❖ Side effects (≥5%): Crying, irritability, fever and diarrhea. No vaccine induced intussusception has been reported.

Rotarix

Rotarix contains live attenuated G1P[8]strain; also provides cross protection against G3, G4 and G9. It has to be reconstituted before use. Given as two doses: 1st at 6 week and 2nd dose is given 4 weeks later.

General Preventive Measures

It includes—(1) measures to improve hygiene and sanitation in the community, and (2) contact precautions, such as strict hand hygiene to prevent transmission from infected persons (Chapter 11).

Norwalk Virus

It is the most important cause of epidemic viral gastroenteritis in adults
❖ It is common in winter months in temperate climates; therefore called as **winter vomiting disease** or gastric flu
❖ **Symptoms** begin 12-48 hours after the exposure; characterized by diarrhea, abdominal pain, nausea and vomiting
❖ **Common food sources** include contaminated salad, fresh fruits, shellfish (such as oysters), or water. Other sources include the infected person; touching contaminated surfaces.

Sapoviruses

They cause sporadic cases and occasional outbreaks of diarrheal illness in infants, young children, and the elderly.

Intestinal Protozoan Infections: Intestinal Amoebiasis, Giardiasis, Coccidian Parasitic Infections

CHAPTER 24

INTRODUCTION

The protozoan parasites which cause intestinal infection include:
- Intestinal amoebae: *Entamoeba histolytica*
- Intestinal flagellate: *Giardia lamblia*
- Opportunistic intestinal coccidian parasites: *Cryptosporidium*, *Cyclospora*, and *Cystoisospora*
- Others: *Balantidium coli*, *Blastocystis hominis*, *Sarcocystis* and Microsporidia (now considered as fungi).

Entamoeba histolytica and *Balantidium coli* produce dysentery, whereas the other intestinal protozoans produce diarrheal disease.

INTESTINAL AMOEBIASIS

Problem Solving Exercise 1

Intestinal Amoebiasis

A 13-year-old girl presented with bloody diarrhea with mucus and pus cells, colicky abdominal pain, fever and prostration. The wet mount examination of the stool sample has been focused (Fig. 24.1A).
1. Identify the structure focused and the etiological agent.
2. What is the host, infective form, pathogenic form, diagnostic form, habitat and mode of transmission of the parasite?
3. What are the various diagnostic modalities?
4. How will you treat this condition?

Explanation

This is a case of amoebic dysentery. Points in favor are:

- History of bloody diarrhea with mucus and pus cells, colicky abdominal pain
- The structure focused (Fig. 24.1A) is round, 12–15 μm size, with 3 to 4 nuclei and a central karyosome—suggestive of cyst of *Entamoeba histolytica* or *E. dispar*
- Cysts of *E. histolytica* and *E. dispar* are morphologically indistinguishable. To differentiate, multiplex polymerase chain reaction (PCR) should be performed targeting specific genes
- *Treatment*: Metronidazole 750 mg thrice a day given for 5–10 days (Table 24.1).

(For answers to the other questions, refer Tables 24.1 and 24.2).

Laboratory Diagnosis of Intestinal Amoebiasis

Stool microscopy is the mainstay of diagnosis of intestinal amoebiasis.
- Repeated stool microscopy is done by wet mount and permanent stains. If fails, then examination is done following stool concentration technique
- The cyst and trophozoites of *E. histolytica* must be differentiated from that of *Entamoeba coli* which is a harmless commensal of gut (Table 24.3 and Figs 24.1 and 24.2)
- The cyst and trophozoites of *E. histolytica* are morphologically similar to that of *E. dispar*,

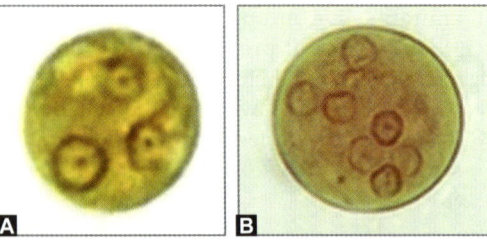

Figs 24.1A and B: Cyst of (A) *Entamoeba histolytica*; (B) *E. coli*.
Source: Swierczynski G, Milanesi B. Atlas of human intestinal protozoa microscopic diagnosis (*with permission*).

Table 24.1: Features/characteristics of *Entamoeba histolytica*.

Host	Humans are the only host
Morphological forms	Trophozoites, precyst and cyst
Infective form	Mature quadrinucleated cyst
Transmission	Feco-oral route (contaminated food and water)
Habitat	Large intestine
Pathogenic form	• Trophozoites • Surface lectin antigen helps in invasion
Major manifestations	*Intestinal amoebiasis:* • Amoebic dysentery • Amoebic appendicitis • Amoeboma • Fulminant colitis *Extraintestinal amoebiasis:* • Amoebic liver abscess—anchovy sauce pus and abscess formation • Other forms—pulmonary, CNS, cutaneous, etc.
Diagnostic form	• Cysts (both mature and immature cyst) are common • Trophozoites are rare
Treatment	*For intestinal amoebiasis:* • Tissue agents— metronidazole (5-10 days) or tinidazole (3 days) **plus** • Luminal agents— Iodoquinol (20 days) or Paromomycin (10 days)

Table 24.2: Laboratory diagnosis *Intestinal amoebiasis*.

Methods	Salient features
Stool microscopy	Detects cysts (most common) and trophozoites (rarely)
Histology	Intestinal biopsies stained with PAS or H&E stains reveal trophozoites
Stool culture	Polyxenic and axenic culture
Stool antigen detection (coproantigen)	ELISA and ICT detecting lectin antigen
Serology	Amoebic antigen—ELISA (170-kDa of lectin Ag) Amoebic antibody—ELISA This is more useful in amoebic liver abscess
Nested PCR	Can differentiate *E. histolytica* and *E. dispar*

Abbreviations: ELISA, enzyme-linked immunosorbent assay; ICT, immunochromatographic test; PCR, polymerase chain reaction.

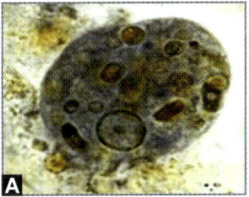 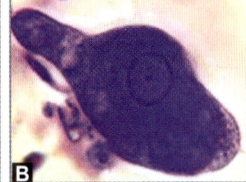

Figs 24.2A and B: Trophozoite of (A) *Entamoeba* coli; (B) *E. histolytica*.
Source: Swierczynski G, Milanesi B. Atlas of human intestinal protozoa microscopic diagnosis (*with permission*).

Table 24.3: Differentiating features between *Entamoeba histolytica* and *E. coli* (Figs 24.1 to 24.4).

Trophozoite	*Entamoeba histolytica*	*Entamoeba coli*
Size	15–20 µm	20–25 µm
Pseudopodia	Pseudopodia with finger-like projection Very active movement	Blunt pseudopodia Sluggish, aimless motility
Cytoplasm	Differentiated to ectoplasm and endoplasm	Not differentiated
Cytoplasmic inclusions	Red blood cell (RBC), leukocytes, tissue debris and bacteria	Same except it does not contain RBC
Nucleus (Figs 24.3A and 24.4A)	Karyosome is small and central Nuclear membrane is thin and lined by fine chromatin granules	Karyosome is large and eccentric Nuclear membrane is thick and lined by coarse chromatin granules
Cyst (Figs 24.3C and 24.4C)		
Size	12–15 µm	15–25 µm
Nucleus	Same as trophozoite	Same as trophozoite
No. of nuclei	1–4	1–8
Chromatoid body	Thick bars with rounded ends	Filamentous and thread-like ends

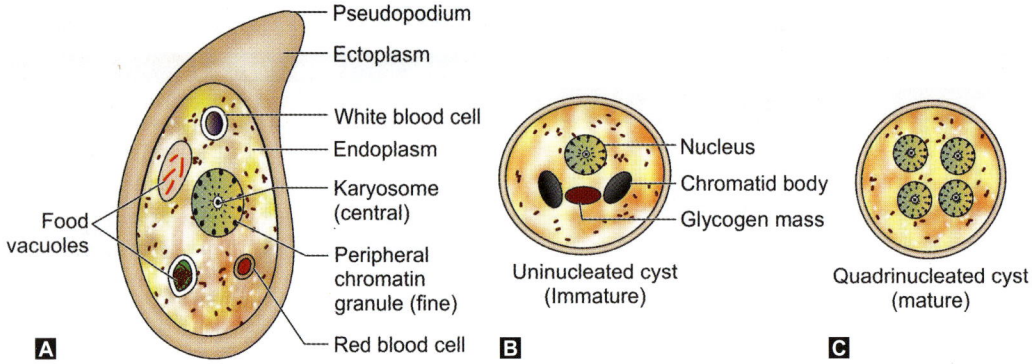

Figs 24.3A to C: *Entamoeba histolytica:* (A) Trophozoite; (B) Immature cyst; (C) Mature cyst.

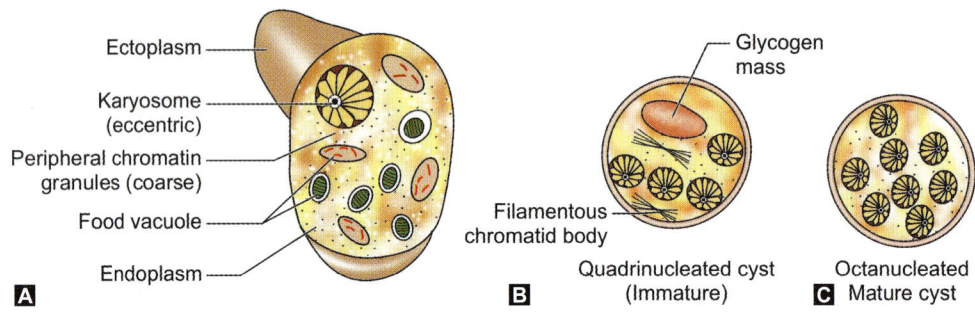

Figs 24.4A to C: *Entamoeba coli:* (A) Trophozoite; (B) Immature cyst; (C) Mature cyst.

which is again a harmless commensal of gut. *E. histolytica* can be differentiated by *E. dispar* by:
- Detection of lection antigen in stool
- Polymerase chain reaction
- Presence of red blood cells (RBCs) inside the trophozoite (sign of invasion)
- Isoenzyme (zymodeme analysis) detecting specific isoenzyme.

GIARDIASIS

Problem Solving Exercise

A 3-year-old boy presented with recurrent episodes of foul smelling diarrhea, foul flatus, sulfurous belching and profound weight loss. The wet mount examination of the stool sample has been focused (Figs 24.5B and C).
1. Identify the structure focused and the etiological agent.
2. What is the host, infective form, pathogenic form, diagnostic form, habitat and mode of transmission of the parasite?
3. What are the various diagnostic modalities?
4. How will you treat this condition?

Explanation

This is a case of giardiasis, caused by *Giardia lamblia* or *G. intestinalis*. Points in favor are:
- History of recurrent episodes of foul smelling diarrhea, foul flatus, sulfurous belching and profound weight loss
- The structure focused (Figs 24.5B and C) is oval cysts measuring 12–15 μm size, having 1–4 number nucleus with central axoneme (axostyle), suggestive of *Giardia lamblia*.
- *Treatment:* Metronidazole or tinidazole.

(For answers to the other questions, refer Tables 24.4 to 24.5).

Laboratory Diagnosis of Giardiasis

Stool microscopy is the mainstay of diagnosis of intestinal amoebiasis; carried out by wet mount (saline and iodine) preparation:

❖ Repeated stool examination (at least three consecutive samples) should be done following concentration techniques for better positivity

CHAPTER 24 ✧ Intestinal Protozoan Infections

Table 24.4: Laboratory diagnosis of *Giardia*.

Methods	Salient features
Stool microscopy	Detects cysts (most common) and trophozoites (rarely) • Sensitivity is 60% to 80% with one stool and >90% after three stools examination • Zinc sulfate flotation or formalin ether sedimentation concentration methods are used to increase the chance of detection
Duodenal sampling	Indicated when stool examination is negative. Direct duodenal samples, such as aspirates (obtained by entero-test) or biopsy (done by endoscopy) used (Fig. 24.7)
Permanent staining	Trichrome stain can be used to demonstrate cysts and trophozoites in stool
Stool culture	In axenic media, such as Diamond's media, not routinely used
Stool antigen detection	Coproantigen detection stool by ELISA, IFA and ICT methods ICT (triage parasite panel) available that simultaneously detects antigen of *Entamoeba histolytica*, *Giardia* and *Cryptosporidium* in stool
Serology (antibody detection)	Formats: ELISA and IFA Cannot differentiate recent and past infection
PCR	Most sensitive and specific

Abbreviations: ELISA, enzyme-linked immunosorbent assay; ICT, immunochromatographic test; IFA, indirect fluorescent antibody test; PCR, polymerase chain reaction.

Table 24.5: Trophozoite and cyst of *Giardia lamblia*.

Forms	Characteristics
Trophozoite (Figs 24.5A and 24.6A)	• Front view: Pear-shaped (or tear drop or tennis racket-shaped) • Lateral view: Spoon shaped • Measures 10–20 µm in length and 5–15 µm in width • Contains two adhesive disks, one pair of nuclei and four pairs of flagella • Has falling leaf-like motility • Presence of trophozoites indicates active stage of the disease
Cyst (Figs 24.5B and C and 24.6B)	• Oval, measuring 11–14 µm in length and 7–10 µm in width • Contains 1–4 nuclei and central axoneme or axostyle (remnant of flagella) • Cysts cannot differentiate active disease from carriers.

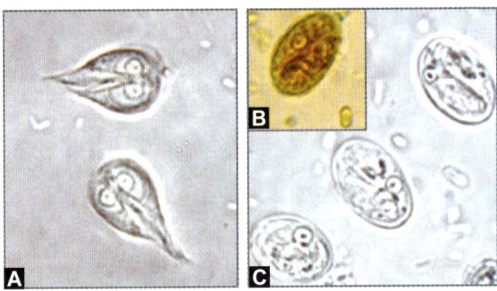

Figs 24.5 A to C: *Giardia lamblia*: (A) Trophozoites in saline mount; (B) Cyst in iodine mount; (C) Cysts in saline mount.
Source: Giovanni Swierczynski, Bruno Milanesi. "Atlas of Human Intestinal Protozoa Microscopic Diagnosis" (*with permission*).

❖ If still fails, direct examination of duodenal content (by performing string test or Entero-test).

Entero-test (or String Test)
It uses a gelatin capsule attached to a thread containing a weight (Fig. 24.7).
- One end of the thread is attached to the outer aspect of the patient's cheek, and then, the capsule is swallowed
- Capsule gets dissolved in stomach releasing the thread which is carried to the duodenum, gets unfolded and takes up the duodenal samples
- Four hours later, the thread is withdrawn and shaken in saline to release trophozoites which can be detected microscopically by wet mount or permanent stained smear
- The entero-test is also useful for other upper intestinal parasites, such as *Strongyloides*, *Cryptosporidium* and *Clonorchis*.

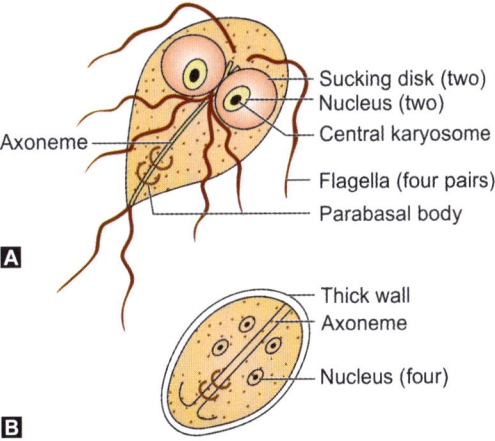

Fig. 24.6: *Giardia lamblia* (schematic diagram): (A) Trophozoite; (B) Cyst.

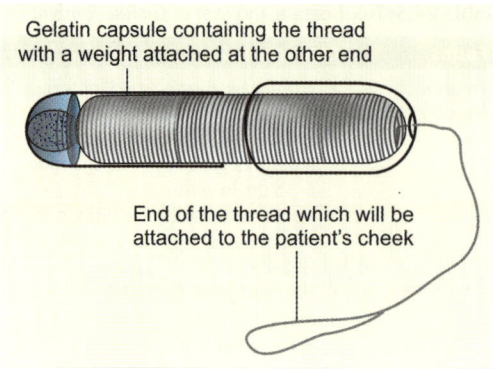

Fig. 24.7: Entero-test equipment showing duodenal capsule.

COCCIDIAN PARASITIC INFECTIONS

Cryptosporidium parvum, Cyclospora cayetanensis and *Cystoisospora belli* (earlier known as *Isospora belli*) are the coccidian parasites that cause diarrhea in immunocompromised host, such as HIV-infected patients.

Differences between properties of *Cryptosporidium, Cyclospora* and *Cystoisospora* is given in Table 24.6 and shown in Figures 24.8 to 24.11. Laboratory diagnosis of intestinal coccidian parasites is given in Table 24.7.

Problem Solving Exercise

A 61-year-old female presented with severe profuse diarrhea (20 times a day) for more than 10 days, weight loss and abdominal pain. The stool specimen was sent to microbiology laboratory for investigation (Fig. 24.8A and B.).
1. Identify the stain and etiological agent based on the smear focused.
2. What is the host, infective form, pathogenic form, diagnostic form, habitat and mode of transmission of this parasite?
3. How will you treat this clinical condition?

Explanation

This is a case of cryptosporidiosis, caused by *Cryptosporidium parvum*.
Points in favor are:
- HIV-infected patient
- Profuse diarrhea
- Modified acid-fast stain and direct fluorescent antibody staining showing round sporulated oocyst (4–6 µm in size), containing four sporozoites (Figs 24.8A and B).

Treatment: Nitazoxanide 500 mg, twice a day for 3 days. For answer to the other questions, refer Tables 24.6 and 24.7.

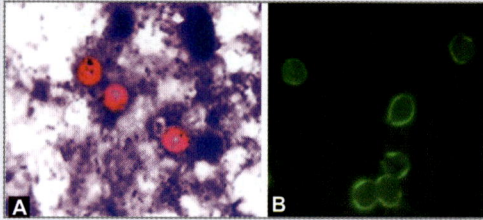

Figs 24.8A and B: *Cryptosporidium* species: (A) Modified acid-fast staining shows red colored (round) oocyst against blue background; (B) Direct fluorescent antibody staining shows brilliant green fluorescent oocysts.
Source: Swierczynski G, Milanesi B. Atlas of human intestinal protozoa Microscopic diagnosis (*with permission*).

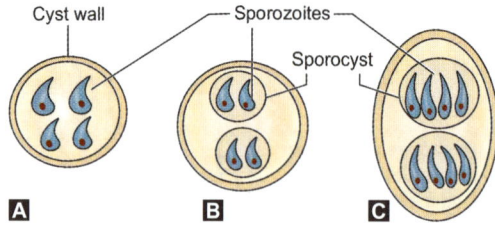

Figs 24.9A to C: Sporulated oocysts (schematic diagram) of (A) *Cryptosporidium*; (B) *Cyclospora*; (C) *Cystoisospora*.

CHAPTER 24 ❖ Intestinal Protozoan Infections

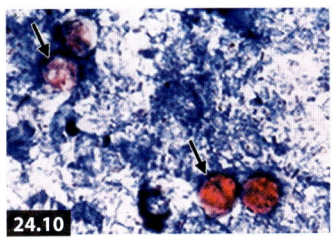 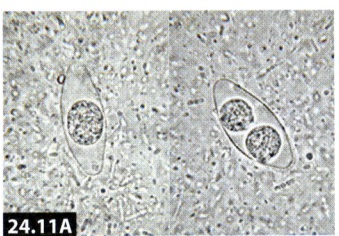 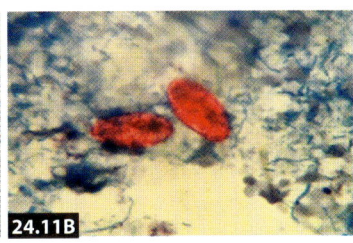

Fig. 24.10: *Cyclospora* species in modified acid-fast staining—shows variable acid-fast oocysts.
Figs 24.11A and B: *Cystoisospora belli*: (A) Saline mount shows unsporulated oocyst (left) and sporulated oocyst (right); (B) Modified acid-fast staining shows unsporulated oocysts.
Source: (Figs. 24.10 and 24.11A) Swierczynski G, Milanesi B. Atlas of human intestinal protozoa microscopic diagnosis (*with permission*).
Source: (Fig. 24.11B) Dr Anand Janagond, Department of Microbiology, S Nijalingappa Medical College, Bagalkot, Karnataka (*with permission*).

Table 24.6: Differences between properties of *Cryptosporidium*, *Cyclospora* and *Cystoisospora*.

Property	*Cryptosporidium*	*Cyclospora*	*Cystoisospora*
Infective form	Sporulated oocyst	Sporulated oocyst	Sporulated oocyst
Diagnostic form	Sporulated oocyst	Unsporulated oocyst	Unsporulated oocyst
Oocyst size	4–6 µm	8–10 µm	23–36 µm
Oocyst shape	Round	Round	Oval
Oocyst contains (Fig. 24.9)	4 sporozoites	2 sporoblasts, each having 2 sporozoites	2 sporoblasts, each having 4 sporozoites (Fig. 24.11A)
Oocyst acid fastness	Uniformly acid-fast (Fig. 24.8A)	Variable acid-fast (Fig. 24.10)	Uniformly acid-fast (Fig. 24.11B)
Autofluorescence	No, but can be stained with fluorescent dye (Fig. 24.8B)	Autofluorescence ++	Autofluorescence +/-
Sporulation of the oocyst	Occurs inside the host cells (enterocytes)	Occurs in soil (environment)	Occurs in soil (environment)
Treatment	Nitazoxanide	Cotrimoxazole	Cotrimoxazole

Table 24.7: Laboratory diagnosis of intestinal coccidian parasites.

Methods	Salient features
Stool examination	It is carried out to detect oocyst. Various methods: • Direct wet mount • Wet mount after stool concentration (Sheather's sugar floatation) • Modified acid-fast stain of stool (1% sulfuric acid as decolorizer) • Direct fluorescent antibody technique
Antigen detection in stool	• Antigen detection in stool by ICT or ELISA • Triage Micro Parasite Panel is an ICT used for simultaneous detection of *Giardia*, *Entamoeba histolytica* and *Cryptosporidium*
Antibody detection	• ELISA and IFA format available • Used for seroepidemiological purposes
Molecular method	Polymerase chain reaction detecting specific genes
Histopathology	Histopathology of intestinal biopsy specimen detecting oocyst

Abbreviations: ELISA, enzyme-linked immunosorbent assay; IFA, immunofluorescence assay; ICT, immunochromatographic test.

CHAPTER 25

Intestinal Helminthic Infections

■ INTRODUCTION

Intestinal helminthic infections contribute a significant proportion of gastrointestinal (GI) infections. Nevertheless, majority of helminths (cestodes, trematodes and nematodes) cause infections of GIT.

- **Intestinal cestodes:** *Diphyllobothrium, Taenia saginata, T. solium, Hymenolepis nana* and *Dipylidium caninum*
- **Intestinal trematodes:**
  - Intestinal fluke, e.g., *Fasciolopsis buski*
  - Blood flukes, such as *Schistosoma mansoni* and *S. japonicum* reside in mesenteric venous plexus of GIT, and cause various GI symptoms including dysentery.
- **Intestinal nematodes:** Include
  - Small intestinal nematodes—*Ascaris*, hookworm and *Strongyloides*
  - Large intestinal nematodes, such as *Trichuris* and *Enterobius*.

Cestodes exist in three morphological forms:
1. **Adult (tapeworm):** Divided into head (scolex), neck and segments called as proglottids or strobila. Some adult worms bear hooklets in scolex and are called as armed tapeworm, e.g., *T. solium, Echinococcus, H. nana*. Proglottids are further grouped into immature, mature and gravid segments (Fig. 25.1A)
2. **Eggs:** All cestodes eggs have an embryophore and an embryo with three pair of hooklets (Fig. 25.1B). The only exception is eggs of *Diphyllobothrium latum* which are operculated (Fig. 25.4)
3. **Larva:** Eggs develop into larva which are called as:
   - Cysticercus—larval stage of *Taenia* (*T. saginata*—Cysticercus bovis, *T. solium*—Cysticercus cellulosae)
   - Hydatid cyst—larval stage of *Echinococcus*
   - Cysticercoid—larval stage of *Hymenolepis*.

INTESTINAL CESTODE INFECTIONS

Cestodes, or tapeworms, are segmented worms. Based on habitat, cestodes are classified into:
- **Intestinal cestodes:**
  - *Diphyllobothrium* spp.
  - *Taenia saginata* and *Taenia solium*
  - *Hymenolepis nana*.
- **Tissue cestodes:**
  - *Echinococcus*—causes hydatid disease; mainly affecting liver (Chapter 27)
  - *Taenia solium*—causes cysticercosis, mainly infecting CNS (Refer Chapter 41).

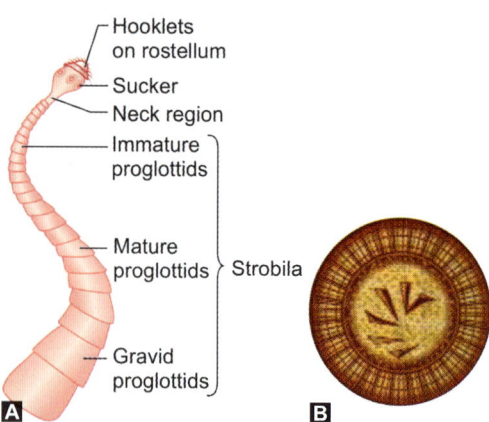

Figs 25.1A and B: (A) Adult worm of cestode (schematic diagram); (B) Egg of cestode (schematic diagram).

INTESTINAL TAENIASIS

Problem Solving Exercise 1

A 10-year-old child came to the pediatric OPD with history of passing segments of a worm. The stool examination revealed segments (Fig. 25.2C) and ova (Fig. 25.1B).
1. Identify the disease and the causative agent.
2. Name the different species which can infect man and how to differentiate them.
3. Which are the hosts, mode of transmission?
4. Name the larval stage of the species found in man and complications caused by the same.

Explanation

This is the case of intestinal taeniasis.
- There are two species of *Taenia* infecting man, *T. saginata* and *T. solium*.
- Figure 25.2C shows *Taenia* adult worm segments, tape-like segments.
- Figure 25.1B shows *Taenia* egg which is round to oval, containing an embryo with three pairs of hooklets, surrounded by an embryophore. The eggs of *T. saginata* and *T. solium* are indistinguishable, except that *T. saginata* eggs are acid-fast.

T. saginata and *T. solium* can be differentiated by:
- Proglottid: The proglottid of *T. saginata* has 15–20 lateral branches from uterus in comparison to that of *T. solium* which has 7–13 lateral branches from uterus
- Scolex: The scolex of *T. saginata* is quadrangular in shape bearing 4 suckers and with no hooklets (Fig. 25.2A). This can be differentiated from that of *T. solium* (globular, 4 suckers, armed with hooklets arising from rostellum (Fig. 25.2B).

Refer Table 25.1 for other details.

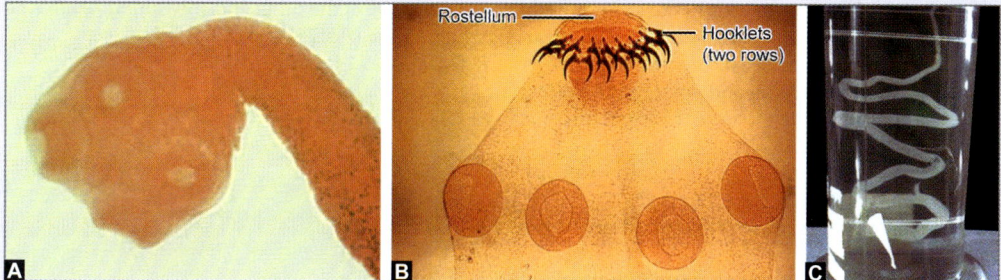

Figs 25.2A to C: (A) Carmine-stained scolex of *T. saginata*; (B) Carmine-stained scolex of *T. solium*; (C) Adult worm of *Taenia* species.
Source: (A) DPDx Image Library, Centers for Disease Control and Prevention (CDC), Atlanta (*with permission*); (B) Public Health Image Library, ID#: 5262, Centers for Disease Control and Prevention (CDC), Atlanta (*with permission*); C. Head, Department of Microbiology, Meenakshi Medical College, Chennai (*with permission*).

HYMENOLEPIASIS

Problem Solving Exercise 2

A 6-year-old child came to the OPD with history of anorexia, abdominal pain, dizziness and diarrhea. On examination, the child was malnourished. The stool specimen was sent for microscopic examination (Fig. 25.3).
1. Identify the parasite based on stool microscopy.
2. Which is the infective stage for man?
3. How the disease is transmitted?
4. Which are the parasites that are transmitted by autoinfection?
5. What are the examples of non-bile stained eggs?

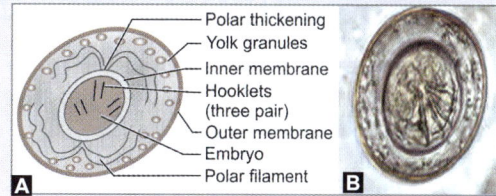

Figs 25.3A and B: Egg of *Hymenolepis nana*: (A) Schematic; (B) In saline mount (non-bile stained).
Source: (B) DPDx Image Library, Centers for Disease Control and Prevention (CDC), Atlanta (*with permission*).

Explanation

The causative agent is *Hymenolepis nana*. The points in favor are:
- Gastrointestinal symptoms—anorexia, abdominal pain, headache, and diarrhea.
- Figure 25.3B reveals non-bile stained eggs, with three pairs of hooklets, polar filaments filling between two membranes (Fig. 25.3A).
- Infective form: Eggs
- Mode of transmission: (i) Ingestion of contaminated food and water containing eggs; (ii) Autoinfection.

Autoinfection is seen in:
- *Cryptosporidium parvum*
- *Hymenolepis nana*
- *Enterobius vermicularis*
- *Strongyloides stercoralis*
- *Taenia solium*

Examples of non-bile stained eggs:
- *Hymenolepis nana*
- *Enterobius vermicularis*
- Hookworm.

Refer Table 25.1 for other details.

DIPHYLLOBOTHRIASIS

Problem Solving Exercise 3

A 16-year-old boy from Russia came to the OPD with complain of abdominal discomfort, diarrhea, vomiting, weakness and weight loss. Peripheral blood smear examination revealed increased mean corpuscular volume, increased mean corpuscular hemoglobin concentration, and enlarged red blood cells. The stool specimen was sent for microscopic examination (Fig. 25.4).

1. Identify the parasite based on the stool microscopy.
2. Which is the infective stage for man?
3. How will you diagnose this condition in the laboratory?
4. Mention two complications caused by the adult worm.

Explanation

This is a case of megaloblastic anemia due to *Diphyllobothrium latum*. Points in favor are:
- Patient from Russia—endemic for *D. latum* infection
- Gastrointestinal symptoms

- Evidence of megaloblastic anemia
- Stool microscopy revealed oval, operculated eggs with knob at the other end; measuring 70 μm × 50 μm in size (Fig. 25.4).

Refer Table 25.1 for other details.

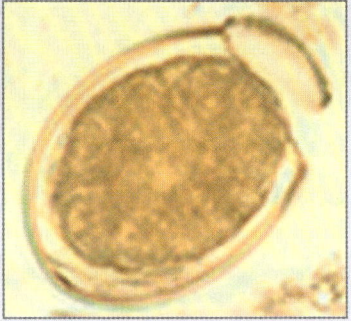

Fig. 25.4: Egg of *Diphyllobothrium latum*.
Source: DPDx Image Library, Centers for Disease Control and Prevention (CDC), Atlanta (*with permission*).

INTESTINAL TREMATODE INFECTIONS

Trematodes (also called as flukes) include the helminths that are unsegmented, flat (flat worms) and leaf like. They are classified based on their habitat into:

- **Blood flukes:**
  - *Schistosoma haematobium*—resides in vesical venous plexus of bladder (Refer Chapter 42)
  - *Schistosoma mansoni, Schistosoma japonicum*—resides in rectal venous plexus and portal venous plexus.
- **Hepatic flukes:** *Fasciola hepatica, Clonorchis* spp., *Opisthorchis* spp (Refer Chapter 27)
- **Intestinal flukes:** *Fasciolopsis buski*
- **Lung flukes:** *Paragonimus westermani* (Refer Chapter 38).

Table 25.1: Features or characteristics of intestinal cestodes.

Properties	Intestinal taeniasis *Taenia saginata/T. solium*	Diphyllobothriasis (*Diphyllobothrium latum*)	Hymenolepiasis (*Hymenolepis nana*)
Definitive host	Man	Man	Man
Intermediate host	*T. saginata*—cattle *T. solium*—pig	1st—cyclopes 2nd—fish	No
Infective form	Larva (cysticercus bovis or cysticercus cellulosae)	L3 larva (pleurocercoid larva)	Eggs
Transmission by ingestion of:	Contaminated beef or pork meat (partially/uncooked)	Fish containing pleurocercoid larva (partially cooked/uncooked)	Contaminated food and water or autoinfection
Habitat	Intestine	Intestine	Intestine
Pathogenic form	Adult	Adult	Adult
Manifestations	Intestinal symptoms only	Intestinal symptoms, megaloblastic anemia	Intestinal symptoms only
Diagnostic form	Demonstration of eggs in feces (Fig. 25.1B)	*Eggs* (Fig. 25.4): • Operculated • Knob at the other end • Shape: Oval • Size: 70 μm x 50 μm	*Eggs* (Fig. 25.3B): • Non-bile stained • Round to oval • Polar filaments
Treatment	• Praziquantel (DOC) • Niclosamide	• Praziquantel • Niclosamide • Parenteral vitamin B_{12}	• Praziquantel • Niclosamide

Abbreviations: ELISA, enzyme-linked immunosorbent assay; DOC, drug of choice.

SCHISTOSOMIASIS

Problem Solving Exercise 4

Schistosoma mansoni Infection

A 62-year-old man from Africa came to the OPD with maculopapular rash, fever and hepatosplenomegaly. Stool sample was sent for wet mount examination (Fig. 25.5).
1. Identify the causative agent based on the stool microscopic findings.
2. Which is the infective stage, host and mode of transmission of the parasite?
3. Mention two complications produced by infection with this parasite.
4. What is the drug of choice for treatment?

Explanation

The causative agent is *Schistosoma mansoni*. Points in favor are:
❑ From Africa—endemic for schistosomiasis
❑ Presented with maculopapular rash, fever and hepatosplenomegaly

❑ Stool microscopy reveals nonoperculated oval elongated eggs with lateral spine (Fig. 25.5)
❑ Drug of choice is praziquantel.
For further details, refer Tables 25.2 and 25.3.

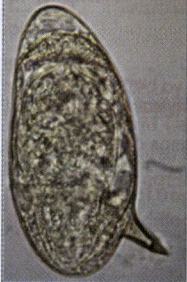

Fig. 25.5: *Schistosoma mansoni* (egg).
Source: ID# 4841. Public Health Image Library, Centers for Disease Control and Prevention (CDC), Atlanta (*with permission*).

FASCIOLOPSIS BUSKI INFECTION

Problem Solving Exercise 5

A 6-year-old child came to the OPD with complaints of vague abdominal pain, passage of greenish-yellow stool. On examination, the child was malnourished. Stool specimen was sent for wet mount examination for detection of ova (Fig. 25.6). The adult form of the causative agent of the condition is also displayed (Fig. 25.7).

1. Identify the causative agent based on the microscopic findings.
2. Which is the infective stage, mode of transmission, hosts for the parasite?

Explanation

The causative agent is *F. buski*. Points in favor are:
- Passage of greenish-yellow stool.
- Stool microscopy reveals large (140 μm × 80–85 μm), oval, operculated, bile-stained eggs (Fig. 25.6).
- Figure 25.7: Adult worm of *F. buski*. Oral and ventral suckers are close to each other and absence of lateral branches from intestinal caeca are the identifying features. For further details, refer Tables 25.2 and 25.3.

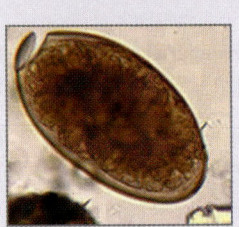 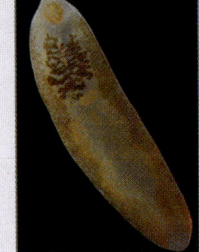

Fig. 25.6: *Fasciolopsis buski* (egg). **Fig. 25.7:** Carmine stained adult worm of *Fasciolopsis buski*.

Source: DPDx Image Library, Centers for Disease Control and Prevention (CDC), Atlanta (*with permission*).

Table 25.2: Features or characteristics of intestinal trematodes.

Properties	*Schistosoma*	*Fasciolopsis buski*
Definitive host	Man	Man
Intermediate host	Snail	1st—Snail 2nd—Aquatic plant
Infective form	Cercaria larva	Metacercaria larva
Transmission	Skin penetration	Ingestion of aquatic plant containing metacercaria
Habitat	Blood vessels of bladder/intestine	Blood vessels of small intestine
Manifestations	*S. mansoni/japonicum* • Cercarial dermatitis • Katayama fever • Egg granuloma formation in intestine, liver and spleen	Malabsorption and protein losing enteropathy with profuse yellowish-green stool
Diagnostic form (Table 25.3)	Eggs (nonoperculated) in stool	Eggs (operculated) in stool
Treatment	Praziquantel	Praziquantel

*S. hematobium resides in blood vessels of urinary bladder, discussed in Chapter 42.

Table 25.3: Eggs of intestinal trematodes (diagnostic forms).

Schistosomes (Nonoperculated eggs)

Schistosoma mansoni
- Size: 110–175 μm in length and 45–70 μm in breadth
- Shape: Elongated oval
- Nonoperculated
- Lateral spine at the posterior end

Schistosoma japonicum
- Size: 70–100 μm in length and 50–70 μm in breadth
- Shape: Spherical
- Nonoperculated
- Rudimentary lateral knob*

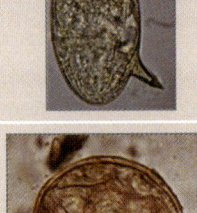

Other trematodes (Operculated eggs)

Fasciolopsis buski
- Large, oval eggs
- Operculated
- Measuring 130–140 μm long and 80–85 μm in breadth

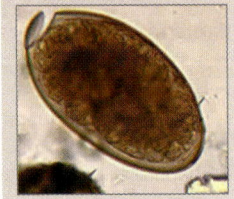

*Source: ID#4842. Public Health Image Library, Centers for Disease Control and Prevention (CDC), Atlanta (*with permission*).

CHAPTER 25 ◆ Intestinal Helminthic Infections

INTESTINAL NEMATODE INFECTIONS

Nematodes are classified into intestinal and tissue or somatic nematodes. Intestinal nematodes are further grouped into:

❖ **Small intestinal nematodes:**
- *Ascaris lumbricoides* (roundworm)
- Hookworm (*Ancylostoma duodenale* and *Necator americanus*)
- *Strongyloides stercoralis*.

❖ **Large intestinal nematodes:**
- *Enterobius vermicularis* (pinworm)
- *Trichuris trichiura* (whipworm).

▮TRICHURIASIS

Problem Solving Exercise 6

A 3-year-old child was brought to the OPD with history of dysentery and growth retardation. The stool specimen was sent for direct microscopy (Fig. 25.8A). The gross specimen of the causative agent obtained through proctoscopy is displayed (Fig. 25.9).
1. Identify the causative agent based on microscopic findings and gross morphology.
2. Draw a labeled diagram of the ova of the causative agent.
3. What is the infective form and mode of transmission?

Explanation

It is a case of trichuriasis; caused by *Trichuris trichiura*. Points in favor are:
❑ History of dysentery and growth retardation.
❑ Figure 25.8A: Stool microscopy showed barrel-shaped egg with mucus plugs.
❑ Figure 25.9: Gross specimen revealed whip-shaped adult worms of 3–5 cm long, anterior 3/5th is thin, hair like, coiled (like a whip), and posterior 2/5th is short and thick (like a handle of a whip). Hence, *Trichuris* is also called as whipworm.
❑ Labeled diagram of ova is shown in Figure 25.8B.
❑ Infective form: Embryonated egg
❑ Mode of transmission: Ingestion of contaminated food and water containing embryonated egg.

For further details, refer Tables 25.4 and 25.5.

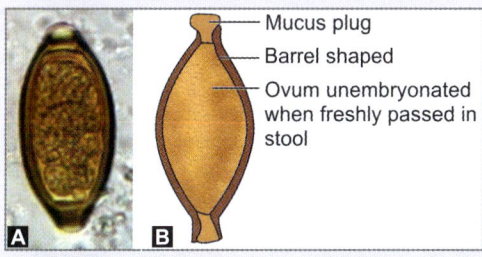

Figs 25.8A and B: *Trichuris* eggs: (A) In saline mount; (B) Schematic diagram.
Source: (A) Dr Anand Janagond, Department of Microbiology, S. Nijalingappa Medical College, Bagalkot, Karnataka (*with permission*).

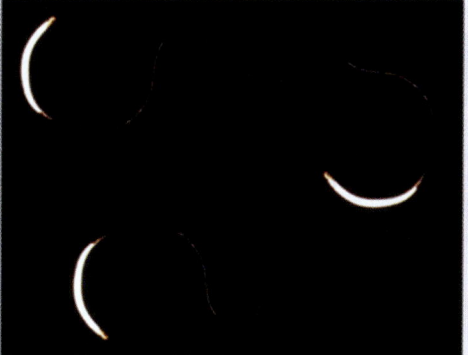

Fig. 25.9: *Trichuris trichiura* (adult worm).
Source: Dr Mae Melvin, Public Health Image Library, Centers for Disease Control and Prevention (CDC), Atlanta (*with pemission*).

▮ENTEROBIASIS

Problem Solving Exercise 7

A 5-year-old child was brought to the OPD with history of repeated episodes of nocturnal enuresis and itching over the perianal region. Perianal swab [NIH (National Institutes of Health) swab] was collected and sent for direct microscopy (Figs 25.10A and 25.11).
1. Identify the causative agent based on the microscopic findings.
2. Draw a labeled diagram of the ova of the causative agent.
3. How will you collect the specimen to diagnose this clinical condition?
4. What is the infective form and mode of transmission?

Explanation

It is a case of enterobiasis; caused by *Enterobius vermicularis*. Points in favor are:
- History of repeated episodes of nocturnal enuresis and itching over the perianal region.
- Figure 25.10A: Perianal swab and stool microscopy showed non-bile stained egg, planoconvex shaped, containing a tadpole shaped larva inside.
- Figure 25.11B: Gross specimen revealed small, white and thread-like worm (hence, named as threadworm) with posterior end pointed and tapering (looks like a pin, hence called as pinworm).
- Labeled diagram of ova is shown in Figure 25.10B.
- Infective form: Embryonated egg.
- Mode of infection: Ingestion of contaminated food and water containing embryonated egg containing larva or by autoinfection.
- Specimen collection: Perianal sampling is collected by cellophane tape (Fig. 25.11A) or specialized swab called as NIH swab (Fig. 25.11C).

For further details, refer Tables 25.4 and 25.5.

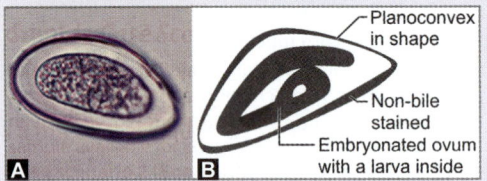

Figs 25.10A and B: *Enterobius* eggs: (A) In saline mount; (B) Schematic diagram.
Source: (A) DPDx Image Library, Centers for Disease Control and Prevention (CDC), Atlanta (*with permission*).

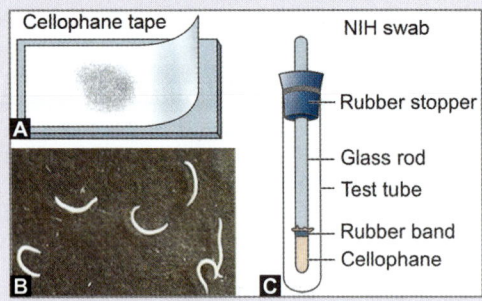

Figs 25.11A to C: *Enterobius vermicularis:* (A) Cellophane tape technique; (B) Adult worms; (C) NIH swab (schematic).
Source: (B) Head, Department of Microbiology, Meenakshi Medical College, Chennai (*with permission*).

ASCARIASIS

Problem Solving Exercise 8

A 4-year-old child came to the OPD with history of severe acute abdominal pain associated with nausea and vomiting. On examination, the child was malnourished. The stool specimen was sent for direct microscopy (Fig. 25.12A). The gross specimen of the causative agent is displayed (Fig. 25.13).
1. Identify the causative agent based on microscopic findings and gross morphology.
2. Draw a labeled diagram of the ova of the causative agent.
3. Which is the infective stage and mode of transmission?
4. How will you diagnose this condition in the laboratory?
5. Mention two complications caused by the adult worm.

Explanation

It is a case of ascariasis; caused by *A. lumbricoides*. Points in favor are:
- History of severe acute abdominal pain, vomiting and malnutrition.
- Figure 25.12A: Stool microscopy showed round to oval bile-stained egg with thick albuminous coat (mammillated)—indicates fertilized egg of *A. lumbricoides*.
- Figure 25.13: Gross specimen revealed cylindrical worm (hence called as roundworm); 15–31 cm long with tapering ends.
- Labeled diagram of ova is shown in Figure 25.12B.
- Infective form: Embryonated egg
- Mode of transmission: Ingestion of contaminated food and water containing embryonated eggs.
- Complications: Small-bowel obstruction and intussusception.

For further details, refer Tables 25.4 and 25.5.

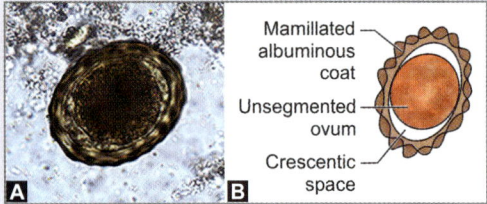

Figs 25.12A and B: *Ascaris fertilized eggs:* (A) In saline mount; (B) Schematic diagram.
Source: DPDx Image Library, Centers for Disease Control and Prevention (CDC), Atlanta (*with permission*).

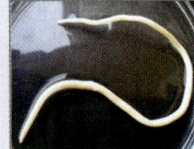

Fig. 25.13: Adult worm of *Ascaris lumbricoides*.
Source: Head, Department of Microbiology, Meenakshi Medical College, Chennai (*with permission*).

CHAPTER 25 ◆ Intestinal Helminthic Infections

Table 25.4: Features or characteristics of intestinal nematodes.

	Trichuris trichiura	Enterobius vermicularis	Ascaris lumbricoides	Hookworm	Strongyloides stercoralis
Host	Humans	Humans	Humans	Humans	Humans
Infective form	Embryonated eggs	Embryonated egg containing larva	Embryonated eggs	Filariform (L_3) larva	Filariform (L_3) larva
Transmission	Ingestion of contaminated food and water containing embryonated eggs	Ingestion of contaminated food and water containing embryonated egg or autoinfection	Ingestion of contaminated food and water containing embryonated eggs	Skin penetration by filariform (L_3) larva	Skin penetration by filariform (L_3) larva or by autoinfection
Habitat	Large intestine	Large intestine	Small intestine	Small intestine	Small intestine
Lung phase	Absent	Absent	Present	Present	Present
Pathogenic form	Adult worm (intestine)	Adult worm (intestine)	Adult worm (intestine) Migrating larva (lungs)	Adult worm (intestine) Migrating larva (lungs, skin)	Adult worm (intestine) Migrating larva (lungs, skin)
Manifestations	• Abdominal pain, anorexia • *Trichuris* dysentery syndrome • Iron deficiency anemia • Recurrent rectal prolapse • Growth retardation and impaired cognitive function	• **Perianal pruritus** often worse at night as a result of the nocturnal migration of the worm liberating eggs in perianal region • Nocturnal enuresis • Abdominal pain and weight loss	**Migratory phase** Eosinophilic pneumonia (Loeffler's pneumonitis) **Intestinal phase** • Malnutrition and growth retardation • Small bowel obstruction • Pain abdomen • Intussusception • Biliary colic • Allergic—fever, urticaria	**Migratory phase** • Ground itch—pruritic rashes • Serpiginous tracks **Intestinal phase** • *Mild worm load:* Epigastric pain • Inflammatory diarrhea *Heavy worm load:* Iron deficiency anemia • Malnutrition	**Migratory phase** *Larva currens*—serpiginous urticarial rash **Intestinal phase** *Mild worm load*—produce epigastric pain, nausea, diarrhea, and blood loss *Heavy larva load*—hyperinfection syndrome—disseminated, central nervous system infection—common in HIV-infected patients
Diagnostic form (Table 25.5)	Unembryonated eggs	Embryonated eggs deposited in perianal area	Unembryonated eggs—fertilized and unfertilized eggs	Segmented eggs with four blastomeres	Rhabditiform larva (L_1) (Table 25.6)
Other methods of laboratory diagnosis	—	**Sample:** • Perianal swabs collected by cellophane tape or special swab called NIH swab (Figs 25.11A and C) • Gravid females may also be detected rarely (Fig.25.11B)	1. Detection of adult worm in intestine (barium meal X-ray) 2. **Serology** (ELISA, IFA)—for pulmonary phase and epidemiological purpose	**Stool culture is done to:** • Differentiate *Necator* and *Ancylostoma* by examining filariform larva (L_3) • To differentiate *Strongyloides* from hookworm (Table 25.6). • Methods: (i) Harada–Mori technique, (ii) Agar plate method **Egg counting** (Kato-Katz method) done for hookworm to know the worm burden	
Treatment	Mebendazole or albendazole	Mebendazole or albendazole	Albendazole	Mebendazole or albendazole	Ivermectin

Abbreviations: ELISA, enzyme-linked immunosorbent assay; NIH, National Institutes of Health; IFA, immunofluorescent antibody.

HOOKWORM INFECTIONS

Problem Solving Exercise 9

A 10-year-old child came to the pediatric OPD for school health check-up. On examination, he had pallor. Peripheral blood smear revealed microcytic, hypochromic anemia. The stool specimen was sent for direct microscopy (Fig. 25.14).
- Identify the causative agent based on stool microscopy findings.
- Which is the infective form of the parasite?
- What is the mode of transmission?
- What further laboratory diagnosis you would like to perform?

Explanation

It is a case of hookworm infection; caused by *A. duodenale* or *N. americanus*. Points in favor are:
- History of pallor and microcytic, hypochromic anemia.
- Figure 25.14: Stool microscopy showed round to oval non-bile stained egg with segmented ovum (four blastomeres)—indicates egg of hookworm.
- Infective form: Filariform larva
- Mode of transmission: Skin penetration by filariform (L_3) larva.
- As eggs of *Ancylostoma* and *Necator* are indistinguishable, hence stool culture (e.g., Harada–Mori) should be performed. Eggs hatch out to develop to filariform larvae (L_3), which can be used to differentiate between *Necator* and *Ancylostoma*.

For further detail, refer Tables 25.4 and 25.5.

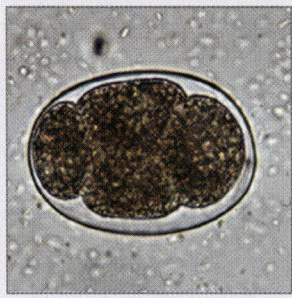

Fig. 25.14: Hookworm: Egg with four blastomeres.
Source: DPDx Image Library, Centers for Disease Control and Prevention (CDC), Atlanta (*with permission*).

STRONGYLOIDIASIS

Problem Solving Exercise 10

A 7-year-old child was brought to the OPD with history of epigastric pain, nausea, diarrhea, and blood loss. On examination, a serpiginous urticarial rash was observed in his lower limb. The stool specimen was sent for direct microscopy (Fig. 25.15).
1. Identify the causative agent based on the stool microscopy finding.
2. Name the infective form and modes of transmission of infection by this parasite.
3. How will you treat this condition?

Explanation

It is a case of strongyloidiasis; caused by *Strongyloides stercoralis*. Points in favor are:
- History of epigastric pain, nausea, diarrhea and blood loss.
- Serpiginous urticarial rash, i.e., larva currens
- Figure 25.15: Stool microscopy revealed larva of 250 μm × 16 μm in size, with short buccal cavity and prominent large genital primordium—indicates rhabditiform larva of *Strongyloides*.
- Infective form: Filariform larva
- Mode of transmission: Skin penetration by filariform larva or by autoinfection.
- Treatment: Ivermectin is the drug of choice.

For further details, refer Tables 25.4 and 25.5.

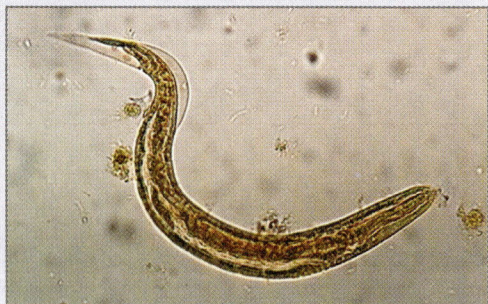

Fig. 25.15: *Strongyloides stercoralis* (rhabditiform larva).
Source: Department of Microbiology, Meenakshi Medical College, Chennai (*with permission*).

CHAPTER 25 ◆ Intestinal Helminthic Infections

Table 25.5: Characteristics or identifying features of eggs of intestinal nematodes.

Diagnostic form	In saline mount	Schematic diagram
Trichuris eggs • Size: 50 μm × 22 μm • Shape: Barrel shaped • Unembryonated ovum • Mucus plugs at both ends • Bile stained		Mucus plug Barrel shaped Ovum unembryonated when freshly passed in stool
Enterobius eggs • Size: 50–60 μm × 20–30 μm • Shape: Planoconvex • Embryonated ovum with a larva inside • Non-bile stained		Planoconvex in shape Non-bile stained Embryonated ovum with a larva inside
Ascaris fertilized eggs • Size: 50–70 μm × 40–50 μm • Shape: Round to oval • Surrounded by a thick mammillated, albuminous coat • Crescentic space at poles • Bile stained • Floats in saturated salt solution • Unembryonated large ovum		Mamillated albuminous coat Unsegmented ovum Crescentic space
Ascaris unfertilized eggs • Size: 90 μm × 45 μm • Shape: Elongated • Albuminous coat is thin/absent • No crescentic space at poles • Bile stained • Does not float in saturated salt solution • Ovum is atrophied with a mass of highly refractile granules		Thin/scanty albuminous coat Ovum atrophied with refractile granules
Hookworm eggs • Size: 60 μm × 40 μm • Oval shaped • Non-bile stained, colorless • Surrounded by thin, hyaline shell • Clear space between the egg shell and ovum • Egg is segmented with four blastomeres Eggs of both *Ancylostoma duodenale* and *Necator americanus* are morphologically indistinguishable; hence stool culture is done for species identification. Both are differentiated by their filariform larva grown in culture.		Four blastomeres Egg shell

Table 25.6: Differences between rhabditiform larva of hookworm and *Strongyloides stercoralis*.

Rhabditiform larva	*Strongyloides stercoralis*	Hookworm
Size	108–380 µm long × 14–20 µm width	100–150 µm long × 16 µm width
Buccal cavity	Shorter	Three times longer
Genital primordium	Prominent and large	Less prominent, small
Anal pore	50 µm from the posterior end	80 µm from the posterior end
Stool microscopy	*Source:* Department of Microbiology, Meenakshi Medical College, Chennai (*with permission*).	*Source:* Department of Microbiology, Pondicherry Institute of Medical Sciences, Puducherry (*with permission*).
Schematic diagram	Genital primordium, Intestine, Double bulb esophagus, Anal pore, Buccal cavity (smaller)	Intestine, Double bulb esophagus, Anal pore, Genital primordium, Buccal cavity (larger)

CHAPTER 26

Viral Hepatitis

HEPATITIS B VIRUS INFECTION

Problem Solving Exercise 1

A 40-year-old male presented with history of loss of appetite, malaise and jaundice of 2 months duration. On examination, there was icterus, hepatomegaly and tenderness in the right hypochondriac region. He gave a history of blood transfusion in the past. Liver enzymes were found to be elevated. His serum specimen was sent for hepatitis B surface antigen (HBsAg) tests as shown in Figures 26.1A and B.
- What are the test formats used and interpret the results?
- What are the investigations you would like to advice further?
- List other hepatitis viruses and their modes of transmission.
- Describe the three morphological forms of this agent seen under electron microscopy.

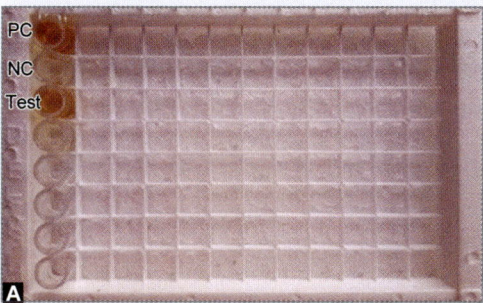

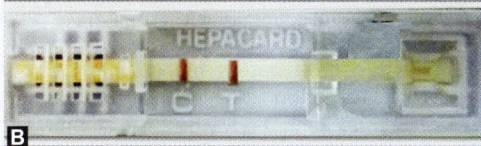

Figs 26.1A and B: Test for detection of hepatitis B surface antigen.
Abbreviations: PC, positive control; NC, negative control
Source: Department of Microbiology, Pondicherry Institute of Medical Sciences, Puducherry *(with permission).*

Explanation

Clinical Diagnosis

History of jaundice, hepatomegaly and tenderness in the right hypochondriac region is suggestive of a case of hepatitis.

Laboratory Diagnosis

It is a case of hepatitis due to hepatitis B virus (HBV). *Test A* is sandwich enzyme-linked immunosorbent assay (ELISA) for detection of HBsAg, and *test B* is immunochromatographic test (ICT) for rapid detection of HBsAg. In both the tests, the sample was found to be positive for HBsAg.

Interpretation

Hepatitis B surface antigen may be present at any stage of hepatitis B infection ranging from carrier to acute and chronic hepatitis. Hence, to determine the stage of the disease further investigations should be done such as:
- **Hepatitis B precore antigen (HBeAg):** If present, indicates active viral replication and high infectivity.
- **Anti-hepatitis B core (HBc) antibody:** Immunoglobulin (Ig) M indicates acute and IgG indicates chronic infection.

Modes of Transmission

There are five hepatitis viruses (Table 26.1).
- Hepatitis A virus (HAV) and hepatitis E virus (HEV) are transmitted by consumption of contaminated food and water (feco-oral route).
- Hepatitis B virus (HBV), hepatitis C virus (HCV) and hepatitis D virus (HDV) are transmitted by blood, sexual and vertical route.

Morphological Forms of HBV

Hepatitis B has three morphological forms; spherical form, tubular form and complete form or Dane particles (Fig. 26.2) These forms can be visualized under electron microscopy.
(For answers to other questions, refer text below.)

Table 26.1: Features of hepatitis viruses.

HAV and HEV	HBV, HCV and HDV
Both HAV and HEV are RNA viruses	HBV is a DNA virus HCV and HDV are RNA viruses
Feco-oral transmission	Blood (common), sexual, and vertical
Incubation period: 15–50 days, onset-abrupt	Incubation period: 30–180 days, insidious onset
No carriers	Carriers seen
No chronicity	Chronicity seen
Not oncogenic	Oncogenic
Fulminant rare (<1%); except HEV in pregnancy (10–20%)	Fulminant rare (1–2%) except HDV (10–20%)
Non-enveloped; icosahedron symmetry	Enveloped; spherical symmetry

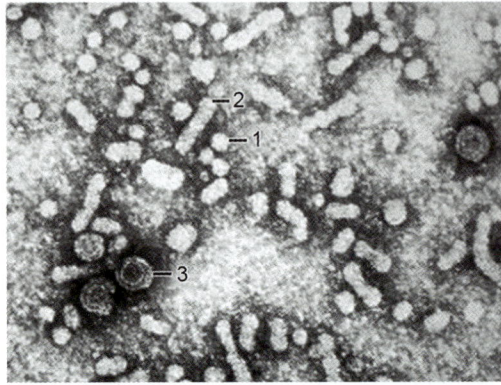

Fig. 26.2: Electron microscopic appearance of hepatitis B virus showing: 1, spherical form; 2, tubular form and 3, Dane particle.
Source: ID# 5631/Public Health Image Library/Centers for Disease Control and Prevention (CDC), Atlanta (*with permission*).

Problem Solving Exercise 2

Acute Hepatitis

In a patient with jaundice and elevated liver enzymes for 2 months, the following serological investigations are done with their results displayed below. Interpret the diagnosis.

HBsAg	Anti-HBs	Anti-HBc	HBeAg	Anti-HBe
+	–	IgM	+	–

Explanation

The stage of the disease is acute HBV infection with active viral replication and high infectivity.
- IgM Anti-HBc antibody indicates—acute hepatitis
- HBeAg indicates—active viral replication and high infectivity.

Problem Solving Exercise 3

Chronic Hepatitis

In a patient with history of jaundice and elevated liver enzymes for 6 months, the following serological investigations are done.
Two patterns of results are displayed below (A and B). Interpret the diagnosis.

A:

HBsAg	Anti-HBs	Anti-HBc	HBeAg	Anti-HBe
+	–	IgG	+	–

B:

HBsAg	Anti-HBs	Anti-HBc	HBeAg	Anti-HBe
+	–	IgG	–	+

Explanation

A: The stage of the disease is chronic active HBV infection with high infectivity (immunoreactive chronic hepatitis).
  - IgG anti-HBc antibody indicates—chronic hepatitis.
  - HBeAg indicates—active viral replication and high infectivity.

  The same set of markers in an asymptomatic individual would suggest the stage as "supercarrier".

B: The stage of the disease is chronic hepatitis B with low infectivity (chronic inactive hepatitis).
  - IgG anti-HBc antibody indicates—chronic HBV infection.
  - HBeAg absent indicates—low infectivity.

  The same set of markers in an asymptomatic individual would suggest the stage as "simple carrier".

Problem Solving Exercise 4

Vaccination/Recovery

A patient is asymptomatic, with normal liver enzymes. He attended a master health check-up; the following serological investigations were done. Two patterns of results are displayed below (A and B). Interpret the diagnosis.

A:

HBsAg	Anti-HBs	Anti-HBc	HBeAg	Anti-HBe
−	+	−	−	−

B:

HBsAg	Anti-HBs	Anti-HBc	HBeAg	Anti-HBe
−	+	+	−	−

Explanation

A: The diagnosis here is post-hepatitis B vaccination. Presence of anti-HBs antibody in the absence of any other viral markers indicates vaccination with HBsAg. Details about the vaccination—discussed later in this chapter.

B: The diagnosis here is post-recovery from hepatitis B infection. Along with anti-HBs antibody, anti-HBc IgG indicates post-recovery.

Problem Solving Exercise 5

Carriers/Incubation Period

A person came to donate blood in a blood donation camp. As a part of routine screening he was tested for HBsAg, which came positive. He is asymptomatic, with normal liver enzymes. The following serological investigations were done and their results shown below. Interpret the results.

A:

HBsAg	Anti-HBs	Anti-HBc	HBeAg	Anti-HBe
+	−	−	−	−

B:

HBsAg	Anti-HBs	Anti-HBc	HBeAg	Anti-HBe
+	−	IgG	−	−

Explanation

A: Presence of HBsAg in the absence of any other hepatitis B viral marker in an asymptomatic individual with normal liver enzymes suggests that he is in *incubation period* of infection with HBV (early acute hepatitis).

B: Presence of HBsAg and anti-HBc IgG in the absence of other hepatitis B viral marker in an asymptomatic individual with normal liver enzymes suggests that he is simple carrier of HBV infection. In additon if HBeAg is also positive, then he will be called as supercarrier.

Laboratory Diagnosis of Hepatitis B

Definitive diagnosis of hepatitis B depends on the serological demonstration of the viral markers, which can be classified as:

- **Antigen markers:** HBsAg and HBeAg
- **Antibody markers:** Anti-HBs, anti-HBe and anti-HBc
- **Molecular markers:** HBV DNA
- **Nonspecific markers:** Elevated liver enzymes and serum bilirubin.

The most useful detection method for HBV antigens and antibodies is ELISA; although various rapid test formats such as ICT are also available.

Viral DNA can be detected by polymerase chain reaction (PCR); real-time PCR is very useful for quantification of HBV DNA. HBV does not grow in any conventional culture system.

Hepatitis B Surface Antigen

It is the first marker to be elevated following infection; within 8–12 weeks.
- It appears during incubation period.
- Presence of HBsAg indicates onset of infectivity.
- It remains elevated in the entire duration of acute hepatitis; rarely persists beyond 6 months if the disease progresses to chronic hepatitis or in carrier state.
- It is used as an epidemiological marker of hepatitis B infection.

Hepatitis B Precore Antigen and HBV DNA

They appear concurrently with or shortly after appearance of HBsAg in serum. They are the markers of active viral replication and high viral infectivity. HBV DNA load is used to monitor the response to treatment.

Hepatitis B Core Antigen

Hepatitis B core antigen (HBcAg) is a hidden antigen, nonsecretory in nature; hence, it cannot be detected in blood. However, can be detected in hepatocytes by immunofluorescence.

Anti-HBc IgM (Hepatitis B Core Antibody)

Anti-HBc IgM is the first antibody to elevate following infection:
- It appears within the first 1-2 weeks after the appearance of HBsAg and lasts for 3-6 months.
- Its presence indicates acute HBV infection.

Anti-HBc IgG (Hepatitis B Core Antibody)

Anti-HBc IgG appears in late acute stage and remains positive indefinitely whether the patient proceeds to—chronic stage or carrier state or recovery. It can also be used as epidemiological marker of HBV infection.

Anti-hepatitis B Precore Antibody

Anti-HBe antibodies appear after the clearance of HBeAg and its presence signifies diminished viral replication and decreased infectivity.

Anti-hepatitis B Surface Antibody

It appears after the clearance of HBsAg and remains elevated indefinitely.
- Its presence indicates recovery, immunity and noninfectivity (i.e., stoppage of transmission).
- It is also the marker of vaccination if rest all markers are negative (Fig. 26.3).

Various outcomes following HBV infection and markers for diagnosis is depicted in Fig. 26.3.

Treatment

Most acute hepatitis B infections are self-limiting; do not require any specific treatment. In contrast, treatment of chronic hepatitis B may require antiviral drugs such as tenofovir and telbivudine.

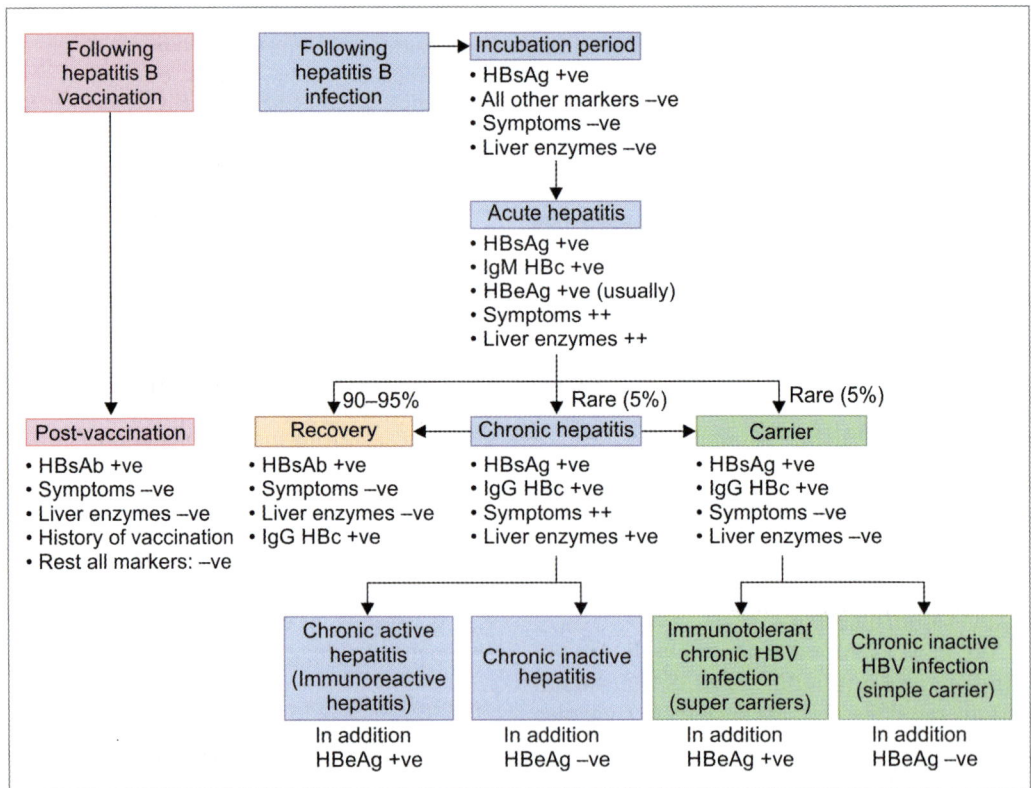

Fig. 26.3: Various outcomes following hepatitis B infection and markers for diagnosis.

Prevention

Hepatitis B Vaccine (Active Immunization)

Hepatitis B vaccine is a recombinant subunit vaccine of HBsAg, prepared in Baker's yeast by DNA recombinant technology.
- **Route:** Administered by intramuscular route over deltoid (in infant—anterolateral thigh)
- **Dosage:** 10–20 µg/dose (half of the dose is given to children below 10 years)
- **Schedule:** Three doses are given at 0, 1 and 6 months. Under National Immunization Schedule, it is given at 6, 10, 14 weeks (along with DPT vaccine)
- **Marker of protection:** Recipients are said to be protected if the anti-HBsAg antibody titer is above 10 mIU/mL.

Hepatitis B Immunoglobulin

Hepatitis B immunoglobulin (HBIG) is used in the following situations where an immediate protection is warranted; given at dose of 0.06 mL/kg or 10–12 IU/kg.
- Acutely exposed to HBsAg positive blood, e.g., surgeons, nurses, laboratory workers
- Sexual partners of acute hepatitis B patients
- Neonates borne to hepatitis B carrier mothers
- Post-liver transplant patients who need protection against HBV infection
- Following accidental exposure.

The post-exposure prophylaxis for HBV is discussed in Chapter 14.

OTHER HEPATITIS VIRUSES

Both ELISA and rapid tests (e.g., immunochromatographic or flow through assay) formats are available for detection of anti-HAV, anti-HCV and anti-HDV antibodies. Apart from molecular methods like PCR and real-time PCR are available for detection of viral RNA in blood (for HCV and HDV) and from stool specimen (HAV and HEV).

Problem Solving Exercise 6

A patient with history of jaundice and elevated liver enzymes, the following serological investigations are done. Three patterns of results are displayed below (A, B and C). Interpret the diagnosis in all test patterns.

A:

HAV	HBV	HCV	HDV	HEV
Anti-HAV IgG +ve	HBsAg –ve	Anti-HCV IgG +ve	Anti-HDV –ve	Anti-HEV –ve

B:

HAV	HBV	HCV	HDV	HEV
Anti-HAV IgM +ve	HBsAg –ve	Anti-HCV –ve	Anti-HDV –ve	Anti-HEV –ve

C:

HAV	HBV	HCV	HDV	HEV
Anti-HAV –ve	HBsAg +ve Anti-HBs –ve Anti-HBc IgM +ve HBeAg +ve Anti-HBe –ve	Anti-HCV –ve	Anti-HDV IgM +ve	Anti-HEV –ve

Explanation

A. Anti-HCV IgG +ve in a patient with jaundice indicates chronic hepatitis C virus infection. Please note that there is no chronic infection in HAV and HEV; hence detection of anti-HAV IgG indicates past infection or recovery.
B. Anti-HAV IgM +ve in patient with history of jaundice indicates acute hepatitis A virus infection.
C. It is a case of **acute HDV coinfection** with acute hepatitis B infection with high infectivity. Points in favor are:
  ➢ Positive for anti-HDV IgM—indicates acute hepatitis D infection
  ➢ Positive for HBsAg, anti-HBc IgM and HBeAg—acute hepatitis B infection with high infectivity.
  Note: However, in case of **superinfection** (HDV infects a hepatocyte which is already infected by HBV)—Positive for HBsAg, anti-HBc (IgG) and anti-HDV (IgM).

Parasitic Infections of Hepatobiliary System: Amoebic Liver Abscess, Hydatid Disease and Others

CHAPTER 27

■ INTRODUCTION

Parasites causing hepatobiliary infections include:
- Protozoa: *Entamoeba histolytica*, causes amoebic liver abscess (ALA)
- Cestode: *Echinococcus*, causes human echinococcosis (e.g., hydatid disease)
- Trematodes such as *Fasciola hepatica, F. gigantica, Clonorchis* and *Opisthorchis*
- Nematode: *Toxocara* causing visceral larva migrans.

■ AMOEBIC LIVER ABSCESS

Invasion of trophozoites lead to various extraintestinal complications. Amoebic liver abscess is the most common complication; others are amoebic appendicitis, ameboma, fulminant colitis and ruptured liver abscess leading to peritonitis.

Problem Solving Exercise 1

A patient with history of dysentery and jaundice for 2 months had a sudden episode of high-grade fever and acute pain in the right hypochondrium was brought to the emergency department. Ultrasound scan of the abdomen revealed enlarged liver with acute peritonitis. He succumbs to death before any intervention. A postmortem sample from the patient is displayed in Figure 27.1.
1. Identify the clinical condition based on the lesion displayed and the most probable causative agent.
2. Name the laboratory tests that can be done to confirm the diagnosis.
3. What are the complications of intestinal amoebiasis?

Explanation

This is a case of ruptured amoebic liver abscess with acute peritonitis. Points in favor are:
❑ Acute onset of pain in the right hypochondrium with high-grade fever, in a patient with chronic dysentery and jaundice, suggest ruptured amoebic liver abscess, leading to acute peritonitis and death of the patient.
❑ The causative agent for this clinical condition is *Entamoeba histolytica*.
(For answers to other questions, refer below).

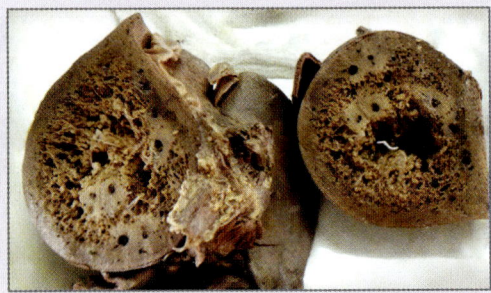

Fig. 27.1: Cross section of liver showing amoebic liver abscess.
Source: Head, Department of Pathology, Meenakshi Medical College, Chennai (*with permission*).

Laboratory Diagnosis of ALA

- Microscopy of liver pus (Anchovy sauce pus)—trophozoites of *E. histolytica* are seen
- Trophozoites may be found only in the last portion of the aspirated material from the abscess wall, not in the necrotic debris obtained from the center of the abscess. Trophozoites measure 15–20 µm, possess a single nucleus; are actively motile, with finger-like pseudopodia (Fig. 24.2B, Chapter 24)
- Lectin antigen detection and antibody detection methods like indirect hemagglutination test, indirect fluorescent antibody test, ELISA, etc., are useful.

- ❖ Histopathological staining of pus aspirate — demonstrates amoebic trophozoites
- ❖ Ultrasonography of liver shows the site and extension of abscess. Posterior superior area of right liver is the most common site affected.

Treatment

- ❖ **Amoebicidal agents:** Treatment of ALA consists of a tissue amoebicidal agent (acts on trophozoites in the liver), followed by luminal amoebicidal agent to eradicate the intestinal carriage
  - *Tissue agents:* Metronidazole (for 5–10 days) or tinidazole/ornidazole (once) and
  - *Luminal agents:* Iodoquinol (for 20 days) or paromomycin (for 10 days).
- ❖ **Aspiration** of the liver abscess content is indicated—(1) risk of impending rupture, (2) left lobe liver abscess of >10 cm, (3) no improvement after anti-protozoan therapy for 5–7 days.

HYDATID DISEASE

Problem Solving Exercise 2

A 40-year-old man presented with complaints of pain in the right hypochondrium. Ultrasonography revealed a single space-occupying lesion in the right lobe of the liver. This was surgically removed (Fig. 27.2) and subjected to histopathological examination (Figs 27.3A and B).
1. Identify the specimen.
2. Draw a neat, labeled diagram of the structure focused in the slide.
3. What is the causative agent of this condition?
4. Name the definitive and intermediate hosts.
5. Which is the infective form of the parasite for man and how does man acquire this infection?
6. What are the various diagnostic modalities?

- ❑ The causative agent—*Echinococcus granulosus*
- ❑ Host: Definitive (dog) and intermediate host (sheep, man)
- ❑ Infective form: Eggs
- ❑ Mode of transmission: Ingestion of food and water contaminated with dog's feces containing eggs.

For answer to the other questions, refer Table 27.1.

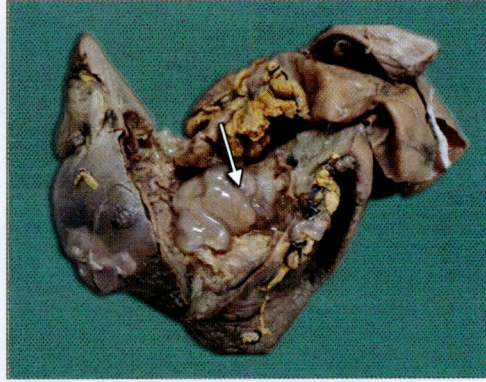

Fig. 27.2: Surgically resected hydatid cyst from liver.
Source: Head, Department of Pathology, Meenakshi Medical College, Chennai (*with permission*).

Explanation

This is a hydatid cyst specimen (Fig. 27.2), obtained surgically from a patient suffering from right hypochondrial pain and cystic lesion in liver detected by ultrasound scan.
- ❑ Figures 27.3A and B show histopathological section of hydatid cyst: (A) All three layers of cyst wall are seen—pericyst, ectocyst and endocyst; (B) Endocyst with attached brood capsules.
- ❑ Labeled diagram of section of hydatid cyst (Fig. 27.3C).

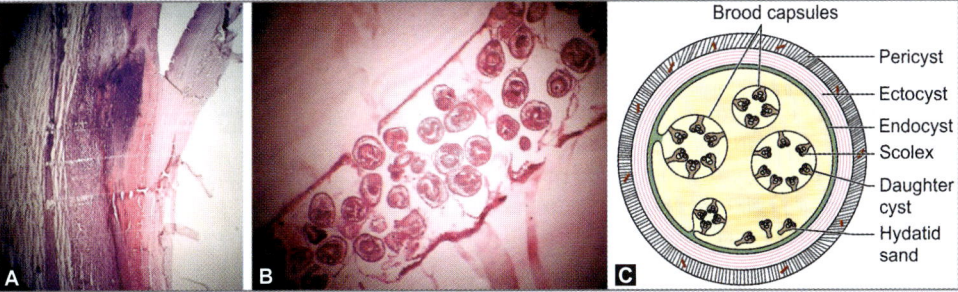

Figs 27.3A to C: Histopathological section of hydatid cyst (hematoxylin and eosin stain). (A) Cyst wall—pericyst, ectocyst and endocyst; (B) Endocyst with attached brood capsules; (C) Schematic diagram of section of hydatid cyst.
Source: Head of Department (Pathology), Meenakshi Medical College, Chennai (*with permission*).

Table 27.1: Hydatid disease (cystic echinococcosis).

Properties	Hydatid diseas
Agent	*Echinococcus granulosus*
Hosts	**Definitive host:** Dog, **Intermediate host:** Sheep, man (accidental)
Infective form	Eggs
Transmission	Consumption of contaminated food and water (ingestion)
Habitat	Tissues: Liver (most common), lungs, brains and others
Pathogenic form	Larva (hydatid cyst)
Manifestations	• **Pressure effect** of the enlarging cyst: leads to palpable abdominal mass, hepatomegaly, abdominal tenderness, portal hypertension and ascites • **Secondary bacterial infection** • **Anaphylactic reactions** due to cyst leakage or rupture
Diagnostic form	• **Hydatid fluid microscopy** (direct mount or staining with acid-fast stain)—detects brood capsules and protoscolices • **Histological examination** (H & E)—demonstrates cyst wall and attached brood capsules • **Antibody detection**—ELISA (using B2t antigen), DIGFA (dot immunogold filtration assay) and western blot • **Imaging methods**—X-ray, USG (demonstrates Water lily sign), CT scan, MRI • **Molecular methods**—PCR, PCR-RFLP and molecular typing (10 genotypes, most common in India is type 1) • **Skin test** (Casoni test)—demonstrates type I hypersensitivity reaction (obsolete now)
Treatment	• Albendazole • Surgery (resection of affected part of liver) • PAIR (percutaneous puncture, aspiration, injection and re-aspiration)

■ TREMATODE INFECTIONS OF LIVER

Fasciola hepatica, Fasciola gigantica, Clonorchis, and *Opisthorchis* are together called as liver flukes.

- **Hosts:** They have three hosts. Humans are the definitive host, snails are the first intermediate host, whereas the second intermediate host is aquatic plant (for *Fasciola*) and cray fish (for *Clonorchis,* and *Opisthorchis*)
- **Transmission:** Man gets infection by ingestion of second intermediate host carrying metacercaria larvae (infective form)
- ***Fasciola hepatica* and *F. gigantica:*** They infect liver; cause fever, right upper quadrant pain, and hepatomegaly. *F. hepatica* is diagnosed by detection of characteristic operculated eggs, measuring 130–150 μm × 63–90 μm in size in stool microscopy (Fig. 27.4A). Eggs of *F. gigantica* are morphologically similar to that of *F. hepatica*, but larger in size
- ***Clonorchis* and *Opisthorchis:*** They infect bile duct and cause mechanical obstruction of the bile duct, leading to fibrosis and **cholangiocarcinoma**. Demonstration of the characteristic flask-shaped eggs (measuring 28–35 μm × 12–19 μm) in the stool establishes the diagnosis (Fig. 27.4B)
- **Treatment of liver fluke infections:**
  - Triclabendazole is the drug of choice for fascioliasis
  - Praziquantel is the drug of choice for clonorchiasis and opisthorchiasis.

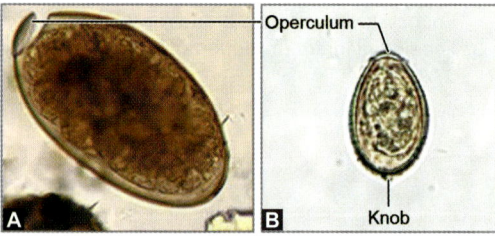

Figs 27.4A and B: Saline mount showing operculated eggs of: (A) *Fasciola hepatica*; (B) *Clonorchis* or *Opisthorchis*.
Source: DPDx Image Library, Centers for Disease Control and Prevention (CDC), Atlanta (*with permission*).

CHAPTER 28
Staphylococcal Infections

Problem Solving Exercise

A 55-year-old male diabetic patient admitted to the hospital with complaints of severe calf pain and pus discharge from the ingrown hair. On physical examination, the local area was found to be red, warm and tender. Pus aspirated was subjected to the following tests: Gram stain (Fig. 28.1A), culture (Fig. 28.2B), biochemical reactions (Figs 28.3A and 28.4A) and antimicrobial susceptibility testing (Fig. 28.5 and Table 28.3).

1. What is the clinical diagnosis and its causative organism?
2. Interpret the antimicrobial susceptibility testing.
3. List the infections caused by this organism.
4. What antibiotic you would like to prescribe?
5. What are the different modalities of laboratory diagnosis?
6. What is MRSA? How will you detect, treat and prevent its transmission?

Explanation
Clinical Diagnosis
Diabetic patient with clinical features of severe calf pain with pus discharge with clinical signs of local inflammation indicates skin and soft tissue infection.

Identification
Gram-positive cocci in cluster with pus cells in Gram-stained smear of pus discharge (Fig. 28.1A), golden yellow hemolytic colonies on blood agar (Fig. 28.2B), mannitol fermented (Fig. 28.3A) and tube coagulase test positive (Fig. 28.4A) indicate that the causative organism is *Staphylococcus aureus*.

Antimicrobial Susceptibility Testing
Antimicrobial susceptibility testing on Mueller Hinton agar (Fig. 28.5 and Table 28.3) showed resistance to penicillin and cefoxitin, and sensitive to clindamycin, doxycycline and linezolid.

As the isolate is resistant to cefoxitin; this isolate is methicillin-resistant *S. aureus* (MRSA).

Treatment
Methicillin-resistant *S. aureus* is resistant to all beta-lactams; hence all beta-lactam drugs should be avoided in this case. Doxycycline, clindamycin or linezolid are the useful options available for this patient (skin and soft tissue infection).
(For answers to other questions, refer below)

■ CLINICAL SPECTRUM

Staphylococcus aureus produces a range of manifestations; which is attributed to production of several virulence factors by the organisms such as:
- Cell wall factors such as peptidoglycan, protein A, clumping factor and teichoic acid
- Hemolysins and leukocidin (panton-valentine toxin)
- **Toxins:** Epidermolytic toxin, enterotoxin and toxic shock syndrome toxin
- *Enzymes*: Coagulase, nucleases, deoxyribonuclease (DNase), etc.

Clinical spectrum of *S. aureus* infections
Skin and soft tissue infections
- Folliculitis, furuncle, carbuncle, impetigo, mastitis and breast abscess (in nursing mothers), surgical site wound infections, cellulitis, etc.

Musculoskeletal infections
- Septic arthritis, osteomyelitis, pyomyositis, psoas abscess and epidural abscess

Respiratory tract infections
- Ventilator-associated pneumonia, post-viral pneumonia (e.g., influenza), empyema, pneumatocele, etc.

Bacteremia and its complications
- Sepsis, central line associated bloodstream infection, infective endocarditis and urinary tract infection (UTI)

Contd...

Contd...

Toxin-mediated illness
- Toxic shock syndrome, food poisoning and staphylococcal scalded-skin syndrome

LABORATORY DIAGNOSIS

Sample Collection

It depends on the site affected (Table 28.1). The discussion in this chapter will be confined to skin and soft tissue (suppurative) infections.

Direct Smear Microscopy

Gram staining of pus or wound swab reveals pus cells with gram-positive cocci in clusters (Fig. 28.1A).

Culture

Specimens are inoculated into various media and incubated overnight at 37°C aerobically. The colony morphology observed is as follows:
- **Blood agar:** Colonies are β-hemolytic with golden yellow in color (due to non-diffusible pigment), 1–3 mm in size, circular, convex and opaque (Fig. 28.2B). However, pigmentation is better appreciated on nutrient agar (Fig. 28.2A).
- **Selective media** are useful when staphylococci are expected to be scanty or outnumbered by other bacteria in the sample (e.g., swabs from carriers, feces); e.g., mannitol salt agar (Fig. 28.2C).

Table 28.1: Specimen collection for *S. aureus* infections.

Infection	Specimen
Suppurative lesion	Pus, wound swab
Respiratory infections	Sputum
Urinary tract infection	Mid-stream urine
Pyrexia of unknown origin (PUO), bacteremia	Blood
Food poisoning	Feces, vomitus, food
Carriers	Nasal and skin swab

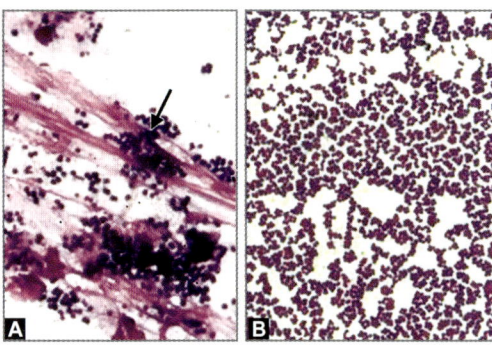

Figs 28.1A and B: (A) Direct smear: arrow showing gram-positive cocci in clusters with pus cells; (B) Culture smear showing gram-positive cocci in clusters.
Source: Department of Microbiology, JIPMER, Puducherry (*with permission*).

Culture Smear Microscopy

Gram staining from the colonies shows gram-positive cocci (1 μm), arranged in clusters (Fig. 28.1B).

Biochemical Tests for Identification

Staphylococci are catalase positive which differentiates them from streptococci (catalase negative). Once genus identification is done, the following tests should be carried out to differentiate *S. aureus* from other *Staphylococcus* species (coagulase-negative staphylococci, CoNS).
- Coagulase test (tube and slide)
- Deoxyribonuclease test
- Phosphatase
- Golden yellow pigmentation
- Hemolysis on blood agar
- Mannitol fermentation: *S. aureus* ferments mannitol, indicating change in the color of the medium from pink to yellow (Fig. 28.3A)
- Protein A detection.

Coagulase Test

It is the most commonly used biochemical reaction for identification of *S. aureus* (Table 28.2). There are two types of coagulase tests.
1. **Tube coagulase test:** It detects free coagulase.
   - Colony of *S. aureus* is emulsified in a broth of *S. aureus* and incubated for 4 hours at 37°C.
   - *Positive test* is indicated by formation of a clot (Fig. 28.4A).
   - The *negative test* is indicated by no clot formation (Fig. 28.4B).
2. **Slide coagulase test:** It detects clumping factor (i.e., bound coagulase).
   - A colony of *S. aureus* is emulsified with a drop of normal saline to form a milky white

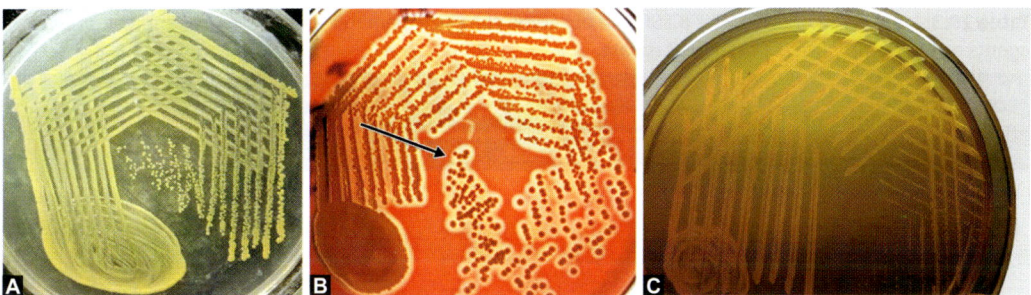

Figs 28.2A to C: Colonies of *S. aureus*: (A) Nutrient agar—shows golden-yellow pigmented colonies; (B) Blood agar—arrow shows zone of beta hemolysis surrounding the colonies; (C) Mannitol salt agar shows yellow-colored colonies of *S. aureus* due to fermentation of mannitol.
Source: Department of Microbiology, Pondicherry Institute of Medical Sciences, Puducherry (*with permission*).

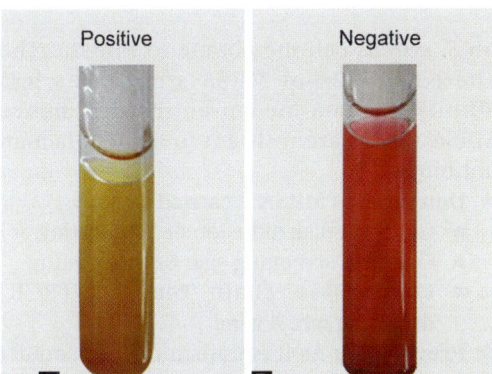

Figs 28.3A and B: Mannitol fermentation test; (A) Positive (mannitol fermented); (B) Negative (mannitol non-fermented).
Source: Department of Microbiology, JIPMER, Puducherry (*with permission*).

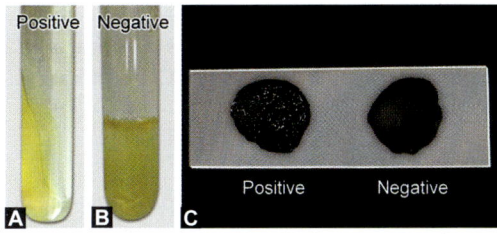

Figs 28.4A to C: Coagulase test: (A) Tube coagulase test (positive); (B) Tube coagulase test (negative); (C) Slide showing coagulase test.
Source: Department of Microbiology, Pondicherry Institute of Medical Sciences, Puducherry (*with permission*).

Table 28.2: Tube coagulase and slide coagulase test.

Tube coagulase	Slide coagulase
Due to coagulase enzyme	Due to clumping factor
Requires CRF in plasma	Does not require CRF in plasma
Done in tube	Done in slide
Positive if clot is formed	Positive if clumps are formed

Abbreviation: CRF, coagulase reacting factor.

suspension. Then a drop of undiluted plasma is added and mixed properly.
- Positive result is indicated by formation of coarse clumps (Fig. 28.4C).

Staphylococci are also identified up to species level by automated identification systems such as MALDI-TOF or VITEK, which detect more accurately and faster than biochemical tests.

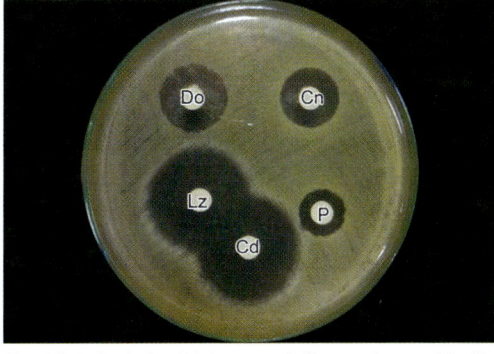

Fig. 28.5: Antimicrobial susceptibility testing on Mueller Hinton Agar [Refer Table 28.3 for Clinical and Laboratory Standards Institute (CLSI) zone interpretation].
Source: Department of Microbiology, Pondicherry Institute of Medical Sciences, Puducherry (*with permission*).

Antimicrobial Susceptibility Test

As *S. aureus* develops resistance to antibiotics readily, drugs should be prescribed according to the antimicrobial susceptibility test (disk diffusion) done on Mueller Hinton agar (Fig. 28.5)

Table 28.3: Interpretative categories (CLSI) and observed zone size diameter (mm) to various antimicrobial agents tested for *Staphylococcus aureus* isolate.

Antimicrobial agents	Disk (µg) strength	CLSI interpretative criteria for *S. aureus* (in mm)			Observed zone size (in mm) (Fig. 28.5)	Interpretation
		Resistant	Intermediate	Sensitive		
Benzyl penicillin (P)	10 units	≤28	–	≥29	12	Resistant
Cefoxitin (Cn)	30	≤21	–	≥22	15	Resistant (MRSA)*
Clindamycin (Cd)	2	≤14	15–20	≥21	22	Sensitive
Linezolid (Lz)	30	≤20	–	≥21	24	Sensitive
Doxycycline (Do)	30	≤12	13–15	≥16	18	Sensitive

Note:
* Methicillin-resistant *S. aureus* (MRSA) is resistant to all beta-lactam antibiotics.
Note: Disk diffusion is not recommended for susceptibility testing of vancomycin to *S. aureus* isolates (as there are no standard interpretative criteria); therefore should only be reported based on MIC testing (e.g., VITEK).

and zone interpretation is done as per Clinical and Laboratory Standards Institute (CLSI) guidelines (Table 28.3).

Treatment

***For MSSA** (methicillin sensitive S. aureus)*: Beta-lactams such as cloxacillin, cefazolin (for serious systemic infections) or cephalexin (for local skin and soft tissue infections) are the preferred drugs. Vancomycin is inferior to beta-lactams for the treatment of MSSA infections.

For MRSA: MRSA strains are resistant to all beta-lactams (except fifth generation cephalosporins such as ceftaroline); hence beta-lactams are contraindicated. Vancomycin is the drug of choice. Alternatively linezolid, daptomycin, clindamycin, doxycycline, etc. are also useful.

Staphylococcus aureus shows resistance to beta-lactam antibiotics; mainly by two mechanisms.
❖ Production of penicillinase enzyme (90% of *S. aureus*).
❖ By alteration of penicillin-binding protein (PBP): It is shown by MRSA strains, which accounts for 30–40% of *S. aureus* isolates.

Methicillin-Resistant *Staphylococcus aureus* (MRSA)

MRSA is mediated by *mec A gene*; which is chromosomally coded. It alters PBP present on *S. aureus* cell membrane to PBP-2a. The altered PBP-2a of MRSA strains has less affinity for beta-lactam antibiotics; hence MRSA strains are resistant to all beta-lactam antibiotics.

❖ **Detection of MRSA** is carried out by:
  ▪ Cefoxitin disk diffusion or MIC testing
  ▪ Oxacillin screening agar or MIC testing
  ▪ Polymerase chain reaction (PCR) detecting *mec A* gene
❖ **Prevention:** As it is transmitted by contact from HCWs and environment; thorough handwashing and other methods of contact precaution (Chapter 11) are the important to prevent its spread.

Coagulase-negative *Staphylococcus*

Most of the coagulase-negative *Staphylococcus* (CoNS) are harmless skin commensals; however, recently their role as pathogens is increasingly been reported.
❖ *Staphylococcus epidermidis:* It causes stitch abscess and prosthetic device-related infections such as endocarditis with insertion of valvular prosthesis and ventricular shunt infections.
❖ *Staphylococcus saprophyticus:* It causes UTI in sexually active young women.

Beta-hemolytic Streptococcal Infections

CHAPTER 29

■ INTRODUCTION

Streptococci are catalase negative gram-positive cocci arranged in pairs or chains (Fig. 29.1A). They can be classified based on the hemolysis produced on 5% sheep blood agar into α, β and γ-hemolytic streptococci.

- ❖ **α-hemolysis:** It is due to partial lysis of red blood cells (RBCs); there is greenish discoloration surrounding the colonies. It is observed with viridans streptococci (Chapter 16) and pneumococci (Chapter 34)
- ❖ **β-hemolysis** or clearing of blood surrounding the colonies: It is due to complete lysis of RBCs. It is observed with *Streptococcus pyogenes* (group A) and *S. agalactiae* (group B)
- ❖ **γ-hemolysis:** There is no hemolysis surrounding the colonies; e.g., *Enterococcus* (Chapter 42).

Problem Solving Exercise 1

Necrotising fasciitis (Group A *Streptococcus*)
A 51-year old male, presented with right foot pain and swelling over 2 weeks, with 10-year history of poorly controlled diabetes mellitus. Clinical examination revealed a gangrenous lateral two toes, with pus discharge and associated warmth and crepitus on the affected area. Following wound debridement, tissue cultures were taken perioperatively and sent to the microbiology laboratory for Gram stain (Fig. 29.1 A), culture (29.2 A), culture smear (Fig. 29.1B) and antimicrobial susceptibility testing (AST) (Fig. 29.2B, 29.3 and Table 29.3).
1. Identify the causative agent based on the microbiological investigations performed.
2. List the infections caused by this organism.
3. Interpret the AST.
4. What antibiotic you would like to prescribe?
5. What are the different modalities of laboratory diagnosis?

Explanation
Clinical Diagnosis
A diabetic patient with gangrenous lateral two toes, with pus discharge and associated warmth and crepitus is suggestive of a case of necrotising fasciitis.

Identification
Gram-positive cocci in chain and pus cells seen on direct smear from specimen, pinpoint colonies on blood agar with wide zone of beta-hemolysis (Fig. 29.2A), gram-positive cocci in chain in culture smear (Fig. 29.1B), Bacitracin sensitive (Fig. 29.2B) are indicative that the causative organism is *Streptococcus pyogenes*.

Antimicrobial Susceptibility Testing
Antimicrobial susceptibility testing on Mueller Hinton blood agar (MHBA) Fig. 29.3 and Table 29.3 showed sensitive to penicillin, azithromycin and clindamycin and intermediate to erythromycin.

Treatment
Surgical debridement (most crucial) along with antibiotics, such as penicillin G plus clindamycin (standard treatment given for necrotising fasciitis).
(For answers to other questions, refer below).

STREPTOCOCCUS PYOGENES INFECTIONS

Clinical Manifestations of *S. pyogenes*

Group A *Streptococcus* (GAS) produces both suppurative and non-suppurative manifestations (Table 29.1).

Laboratory Diagnosis

Specimen Collection and Transport

Commonly collected specimens are throat swab, pus swab, exudates and blood, based on the clinical manifestation.

Direct Smear Microscopy

Gram staining of pus or wound swab reveals pus cells with gram-positive cocci in short chains (Fig. 29.1A). However, direct microscopy is not much useful when *S. pyogenes* is a part of normal flora in the sample (e.g., throat swab).

Culture

Streptococcus pyogenes is fastidious, does not grow in basal media. On blood agar colonies

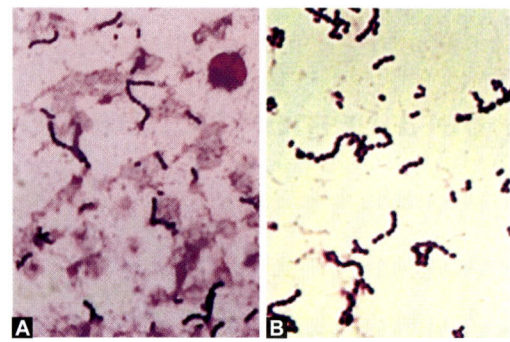

Figs 29.1A and B: Streptococci: (A) In Gram stained smear of pus; (B) In culture smear showing gram-positive cocci in chains.
Source: Department of Microbiology, Pondicherry Institute of Medical Sciences, Puducherry (with permission).

are small, pinpoint, circular, with a wide zone of β-hemolysis (Fig. 29.2A).

Culture Smear Microscopy

Gram-stained smear from the colonies shows gram-positive spherical cocci, arranged in short chains (Fig. 29.1B).

Biochemical Tests for Identification

Catalase test: Streptococci are catalase negative; in contrast to staphylococci which are catalase positive.

Table 29.1: Suppurative and nonsuppurative manifestations of *Streptococcus pyogenes*.

Suppurative	Nonsuppurative
Respiratory infections (Refer Chapter 33): • Pharyngitis/sore throat • Scarlet fever • Others (rare): Pneumonia, empyema, quinsy, sinusitis and otitis media	Acute rheumatic fever (Refer Chapter 16) Acute glomerulonephritis
Skin and soft tissue infections (superficial): • Impetigo (pyoderma) • Cellulitis and erysipelas	Guttate psoriasis Reactive arthritis
Deep soft tissue infections: • Necrotizing fasciitis • Streptococcal myositis	PANDAS (Pediatric Autoimmune Neuropsychiatric Disorders Associated with Streptococcal infections)
Bacteremia leading to endocarditis, osteomyelitis, septic arthritis, meningitis, etc.	
Toxic shock syndrome	
Puerperal sepsis (rare)	

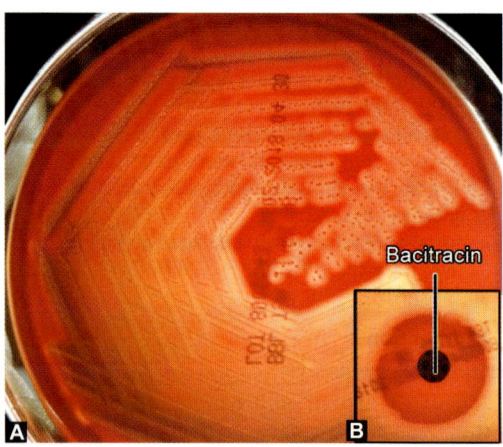

Figs 29.2A and B: *Streptococcus pyogenes*: (A) Growth on blood agar with wide zone of beta-hemolysis around the pin point colonies; (B) Bacitracin sensitive.
Source: Department of Microbiology, Pondicherry Institute of Medical Sciences, Puducherry (with permission).

Table 29.2: Tests to differentiate *Streptococcus pyogenes* and *Streptococcus agalactiae*.

Characters	S. pyogenes	S. agalactiae
Lancefield group	A	B
Bacitracin	Sensitive	Resistant
CAMP test*	Negative	Positive
β-hemolytic colonies	0.5–1 mm, pinpoint	Mucoid, larger (2 mm)

*CAMP, Christie–Atkins–Munch-Peterson test.

Bacitracin sensitivity testing: GAS is sensitive to bacitracin 0.04 U disk (any zone of inhibition around the disk is considered as sensitive), which differentiates it from group B streptococci (resistant) (Fig. 29.2B and Table 29.2).

Serology

Nonsuppurative streptococcal infections such as acute rheumatic fever and glomerulonephritis [post-streptococcal glomerulonephritis (PSGN)] usually develop in patients with a past history of streptococcal sore throat and skin infection (pyoderma), respectively. Hence, in these conditions antibodies in patient's serum is detected to establish retrospective diagnosis of past streptococcal infections.

- **ASO (antistreptolysin O) antibodies** titer is elevated >200 Todd unit/mL in most of the streptococcal infections except pyoderma and PSGN
- **Anti-DNase-B antibodies:** Titer >300–350 units/mL is diagnostic of PSGN and pyoderma.

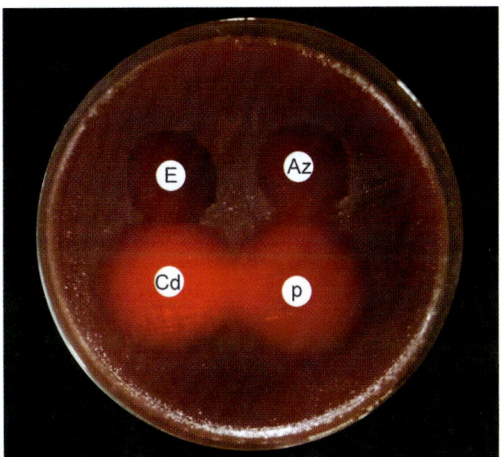

Fig. 29.3: Antimicrobial susceptibility testing on Mueller Hinton blood agar (zone interpretation is given in Table 29.3).
Abbreviations: P, penicillin; E, erythromycin; Cd, clindamycin; Az, azithromycin.
Source: Department of Microbiology, Pondicherry Institute of Medical Sciences, Puducherry *(with permission)*.

Antimicrobial Susceptibility Test

It is carried out on MHBA by disk diffusion test (Fig. 29.3) and reported as per Clinical and Laboratory Standards Institute (CLSI) zone interpretation criteria (Table 29.3).

Treatment

Penicillin is the drug of choice for pharyngeal infections as well as for suppurative complications. Resistance to penicillin is not reported yet.

Table 29.3: Interpretative categories (CLSI) and observed zone size diameter (mm) to various antimicrobial agents tested for *Streptococcus pyogenes* isolate.

Antimicrobial agents	Disk strength (µg)	CLSI interpretative criteria for *Streptococcus pyogenes* (in mm)			Observed zone size (in mm) (Fig. 29.3)	Interpretation
		Resistant	Intermediate	Sensitive		
Penicillin (P)	10 units	—	—	≥24	30	Sensitive
Erythromycin (E)	15	≤15	16–20	≥21	18	Intermediate
Clindamycin (Cd)	2	≤15	16–18	≥19	30	Sensitive
Azithromycin (Az)	15	≤13	14–17	≥18	19	Sensitive

Abbreviation: CLSI, Clinical and Laboratory Standards Institute.

- For outpatients with upper respiratory infections, oral cefepime or azithromycin can be given
- Surgical debridement (most crucial) + Penicillin G + Clindamycin is the standard treatment given for necrotizing fasciitis.

GROUP B STREPTOCOCCI (STREPTOCOCCUS AGALACTIAE)

Problem Solving Exercise 2

Group B Streptococcal Cellulitis

A 13-year-old boy presented to surgery OPD with tender, bright red, subcutaneous swelling on malar area of the face with indurated peau d'orange texture of involved skin along with fever and chills. A clinical diagnosis of cellulitis was made. The aspirated pus specimen was sent to microbiology laboratory for culture (Fig. 29.4A and 29.5) and antimicrobial susceptibility testing (Fig. 29.6 and Table 29.5).
1. Identify the causative agent based on the microbiological investigations performed.
2. List the infections caused by this organism.
3. Interpret the AST.
4. What antibiotic you would like to prescribe?

Explanation

Clinical Diagnosis

History of tender, bright red, subcutaneous swelling on malar indicates that it is a case of cellulitis.

Identification

Beta hemolytic colonies (29.4A), CAMP test positive (Fig. 29.5), bacitracin resistant (Fig. 29.6). These findings are indicative that the causative organism is *Streptococcus agalactiae*.

Antimicrobial Susceptibility Testing

Antimicrobial susceptibility testing on MHBA (Fig. 29.6 and Table 29.5) showed sensitive to penicillin, cefotaxime and resistant to erythromycin.

Treatment

Penicillin would be preferred choice of treatment for streptococcal cellulitis. (if patient is not allergic to penicillin).
(For answers to other questions, refer below)

Clinical Manifestations

Approximately 30% of women are vaginal or rectal carriers of group B *Streptococcus* (GBS). Hence, the GBS infection is common in neonates and in pregnancy. Common infections caused by GBS are:
- Neonatal sepsis and meningitis: two types—early onset and late onset type (Table 29.4)
- Peripartum fever in women
- Cellulitis and soft tissue infections, urinary tract infection, pneumonia, and endocarditis, (commonly occurs among diabetics and elderly people).

Laboratory Diagnosis

GBS is catalase negative and β-hemolytic like GAS, but differs from it by (Table 29.2):
- β-hemolytic colonies are mucoid and slightly larger (Fig. 29.4A)
- Bacitracin resistant (Figs 29.4B and 29.6)

Table 29.4: Early and late onset group B *Streptococcus* disease in neonates.

Characteristics	Early-onset disease	Late-onset disease
Age of onset	0–6 days of birth	7–90 days of birth
Obstetric risk	Prematurity and prolonged labor	Not associated with obstetric risk
Mode of transmission to the baby	During or before birth from the colonized maternal genital tract	Contact with a colonized mother and nursing personnel
Common clinical manifestations	Pneumonia and/or respiratory distress syndrome followed by meningitis	Bacteremia and meningitis (most common)

- **CAMP positive:** CAMP factor (named after the discoverers: *C*hristie-*A*tkins-*M*unch-*P*etersen)

CHAPTER 29 ❖ Beta-hemolytic Streptococcal Infections

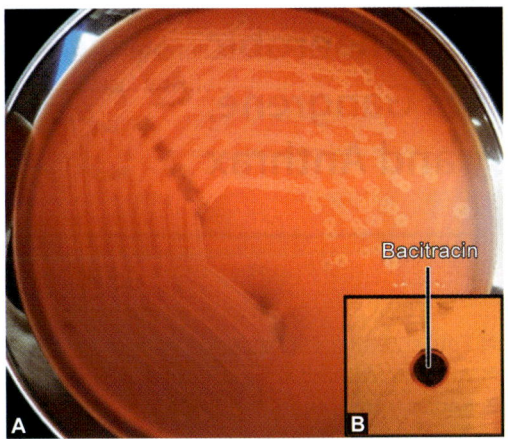

Figs 29.4 A and B: *Streptococcus agalactiae*: (A) Growth on blood agar with wide zone of beta-hemolysis around the colonies; (B) Bacitracin resistant.
Source: Department of Microbiology, JIPMER, Puducherry (*with permission*).

is a phospholipase produced by GBS that causes synergistic hemolysis with β-hemolysin produced by *S. aureus*. When GBS is streaked on blood agar plate perpendicular to *S. aureus*, an enhanced arrow head-shaped hemolysis is produced at their junction (Fig. 29.5).

❖ **AST:** Antimicrobial susceptibility test: It is carried out on MHBA by disk diffusion test (Fig. 29.6) and reported as per CLSI zone interpretation criteria (Table 29.5).

Treatment

Penicillin is the drug of choice for all GBS infections. GBS is less sensitive to penicillin than GAS, hence a higher dose of penicillin is recommended.

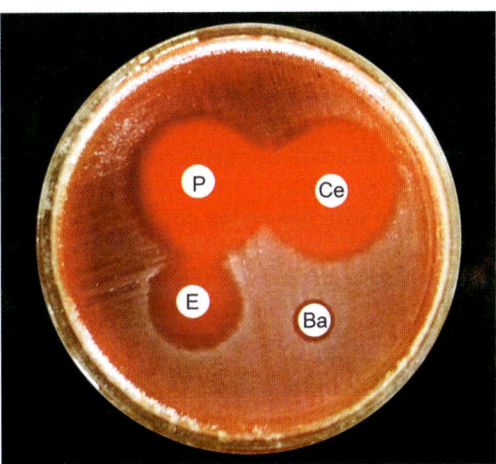

Fig. 29.6: Antimicrobial susceptibility testing on Mueller Hinton blood agar (for zone size interpretation, refer Table 29.5).
Abbreviations: P, penicillin; E, erythromycin; Ce, Cefotaxime; Ba, bacitracin.
Source: Department of Microbiology, Pondicherry Institute of Medical Sciences, Puducherry (*with permission*).

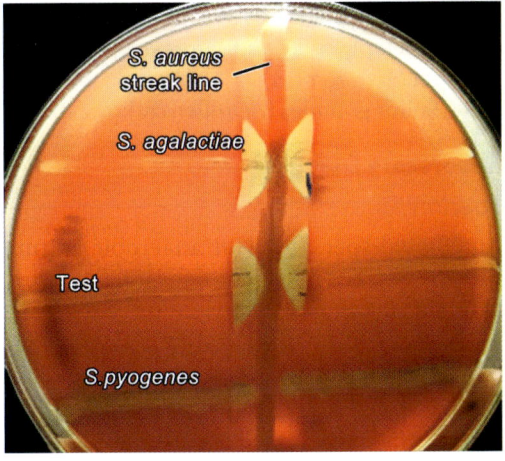

Fig. 29.5: CAMP test positive, indicates the test isolate is *Streptococcus agalactiae*.
Source: Department of Microbiology, JIPMER, Puducherry (*with permission*).

Table 29.5: Interpretative categories (CLSI) and observed zone size diameter (mm) to various antimicrobial agents tested for *Streptococcus agalactiae* isolate.

Antimicrobial agents	Disk strength (µg)	CLSI interpretative criteria for *Streptococcus agalactiae* (in mm)			Observed zone size (in mm) (Fig. 29.6)	Interpretation
		Resistant	Intermediate	Sensitive		
Penicillin (P)	10 units	—	—	≥24	27	Sensitive
Erythromycin (E)	15	≤15	16–20	≥21	15	Resistant
Cefotaxime (Ce)	2	—	—	≥24	28	Sensitive

Abbreviation: CLSI, Clinical and Laboratory Standards Institute.

Miscellaneous Bacterial Infections of Skin and Soft Tissues: Anaerobic Infections including Gas Gangrene, Leprosy and Anthrax

CHAPTER 30

ANAEROBIC INFECTIONS

Obligate anaerobes cannot grow in presence of oxygen. They need special requirements to grow in culture such as:
- **Anaerobic condition:** This can be achieved by various methods such as (Refer Chapter 3.6):
    - McIntosh and Filde's anaerobic jar
    - GasPak system
    - Anoxomat system
    - Anaerobic glove box workstation
    - Pre-reduced anaerobically sterilized (PRAS) media.
- **Medium with low redox potential:** This can be achieved by adding to the media with reducing substances such as unsaturated fatty acid, ascorbic acid, glutathione, cysteine, glucose, sulfites and metallic iron.

Examples of obligate anaerobes include:
- Spore bearing anaerobes (e.g., *Clostridium*): Clostridia are gram-positive bacilli, having bulging spores; found as saprophytes in environment as well as commensal in human and animal gut. However, few members are pathogenic to man such as *C. perfringens, C. tetani, C. botulinum* and *C. difficile*
- Non-sporing anaerobes (e.g., *Bacteroides*).

Clinical Presentations

Anaerobic infections are associated with various clinical clues, such as:
- Infections adjacent to mucosal surfaces that bear anaerobic flora
- Predisposing factors such as ischemia, tumor, penetrating trauma, foreign body, or perforated viscus
- Spreading gangrene involving skin, subcutaneous tissue, fascia, and muscle
- Foul smelling putrid pus
- Abscess formation
- Septic thrombophlebitis
- Toxemia and fever not marked
- Failure to respond to antibiotics that do not have significant anaerobic activity
- Organisms are seen under Gram stain, but fail to grow in routine aerobic culture
- **Special features** may be observed such as:
    - Gas in specimen (gas gangrene)
    - Black pigment that fluoresce (*Prevotella melaninogenica*)
    - Sulfur granules (*Actinomyces*).

Laboratory Diagnosis

Specimens

All clinical specimens for anaerobic culture must be handled meticulously as brief exposure to oxygen may kill obligate anaerobes and result in failure to isolate them in the laboratory.
- Accepted specimens: Tissue bits, necrotic materials, aspirated body fluids or pus in syringes
- Unacceptable specimens: All swabs, sputum or voided urine
- Specimens should be immediately put into RCM broth or other anaerobic transport media and brought to the laboratory as soon as possible.

> **Robertson's cooked meat (RCM) broth**
> It is the most commonly used anaerobic media. It contains chopped meat particles (beef heart), which provide glutathione and unsaturated fatty acids, which take up oxygen and create lower redox potential and thus permit the growth of obligate anaerobes (Fig. 30.1A). *C. perfringens* turns meat particles pink and broth turbid (30.1B); whereas *C. tetani* turns the color black and turbid (30.1C).

CHAPTER 30 ❖ Miscellaneous Bacterial Infections of Skin and Soft Tissues

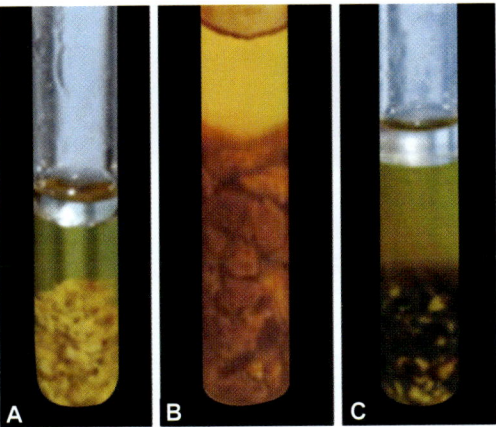

Figs 30.1A to C: Robertson cooked meat broth: (A) Uninoculated; (B) Pink and turbid (*C. perfringens*); (C) Black and turbid (*C. tetani*).
Source: Department of Microbiology, JIPMER, Puducherry (with permission).

Microscopy

All clinical specimens from suspected anaerobic infections should be Gram stained and examined for the characteristic morphology.

Cultural Identification

Samples should be processed immediately under anaerobic condition which can be created by various methods as described earlier.

- ❖ **Culture:** Various culture media can be used for the isolation of anaerobes, such as:
  - Anaerobic blood agar and neomycin blood agar
  - Egg yolk agar and phenylethyl agar (PEA)
  - BHIS agar: Brain–heart infusion agar added with supplements, such as vitamin K and hemin
  - *Bacteroides* bile esculin agar (BBE agar).
- ❖ **Identification of anaerobes** is based on:
  - Biochemical tests
  - Susceptibility to antibiotic disks
  - Gas liquid chromatography
  - Automated systems such as MALDI-TOF.

Treatment

Common antibiotics given for anaerobic infections are:
- ❖ Metronidazole plus penicillin-DOC for odontogenic infections
- ❖ Carbapenems (e.g., meropenem)
- ❖ β-lactam/β-lactamase inhibitor combination (amoxicillin-clavulanate, piperacillin-tazobactam)
- ❖ Clindamycin (in case of penicillin allergy).

Antimicrobial resistance in anaerobic bacteria is an increasing problem.

Problem Solving Exercise 1

Gas gangrene (*Clostridium perfringens*)

Three days after a road traffic accident, a 30-year-old man presented to hospital with sudden onset of excruciating pain at left leg with wound oozing foul-smelling thin serosanguineous discharge. On examination, the wound was found to be bandaged with a soiled gauze, appeared to be heavily contaminated with soil, there was edema and pain at the site and crepitus was felt on palpation. Gram-stained smear of exudate specimen from deeper part of the wound is shown in Figure 30.3.
1. What is the clinical diagnosis and its causative organism?
2. List other infections caused by this organism?
3. What are the various modalities of laboratory diagnosis?
4. How will you treat this condition?

Explanation

Clinical Diagnosis

The history is suggestive of gas gangrene. Points in favor are:
- ❑ Road traffic accident, wound heavily contaminated with soil
- ❑ Five days later, develops painful wound oozing foul-smelling serosanguineous discharge
- ❑ On examination, edema and pain at the site and crepitus on palpation.

Identification

Thick, *boxcar-shaped* gram-positive bacilli without spore in direct smear from deeper exudate specimen (Fig. 30.3) indicates that causative agent is *C. perfringens*.
(For answers to other questions, refer below.)

Gas Gangrene

Gas gangrene is defined as a rapidly spreading, edematous myonecrosis, occurring in association with severely crushed wounds contaminated with pathogenic clostridia, particularly with *C. perfringens*.

Etiological Agents

Gas gangrene is always polymicrobial and is caused by many clostridial species.
- **Established agents:** *Clostridium perfringens* (most common, 60% of the total cases) and *C. novyi* and *C. septicum* (20–40%)
- **Probable agents:** They are less commonly implicated, e.g., *C. histolyticum, C. sporogenes, C. fallax, C. bifermentans, C. sordellii, C. aerofoetidum,* and *C. tertium*.

Pathogenesis

The development of gas gangrene requires:
- **Anaerobic environment:** Crushing injuries of muscles such as road traffic accidents, bullet injuries leads to interruption in the blood supply and tissue ischemia
- **Contamination of wound** with clostridial spores present in the soil (during war or road traffic accident) or clothes
- **Toxin production:** Once introduced, *C. perfringens* proliferates locally and elaborates exotoxins, chiefly α-toxin and θ-toxin. **α-toxin** is the principle virulence factor. It has both phospholipase C and sphingomyelinase activities.

Clinical Manifestations

The **incubation period** is variable. Depending upon the nature of injury, the amount of wound contamination and the type of clostridial species involved, the incubation period varies. For example:
- 10–48 hours for *C. perfringens*
- 2–3 days for *C. septicum*
- 5–6 days for *C. novyi*.

Various manifestations include:
- Sudden onset of excruciating pain at the affected site
- Rapid development of a foul-smelling thin serosanguineous discharge
- Gas bubbles **(crepitus)** in the muscle planes (Fig. 30.2)

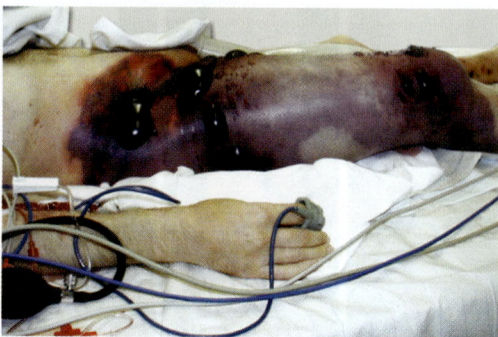

Fig. 30.2: Gas gangrene of the right leg showing swelling and discoloration of the right thigh with bullae, and palpable crepitus.
Source: Wikipedia/Cases/Engelbert Schröpfer, Stephan Rauthe and Thomas Meyer (*with permission*).

- Brawny edema and induration
- Such gangrenous tissues later may become liquefied and sloughed off
- Shock and organ failure develop later
- Associated with higher mortality rate (50%).

Laboratory Diagnosis of Gas Gangrene

Based on the clinical diagnosis of gas gangrene, treatment should be started as early as possible. Laboratory diagnosis has role only for (1) confirmation of the clinical diagnosis, (2) species identification.

Specimen

Ideal specimens are necrotic tissues, muscle fragments and exudates from deeper part of the wound, where the infection appears to be more active.
- Blood culture may be positive for *C. perfringens* and *C. septicum*. However, *C. perfringens* bacteremia can occur even in the absence of gas gangrene
- Swabs rubbed over the wound surface or soaked in exudates are not satisfactory
- Specimens should be put into Robertson's cooked meat broth and transported immediately to the laboratory.

Direct Microscopy

Gram stained films provide clues about the species of clostridia present. Absence of neutrophils in the infected tissues is a characteristic feature.
- Thick, stubby, boxcar-shaped, gram-positive bacilli without spore—suggestive of *C. perfringens* (Fig. 30.3)

CHAPTER 30 ❖ Miscellaneous Bacterial Infections of Skin and Soft Tissues

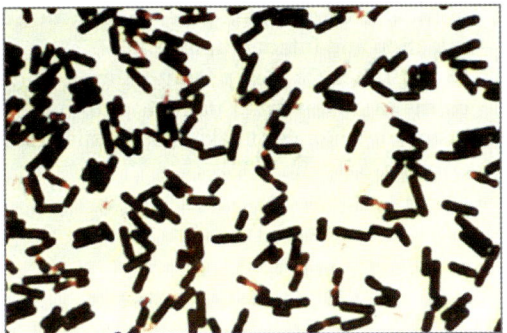

Fig. 30.3: Gram stained smear of *Clostridium perfringens*.
Source: Public Health Image Library/ID# 11196, Don Stalons/ Centers for Disease Control and Prevention (CDC), Atlanta (*with permission*).

- Spore bearing gram-positive bacilli suggest other clostridia species
  - Citron bodies (boat or leaf-shaped pleomorphic irregularly stained bacilli with spores)—suggest *C. septicum*
  - Large rods with oval sub-terminal spores—suggest *C. novyi*.

Identification

C. perfringens can be further identified by the following properties. Culture plates should be incubated anaerobically at 37°C for 2 days.

- **Target hemolysis** (double zone hemolysis, Fig. 30.4A): On blood agar, *C. perfringens* produce an inner narrow zone of complete hemolysis (due to θ-toxin), surrounded by a much wider zone of incomplete hemolysis (due to the alpha toxin)
- **Nagler's reaction:** *C. perfringens* produces an opalescence surrounding the streak line on egg yolk agar or media containing 20% human serum (due to lecithinase activity of α-toxin). Opalescence can be inhibited by incorporating anti-α-toxin to the medium (30.4B). The test is also positive for *C. bifermentans, C. baratti* and *C. sordellii* (all produce α-toxin)
- **Reverse CAMP test:** *C. perfringens* is streaked over the center of blood agar plate and *Streptococcus agalactiae* is streaked perpendicular to it. Presence of enhanced zone of hemolysis (arrow-shaped) pointing towards *C. perfringens* indicates the test is positive (Fig. 30.4C).

Automated methods such as MALDI-TOF is currently the method of choice of rapid and accurate identification of various clostridia species.

Treatment (Gas Gangrene)

- **Early surgical debridement** is the most crucial step in the management of gas gangrene. All devitalized tissues should be widely resected so as to remove conditions that produce anaerobic environment. Closure of wounds should be delayed for 5–6 days until the sites are free from infection
- **Antibiotics:** Combination of penicillin and clindamycin is recommended for 10–14 days
- **Hyperbaric oxygen:** It may kill the obligate anaerobic clostridia such as *C. perfringens*; however, it has no effect on aerotolerant clostridia (*C. septicum*)
- **Passive immunization** with anti-α-toxin antiserum.

Other pathogenic clostridia include:

- ***C. tetani:*** Causes **tetanus**; mediated by a neurotoxin (tetanus toxin) which causes

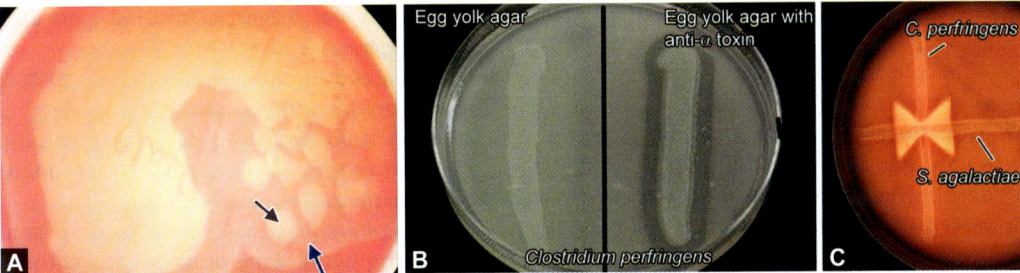

Figs 30.4A to C: (A) Target hemolysis of *C. perfringens*-zone of incomplete hemolysis (blue arrow) and zone of complete hemolysis (black arrow); (B) Nagler's reaction; (C) Reverse CAMP test.
Source: (A and B) Department of Microbiology, JIPMER, Puducherry; (C) Dr Padmaja A Shenoy, Department of Microbiology, Kasturba Medical College, Manipal, Karnataka (*with permission*).

skeletal muscle spasm and autonomic nervous system disturbance
- ❖ **C. botulinum:** Produces a powerful neurotoxin called botulinum toxin that causes **botulism**; characterized by flaccid paralysis of muscles. It presents in three clinical forms—food poisoning, wound infection and infant botulism
- ❖ **C. difficile:** Causes pseudomembranous colitis in hospitalized patients who have a history of prolonged intake of broad spectrum antibiotics (Chapter 22).

LEPROSY

Problem Solving Exercise 2

A 37-year-old village lady presented with complaints of numerous hypopigmented skin lesions on her arms, cheeks, abdomen, back and legs for last 5 years. Her eyebrows had started thinning and she had numbness in her forearm. Specimen collected from the skin lesion was subjected to microscopy (Fig. 30.5).
- ❑ What is the clinical diagnosis and its causative organism?
- ❑ What are the various modalities of laboratory diagnosis?
- ❑ How will you treat this condition?

Explanation
Clinical Diagnosis
The history of numerous hypopigmented skin lesions, numbness in her forearm and eyebrows started thinning is suggestive of leprosy.

Identification
The modified acid-fast smear (Fig. 30.5) demonstrating globi (arrow) filled with acid-fast bacilli arranged singly or in cigar-like bundles. This suggests that the causative agent is *Mycobacterium leprae*. (For answers to other questions, refer below).

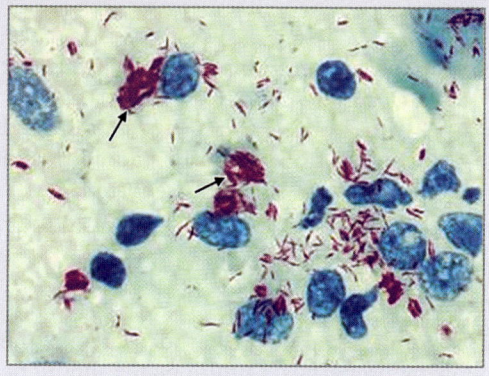

Fig. 30.5: Microscopy of specimen (slit skin smear) collected from the skin lesion.
Source: Dr Isabella Princess, Apollo Hospital, Chennai (with permission).

Laboratory Diagnosis of Leprosy

Smear Microscopy

- ❖ **Specimen collection:**
  - Total six samples are collected; four from skin (forehead, cheek, chin and buttock), one from ear lobe and nasal mucosa by nasal blow or scraping
  - Slit skin smear is the technique followed to collect the skin and ear lobe specimens from the edge of the lesion.
- ❖ **Procedure:** The smears are stained by ZN technique by using 5% sulfuric acid for decolorization
- ❖ **Interpretation:** Under oil immersion objective, red acid-fast bacilli are seen, arranged singly or in groups, bound together by lipid-like substance, the *glia* to form *globi* (called as *cigar bundle* appearance). The globi are present inside the foamy macrophages called as Virchow's "lepra cells" or "foamy cells" (Fig. 30.5).
  - *Live bacilli* will be uniformly stained with parallel sides and round ends and length is five times the width
  - *Dead bacilli* are less uniformly stained and have *fragmented and granular* appearance.
- ❖ **Grading of the smear:** The smears are graded, based on the number of bacilli
  - *Bacteriological index (BI)* is based on the total number of bacilli (live and dead) seen per oil immersion field
  - *Morphological index (MI)* is expressed as the percentage of uniformly stained bacilli out of the total number of bacilli counted.

1–10 bacilli in 100 OIF	= 1+
1–10 bacilli in 10 OIF	= 2+
1–10 bacilli per OIF	= 3+
10–100 bacilli per OIF	= 4+
100–1,000 bacilli per OIF	= 5+
>1,000 bacilli or bacilli in clumps and globi in each OIF	= 6+

Other tests include:
- **Mouse foot pad cultivation:** *M. leprae* is not cultivable either in artificial culture media or in tissue culture. It can be cultivated only by inoculating the specimens into foot pad of mice keeping at 20°C for 6–9 months. Other animals such as nine-banded armadillo can also be used
- **Lepromin test:** It demonstrates the delayed hypersensitivity reaction and an intact cell-mediated immunity against the lepra antigen.

Treatment

WHO recommends multidrug therapy for treatment of leprosy. Dapsone, rifampicin and clofazimine are the recommended drugs.

ANTHRAX

Problem Solving Exercise 3

A 35-year-old male who is a worker in a wool factory, was admitted into hospital with prolonged fever, with chills, night sweats and chest discomfort with blood-stained sputum. Sputum specimen was collected and was subjected to Gram staining (Fig. 30.6).
1. What is the clinical diagnosis and its causative organism?
2. List the virulence factors and other infections caused by this organism?
3. What are the various modalities of laboratory diagnosis?
4. What antibiotic you would like to prescribe?

Explanation
Clinical Diagnosis
History of fever and blood-stained sputum in wool factory worker is suggestive of respiratory anthrax (wool sorter's disease). Occupational exposures, leading to infection among farmer, butcher, abattoir, etc., are common in anthrax.

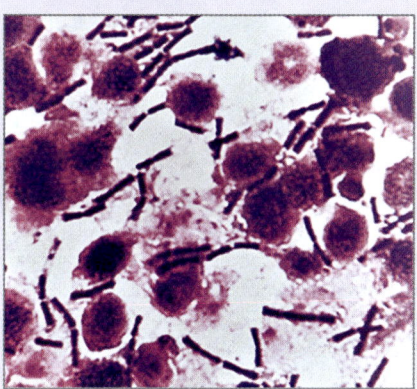

Fig. 30.6: Gram stain of *B. anthracis* showing gram-positive, large rectangular bacilli and pus cells.
Source: A. Public Health Image Library/ID#: 1811, Centers for Disease Control and Prevention (CDC), Atlanta *(with permission).*

Identification
Direct Gram staining (Fig. 30.6) shows gram-positive large rectangular rods arranged in chain. This suggests that the causative agent as *Bacillus anthracis*. (For answers to other questions, refer below).

Clinical Manifestations

Anthrax is primarily a zoonosis affecting herbivorous animals such as cattle and sheep. Human beings acquire infection by: (1) direct contact by spores entering through the abraded skin among people with occupational exposure to animals; (2) by inhalation of spores and (3) ingestion of carcasses.

Types of human anthrax are:
- **Cutaneous anthrax (hide porter's disease):** It is characterized by necrotic eschar surrounded by non-pitting indurated edema, called as malignant pustule
- **Pulmonary anthrax or Wool sorter's disease:** It is characterized by hemorrhagic pneumonia with blood stained sputum
- Intestinal anthrax.

Virulence factors of B. anthracis are:
- **Anthrax toxin:** Tripartite toxin consists of edema factor, protective factor and lethal factor
- **Anthrax polypeptide capsule.**

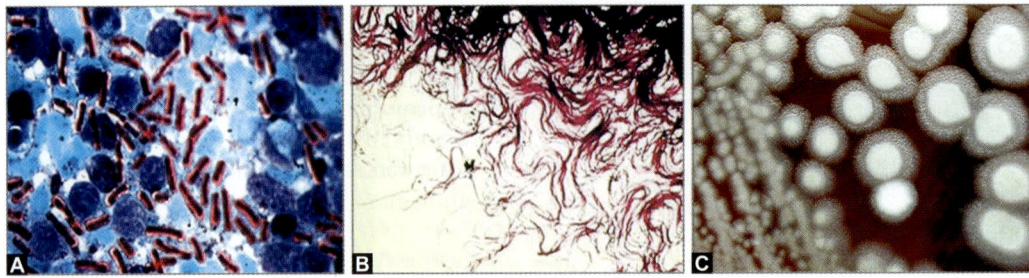

Figs 30.7A to C: (A) McFadyean's reaction—amorphous purple capsule surrounding blue bacilli (polychrome methylene blue stain); (B) Medusa head colonies of *Bacillus anthracis* on nutrient agar (10x magnification); (C) Non-hemolytic dry wrinkled colonies of *Bacillus anthracis* on blood agar.

Source: (A) Department of Pathobiology, University of Guelph, Canada; (B) Dr J Glenn Songer, Iowa State University, USA; (C) Public Health Image Library/ID#: 1897/Dr Larry Stauffer, Centers for Disease Control and Prevention (CDC), Atlanta (*with permission*).

Laboratory Diagnosis

As there is high-risk of laboratory-acquired infection of anthrax, hence specimens should be processed in appropriate biological safety cabinets.

Specimen

The following specimens to be collected—pus or swab from malignant pustule, sputum (in pulmonary anthrax), blood (in septicemia) and CSF (in hemorrhagic meningitis).

Direct Demonstration

- **Gram staining:** Reveals gram-positive, large rectangular rods; spores are usually not seen in clinical samples (Fig. 30.6)
- **McFadyean's reaction:** Polypeptide capsule can be demonstrated by staining with polychrome methylene blue stain for 30 seconds. Capsule appears as amorphous purple material surrounding blue bacilli (Fig. 30.7A).

Culture

Bacillus anthracis is obligate aerobic and non-fastidious.
- **Medusa head appearance:** When colonies are viewed under low power microscope, the edge of the colony is composed of long interlacing chains of bacilli, appears as locks of matted hair (Fig. 30.7B)
- **Blood agar:** Dry wrinkled, *nonhemolytic* colonies are produced (Fig. 30.7C)
- **Culture smear:** Gram staining reveals *bamboo stick appearance*, i.e., long chain of gram-positive bacilli with nonbulging spores (appear as empty space) (Fig. 30.8).

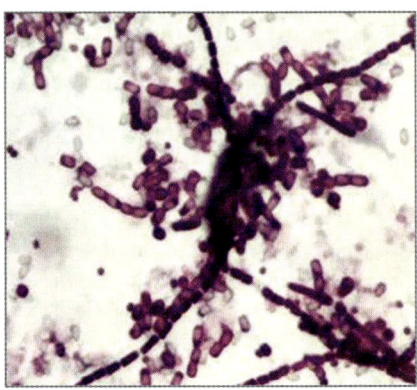

Fig. 30.8: Gram stained culture smear-shows gram-positive bacilli with spores (bamboo stick appearance).
Source: Department of Microbiology, JIPMER, Puducherry.

Treatment

Treatment should be started early; consists of ciprofloxacin or doxycycline plus clindamycin for 60 days.

Viral Exanthems and Other Cutaneous Viral Infections

CHAPTER 31

INTRODUCTION

An exanthem is an eruption or rash on the skin, that may be associated with fever or other systemic symptoms. Majority of exanthems have an infectious etiology; most commonly by viruses. Exanthems may also be seen due to drug reactions. The viruses that can cause exanthematous and other types of skin lesions are enlisted in Table 31.1.

HERPES SIMPLEX VIRUS INFECTIONS

Introduction

Herpes simplex viruses belong to α-subfamily of Herpesviridae.
- They are extremely widespread and exhibit a broad host range; can infect many types of cells and different animals. However, the human herpesviruses infect exclusively man
- They replicate fast (12–18 hours cycle), spread fast and are cytolytic
- They can cause a spectrum of diseases, involving skin, mucosa and various organs
- They undergo **latency in nerve cells**; reactivate later causing recurrent lesions.

Herpes simplex viruses (HSV) are of two distinct types: HSV-1 and HSV-2. They differ from each other in many aspects (Table 31.2).

Pathogenesis

Primary Infection

- **Transmission** occurs through abraded skin or mucosa from any site, but more commonly by:
  - **HSV-1:** Oropharyngeal contact with infected saliva or direct skin contact
  - **HSV-2:** Sexual contact or rarely vertical mode (from mother to fetus).

Table 31.1: Viral exanthems and other cutaneous viral infections.

Viruses	Viral exanthems/other skin lesions
Herpesviruses	
Herpes simplex virus	Vesicular lesions
Varicella-zoster virus	Chickenpox and zoster
Epstein–Barr virus	Following ampicillin therapy
Human herpesvirus-6	Roseola infantum (exanthem subitum or sixth disease)
Other DNA viruses	
Poxviruses	Smallpox Molluscum contagiosum*
Parvovirus	Erythema infectiosum (fifth disease) Papular-purpuric gloves and socks syndrome*
Human papillomavirus (HPV)	Warts*: Common warts, flat warts, plantar warts, anogenital warts (condyloma acuminatum)
RNA viruses	
Measles virus	Rashes, Koplik's spots
Rubella virus	Rashes
Coxsackie viruses	Hand-foot-mouth disease
Agents of viral hemorrhagic fever	Dengue, Ebola and others

*These viruses produce non-exanthematous skin lesions.

- **Site of infection:** HSV replicates at the local site of infection and produces lesions anywhere, but more commonly in:
  - HSV-1 lesions are confined to areas above the waist (most common site—around mouth)
  - HSV-2 produces lesions below the waist (most common site—genital area).
- **Spread via nerve:** Virus then invades the local nerve endings and is transported by retrograde

Problem Solving Exercise 1

Herpes

A 7-year-old boy had developed multiple painful vesicles over the lips, tongue and buccal mucosa (Fig. 31.1A). His parents revealed that two children of his school had a similar presentation few days back. Scrapings obtained from the base of the lesion is subjected to staining with Wright's or Giemsa (Tzanck preparation) (Fig. 31.2A).
a. What is the most probable diagnosis and etiological diagnosis?
b. What are the various cutaneous and mucosal infections produced?
c. How is this infection diagnosed in the laboratory?

Explanation

It is a case of Herpes labialis and the etiological agent is herpes simplex virus
- Multiple painful vesicles over the lips, tongue and buccal mucosa (Fig. 31.1A).
- Scrapings obtained from the base of the lesion is subjected to staining with Wright's or Giemsa [Tzanck preparation)which revealed multinucleated giant cell (Tzanck cell) in the center (arrow showing) (Fig. 31.2A)].

(For answers to other questions, refer below).

Table 31.2: Differences between HSV-1 and HSV-2.

Properties	Herpes simplex virus 1	Herpes simplex virus 2
Common modes of transmission	Direct contact with mucosa or abraded skin	Sexual mode or vertical mode
Latency in	Trigeminal ganglia	Sacral ganglia
Age affected	Young children	Young adults
Common manifestations	• Oral-facial mucosal lesions • Encephalitis and meningitis • Ocular lesions • Skin lesions—above the waist	• Genital lesions • Skin lesions—below the waist • Neonatal herpes

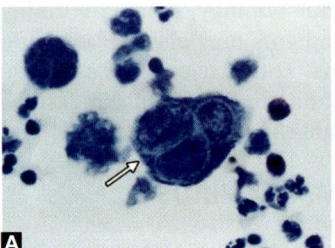
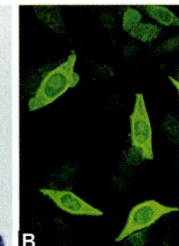

Figs 31.2A and B: (A) Tzanck smear of a tissue scraping showing multinucleated giant cell (Tzanck cell) in the center (arrow showing); (B) Indirect IF for HSV1/2 antibody detection.
Source: (A) Public Health Image Library, ID# 14428/Centers for Disease Control and Prevention (CDC), Atlanta; (B) Euroimmun (*with permission*).

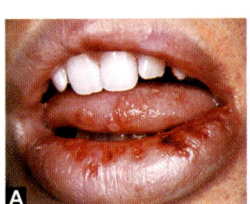
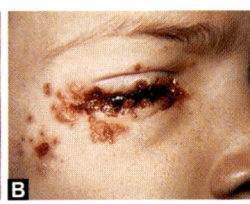

Figs 31.1A and B: (A) Vesicular lesions on lips and tongue due to HSV-1 infection; (B) Periocular vesicular lesions due to HSV-1 infection.
Source: Public Health Image Library, (A) ID# 12616 (Robert E Sumpter); (B) ID# 6492 (Dr KL Hermann)/Centers for Disease Control and Prevention (CDC), Atlanta (*with permission*).

axonal flow to the dorsal root ganglia, where it replicates further, and then undergoes latency
❖ Primary HSV infections are usually mild; in fact, most are asymptomatic
❖ However, in immunocompromised hosts, viremia occurs that leads to widespread organ involvement and systemic manifestations.

Clinical Manifestations

Both HSV-1 and 2 have been isolated from nearly all mucocutaneous sites and viscera; however, in general, oral-facial infections are common with HSV-1, whereas HSV-2 frequently causes genital infections and intrauterine infections. The incubation period ranges from 1 to 26 days (median, 6–8 days).

Oral-facial Mucosal Lesions

Oral-facial mucosal lesions are the most common manifestation of HSV infections (Figs 31.1A and B).
❖ Most common affected site is buccal mucosa
❖ Most frequent primary lesions are gingivostomatitis and pharyngitis

- Most frequent recurrent lesion is herpes labialis (painful vesicles near lips) (Fig. 31.1A)
- Other lesions produced are—ulcerative stomatitis, tonsillitis and vesicular lesions on the eyelids (Fig. 31.1B)
- Many cases are asymptomatic but can predispose to secondary bacterial infection.

Cutaneous Lesions

HSV usually infects through abraded skin and causes various cutaneous lesions.
- **Herpetic whitlow:** Lesions present on the fingers of dentists and hospital personnel
- **Febrile blisters** (herpes febrilis): Fever due to any other cause can provoke HSV to cause recurrent blisters
- **Herpes gladiatorum:** Mucocutaneous lesions present on the body of wrestlers
- Skin lesions are often severe on underlying eczema or burns which permit extensive local viral replication and spread
- **Eczema herpeticum:** Caused by HSV-1 in patients with chronic eczema
- **Erythema multiforme:** HSV is commonly associated with this condition.

Other Infective Syndromes of HSV

- **CNS infections:** Such as encephalitis, meningitis
- **Ocular manifestations:** such as keratoconjunctivitis, corneal ulcer and blindness
- **Genital lesions:** described as bilateral, painful, multiple, tiny vesicular ulcers (HSV-2 is more common than HSV-1)
- **Visceral and disseminated herpes**
- **Neonatal herpes.**

Laboratory Diagnosis

The sensitivity of all the methods to diagnose HSV infection depends on the type of specimen, as well as the type of infection. The sensitivity is more for vesicular lesions and primary infection than for ulcerative lesions and recurrent infections.

Cytopathology

Scrapings obtained from the base of the lesion can be stained with Wright's or Giemsa (Tzanck preparation), or Papanicolaou stain. Sensitivity of staining is low (<30% for mucosal swabs). It cannot differentiate between HSV-1, HSV-2, and varicella-zoster virus; as all of them produce similar but characteristic cytopathological changes such as:
- Production of Cowdry type A intranuclear inclusion bodies (Lipschultz body)
- Formation of multinucleated giant cells with faceted nuclei and ground glass chromatin (Tzanck cells) (Fig. 31.2A)
- Ballooning of infected cells, margination of chromatin.

Virus Isolation

It remains the most definitive tool for HSV diagnosis. McCoy cell lines are preferred for isolation of HSV. Viral growth can be detected in 2–4 days by:
- **Characteristic cytopathic effect:** Diffuse rounding and ballooning of the infected cells
- Viral antigen detection by neutralization test or immunofluorescence staining with specific antiserum
- Shell vial technique can be followed to decrease the detection time to <24 hours.

Viral Antigen Detection by Immunofluorescence

Viral antigen detection (targeting cell surface glycoprotein antigens) by direct IF is also a sensitive and specific assay. It can differentiate HSV-1 from HSV-2.

HSV DNA Detection

Molecular methods such as polymerase chain reaction (PCR), real-time PCR (can quantitate the viral load in specimens) and BioFire FilmArray (automated nested mulitplex PCR) are useful; can also be used to differentiate between HSV-1 and 2.

Antibody Detection

Antibodies appear in 4–7 days after the infection and peak in 2–4 weeks. IgM appears first and is replaced by IgG, which persists for life.
- Most available tests usually detect IgG or total antibodies, hence cannot differentiate

between recent and past infections. Seroconversion or a rise in titer is more meaningful
- Serologic assays (e.g., ELISA) based on the type-specific antigens such as glycoprotein G antigens (gG1 and gG2) can differentiate between HSV-1 and HSV-2. Western blot is more accurate, with 98% sensitivity and specificity
- Both ELISA and indirect IF formats are available (Fig. 31.2B).

Treatment

For mucocutaneous infections, acyclovir, famciclovir and valacyclovir have been the mainstay of treatment.

Prevention

Infection control measures: Patients with mucocutaneous herpes in hospitals, should be kept on contact precautions until lesions are dry and crusted (Refer Chapter 11).

VARICELLA-ZOSTER VIRUS INFECTIONS

Problem Solving Exercise 2

A child presents with vesicular rashes (Fig. 31.3), which appeared first on the face and trunk, spread rapidly to involve flexor surfaces; sparing distal part of the limbs. Rashes are bilateral and diffuse in distribution, appear in multiple crops. Fever appears with each crop of rashes.
- What is the clinical diagnosis?
- What are the complications seen?
- Discuss about the infection control measures to be taken when giving care to this patient.

- Fever appears with each crop of rashes. Refer text below for the answer to other questions.

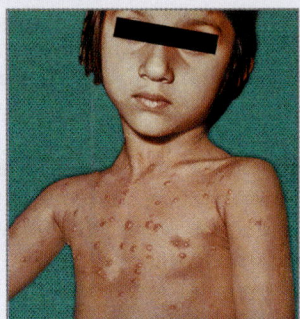

Fig. 31.3: Vesicular rashes of Chickenpox.
Source: Public Health Image Library, ID#/2882/JD Millar/ Centers for Disease Control and Prevention (CDC), Atlanta (*with permission*).

Explanation

The clinical presentation is suggestive of chickenpox:
- Vesicular rashes (Fig. 31.3), on the face and trunk of child, which spread rapidly to involve flexor surface.
- Rashes are bilateral and diffuse in distribution, appear in multiple crops.

Introduction

Varicella-zoster virus (VZV) produces vesicular eruptions (rashes) on the skin and mucous membranes in the form of two clinical entities:
1. **Chickenpox:** It is characterized by generalized diffuse bilateral vesicular rashes which occur following primary infection, usually affecting children
2. **Zoster or shingles:** It occurs following reactivation of latent VZV, present in the trigeminal ganglia that occurs mainly in adult life. Vesicular rashes are unilateral and segmental (confined to the skin innervated by a single sensory ganglion).

Chickenpox

Pathogenesis

VZV enters through the upper respiratory mucosa or the conjunctiva by aerosol (most common) and contact transmission. From the local site, it spills over to blood and then is carried through the infected mononuclear cells to target sites such as:
- Skin (produces rashes)
- Respiratory tract (shed in respiratory secretions)
- Neurons (undergoes latency).

Clinical Manifestations

- Incubation period is about 10–21 days (2–3 weeks)
- **Rashes** are the main manifestation of chickenpox
  - Rashes are vesicular (Fig. 31.3)
  - Centripetal in distribution: Usually start on the face and trunk, spread rapidly to involve flexor surfaces; sparing distal part of the limbs

- Bilateral and diffuse in distribution
- Rashes appear in multiple crops: Lesions in various stages of evolution, such as maculopapules, vesicles, pustules, and scabs can be found in one area at the same time
- Fever appears with each crop of rashes.
❖ Chickenpox is a disease of childhood
❖ When occurs in adults, it is more severe with bullous and hemorrhagic rashes leaving behind pitted scars on skin after recovery.

Complications

Complications are more common in adults and in immunocompromised individuals.
❖ **Most common complications:** Secondary bacterial infections of the skin and CNS involvement (cerebellar ataxia, encephalitis and aseptic meningitis)
❖ **Other complications:** (1) Varicella pneumonia—serious complication, seen in adults and (2) Reye's syndrome—fatty degeneration of liver, occurs following aspirin intake
❖ **Chickenpox in pregnancy:** Chickenpox in pregnancy can affect both mother and the fetus
  - Mothers are at high-risk of developing varicella pneumonia
  - Fetus is at higher risk of developing **congenital varicella syndrome** (in early pregnancy); characterized by cicatricial skin lesions and limb hypoplasia.

Zoster or Shingles or Zona

Zoster usually occurs due to reactivation of latent VZV in old age (>60 years of age), in immunocompromised individuals or occasionally in healthy adults.
❖ It usually starts with severe pain in the area of skin or mucosa supplied by one or more groups of sensory nerves and ganglia
❖ **Rashes:** They are unilateral and segmental, confined to the area of skin supplied by the affected nerves
❖ **Most common nerve involved** is ophthalmic branch of trigeminal nerve. Head, neck and trunk are the most common affected sites.

Vaccine

Live attenuated vaccine using Oka strain of VZV is available. It is given to children after 1 year of age; 2 doses, first dose is given at 12–15 months and second at 4–6 years.

Varicella-zoster Immunoglobulin (VZIg)

❖ It is useful for **post-exposure prophylaxis;** given within 96 hours (preferably within 72 hours) of exposure
❖ It is also indicated for **neonates born to mothers** suffering from chickenpox.

Infection Control Measures

Patients infected with VZV should be kept in isolation. Airborne precautions (e.g., negative air-flow rooms, and PPE such as N95 respirator) plus contact precautions must be followed until lesions are dry and crusted (Refer Chapter 11). For localized zoster in an immunocompetent host, contact precaution alone need to be followed.

HPV INFECTIONS

Human papillomavirus (HPV) is a DNA virus, belongs Papillomaviridae family. It has selective tropism for epithelium of skin and mucous membranes. It has >100 serotypes, which produce an array of infections ranging from benign warts, to malignant neoplasia of cervix.

Benign warts: They are small, hard, rough growth on the skin (Fig. 31.4). They are of following types:
❖ **Common skin warts** (verruca vulgaris) and flat warts (verruca plana) are common in children (seen with serotypes 2, 4, 27, 57)
❖ **Plantar warts** (verruca plantaris)—benign lesion, widely prevalent among adolescents (seen with serotype 1)
❖ **Anogenital warts** (condyloma acuminatum): It is a sexually transmitted infection, seen

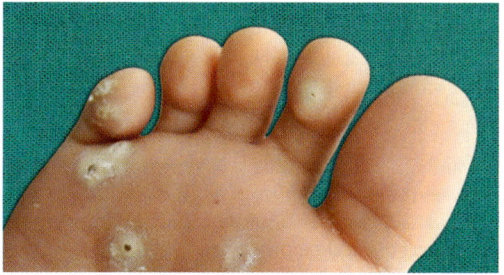

Fig. 31.4: Plantar warts.
Source: Wikipedia (*with permission*).

among adults and is associated with HPV serotypes 6 and 11.

Molluscum Contagiosum

Molluscum contagiosum virus is an obligate human poxvirus that produces characteristic skin lesions.
- **Lesions:** It produces dome-shaped, pink pearly wart-like lesions (2–5 mm size), umbilicated, with a dimple at the center (Fig. 31.5A). Lesions are found singly or in clusters, anywhere on the body except on the palms and soles. Genital lesions are seen in adults
- **Transmission:** Children are commonly affected, acquire infection by direct and indirect contact
- **Self-limiting** but more generalized and severe in HIV-infected patients
- **Laboratory diagnosis:** Molluscum bodies are the intracytoplasmic eosinophilic inclusions seen in skin scrapings stained with histopathological stains (Fig. 31.5B)
- **Treatment:** Surgical removal of the lesions by ablation (by cryotherapy or laser therapy) is the mainstay of treatment.

MEASLES

Clinical Manifestations

Measles is an acute, highly contagious childhood disease, characterized by fever and respiratory symptoms, followed by rashes. It is transmitted by droplet and aerosol routes.

Incubation period is about 10 days. Disease can be divided into three stages.

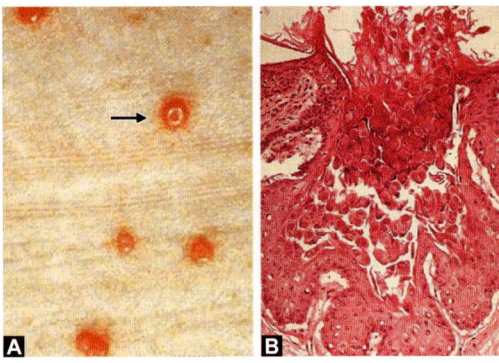

Figs 31.5A and B: (A) Molluscum contagiosum lesions on skin; (B) Histopathology of skin showing molluscum bodies.
Source: (A) CDC/ L Sperling, MD, Walter Reed Army Medical Center; (B) Public Health Image Library, ID# 860/Centers for Disease Control and Prevention (CDC), Atlanta/Dr Edwin P Ewing, Jr (*with permission*).

1. Prodromal Stage

This stage lasts for 4 days (i.e., from 10th to 14th day of infection) and is characterized by manifestations such as:
- **Fever** is the first manifestation, occurs on day 1 (i.e., on 10th day of infection)
- **Koplik's spots** are pathognomonic of measles, appear after two days following fever (i.e., on 12th day of infection) and are characterized by:
  - White to bluish spot surrounded by an erythema
  - Appear first on buccal mucosa near second lower molars (Fig. 31.6A)
  - Rapidly spread to involve the entire buccal mucosa and then fade with the onset of rash.

Problem Solving Exercise 3

Measles

A 3-year-old child developed fever, cough, coryza and conjunctivitis followed by the appearance of a maculopapular rash behind the ears, soon progressed all over the body (Fig. 31.6B). On examination, small bluish white spot surrounded by erythema was found in the buccal mucosa (Fig. 31.6A) and on inquiry mother gave history of incomplete vaccination.
1. What is the most probable of clinical diagnosis?
2. What are the different modalities of laboratory diagnosis?
3. How the disease can be prevented?

Explanation

Clinical Diagnosis

The symptoms of fever, cough, coryza and conjunctivitis, maculopapular rash (first to appear behind ears, then spreads; Fig. 31.6B), with a Koplik spot (small bluish white spot in the buccal mucosa, Fig. 31.6A) in a 3-year-old child with incomplete vaccination, are all suggestive of measles as first differential diagnosis.

(For answers to other questions, refer below.)

- **Non-specific symptoms** may be present such as cough, coryza, nasal discharge, redness of eye, diarrhea or vomiting.

2. Eruptive Stage

Maculopapular dusky red rashes appear after 4 days of fever (i.e., on 14th day of infection).
- Rashes typically appear first **behind the ears**
  → then spread to face, arm, trunk and legs
  → then fade in the same order after 4 days of onset (Fig. 31.6B)
- Rashes are typically absent in HIV infected people.

Fever (10th day) → Koplik's spot (12th day) → rash (14th day)

3. Post-measles Stage

It is characterized by weight loss and weakness. There may be failure to recover and gradual deterioration into chronic illness.

Complications

Complications following measles include:
- Secondary bacterial infections such as otitis media
- Giant-cell pneumonitis (Hecht's pneumonia)
- Acute laryngotracheobronchitis (croup)
- Diarrhea, leads to malnutrition
- Subacute sclerosing panencephalitis (SSPE): Rare, but most severe.

Laboratory Diagnosis

Specimens

Nasopharyngeal swab, conjunctival swab, blood, respiratory secretions, and urine are the ideal specimens. Synthetic swabs are recommended.

Antigen Detection

Measles antigens in the infected cells can be detected directly by using anti-nucleoprotein antibodies (direct immunofluorescence test).

Virus Isolation

Monkey or human kidney cell lines are used. Cytopathic effect observed—multinucleated giant cells (**Warthin-Finkeldey cells**) containing both intranuclear and intracytoplasmic inclusion bodies (*see* Fig. 31.6C).

Antibody Detection

- Detection of measles-specific IgM antibody in serum or oral fluid or four-fold rise of IgG antibody titer between acute and convalescent-phase sera is taken as significant
- Demonstration of raised titers of anti-measles antibody in the CSF is diagnostic of SSPE
- ELISA is the most recommended test that uses recombinant measles nucleoprotein (NP) antigen.

Reverse-transcription PCR

RT-PCR is extremely sensitive and specific; measles RNA can be detected in specimens up to 10–14 days post rashes.

Prevention

General Preventive Measures

Airborne precaution such as isolation in negative pressure room, use of PPEs such as N95 respirator, etc., must be followed while handling measles cases (Refer Chapter 11 for detail).

Measles Vaccine

Live attenuated vaccine is available for measles; using Edmonston–Zagreb strain. Under national

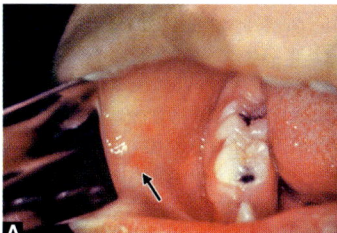
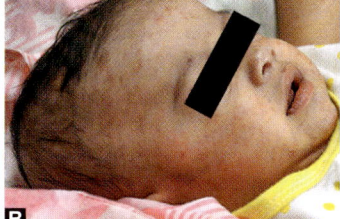
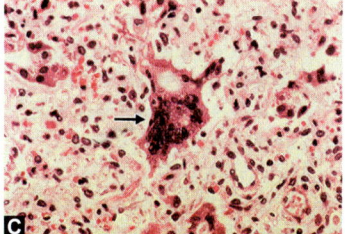

Figs 31.6A to C: (A) Koplik spot in buccal mucosa (measles) (arrow showing); (B) Measles rashes (on face); (C) Multinucleated giant cell of measles infected cell lines (arrow showing).
Source: (A) Public Health Image Library, ID# 6111; (B) ID# 17980; C. ID# 859/Centers for Disease Control and Prevention (CDC), Atlanta (*with permission*).

immunization schedule of India, measles-rubella (MR) vaccine is given at 9 completed months to 12 months along with vitamin A supplements and second dose of MR vaccine at 16–24 months.

RUBELLA

Problem Solving Exercise 4

A 5-month-old infant was brought to the neonatal care unit with history of preterm delivery, low birth weight, hearing and visual impairment. On detail investigations baby was found to have hearing impairment, congenital heart defects, hyperpigmented skin lesions, bilateral cataract and cerebral edema. The blood sample of the infant was sent for rubella-specific IgM ELISA and the test result is displayed in Figure 31.7.
1. Interpret the test result and etiological agent.
2. What are the different modalities of laboratory diagnosis?
3. How can you prevent this clinical condition?

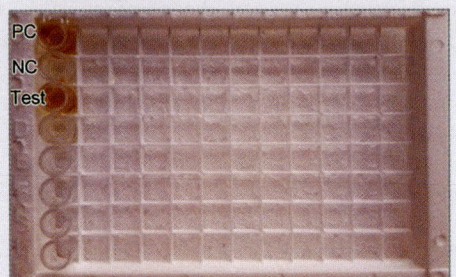

Fig. 31.7: Rubella-specific IgM ELISA test.
Source: Pondicherry Institute of Medical Sciences, Puducherry (*with permission*).

Introduction

Rubella virus produces a childhood exanthema similar to that of measles. Therefore, rubella is also known as **German measles**. However, unlike measles, it is highly teratogenic; can cause congenital rubella syndrome. Rubella may present in two clinical forms—postnatal infection and congenital infection.

Postnatal Rubella

Postnatal rubella may occur during neonatal age, childhood, and adult life. It spreads from person-to-person by respiratory droplets via upper respiratory mucosa.

Clinical Manifestations

- Incubation period is about 14 days (range, 12–23 days)
- **Rashes** are generalized and maculopapular in nature, start on the face, extend to trunk and extremities, and disappear in 3 days (Fig. 31.8A)
- **Lymphadenopathy** (occipital and postauricular) is the most striking feature
- **Forchheimer spots** may be seen in some cases. They are pin-head sized petechiae; develop on the soft palate and uvula; usually start with the onset of rash.

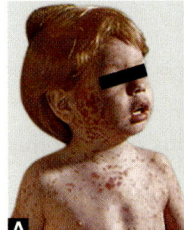 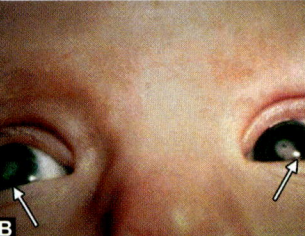

Figs 31.8A and B: (A) Child with rubella rash; (B) Cataract seen in congenital rubella infection (arrows showing).
Source: Public Health Image Library, A. ID# 10146; B. ID#4284/Centers for Disease Control and Prevention (CDC), Atlanta (*with permission*).

Laboratory Diagnosis

- **Isolation of virus:** Nasopharyngeal or throat swabs taken 6 days before and after the onset of rash. Monkey or rabbit origin cell lines are preferred
- **Serology (antibody detection):**
  - ELISA is the preferred method for rubella diagnosis (Fig. 31.7). It detects both IgM and IgG separately. Various antigens employed are whole virus lysate or recombinant E1/E2 antigens
  - Results need to be confirmed by **IgG avidity test** to differentiate active infection from the past infection or vaccination.

- **Molecular test:** RT-PCR is available for detecting rubella specific RNA (nucleoprotein N gene) in clinical specimens.

Congenital Rubella Syndrome

The most serious consequence of rubella virus infection is congenital rubella syndrome. Rubella is highly teratogenic; affects ear (deafness), eyes (cataract, Fig. 31.8B), and heart (patent ductus arteriosus). The severity is maximum in first trimester.

Prevention

General Preventive Measures

Airborne precaution must be followed while handling rubella cases (Refer Chapter 11).

Rubella Vaccine

RA 27/3 is a live attenuated vaccine for rubella, prepared from human diploid fibroblast cell line.
- It is available singly or in combination with vaccines of mumps and measles (MMR vaccine)
- **Indication:** In India, rubella vaccine is indicated to all women of reproductive age (first priority group) followed by all children (1–14 years). Under national immunization schedule, rubella vaccine is given along with measles (MR vaccine) at 9–12 months of age and second dose at 16–24 months in selected states
- **Precautions:**
  - Vaccine is contraindicated in pregnancy
  - As it is teratogenic, pregnancy should be avoided at least for 4 weeks (28 days) following vaccination
  - Infants below 1 year should not be vaccinated due to possible interference from persisting maternal antibody.

HAND-FOOT-AND-MOUTH (HFM) DISEASE

HFM disease usually affects children; is characterized by ulcerations on oral and pharyngeal mucosa and vesicular rashes on the palms and soles, which heal without crusting (Figs 31.9A to C). Fever and sore throat with flu-like symptoms are the other manifestations.
- **Agents:** It is mainly caused by Coxsackieviruses, rarely by other enteroviruses. Coxsackievirus A16 is the most common cause
- Transmission occurs through contact (direct or indirect) and droplets.

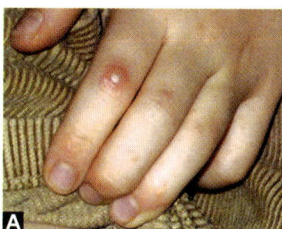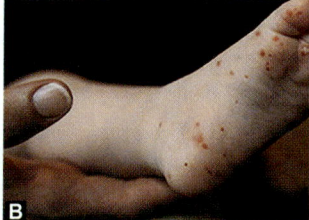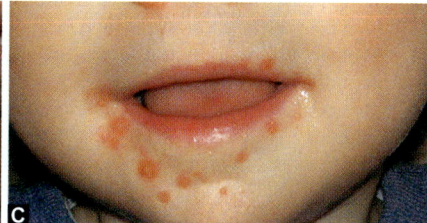

Figs 31.9A to C: Vesicular eruptions in hand-foot-and-mouth (HFM) disease: (A) Hand; (B) Foot; (C) Mouth.
Source: A and B. Centers for Disease Control and Prevention (*with permission*); C. Wikipedia, Mr Midgley (*with permission*).

Superficial and Subcutaneous Fungal Infections

CHAPTER 32

■ SUPERFICIAL MYCOSES

Dermatophytoses

Dermatophytoses (tinea or ringworm) is the commonest superficial mycoses affecting skin, hair and nail; caused by a group of related fungi (called dermatophytes).
- ❖ *Trichophyton* species: Infect skin, hair and nail
- ❖ *Microsporum* species: Infect skin and hair
- ❖ *Epidermophyton* species: Infect skin and nail.

Problem Solving Exercise 1

Dermatophytoses

A 6-year-old girl presented to the dermatology clinic with scaly patches on her scalp for one month. On speaking with her parents, it was discovered that there were several pets in the household. Her scalp hair and scaly scrapings were sent for fungal culture and identification (Figs 32.1A and B).
1. What is the clinical diagnosis and its probable causative organisms?
2. Identify the causative agent based on fungal culture on Sabouraud's dextrose agar (SDA) and lactophenol cotton blue (LPCB) mount.
3. What are the clinical features seen in this disease?
4. What are the various modalities of laboratory diagnosis?
5. Mention about the treatment for the same clinical condition.

Explanation

Clinical Diagnosis

A 6-year-old child with scaly lesions on scalp (involving hair and scalp), with contact history of pets at residence, is suggestive of tinea capitis (dermatophytic infection of scalp) due to a zoophilic dermatophyte. Infection of hair and skin can be caused by either *Trichophyton* species or *Microsporum* species.

Identification

SDA culture revealed cottony growth, with orange pigment on reverse (Fig. 32.1A).
LPCB mount showed abundant, thick-walled, spiny, spindle-shaped (up to 15 septa), pointed ends macroconidia and hence the causative agent is *Microsporum canis* (Fig. 32.1B).
(For answers to the other questions, refer below).

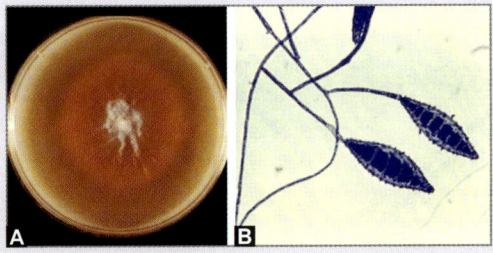

Figs 32.1A and B: *Microsporum canis:* (A) Culture on Sabouraud's dextroseagar (SDA); (B) Lactophenol cotton blue (LPCB) mount.
Source: Public Health Image Library, Centers for Disease Control and Prevention (CDC), Atlanta; (A) ID #15474, (B) ID #15472.

Pathogenesis

Dermatophyte infection is acquired by direct contact of soil, animals or humans infected with fungal spores.
- ❖ **Skin:** Characteristic well-demarcated *annular* or *ring-shaped* pruritic scaly skin lesions with central clearing and raised edges
- ❖ **Nails:** They invade the nails through the lateral or superficial nail plates
- ❖ **Hair shafts:** Hairs become brittle and areas of alopecia may appear.

Clinical Types

Depending on the site of involvement, various clinical types of tinea/ringworm infections

Table 32.1: Clinical types of dermatophytoses/tinea infection.

Clinical types	Area involved
Tinea capitis (Fig. 32.2A)	Infection of the scalp
Tinea faciei (Fig. 32.2B)	Infection of the nonbearded area of face
Tinea pedis (Athlete foot) (Fig. 32.2C)	Infect first the webs between the toes, then spread to the sole in a "moccasin" pattern
Tinea corporis (Fig. 32.2D)	Infection of the nonhairy skin of the body
Tinea cruris (or jock itch)	Infection of the groin area

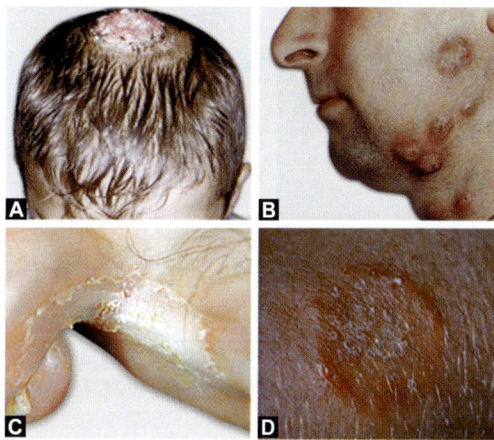

Figs 32.2A to D: Ringworm infections (Tinea): (A) Tinea capitis; (B) Tinea faciei; (C) Tinea pedis; (D) Tinea corporis.
Source: Public Health Image Library, Centers for Disease Control and Prevention (CDC), Atlanta; (A) ID #2936, (B) ID #4807, (C) ID #2939 and (D) ID #2938 (*with permission*).

are produced (Table 32.1) (Figs 32.2A to D). Incubation period is about 1–2 weeks.

Laboratory Diagnosis

Wood's Lamp Examination

Certain dermatophytes fluoresce when the infected lesions are viewed under Wood's lamp (due to presence of pteridine pigment in cell wall). It is usually positive for various *Microsporum* species and *Trichophyton schoenleinii*.

Specimen Collection

Skin scrapings, hair plucks (broken or scaly ones) and nail clippings are obtained from the active margin of the lesion and are kept in folded black paper. Hairs should be plucked and not cut.

Direct Examination

KOH mount examination with 10% for skin scrapings or hair, 20% for nail clippings or **calcofluor-white mount** shows presence of thin septate hyaline hyphae with arthroconidia; arthroconidia can be found on the periphery of the hair shaft (ectothrix) or within the shaft (endothrix).

Culture

Specimens should be inoculated onto SDA containing cycloheximide (actidione) and incubated at 26–28°C for 4 weeks. Potato dextrose agar is used to stimulate the sporulation. Identification is made by:
- **Macroscopic appearance** of the colonies such as rate of growth, texture, pigmentation, colony topography
- **Microscopic appearance:**
  - *Hyphae:* Dermatophytes possess thin septate hyaline hyphae
  - *Two types of spores are observed:* Small unicellular microconidia and large septate macroconidia; both are used for identification of species (Table 32.2) (Fig. 32.3).

Identification features (macroscopic and microscopic) of commonly encountered dermatophytes are given in Table 32.3.

Other Methods of Diagnosis

- **Hair perforation test:** It is positive for *Trichophyton mentagrophytes* and *Microsporum canis*
- **Urease test:** *Trichophyton mentagrophytes* is urease positive
- Dermatophyte test medium and dermatophyte identification medium

Table 32.2: Distribution of conidia of dermatophytes.

Dermatophytes	Macroconidia	Microconidia
Trichophyton	Rare, thin, walled, smooth, pencil shaped	Abundant, round to tear drop shaped
Microsporum	Numerous, thick walled, rough, spindle shaped	Rare
Epidermophyton	Numerous, smooth, walled, club-shaped	Absent

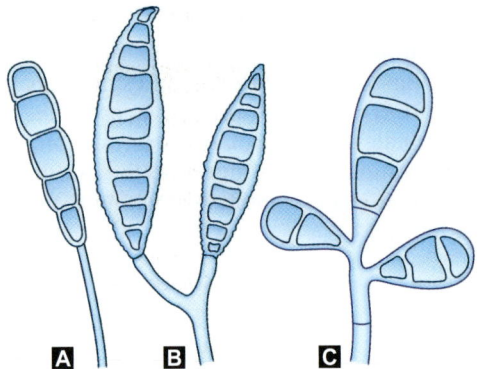

Figs 32.3A to C: Macroconidia of various dermatophyte species: (A) *Trichophyton mentagrophyte*; (B) *Microsporum canis*; (C) *Epidermophyton floccosum*.

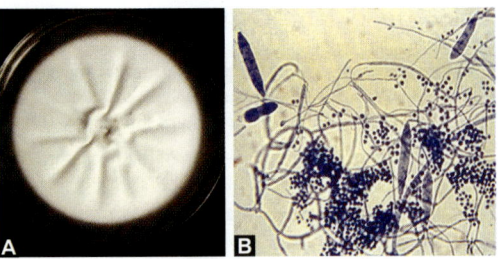

Figs 32.4A and B: *Trichophyton mentagrophyte:* (A) Colony on SDA; (B) LPCB mount.
Source: Public Health Image Library, Centers for Disease Control and Prevention (CDC), Atlanta; (A) ID #14717, (B) ID #15105 *(with permission).*

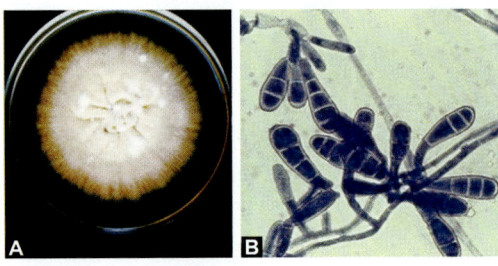

Figs 32.5A and B: *Epidermophyton floccosum:* (A) Culture on SDA; (B) LPCB mount.
Source: Public Health Image Library, Centers for Disease Control and Prevention (CDC), Atlanta; (A) Dr Lucille KG/ID #2937, (B) ID #14588 *(with permission).*

Table 32.3: Identification features of commonly encountered dermatophytes.

Dermatophytes	Macroscopic appearance	Microscopic appearance
Trichophyton mentagrophytes (Figs 32.4A and B)	White to tan powdery Pigment variable	Microconidia—numerous, round to pyriform Macroconidia—cigar-shaped Spiral hyphae seen
Microsporum canis (Figs 32.1A and B)	Cottony, orange pigment on reverse	Macroconidia—abundant, thick walled, spiny, spindle shaped, up to 15 septa, pointed ends Microconidia—rare
Epidermophyton floccosum (Figs 32.5A and B)	Powdery, folded, yellowish-green	Macroconidia—club or clavate shaped in clusters, 4–6 septa Microconidia—absent

- ❖ **Molecular methods:** PCR can be used to detect species specific genes (e.g., chitin synthase gene).

Treatment
- ❖ Oral terbinafine or itraconazole, used for 1–2 weeks for skin lesions, 6 weeks for hair infection, 3 months for onychomycosis
- ❖ Alternatively: Oral griseofulvin or topical lotion such as Whitfield ointment or tolnaftate can be applied.

Mucocutaneous Candidiasis
Candida species (Chapter 21) are the most common fungal agent to cause lesions of skin and mucosa.

Mucosal Candidiasis
The various mucosal manifestations include:
- ❖ Oropharyngeal candidiasis (oral thrush): It presents as white, adherent, painless patches in the mouth
- ❖ Vulvovaginitis
- ❖ Balanitis and balanoposthitis (occurring in uncircumcised males)
- ❖ Esophageal candidiasis
- ❖ Angular stomatitis and denture stomatitis
- ❖ **Chronic mucocutaneous candidiasis:** It is seen in children with deficient CMI.

CHAPTER 32 ◆ Superficial and Subcutaneous Fungal Infections

Cutaneous Candidiasis

The following cutaneous manifestations are produced in candidiasis:
- **Intertrigo:** It is characterized by erythema and pustules in the skin folds; associated with tight fitting undergarments and sweating
- **Paronychia** (involving nail-skin interface) and onychomycosis (fungal infection of nail)
- **Diaper candidiasis:** Pustular rashes, associated with use of diapers in infants
- Perianal candidiasis
- **Erosio interdigitalis blastomycetica:** It is an infection affecting the web spaces of hands or toes
- Generalized disseminated cutaneous candidiasis, seen in infants.

For laboratory diagnosis, refer Chapter 21.

SUBCUTANEOUS MYCOSES

The agents of subcutaneous mycoses usually inhabit soil and they enter the skin by traumatic inoculation with contaminated material and tend to produce the granulomatous lesions in the subcutaneous tissue.

Mycetoma

Mycetoma is a chronic, slowly progressive granulomatous infection of the skin and subcutaneous tissues.

Types of Mycetoma and Causative Agents

Mycetoma can be of two types. It can be caused by either fungal agents (eumycetoma) or bacterial agents (actinomycetoma). They differ from each other by various properties (Tables 32.4 and 32.5).

Table 32.4: Agents of mycetoma and the types of grains they produce.

Eumycetoma	Actinomycetoma
Black granules: • Madurella mycetomatis • Madurella grisea • Exophiala jeanselmei • Curvularia species	**White to yellow granules:** • Nocardia species Streptomyces somaliensis • Actinomadura madurae
White granules: • Pseudallescheria boydii • Aspergillus nidulans • Acremonium species • Fusarium species	**Pink to red granules:** • Actinomadura pelletieri

Table 32.5: Clinical manifestations of eumycetoma and actinomycetoma.

	Eumycetoma	Actinomycetoma
Tumor	Single, well defined margins	Multiple tumor masses, ill-defined margins
Sinuses	Appear late, few in number	Appear early, numerous with raised inflamed opening
Discharge	Serous	Purulent
Grains	Black/white	White/red
Grains contain	Fungal hyphae (>2 μm)	Filamentous bacteria (<2 μm)

Clinical Manifestations

Clinical triad consists of (Fig. 32.6):
- Tumor-like swelling, i.e., tumefaction

Problem Solving Exercise 2

Mycetoma

A 35-year-old farmer, with history of thorn prick injury 20 days back presented to the hospital with swelling of the right foot, 2–3 sinuses, discharging black granules for 1 week (Fig. 32.6). Granules were collected in a sterile gauge and sent to the laboratory for diagnosis. Histopathogical examination of the granules is given in Figure 32.7A.
1. What is the clinical diagnosis?
2. List the probable causative organisms.
3. What are the various modalities available to confirm the diagnosis?
4. Mention about the treatment for the same clinical condition.

Explanation

Clinical Diagnosis

A farmer, with thorn prick injury developed swelling of the right foot, 2–3 discharging sinuses, gives a clue to the diagnosis of eumycetoma (Fig 32.6).

Identification

As the discharging granules were black in color probable causative agents are *Madurella mycetomatis*, *Madurella grisea*, *Exophiala jeanselmei* and *Curvularia* (Fig. 32.7A).
(For answers to the other questions, refer below.)

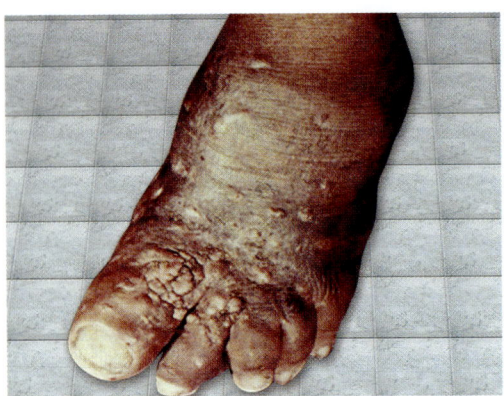

Fig. 32.6: Mycetoma of foot
Source: Public Health Image Library, Centers for Disease Control and Prevention (CDC), Atlanta; ID #14816 (*with permission*).

- Discharging sinuses
- Discharge oozing from sinuses containing granules.

Laboratory Diagnosis

Specimen Collection

The lesions should be thoroughly cleaned with antiseptics and the grains should be collected on sterile gauze by pressing the sinuses from periphery or by a loop.

Direct Examination

Granules are thoroughly washed in sterile saline; crushed between the slides and examined.
- **Macroscopic appearance of granules** such as color and size

- **If eumycetoma is suspected** then grains are subjected to KOH mount, which reveal fungal hyphae
- **If actinomycetoma is suspected**, grains are subjected to Gram staining which reveals filamentous gram-positive bacilli (0.5–1 μm wide). Modified acid-fast stain is performed if *Nocardia* is suspected, as it is partially acid-fast
- **Histopathological staining** of the granules
  - Eumycetoma: Reveals granulomatous reaction with palisade arrangement of hyphae in the cement substance (Fig. 32.7A)
  - Actinomycetoma: Shows granulomatous reaction with filamentous bacteria at the margin (Fig. 32.7B).

Treatment

Treatment of mycetoma consists of surgical removal of the lesion followed by use of:
- For eumycetoma, itraconazole or amphotericin B for 8–24 months, or
- For actinomycetoma, amikacin plus cotrimoxazole.

Sporotrichosis

Sporotrichosis or rose gardener's disease is characterized by subcutaneous noduloulcerative lesions along the lymphatics; caused by a thermally dimorphic fungus, *Sporothrix schenckii*.

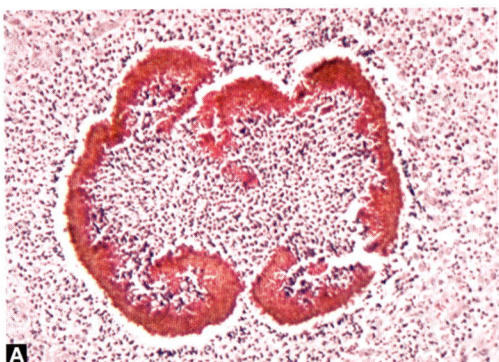 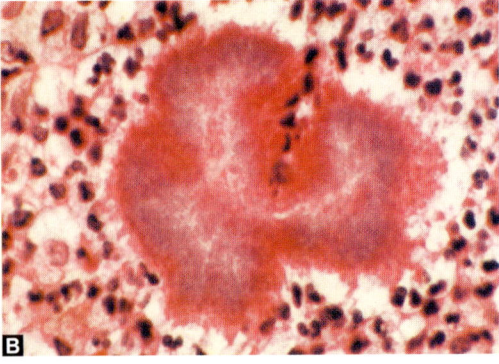

Figs 32.7A and B: (A) Eumycetoma (black grain and cement-like substance); (B) Actinomycetoma caused by *Nocardia brasiliensis* (hematoxylin-eosin staining).
Source: (A) ID: #4331; (B) ID: #15055, Public Health Image Library, Centers for Disease Control and Prevention (CDC), Atlanta (*with permission*).

Laboratory Diagnosis

Direct Microscopy

- Specimens such as pus, aspirate from nodules, are subjected to KOH mount or calcofluor staining which demonstrate elongated yeasts cells of 3–5 μm in diameter
- Histopathological staining of tissue sections reveals cigar-shaped asteroid bodies. *Asteroid body* consists of a central basophilic yeast cell surrounded by radiating extensions of eosinophilic mass, composed of antigen-antibody complexes (Fig. 32.8A).

Culture

The most definitive tool for diagnosis is culture. Specimens are inoculated on SDA and blood agar in duplicate and incubated at 25°C and 37°C as *S. schenckii* is a dimorphic fungus.

- **At 25°C:** It produces mycelial form, consisting of hyphae with conidia arranged in *flower-like pattern* (Fig. 32.8B)
- **At 37°C:** It produces yeast form, with creamy-white colonies.

Treatment

Itraconazole is the drug of choice for all forms of sporotrichosis, except for disseminated form where amphotericin B is recommended.

Rhinosporidiosis

Rhinosporidiosis is a chronic granulomatous disease, characterized by large friable polyps in the nose (most common site), conjunctiva and occasionally in ears, larynx, bronchus and genitalia.

- **Agent:** It is caused by *Rhinosporidium seeberi*, a lower aquatic fungus
- **Source:** Fungal spores are inhaled while taking bath in contaminated ponds and rivers
- **Diagnosis** is made by histopathology of the polyps that demonstrates *spherules* (large sporangia up to 350 μm size that contain numerous endospores, each 6–9 μm in size) (Fig. 32.9). It is stained better with mucicarmine stain. *R. seeberi* has not been cultivated yet
- **Treatment:** Radical surgery with cauterization is the mainstay of treatment. Dapsone has been found to be effective.

Penicillium marneffei

Penicillium marneffei is a thermally dimorphic fungus that causes opportunistic infection in HIV-infected patients. It is endemic in Thailand, Vietnam and India (Manipur).

Clinical Manifestations

P. marneffei produces two types of clinical manifestations:

- Systemic infection mimicking that of disseminated histoplasmosis—such as fever, weight loss, dyspnea, lymphadenopathy and hepatosplenomegaly
- *Skin lesions:* Warty lesions mimicking that of molluscum contagiosum are seen.

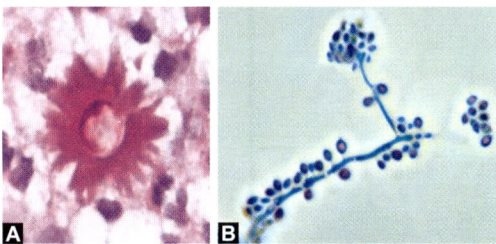

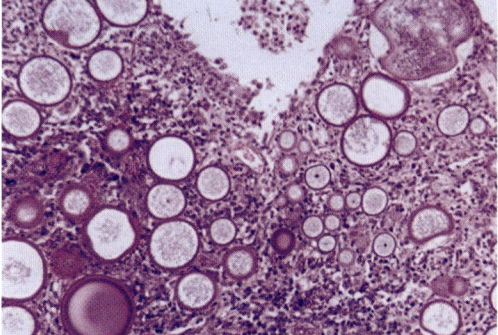

Figs 32.8A and B: *Sporothrix schenckii.* (A) Yeast form (asteroid body); (B) Mold form showing thin septate hyphae with flower-like sporulation.
Source: (A) Dr Manoj Singh and Dr M Ramam, All India Institute of Medical Sciences, New Delhi; (B) Public Health Image Library, Centers for Disease Control and Prevention (CDC), Atlanta; Dr Libero Ajello, ID #4208 (*with permission*).

Fig. 32.9: *Rhinosporidium seeberi*—spherules containing sporangia filled with endospores.
Source: Public Health Image Library, Centers for Disease Control and Prevention (CDC), Atlanta; Dr Martin Hicklin, ID #3107 (*with permission*).

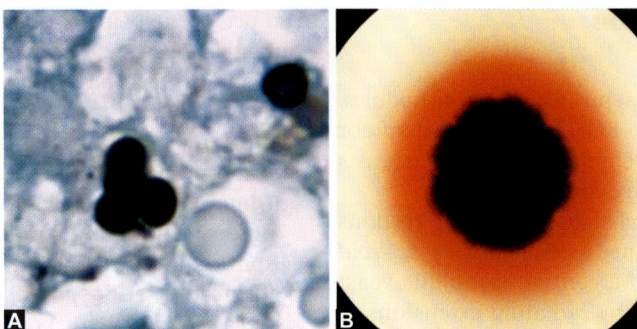

Figs 32.10A and B: *Penicillium marneffei*: (A) Methenamine silver staining shows yeast cells with central septations; (B) Red pigmented colony (mold form).
Source: Public Health Image Library/Dr Libero Ajello, (A) ID#: 11959; (B) ID#: 11967/Centers for Disease Control and Prevention (CDC), Atlanta (*with permission*).

Laboratory Diagnosis

- **Histopathological staining** of tissue sections shows oval or elliptical yeast cells with central septation (Fig. 32.10A)
- **Culture:** *P. marneffei* being dimorphic produces yeast-like colonies at 37°C and mold form at 25°C (Fig. 32.10B)
- The mold form has a characteristic *brick red pigment,* but the microscopic appearance is similar to other *Penicillium* species.

Treatment

Patients with HIV/AIDS suffering from severe penicilliosis are treated with amphotericin B and in mild cases, itraconazole is recommended.

Bacterial Pharyngitis: Streptococcus pyogenes Pharyngitis and Diphtheria

CHAPTER 33

▇ INTRODUCTION

Pharyngitis (or sore throat) is one of the most common upper respiratory tract infections (URTI). Viral pharyngitis accounts for the vast majority of cases, and is usually self-limited. Bacteria are also important etiologic agents of pharyngitis, require specific antibiotic treatment; if not given, can lead to serious complications and sequelae. The common etiological agents of bacterial pharyngitis include:
- *Streptococcus pyogenes* (most common)
- *Corynebacterium diphtheriae*

- Other rare causes include:
  - Other β-hemolytic streptococci (group C and G)
  - *Arcanobacterium hemolyticum*
  - *Fusobacterium necrophorum*
  - *Mycoplasma pneumoniae*
  - *Neisseria gonorrhoeae.*

▇ STREPTOCOCCAL PHARYNGITIS

Streptococcus pyogenes (or group A *Streptococcus*) is the most common bacterial cause of pharyngitis in children and accounts

Problem Solving Exercise 1

Streptococcal pharyngitis

A 7-year-old child with history of pain in the throat and fever for 2 days was brought to ear, nose, and throat (ENT) out-patient department (OPD). On examination, he was febrile and throat examination revealed pustules over the tonsils (Fig. 33.1). His throat swab was sent to the microbiology laboratory and was subjected to culture (Fig. 29.2A, Chapter 29), and antimicrobial susceptibility testing (AST) (Figs 29.2B, 29.3 and Table 29.3, Chapter 29).
1. Identify the causative agent based on the microbiological investigations performed.
2. List the infections caused by this organism.
3. Interpret the AST.
4. What antibiotic you would like to prescribe?
5. What are the different modalities of laboratory diagnosis?

Explanation

Clinical Diagnosis

Child with sore throat and fever for 2 days, with enlarged tonsils covered with white fibrinous exudate (Fig. 33.1) indicate acute pharyngitis.

Identification

Pinpoint colonies on blood agar with wide zone of beta-hemolysis (Fig. 29.2A), gram-positive cocci in chain in culture smear (Fig. 29.1B), bacitracin sensitive (Fig. 29.2B and 29.3) are indicative that the causative organism is *Streptococcus pyogenes*.

Antimicrobial susceptibility testing

Antimicrobial susceptibility testing on Mueller Hinton blood agar (MHBA) (Fig. 29.3 and Table 29.3) showed sensitive to penicillin, azithromycin and clindamycin, and intermediate to erythromycin.

Treatment

As patient is a child and from OPD, azithromycin can be used for treatment.
(For answers to other questions, refer below).

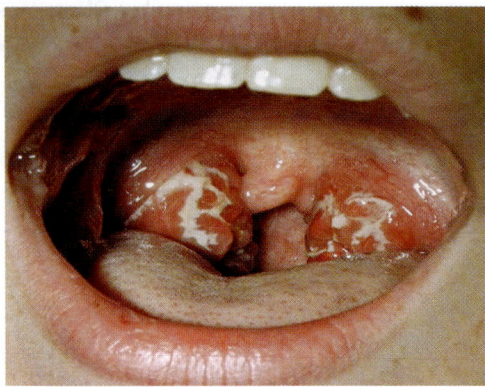

Fig. 33.1: Streptococcal sore throat, with enlarged tonsils covered with white fibrinous exudate.
Source: James Heilman, Wikipedia *(with permission).*

for 5–15% of all sore throats in adults. Infection occurs through respiratory droplets. In addition, it causes skin and soft tissue infections (Refer Chapter 29).

Clinical Manifestations

Streptococcal sore throat presents as either localized (tonsillitis) or diffuse (pharyngitis).
- **Symptoms:** Manifests as erythema and swelling of pharyngeal mucosa with purulent exudate formation (Fig. 33.1); commonly affects children
- **Suppurative complications:** May occur due to direct extension to deeper tissues causing peritonsillar abscess (or quinsy) and retropharyngeal abscess, or spillover to blood (bacteremia)
- **Non-suppurative complications** may develop 2–3 weeks following streptococcal sore throat, such as acute rheumatic fever (ARF) and post-streptococcal glomerulonephritis (PSGN)
- **Differential diagnosis** of streptococcal sore throat include:
  - *Diphtheria:* It can be differentiated from streptococcal pharyngitis by presence of membrane over the tonsil
  - *Viral pharyngitis:* It is differentiated from streptococcal pharyngitis by presence of concomitant rhinorrhea, oral ulcers, cough and/or hoarseness.
- **Scarlet fever:** It is mediated by streptococcal pyrogenic exotoxins (e.g., SPE-A, B, and C) It is characterized by pharyngitis and rashes (with sandpaper feel), strawberry tongue. It has become less common now a days.

Laboratory Diagnosis

Culture

Throat (oropharyngeal) swabs should be collected by vigorous rubbing of a sterile cotton swab over both tonsillar pillars. Two swabs may be collected, one for direct smear and the other for culture.
- **Culture:** On blood agar, *S. pyogenes* forms small pinpoint colonies of 0.5–1 mm size with a wide zone of β-hemolysis (Fig. 29.2A, Refer Chapter 29)
- **Culture smear:** Gram-stained smear from the colonies show gram-positive spherical cocci (0.5–1 µm), arranged in short chains (Fig. 29.1B, Refer Chapter 29)
- **Identification:** *S. pyogenes* is identified by conventional biochemical tests (catalase negative and susceptible to bacitracin, Fig. 29.2B) or by automated identification systems such as MALDI-TOF or VITEK.

Rapid Antigen Detection Test

Rapid antigen detection test (RADT) is available commercially, which detects group A carbohydrate antigens from throat swab by latex agglutination or enzyme immunoassay for the diagnosis of pharyngitis.

ASO Titer

Anti-streptolysin O (ASO) antibodies appear late; therefore, a retrospective diagnosis of streptococcal infection may be established by detecting ASO antibodies in patient's serum. ASO titer is elevated >200 Todd unit/mL in most of the streptococcal infections. This was used in the past for establishing rheumatic fever.

Molecular Test

Commercial PCR assay is available for the detection of *S. pyogenes* in throat swab. It is a rapid point of care test (turnaround time of 15 minutes), claims to be more sensitive.

Treatment

Streptococcal pharyngitis is treated with benzathine penicillin G, IM single dose or oral penicillin V for 10 days.

DIPHTHERIA

Introduction

Diphtheria is a highly infectious childhood disease caused by the bacterium *Corynebacterium diphtheriae*, which primarily infects the throat and produces toxin (diphtheria toxin) that causes an exudative pharyngitis and membranous tonsillitis. If not promptly treated, it can be life-threatening.

❖ The genus *Corynebacterium* is a gram-positive, non-capsulated, non-sporing, non-motile bacillus. It is irregularly stained and frequently shows **club-shaped swellings** (Fig. 33.2A) (Greek word *koryne*, meaning club)
❖ It has several species; the most important pathogenic being *C. diphtheriae*. The other *Corynebacterium* species (called as diphtheroids) are usually found as commensals of throat and skin in man, can occasionally cause infections
❖ ***Corynebacterium diphtheriae*** typically shows two characteristic features, which differentiates it from other *Corynebacterium* species
   1. **Chinese letter or cuneiform** arrangement: They appear as V- or L-shaped in smear,

Problem Solving Exercise 2

Diphtheria

A 2-year-old baby presented with pain in throat. On examination a white patch over the tonsil was found which bled on touch (Fig. 33.3A). His mother revealed that the baby has not taken immunization properly. Throat swab collected was subjected to staining (Figs 33.2B and 33.2C) and culture (Fig. 33.4B).
1. What is the clinical diagnosis and its causative organism; and what further test you would like to do?
2. List the virulence factors and other infections caused by this organism.
3. What are the various modalities of laboratory diagnosis?
4. What antibiotic you would like to prescribe?
5. How will you prevent this condition?

Explanation

Clinical Diagnosis

History of white patch over the tonsil (Fig. 33.3A), which bled on touch (pseudomembrane) and absence of childhood immunization is suggestive of respiratory diphtheria. However, streptococcal pharyngitis and candidalpharyngitis are other possibilities.

Identification

Gram-positive bacilli in cuneiform arrangement on direct Gram staining (Fig. 33.2B), green bacilli with metachromatic granules at the ends on Albert staining (Fig. 33.2C) and black colonies on potassium tellurite agar (Fig. 33.4B)—all confirms the causative agent as *C. diphtheriae*.

Toxigenicity test should be carried out further to find out the *C. diphtheriae* isolated is just a commensal or is responsible for the clinical condition (Fig. 7.3, Chapter 7).

(For answers to other questions, refer below).

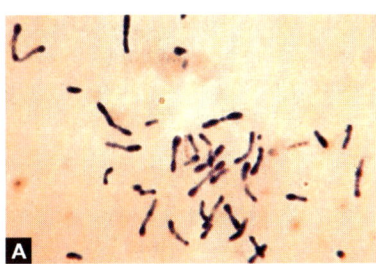 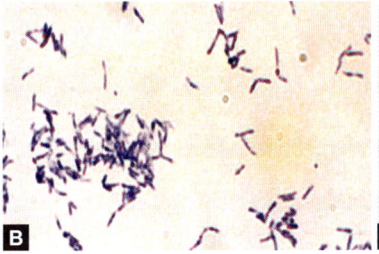 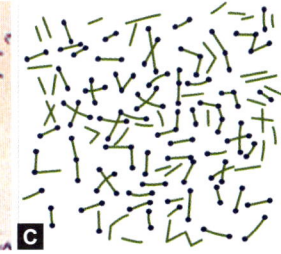

Figs 33.2A to C: *Corynebacterium diphtheriae*: (A) Club-shaped bacilli in methylene blue-stained smear; (B) Gram-stained smear shows V- or L-shaped bacilli with cuneiform arrangement; (C) Albert's stain shows dark blue metachromatic granules at the ends of the green bacilli (schematic).
Source: Public Health Image Library, (A) ID# /7323/P.B. Smith; (B) ID# /1943, Centers for Disease Control and Prevention (CDC), Atlanta (*with permission*).

because the bacterial cells divide and daughter cells tend to lie at acute angles to each other. This type of cell division is called **snapping type of division** (Fig. 33.2B).
2. **Metachromatic granules:** They are present at ends or poles of the bacilli.

Metachromatic Granules

Also called polar bodies or Babes–Ernst bodies or volutin granules).
- They are storage granules of the organism, composed of polymetaphosphates
- Granules are stained strongly gram-positive compared to remaining part of the bacilli. The granules take up bluish purple metachromatic color when stained with Loeffler's methylene blue
- However, they are better stained with special stains, such as Albert's, Neisser's and Ponder's stain (Fig. 33.2C)
- Granules are well developed on enriched media, such as blood agar or Loeffler's serum slope
- Volutin granules can also be possessed by other organisms such as—by *Corynebacterium xerosis* and *Gardnerella vaginalis*.

Virulence Factors (Diphtheria Toxin)

Diphtheria toxin (DT) is the primary virulence factor responsible for diphtheria. It is encoded by genome of a bacteriophage.
- Toxin is a polypeptide chain, comprises of two fragments—A (active) and B (binding)
- Fragment B binds to the host cell receptors and helps in entry of fragment A
- Fragment A gets internalized into the cell and then acts by the mechanism given below.

Mechanism of Diphtheria Toxin

- Fragment A is the active fragment, which causes ADP ribosylation of elongation factor 2 (EF-2) → leads to inhibition of EF-2 → leads to inhibition of translation step of protein synthesis
- Exotoxin A of *Pseudomonas* has a similar mechanism like that of DT.

Pathogenicity and Clinical Features

Pathogenesis of diphtheria is toxin mediated.
- Diphtheria is toxemia but never a bacteremia
- Bacilli are noninvasive, present only at local site (pharynx), secrete the toxin which spreads via bloodstream to various organs
- It is the toxin which is responsible for all types of manifestations including local (respiratory)

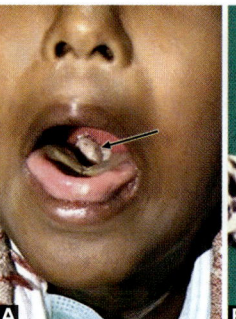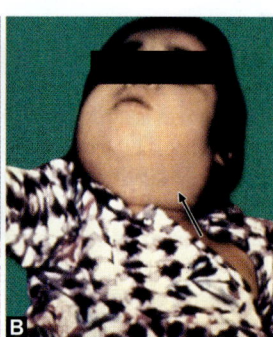

Figs 33.3A and B: (A) Pseudomembrane covering the tonsils classically seen in diphtheria; (B) Bull neck appearance (arrow showing).
Source: (A) Department of Microbiology, JIPMER, Puducherry; (B) Public Health Image Library/ID#5325, Centers for Disease Control and Prevention (CDC), Atlanta (*with permission*).

and systemic complications (except the skin lesions, which is caused due to the organism, not toxin).

Respiratory Diphtheria

This is the most common form of diphtheria. Tonsil and pharynx (faucial diphtheria) are the most common sites followed by nose and larynx. Incubation period is about 3–4 days.
- **Faucial diphtheria:** Characterized by formation of a tough leathery greyish white **pseudomembrane** over tonsil (Fig. 33.3A). It is so named as it is adherent to the mucosal base and bleeds on removal, in contrast to the true membrane which can be easily separated
- **Extension of pseudomembrane:** In severe cases, it may extend into the larynx and bronchial airways, which may result in fatal airway obstruction leading to asphyxia. This mandates immediate tracheostomy
- **Bull-neck appearance:** It is characterized by massive tonsillar swelling and neck edema. Patients present with foul breath, thick speech, and stridor (noisy breathing) (Fig. 33.3B).

Laboratory Diagnosis

The diagnosis of diphtheria is based on the clinical signs and symptoms plus laboratory confirmation.
- Because of the risk of respiratory obstruction, specific treatment should be instituted immediately on clinical suspicion without waiting for laboratory reports

- Laboratory diagnosis is necessary only for:
  - Confirmation of clinical diagnosis
  - Initiating the control measures
  - Epidemiological purposes.

Laboratory diagnosis consists of isolation of the bacilli and toxin demonstration.

Isolation of Diphtheria Bacilli

Specimen

Useful specimens include: (1) throat swab (one or two) containing fibrinous exudates, (2) a portion of pseudomembrane, (3) nose or skin specimens (if infected).

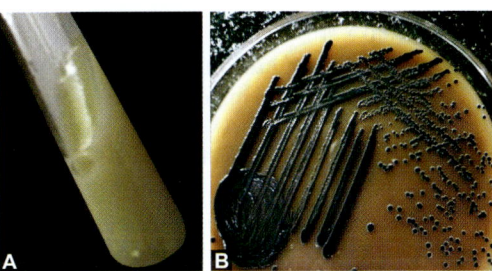

Figs 33.4A and B: (A) Loeffler's serum slope; (B) Potassium tellurite agar shows black colonies.
Source: (A) Department of Microbiology, JIPMER, Puducherry; (B) Department of Microbiology, Pondicherry Institute of Medical Sciences, Puducherry (*with permission*).

Direct Smear Microscopy

- **Gram stain:** *C. diphtheriae* appear as irregularly stained club-shaped gram-positive bacilli of 3–6 μm length, typically arranged in **Chinese letter** or **cuneiform** arrangement (V- or L-shaped). It is difficult to differentiate them from other commensal coryneforms found in the respiratory tract (*see* Fig. 33.2B)
- **Albert's stain:** It is more specific for *C. diphtheriae*; they appear as green bacilli with bluish black metachromatic granules at the poles. Details of Albert's staining procedure is given in Chapter 3.5 (*see* Fig. 33.2C).

Culture Media

Enriched Medium

C. diphtheriae is fastidious, aerobe and facultative anaerobe; does not grow on ordinary medium. It grows best in enriched medium such as blood agar, chocolate agar and Loeffler's serum slope. Plates are incubated at 37°C aerobically.

- **Blood agar:** Colonies are small circular, white and sometimes hemolytic (mitis biotype)
- **Loeffler's serum slope:** Colonies appear as small, circular, glistening, and white with a yellow tinge in 6–8 hours (Fig. 33.4A).
  - *Advantages:* (1) Growth can be detected as early as 6–8 hours. (2) Best medium for metachromatic granules production
  - *Disadvantages:* Being an enriched medium, if incubated beyond 6–8 hours, it supports growth of other throat commensals also.

Selective Medium

Selective media are best for isolation of *C. diphtheriae* from cases as well as from carriers, as the normal flora will be inhibited.

Potassium tellurite agar (PTA): *C. diphtheriae* reduces tellurite to metallic tellurium which gets incorporated into the colonies giving them black color (Fig. 33.4B). *C. ulcerans* and *C. pseudotuberculosis* can also grow on PTA producing black colored colonies.

- *Advantage:* Throat commensals are inhibited
- *Disadvantage:* Colonies appear only after 48 hours of incubation.

Identification

Identification of *C. diphtheriae* is made by:

- **Biochemical tests** such as—(i) Sugar fermentation test using Hiss's serum sugar media, (ii) Pyrazinamidase test, and (iii) Urease test. The latter two tests are negative for *C. diphtheriae*
- **Automated identification systems** such as MALDI-TOF or VITEK.

Toxin Demonstration

As the pathogenesis is due to diphtheria toxin, mere isolation of bacilli does not complete the diagnosis. Toxin demonstration should be done following isolation, which can be performed by in vivo and in vitro methods.

In Vivo Tests (Animal Inoculation)

In vivo toxin demonstration can be done by inoculation of culture broth into **guinea pig**. With the advent of other techniques, this method is rarely followed nowadays.

In Vitro Test

- **Elek's gel precipitation test:** This is a type of immunodiffusion in gel described by Elek (1949)
  - The strain isolated is streaked onto a media containing a filter paper soaked with antitoxin
  - If the strain is toxigenic, it liberates the toxin which diffuses in the agar and meets with the antitoxin to produce an arrow-shaped precipitation band
  - This test can also be used to know the relatedness between the strains isolated during an outbreak. The precipitate bands of outbreak isolates (streaked adjacent) when meet with each other, three patterns may be observed (Fig. 7.3, Chapter 7)
    1. Cross-over with each other—indicates unrelated strain
    2. Spur formation—indicates partially related strain
    3. Fused with each other—indicates identical strain.
- **Other in vitro tests** include:
  - Detection of *Tox* gene by PCR
  - Detection of diphtheria toxin by ELISA or immunochromatographic test (ICT)
  - Cytotoxicity produced on cell lines.

Typing of C. diphtheriae

Typing methods are useful for epidemiological studies, to know the relatedness between the isolates. Biotyping was in use in the past, based on which there are four biotypes of *C. diphtheriae*—gravis, intermedius, mitis and belfanti. They vary in virulence and toxin production; gravis being 100% toxigenic and more virulent.

Treatment

Treatment should be started immediately on clinical suspicion of diphtheria.

- **Antidiphtheritic serum or ADS (antitoxin):** Passive immunization with antidiphtheritic horse serum is the treatment of choice as it neutralizes the toxin
- **Antibiotics:** Penicillin or erythromycin is the drug of choice. Antibiotic plays a minor role as it is of no use once the toxin is secreted. However, antibiotics are useful:
  - If given early (<6 h of infection), before the toxin release
  - Prevent further release of toxin by killing the bacilli
  - Treatment of cutaneous diphtheria
  - Treatment of carriers: Drug of choice is erythromycin.

Prophylaxis

Infection Control Measures

Patient should be placed in isolation room and all the steps of **droplet precaution** should be followed for the prevention of transmission of *C. diphtheriae* in hospitals (Refer Chapter 11).

Post-exposure Prophylaxis

For close contacts (e.g., household), booster dose of diphtheria vaccine + penicillin G (single dose) or erythromycin (7–10 days) is recommended.

Vaccination

Diphtheria toxoid is used for vaccination as it induces antitoxin production in the body. A protective titer of more than 0.01 Unit/mL of antitoxin can prevent all forms of diphtheria. However, vaccine is not effective for:

- Prevention of cutaneous diphtheria
- Elimination of carrier state.

Types of Vccine

- **Single vaccine:** Diphtheria toxoid (DT) is prepared by incubating toxin with formalin and then the toxoid is adsorbed on to alum. Alum acts as adjuvant and increases the immunogenicity of toxoid
- **Combined vaccine:** Various vaccines available are:
  - **DPT:** Contains **D**T (diphtheria toxoid), **P**ertussis (whole cell) and **T**T (tetanus toxoid). **Pertussis** component acts as **adjuvant** and increases the immunogenicity of DT and TT
  - **DaPT:** Contains DT, TT and acellular pertussis (aP)
  - **Td:** It contains tetanus toxoid and adult dose (2 Lf) of diphtheria toxoid
  - **Pentavalent vaccine:** DPT can also be given along with hepatitis B and *Haemophilus influenzae* type b.

Administration of Diphtheria Vaccine

- ❖ **Schedule:** Under National Immunization Schedule (NIS) of India 2020:
  - ■ **Children:** Total seven doses are given; three doses of pentavalent vaccine at 6, 10 and 14 weeks of birth, followed by two booster doses of DPT at 16–24 months and 5 years and another two booster doses of Td at 10 years and 16 years
  - ■ **Pregnant woman** also should receive two doses of Td at one month interval.
- ❖ **Site:** DPT is given deep intramuscularly (IM) at anterolateral aspect of thigh.

Diphtheroids

Diphtheroids or coryneforms are the nondiphtherial corynebacteria, that usually exist as normal commensals in the throat, skin, conjunctiva and other areas. However, they have been associated with invasive disease, particularly in immunocompromised patients. They can be differentiated from *C. diphtheriae* by many features such as:

- ❖ Stains more uniformly than *C. diphtheriae*
- ❖ Palisade arrangement: Arranged in parallel rows rather than cuneiform pattern (Fig. 33.5)
- ❖ Absence of metachromatic granules (except *C. xerosis*).

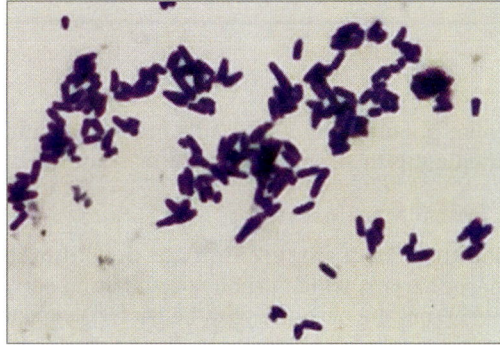

Fig. 33.5: Diphtheroids—palisade arrangement of gram-positive bacilli.
Source: Department of Microbiology, JIPMER, Puducherry (*with permission*).

Bacterial Pneumonia

CHAPTER 34

■ INTRODUCTION

Bacterial pneumonia is classified into two groups; typical (lobar) and atypical or (interstitial) pneumonia.
- ❖ **Lobar or typical pneumonia:** It involves infection of the lung parenchyma and its alveoli. It is characterized by consolidation (gives a dull note on percussion) and productive cough with purulent sputum. It is mostly caused by pyogenic organisms, such as:
    - *Streptococcus pneumoniae*
    - *Haemophilus influenzae*
    - *Staphylococcus aureus*
    - Gram-negative bacilli.
- ❖ **Interstitial or atypical pneumonia** occurs in the interstitial space of lungs. Cough is characteristically non-productive. It is mostly caused by bacteria, such as *Mycoplasma, Chlamydia, Legionella* species, etc.

■ PNEUMOCOCCAL PNEUMONIA

Introduction

Streptococcus pneumoniae (commonly referred to as pneumococcus) is the leading cause of lobar pneumonia, otitis media in children and meningitis in all ages.

Clinical Manifestations

Pneumococci first colonize the human nasopharynx, which usually occurs at an early age. From the nasopharynx, the bacteria spread either via the bloodstream to distant sites (e.g., brain, joint, bones and peritoneal cavity) or spread locally to cause otitis media or pneumonia.

Table 34.1: Differences between *Streptococcus pneumoniae* and viridans streptococci.

Features	*S. pneumoniae*	Viridans streptococci
Arrangement	Gram-positive cocci in pairs	Gram-positive cocci in long chains
Morphology	Lanceolate shaped	Round/oval
Capsule	Present	Absent
On blood agar	Draughtsman or carrom coin colony	Minute colony
Bile solubility	Soluble in bile	Insoluble in bile
Inulin	Fermented	Not fermented
Optochin	Sensitive	Resistant

Problem Solving Exercise 1

Pneumococcal Pneumonia

A 15-year-old boy presented to emergency department with complaints of high grade fever, productive cough, chest pain and dyspnea for past 3 days. Physical examination revealed dull note on percussion. Chest X-ray revealed consolidation over right lower lobe.

Sputum sample was collected and sent to microbiology laboratory for Gram stain (Fig. 34.1), culture (Figs 34.2A and C), biochemical reactions (Figs 34.2B and D) and antimicrobial susceptibility test (AST) (Fig. 34.3 and Table 34.2).

1. What is the clinical diagnosis and its causative organism?
2. List the virulence factors and infections caused by this organism.
3. Briefly discuss the laboratory diagnosis.
4. Interpret the AST.
5. What antibiotic you would like to prescribe?

Explanation

Clinical Diagnosis

High grade fever, productive cough, chest pain and dyspnea with dull note on percussion and consolidation over right lower lobe (on chest X-ray) are clinically suggestive of lobar pneumonia.

Identification

Gram-positive cocci in pair (lanceolate shaped) (Fig. 34.1), α-hemolytic colonies on blood agar (Fig. 34.2A), bleaching on chocolate agar (Fig. 34.2C), soluble in bile (Fig. 34.2D), sensitive to optochin (Figs 34.2B and 34.3) are suggestive of identification of the etiological agent as *Streptococcus pneumoniae*.

Antimicrobial Susceptibility Testing

AST on Mueller Hinton blood agar (Fig. 34.3 and Table 34.2) showed resistant to levofloxacin, ofloxacin and sensitive to penicillin, erythromycin and vancomycin. Oxacillin is a surrogate marker of penicillin susceptibility for pneumococcus.

Treatment

As it is a pneumonia isolate, oral erythromycin can be given for treatment. If it was a meningitis isolate, penicillin or other beta-lactam antibiotics, such as ceftriaxone would have been the drug of choice. (For answers to other questions, refer below).

Various manifestations include:
- **Lobar pneumonia:** *S. pneumoniae* is the most common cause of lobar (alveolar) pneumonia. Patients present with productive purulent cough, fever and chest pain. Important signs are dullness on percussion due to consolidation and crackles on auscultation
- **Empyema and parapneumonic effusion** may occur as complications of pneumococcal pneumonia
- **Invasive pneumococcal disease (IPD):** Defined as an infection confirmed by isolation of pneumococci from a normally sterile site. Various examples include:
  - Bloodstream infection
  - Pyogenic meningitis: *S. pneumoniae* is the leading cause of meningitis in all ages (Refer Chapter 39)
  - Other invasive manifestations: *S. pneumoniae* can cause osteomyelitis, septic arthritis, endocarditis, pericarditis, primary peritonitis; rarely, brain abscess and hemolytic-uremic syndrome.
- **Noninvasive infections**—otitis media (most common) and sinusitis.

Laboratory Diagnosis

General laboratory diagnosis of various pneumococcal infections is discussed below.

Specimen Collection

Depending on the site of infection, specimens, such as sputum, cerebrospinal fluid (CSF), pleural fluid and other sterile body fluids are collected. Automated blood culture is useful for invasive infection. Other specimens include aspiration of sinus material and ear discharge/aspirate.

Direct Smear Microscopy

Direct microscopy of smears made from specimens show numerous pus cells and **lanceolate or flame**-shaped gram-positive cocci (1 μm) in pairs, surrounded by a clear halo (due to capsule). Direct microscopy is extremely useful especially for meningitis, as empirical treatment (antibiotics) can be started early (Fig. 34.1).

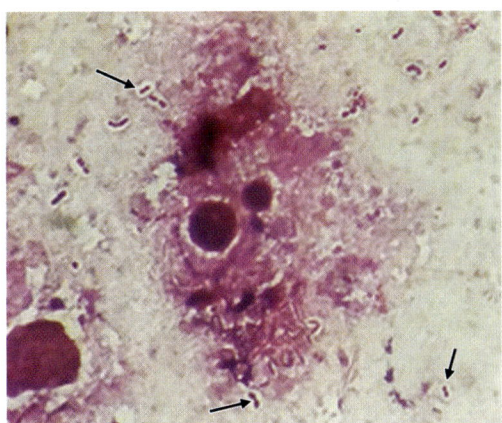

Fig. 34.1: Pneumococci in gram-stained smear of sputum [lanceolate shaped gram-positive cocci in pair surrounded by clear halo (capsule)].
Source: Department of Microbiology, JIPMER, Puducherry (*with permission*).

Antigen Detection

- **Capsular antigens:** Detection of capsular antigens in CSF is more sensitive than microscopy. It is done by latex agglutination test using latex beads coated with anticapsular antibodies
- **C-antigens:** Detection of C-polysaccharide antigen in urine by immunochromatographic test (ICT) is useful for diagnosis of pneumonia; however, it gives positive results even for nasopharyngeal carriers. Therefore, it is not useful in children where the carriage rate is high. This ICT is also available for antigen detection from CSF in meningitis cases.

Culture

S. pneumoniae is fastidious, does not grow in basal media like nutrient agar or nutrient broth. Specimens are inoculated onto enriched media, such as blood agar, and chocolate agar and incubated for 24 hours at 37°C in presence of 5–10% of CO_2.

- **Blood agar:** Colonies are initially small dome shaped, surrounded by green zone of α-hemolysis. Colonies on prolonged incubation, undergo autolysis, and therefore have a central depression with an elevated rim; giving rise to **draughtsman**-shaped or **carrom coin**-shaped appearance (Fig. 34.2A).
- **Chocolate agar:** It produces greenish discoloration (described as bleaching effect) (Fig. 34.2C).

Culture Smear

Gram stained smear of the colonies reveals lanceolate or flame-shaped gram-positive cocci (1 μm) in pairs.

Identification

Pneumococci are catalase negative and can be differentiated from viridans streptococci (which are also α-hemolytic, found as oral commensals in sputum specimens) in various ways (Table 34.1).

- **Bile solubility:** Pneumococci are soluble in bile (sodium deoxycholate) due to their enhanced autolytic activity in presence of bile. Viridans streptococci are insoluble in bile (Fig. 34.2D)
- **Optochin sensitivity:** Pneumococci are sensitive to optochin disk and produce wider zone of inhibition (14 mm or more) (Fig. 34.2B). Viridans streptococci are resistant to optochin
- **Inulin fermentation:** Pneumococci can ferment inulin to form acid, but not viridans streptococci
- **Automated methods,** such as MALDI-TOF and VITEK can also be used for early and

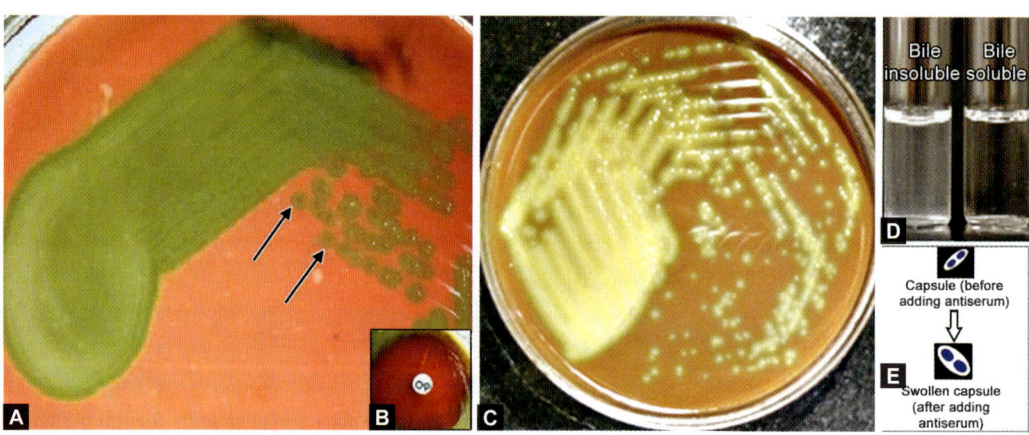

Figs 34.2A to E: Properties of pneumococci: (A) α-hemolytic draughtsman-shaped colonies on blood agar; (B) Sensitive to optochin; (C) Bleaching effect on chocolate agar; (D) Bile solubility test (left-viridans streptococci, not soluble in bile; right—pneumococcus, soluble in bile); (E) Quellung reaction.

Source: (A) Department of Microbiology, Pondicherry Institute of Medical Sciences, Puducherry; (B to D) Department of Microbiology, JIPMER, Puducherry (*with permission*).

Typing of S. pneumoniae

- **Quellung or Neufeld reaction**: This test was routinely done in the past at bedside, directly from sputum samples from pneumonia cases. When specimen is treated with type-specific antiserum, along with methylene blue dye; capsule becomes swollen, sharply delineated and refractile (Fig. 34.2E)
- Currently, serotyping is done by latex agglutination test using type specific antisera.

Molecular Methods

Molecular methods, such as PCR are highly sensitive, more useful when organism load is scanty (e.g., CSF), detect earlier than culture and also help in serotype identification.
- **Real-time PCR** is even more sensitive, specific, takes less time and is quantitative
- **Multiplex PCR** (e.g., BioFire FilmArray, bioMérieux) and Multiplex real-time PCR can be used for simultaneous detection of common agents of lobar pneumonia from sputum or bronchoalveolar lavage
- **Common genes** targeted include: *lytA* (autolysin gene), *ply* (pneumolysin) and *psaA* (pneumococcus surface antigen A).

Nonspecific Findings

- Elevated acute phase reactant proteins, such as C-reactive protein, procalcitonin
- Leukocytosis
- Chest X-ray shows infiltrates and lobar consolidation (In children-distinctly spherical consolidation is seen in upper part of the lower lobe, called round pneumonia).

Antimicrobial Susceptibility Test (AST)

AST is necessary for institution of appropriate antibiotic treatment. It can be performed by disk diffusion test on Mueller Hinton blood agar (Fig. 34.3) or by automated MIC detection method by microbroth dilution (e.g., VITEK). The latter is the preferred method as disk diffusion break points of several antibiotics (e.g., penicillin, ceftriaxone) are not available for pneumococcus. AST should be reported according to CLSI interpretation criteria (Table 34.2).

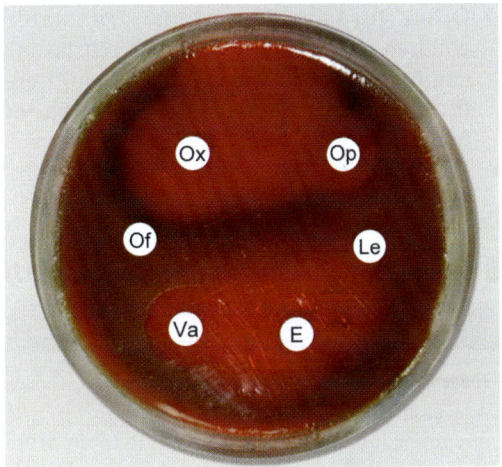

Fig. 34.3: Antimicrobial susceptibility testing on Mueller Hinton blood agar (Pneumococcus) (Refer Table 34.2 for CLSI zone interpretation).

Abbreviations: Op, optochin; Ox, oxacillin; Le, levofloxacin; Of, ofloxacin; E, erythromycin; Va, vancomycin.

Source: Department of Microbiology, Pondicherry Institute of Medical Sciences, Puducherry *(with permission)*.

Table 34.2: Interpretative categories (CLSI) and observed zone size diameter (mm) to various antimicrobial agents tested for pneumococcus isolates.

Antimicrobial agents	Disk strength (µg)	CLSI interpretative criteria for *Streptococcus pneumoniae* (in mm)			Observed zone size (in mm) (Fig. 34.3)	Interpretation
		Resistant	Intermediate	Sensitive		
Optochin (Op)		<14	—	≥14	14	Sensitive
Oxacillin (Ox)*	1	—	—	≥20	22	Sensitive
Levofloxacin (Le)	5	≤13	14–16	≥17	6	Resistant
Ofloxacin (Of)	5	≤12	13–15	≥16	6	Resistant
Erythromycin (E)	15	≤15	16–20	≥21	25	Sensitive
Vancomycin (Va)	30	—	—	≥17	17	Sensitive

*Note: Oxacillin is a surrogate marker of penicillin susceptibility for pneumococcus.

Treatment

The treatment regimen for pneumococci varies depending upon the type of infective syndrome.
- **Pneumonia:** Oral therapy with amoxicillin for five days remains the standard treatment among outpatients. Alternative drugs include IV penicillin or ceftriaxone, oral quinolone (levofloxacin or moxifloxacin), clindamycin or azithromycin
- **Meningitis:** As mortality is very high (~20%), treatment should be initiated as early as possible. Ceftriaxone/cefotaxime ± vancomycin is given for 10–14 days
- **Other invasive infections:** For stable children, penicillin, cefotaxime or ceftriaxone can be instituted. In critically ill children, the treatment should be same as that of meningitis
- **Otitis media:** Oral amoxicillin for 7–10 days is the drug of choice.

Prevention and Vaccination

Measures to prevent pneumococcal disease include vaccination, treatment of underlying diseases (that increase the risk of pneumococcal disease), infection control measures (**droplet precautions**, refer Chapter 11), and prevention of antibiotic overuse.

Pneumococcal Vaccines

There are two vaccines available for pneumococcus: (i) 23-valent pneumococcal polysaccharide vaccine (PPSV23), and (ii) pneumococcal conjugate vaccine (PCV13). The indications include:
- **After birth:** PCV13 is given in infants after birth; three primary doses at 6th, 10th and 14th week of age and a booster at 15 months
- **In adults** (≥65 year, or in presence of risk factors): Either PPSV23 only can be given or PCV13 is given first followed by PPSV23 at a gap of ≥1 year.

HAEMOPHILUS INFLUENZAE PNEUMONIA

Problem Solving Exercise 2

Haemophilus influenzae Pnuemonia

A 4-year-old orphan girl was brought to the emergency room by her parents due to an acute onset of fever, productive cough and dyspnea for past two days. Physical examination revealed dull note on percussion. Chest X-ray showed consolidation over left lower lobe. Sputum sample was sent to microbiology laboratory for Gram stain (Fig. 34.5A) and culture (Fig. 34.5B).
1. What is the clinical diagnosis and its causative organism?
2. List the clinical conditions caused by this organism.
3. How will you treat this condition?
4. How this disease can be prevented?

Explanation

Clinical Diagnosis

Fever, productive cough and dyspnea with dull note on percussion and consolidation over left lower lobe (on chest X-ray) are clinically suggestive of lobar pneumonia.

Identification

The causative agent here is *H. influenzae*. Points in favor are:
- Pleomorphic gram-negative bacilli shown in sputum Gram stain (Fig. 34.5A)
- Presence of satellitism surrounding *Staphylococcus aureus* streak line on blood agar (Fig. 34.5B).

(For answers to other questions, refer below).

Introduction

Haemophilus species are oxidase positive, capsulated pleomorphic gram-negative bacilli that require special growth factors present in blood, such as factor X and V. *H. influenzae* is the most pathogenic species, which causes pneumonia and meningitis in children.

Serotyping

Based on the capsular polysaccharide of *H. influenzae*, it can be typed into six serotypes (a to f). However, some strains lack capsule and are referred to as nontypeable strains. ***H. influenzae* serotype b (Hib)** is the most virulent among all types and accounts for most of the invasive infections.

Clinical Manifestations

H. influenzae Type b (Hib)

H. influenzae type b is the most common and most invasive serotype of *H. influenzae*. It causes systemic disease by invasion and hematogenous spread from the respiratory tract to distant sites, such as the meninges, bones, and joints.

* **Central nervous system infections:** It can cause pyogenic meningitis and subdural effusion. Mortality rate is high if untreated (Refer Chapter 39)
* **Epiglottitis:** Affects children, can lead to acute airway obstruction
* **Community acquired bacterial pneumonia:** Hib causes pneumonia in infants, which is clinically similar to other types of bacterial pneumonia except that, pleural involvement is more common in Hib infection

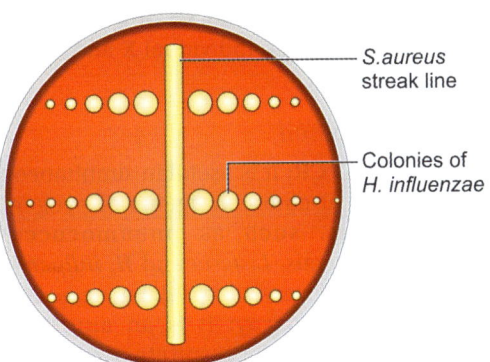

Fig. 34.4: Satellitism of *Haemophilus influenzae* (schematic diagram).

* **Parameningeal focus** of infection is often present in adults (such as sinusitis and otitis), from which the infection may spread to meninges.

Nontypeable H. influenzae

Next to Hib, nontypeable strains are the most common group encountered clinically. They cause disease by local invasion of mucosal surfaces, such as otitis media, sinusitis etc.

Laboratory Diagnosis

Specimen Collection and Transport

Depending upon the site of infection, various specimens may be collected, such as CSF, blood, sputum, pus, aspirates from joints, middle ears or sinuses

* As *H. influenzae* is highly sensitive to low temperature, the specimens for culture **should never be refrigerated**
* The specimens should be transported to the laboratory without any delay and processed immediately.

Direct Detection

* **Gram staining** of CSF and other specimen shows pleomorphic gram-negative coccobacilli (Fig. 34.5A)
* **Capsule detection** (Quellung reaction): Capsular swelling occurs when a drop of CSF is mixed with type b antiserum and methylene blue and observed under the microscope
* **Antigen detection:** The type b capsular antigen can be detected in CSF, urine or other

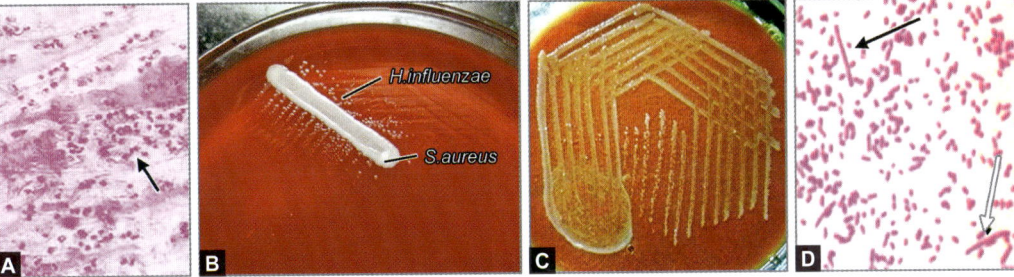

Figs 34.5A to D: (A) Gram-stained smear showing pleomorphic gram-negative bacilli; (B) Satellitism of *H. influenzae* around *S. aureus* streak line; (C) Colonies of *H. influenzae* on chocolate agar; (D) Colony smear of *H. influenzae* showing pleomorphic gram-negative bacilli.
Source: (A) Department of Microbiology JIPMER, Puducherry; (B to D) Department of Microbiology, Pondicherry Institute of Medical Sciences, Puducherry (*with permission*).

body fluids by latex agglutination test using latex particles coated with antibody to type b antigen.

Culture

H. influenzae is highly fastidious, requires two accessory growth factors (factor X and V) in blood for their growth.
- Factor X is a hemin, present freely in blood
- Factor V is nicotinamide adenine dinucleotide (NAD), which is present inside RBCs. It is also produced by some bacteria, such as *Staphylococcus aureus*.

The growth of *H. influenzae* may vary in different media depending upon the availability of X and V factors.
- **No growth on basal media:** Nutrient agar and peptone water lack X and V factors, therefore, they do not support the growth of *H. influenzae*
- **Growth is scanty on blood agar:** It is because only factor X is available freely in blood agar and factor V is largely intracellular, present only inside the RBCs. It is available in very minute quantities freely in the medium
- **Grows well on chocolate agar:** While preparing chocolate agar, blood is poured into molten agar at 75°C which lyses RBCs releasing excess of factor V. Hence, it supports the growth of *H. influenzae* (Fig. 34.5C)
- **Grows well on blood agar with *S. aureus* streak line:** Colonies of *H. influenzae* grow adjacent to *S. aureus* streak line—a phenomenon called as satellitism

> **Satellitism**
> *H. influenzae* can grow on blood agar if the source of V factor is provided (Figs 34.4 and 34.5B)
> - When *S. aureus* is streaked across a blood agar plate perpendicular to the *H. influenzae* streak line, factor V is released from *S. aureus*
> - Therefore, it forms larger colonies adjacent to *S. aureus* streak line and size of the colonies decreases gradually away from the *S. aureus* streak line
> - This phenomenon is called satellitism, a property that is routinely employed for the isolation of *H. influenzae*.

- **Special media**, such as Fildes agar and Levinthal's agar; containing factor X and V
- *Haemophilus* **selective medium** containing bacitracin and sucrose, is useful for sputum specimen

- It is largely aerobic and growth is poor anaerobically. Culture plates are incubated at 37°C in candle jar. Growth is enhanced by 5–10% CO_2.

Culture Smear and Motility Testing

Gram staining of culture isolates reveals pleomorphic gram-negative bacilli (Fig. 34.5D) and hanging drop reveals nonmotile bacilli.

Biochemical Tests

- Catalase positive and oxidase positive
- **Disk test for X and V requirement:** *Haemophilus* species vary in their X and V requirement. This property can be exploited for speciation by inoculating the isolate onto medium lacking X and V factors and then placing the X, V, and combined XV disks on the medium for demonstrating the growth requirements. *H. influenzae* produces growth surrounding combined XV disk, but fails to grow surrounding individual X and V disks (Fig. 34.6).

Molecular Method

- **Multiplex PCR:** It is useful in simultaneous detection of common agents of pyogenic meningitis, such as pneumococcus, meningococcus, *Listeria* and *H. influenzae* (targeting conserved capsular gene *bexA*)
- **BioFire FilmArray:** It is an automated multiplex PCR; the respiratory panel can simultaneously detect 33 pathogens including *H. influenzae*.

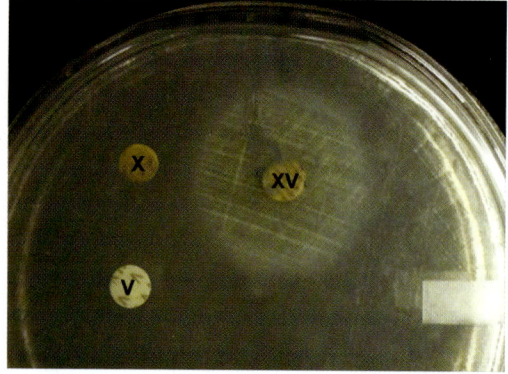

Fig. 34.6: *H. influenzae* showing growth around combined XV disk only, but not around X and V disks.
Source: Department of Microbiology, Pondicherry Institute of Medical Sciences, Puducherry (*with permission*).

Antimicrobial Susceptibility Testing (AST)

AST is performed by disk diffusion method (on *Haemophilus* test medium or chocolate agar) or by automated MIC detection method by microbroth dilution (e.g., VITEK).

Treatment

- For invasive infections due to *H. influenzae* type b, cephalosporins, such as ceftriaxone, cefotaxime (for 1–2 weeks) are the drug of choice
- Nontypeable strains of *H. influenzae* are often resistant to β-lactams. Those strains are usually susceptible to quinolones (levofloxacin) and macrolides (azithromycin).

Hib Conjugate Vaccine

The capsular antigen of *H. influenzae* type b is used for vaccination. To increase its immunogenicity, the capsular antigens are conjugated with adjuvants, such as diphtheria. **Schedule:** Under national immunization program, Hib vaccine is given in combination with DPT, hepatitis B (pentavalent vaccine) at 6, 10 and 14 weeks of birth. It is administered in IM route, at anterolateral side of mid-thigh.

STAPHYLOCOCCAL PNEUMONIA

Staphylococcus aureus causes pneumonia in selected clinical settings.

- **Infant pneumonia:** *S. aureus* is a leading cause of pneumonia in newborns and infants; presents with dyspnea, fever, and respiratory failure
  - Chest X-ray reveals characteristic **pneumatocele** (shaggy, thin-walled cavities)
  - Complications, such as pneumothorax and empyema may be developed subsequently.
- **VAP in adults:** *S. aureus* can cause pneumonia in hospitalized patients who are on mechanical ventilation, called ventilator-associated pneumonia (VAP). Patients who are nasal carriers are at increased risk to develop VAP
- **Post-viral pneumonia:** *S. aureus* can cause pneumonia secondary to viral infections—most commonly influenza
- **CA-MRSA:** Community-associated MRSA strains can be more virulent and can cause necrotizing pneumonia.

Staphylococcus aureus mainly causes skin and soft tissue infections, discussed in Chapter 28.

GRAM-NEGATIVE BACILLI PNEUMONIA

Problem Solving Exercise 3

Klebsiella pneumoniae Pneumonia

A 70-year-old male is admitted with high grade fever and productive cough. Chest X-ray showed consolidation over left lower lobe. Sputum sample was collected and sent to microbiology laboratory for Gram stain (Fig. 34.7A), culture (Fig. 34.7B), biochemical reactions (Fig. 34.8) and AST (Fig. 34.9 and Table 34.3).
1. What is the clinical diagnosis and its causative organism?
2. What is hypervirulent strains of this organism.
3. How will you treat this condition?

Explanation

Clinical Diagnosis

Fever, productive cough with consolidation over left lower lobe (on chest X-ray) are clinically suggestive of lobar pneumonia.

Identification

The causative agent is *Klebsiella pneumoniae*. Points in favor are:

- Short, plump, straight capsulated gram-negative rods in sputum Gram stain (Fig. 34.7A)
- Presence of large dome shaped mucoid sticky, pink color, lactose fermenting colonies on MacConkey agar (Fig. 34.7B)
- Biochemical reaction (Fig. 34.8) shows indole (negative), citrate (positive), urease (positive), TSI shows acid/acid, gas(+) and no H_2S.

Antimicrobial Susceptibility Testing

Antimicrobial susceptibility test on Muller Hinton agar (Fig. 34.9) with zone interpretation chart (Table 34.3) shows that the pathogen is resistant to ceftriaxone, gentamicin, ciprofloxacin and sensitive to amikacin, meropenem, or piperacillin-tazobactam and ceftazidime.

The drug of choice would be **ceftazidime** as it is the narrowest spectrum among the susceptible antibiotics.

(For answers to other questions, refer below).

Gram-negative bacilli are increasingly associated to cause lobar pneumonia, particularly VAP in the healthcare facility. Most of these agents are multidrug resistant (MDR) pathogens found in the hospital environment.

- ❖ **Non-fermenters,** such as *Pseudomonas aeruginosa, Acinetobacter, Burkholderia cepacia.* They are the major cause of ventilator-associated pneumonia
- ❖ **Enterobacteriaceae:** Various members of the family Enterobacteriaceae can cause pneumonia, such as *Escherichia coli, Klebsiella pneumoniae, Enterobacter* species and *Serratia marcescens.*

Klebsiella pneumoniae Pneumonia

K. pneumoniae causes various infections.
- ❖ It is responsible for severe lobar pneumonia, urinary tract infections, meningitis (neonates), septicemia and pyogenic infections, such as abscesses and wound infections
- ❖ It frequently colonizes the oropharynx of the hospitalized patients and is a common cause of nosocomial infections. Most of the hospital strains are multidrug resistant
- ❖ **Pneumonia** tends to be destructive with production of thick, mucoid, brick red sputum. Some time, the sputum has a thin and currant jelly-like appearance.

Hypervirulent Strains of *K. pneumoniae* (hvKp)
It is a strain of *K. pneumoniae,* which is recently emerged as a pathogen of global concern.
- ❑ **It is more virulent than the classical type,** capable of causing various community-acquired infections, such as:

Contd...

Contd...
- ➢ Pyogenic liver abscess (most common)
- ➢ Metastasize from liver to distant sites, such as eye, lung and CNS
- ➢ It can also cause primary extrahepatic infections including bacteremia, pneumonia and soft tissue infections
- ❑ **Identification:** hvKp strains are hypermucoid—a viscous string is formed when a loop is used to stretch the colony on an agar plate (Fig. 34.7C).

Laboratory Diagnosis

Klebsiella belongs to the family Enterobacteriaceae. Similar to *E. coli, Klebsiella* species are also lactose fermenters; however, they differ in being non-motile and capsulated (possess capsular polysaccharide).

Specimens collected depend upon the site of infection, such as sputum, endotracheal aspirate, urine, blood, exudate specimen.

K. pneumoniae shows the following properties:
- ❖ **Gram staining:** It is short, plump, straight capsulated gram-negative rods (Fig. 34.7A)
- ❖ **Culture:** On MacConkey agar, it produces large dome-shaped mucoid (due to capsule) sticky, pink color, lactose fermenting colonies (Fig. 34.7B)
- ❖ **Identification:** Identification of *K. pneumoniae* from colonies is made either by automated identification systems, such as MALDI-TOF or VITEK; or by conventional biochemical tests as described below
    - ■ It is catalase positive and oxidase negative
    - ■ **ICUT tests:** Indole test (negative), citrate test (positive), urease test (positive) and

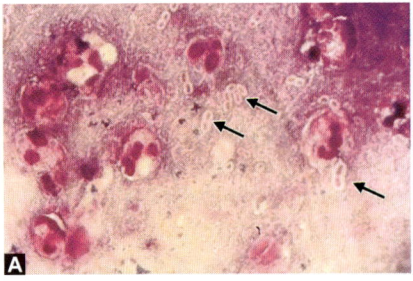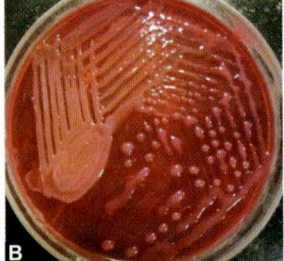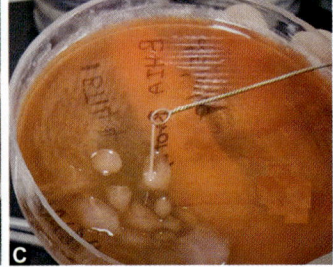

Figs 34.7A to C: (A) Direct smear (sputum) of *Klebsiella pneumoniae;* showing pus cells with gram-negative bacilli with clear halo (capsule) (arrows showing); (B) *Klebsiella* on MacConkey agar (Mucoid dome-shaped pink-colored lactose-fermenting colonies); (C) Hypervirulent *Klebsiella* showing string test positive.
Source: (A) Department of Microbiology, JIPMER, Puducherry (*with permission*); (B and C) Department of Microbiology, Pondicherry Institute of Medical Sciences, Puducherry (*with permission*).

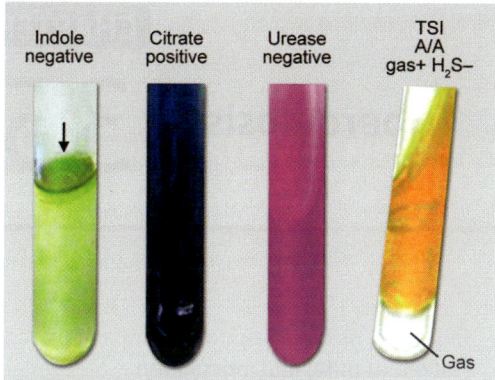

Fig. 34.8: Biochemical reactions of *Klebsiella* species.
Source: Department of Microbiology, JIPMER, Puducherry (with permission).

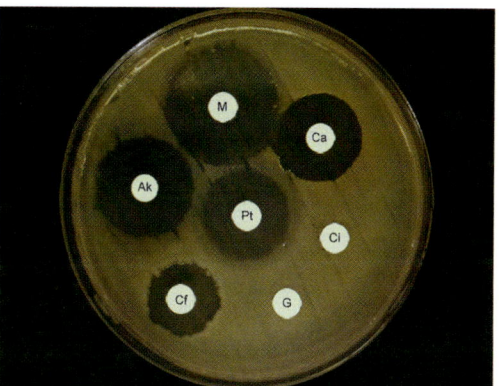

Fig. 34.9: Antimicrobial susceptibility testing on Mueller-Hinton Agar for *Klebsiella* [observed zone size diameter (mm) and zone interpretation to various antimicrobial agents tested are given in Table 34.3].
Abbreviations: Cf, ciprofloxacin; Ak, amikacin; G, gentamicin; Ci, ceftriaxone; Pt, piperacillin/tazobactum; M, meropenem; Ca, ceftazidime.
Source: Department of Microbiology, Pondicherry Institute of Medical Sciences, Puducherry (with permission).

TSI (triple sugar iron agar) test shows acid/acid, gas present, H_2S absent (Fig. 34.8).

❖ **AST:** It is carried out by disk-diffusion test (on Mueller-Hinton agar, Fig. 34.9) or by automated MIC based method (by VITEK) and reported according to CLSI interpretation criteria (Table 34.3).

Treatment

Treatment of *Klebsiella* is global challenge owing to marked drug resistance, which is much higher than that of *E. coli*.

❖ In healthcare facilities with high prevalence of MDR *K. pneumoniae*, empirical treatment should be started with higher spectrum antimicrobial. The therapy can be tailored based on the susceptibility report

❖ Carbapenems, amikacin or β-lactam/β-lactamase inhibitor combinations (BL/BLIs), such as piperacillin-tazobactam or cefoperazone-sulbactam are usually the agents of choice for hospital acquired MDR infections. Polymyxins or tigecycline are the next line antimicrobials, used for carbapenem resistant isolates.

Table 34.3: Interpretative categories (CLSI) and observed zone size diameter (mm) to various antimicrobial agents tested for *Klebsiella pneumoniae*.

Antimicrobial agents	Disk strength (μg)	CLSI interpretative criteria for Enterobacteriaceae (in mm)			Observed zone size (in mm) (Fig. 34.9)	Interpretation
		Resistant	Intermediate	Sensitive		
Ciprofloxacin (Cf)	5	≤21	22–25	≥26	16	Resistant
Amikacin (Ak)	30	≤14	15–16	≥17	24	Sensitive
Gentamicin (G)	10	≤12	13–14	≥15	6	Resistant
Ceftriaxone (Ci)	30	≤21	20–24	≥25	6	Resistant
Piperacillin/Tazobactam (Pt)	100/10	≤17	18–20	≥21	22	Sensitive
Meropenem (M)	10	≤19	20–22	≥23	28	Sensitive
Ceftazidime (Ca)	30	≤17	18–20	≥21	21	Sensitive

Abbreviation: CLSI, Clinical and Laboratory Standards Institute.

CHAPTER 35

Tuberculosis

■ TUBERCULOSIS

Tuberculosis is one of the oldest disease of mankind affecting lungs and other organs. It is caused by **M. tuberculosis complex**, which includes several species, of which the most important ones are *M. tuberculosis* (the most common species) and *M. bovis*.

Mode of Transmission

- **Air-borne:** *M. tuberculosis* is mainly transmitted by inhalation of **aerosols**, generated while coughing, sneezing, or speaking of infected patients. At least 10^4 bacilli/mL in sputum is required for an effective transmission
- **Other modes** of transmission are rare, such as **ingestion** [swallowing of sputum (seen in infant) or consumption of unpasteurized (infected) milk] and inoculation.

Clinical Manifestations

Tuberculosis (TB) is classified as pulmonary and extrapulmonary forms.
- **Pulmonary tuberculosis (PTB):** It accounts for 60–90% of all cases of tuberculosis (TB). It can be further categorized into primary or postprimary (secondary) types (Table 35.1)
- **Extrapulmonary tuberculosis (EPTB):** It results from hematogenous dissemination of tubercle bacilli to various organs
- Though EPTB constitute about 10–40% of all cases of TB. In HIV-positive patients, the frequency is much higher accounting up to two-thirds of all cases of tuberculosis

Problem Solving Exercise

A 29-year-old lady was admitted with complaints of cough with expectoration, chest pain, evening rise of temperature and loss of weight for more than 1 month. Clinical examination revealed crepitations and rales with reduced breath sounds over left upper lobe of lungs on auscultation. Chest X-ray showed cavity measuring 18 mm × 11 mm in the left upper lobe. Her sputum was collected and subjected to microscopy (Fig. 35.1A) and culture (Fig. 35.2A).
1. What is the clinical diagnosis and its causative organism?
2. What are the newer modalities of laboratory diagnosis?
3. How will you perform drug susceptibility test?
4. What are the infection control measures need to be followed while giving care to this patient?

Explanation
Clinical Diagnosis
The history is suggestive of pulmonary tuberculosis (PTB). Points in favor are:

- Cough with expectoration for 1 month
- Chest pain, evening rise in temperature and loss of weight for 1 month
- Crepitations and rales with reduced breath sounds over left upper lobe of lungs
- Chest X-ray showed cavity measuring 18 mm × 11 mm in the left upper lobe.

Identification
The causative agent is *Mycobacterium tuberculosis*. Points in favor are:
- The acid-fast stained sputum smear (Fig. 35.1A) showing pus cells and long slender and beaded acid-fast bacilli. Revised National Tuberculosis Control Program (RNTCP) grading is found to be grade 3+.
- Culture on Löwenstein–Jensen (LJ) medium shows rough, tough and buff colored colonies (Fig. 35.2A).

(For answers to other questions, refer text below).

Table 35.1: Comparison of primary and secondary pulmonary tuberculosis.

Features	Primary pulmonary tuberculosis	Postprimary (adult-type)/secondary pulmonary tuberculosis
Results due to	Initial exogenous infection with tubercle bacilli	• Exogenous reinfection • Endogenous—reactivation of the latent primary lesion
Age group affected	Children	Adults
Parts of the lungs commonly affected	Subpleural lesion affecting, middle and lower lung lobes	Apical and posterior segments of the upper lobes (areas of high oxygen tension)
Lesions formed at the initial sites	Fibrotic nodular lesions are formed (**Ghon focus**)	Hematogenous seedling in the apex of lungs called **Simon's focus** Reactivated Simon focus with central caseation (**Assmann focus**)
Lymph node	Ghon focus with associated hilar lymphadenopathy is common (called **primary complex**)	Lymph node involvement is unusual
Clinical features	It may be asymptomatic or may present with fever, productive cough (with or without hemoptysis) and occasionally pleuritic chest pain, night sweating, weight loss	Lesions undergoing necrosis and tissue destruction, leading to cavity formation Symptoms are similar, but more pronounced

❖ Virtually all organ systems may be affected however, the sites commonly involved (in order of frequency) are lymph node (most common), pleura, genitourinary form, skeletal form, CNS, etc.

Laboratory Diagnosis

Laboratory diagnosis of active tuberculosis can be established by various methods described below. The diagnosis of latent tuberculosis is explained later in this chapter.

Specimen Collection

In PTB, *two sputum* samples are recommended—**spot sample** (collected on the same day under supervision) and **early morning sample** (collected on the next day). Alternatively 2 spot samples at least one hour apart can be collected.

❖ **Sputum collection booths** should be located away from other people, outside in an open well-ventilated space; as air dilutes the aerosols generated during coughs
❖ **Early morning sputum specimen** should be collected in empty stomach, after rinsing the mouth well; so as to remove any food remnants, as they interfere with smear examination
❖ **Inhale deeply:** Patient should be advised to inhale deeply (2–3 times) and cough out deep from the chest during exhalation and then to spit the sputum into the wide mouthed screw capped container
❖ **Quality:** Sputum should be at least 3–5 mL in quantity; thick and purulent (yellowish mucus). Salivary specimens that appear watery should be rejected.

The extrapulmonary specimens vary depending on the site involved, which can be divided into two categories (Table 35.2).

Digestion, Decontamination and Concentration

Sputum and specimens from non-sterile sites subjected to smear microscopy and culture need prior treatment for digestion (to liquefy the thick pus cells and homogenization), decontamination (to inhibit the normal flora) and concentration (to increase the yield). However, this step is not required for molecular methods and also for processing of extrapulmonary specimens collected aseptically from sterile sites. Commonly used methods are:

❖ **Modified Petroff's method (4% NaOH):** Sputum is mixed with 4% sodium hydroxide, centrifuged and the sediment is neutralized with phosphate buffer saline. This method is recommended for LJ culture
❖ **NALC (N-acetyl-L-cysteine) + 2% NaOH:** This is superior to Petroff's method for isolation. NALC liquefies the sputum and NaOH kills the

normal flora. This method is more compatible with automated culture systems.

Table 35.2: Extrapulmonary specimens.

Sterile site specimens collected aseptically	
Optimum specimens	CSF, pericardial fluid, synovial fluid and ascitic fluid
Suboptimal specimens (organism load is less)	Pleural fluid (20–50 mL is collected and centrifuged) Blood (indicated only for disseminated TB and co-infected with HIV)
Specimens containing normal flora	
Swabs	Considered suboptimal specimen. The only recommended swabs are: • *Laryngeal swabs:* Collected early morning in empty stomach or • Swab from discharging sinus
Urine	Three early morning specimens collected (500 mL/specimen, centrifuged) on different days as TB bacilli in urine are shed intermittently
Stool	For disseminated TB in HIV infected patients and infants
Other respiratory specimens	Bronchial secretions (2–5 mL) Bronchoalveolar lavage (20–50 mL) Transbronchial and other biopsies (collected in sterile normal saline)
Gastric lavage	Recommended for children (tend to swallow sputum), or ICU patients (aspiration) Early morning lavage should be collected and processed early (<4 hours)

Note: Samples for culture should never be collected in formalin. If histopathological examination is required, two samples should be collected.

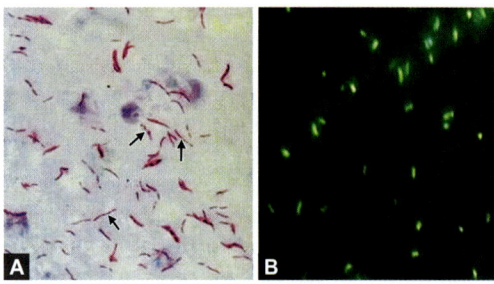

Figs 35.1A and B: (A) ZN staining of sputum smear showing long, slender and beaded red colored acid–fast bacilli; (B) Auramine phenol staining of sputum smear—tubercle bacilli appear bright brilliant green against the dark background.
Source: Department of Microbiology, JIPMER, Puducherry (with permission).

Direct Microscopy by Acid-fast Staining

Ziehl–Neelsen (ZN) Technique (Hot Method)

Smears are prepared from thick mucopurulent part of sputum or with the sediment obtained after concentration. Optimum thickness of the smear can be assessed by placing the smear on printed matter. The print should be just readable through the smear. Then the smear is stained by acid-fast stain (for procedure, refer 'acid-fast staining' in Chapter 3.5).

❖ **Interpretation**
  ▪ *Negative result:* At least 100 oil immersion fields should be examined for 10–15 minutes before giving a negative report
  ▪ *Positive result:* M. tuberculosis appears as long slender, beaded, less uniformly stained red colored acid-fast bacilli (AFB) (Fig. 35.1A).
❖ **Presumptive diagnosis:** Microscopy provides only presumptive diagnosis. If typical beaded appearance is seen, then it should be reported as '*acid-fast bacilli resembling M. tuberculosis are seen by smear microscopy by ZN stain*'
❖ **Advantages:** Smear microscopy is rapid, easy to perform at peripheral laboratories and is cheaper
❖ **Disadvantages:** (i) Smear microscopy is less sensitive than culture, (ii) low sensitivity with a detection limit of 10,000 bacilli/mL of sputum, (iii) it cannot determine the viability of bacilli
  ▪ It is difficult to differentiate *M. tuberculosis* from saprophytic mycobacteria present in tap water or even as commensal in clinical samples such as gastric aspirate, and urine
  ▪ *Acid alcohol* (3% hydrochloric acid + 95% ethyl alcohol) can be used to differentiate *M. tuberculosis* (acid and alcohol-fast) from *M. smegmatis* (only acid-fast, but not alcohol-fast) in urine sample.

RNTCP Guidelines for Grading of Sputum Smear

Revised National Tuberculosis Control Programme (RNTCP) of India has given guidelines for grading of **ZN stained sputum smears** (Table 35.3).
RNTCP grading is useful for:
❑ Monitoring the treatment response of the patients
❑ Assessing the severity of disease

Contd...

Contd...

- Assessing the infectiousness of the patient: Higher the grade more is the infectiousness. Smear negative patients (<10,000 bacilli/mL of sputum) are less infectious.
However, grading of the sputum smear depends upon the quality of sputum collected.
Note: In 2020, RNTCP has been renamed as National Tuberculosis Elimination Programme (NTEP).

Table 35.3: RNTCP guidelines for grading of ZN stained sputum smears.

No. of AFB seen	OIF to be screened	Grading	Result
No AFB in 100 OIF	100	0	Negative
1–9/ 100 OIF	100	Scanty*	Positive
10–99/100 OIF	100	1+	Positive
1–10/ OIF	50	2+	Positive
>10/ OIF	20	3+	Positive

Abbreviations: AFB, acid-fast bacilli; OIF, oil immersion fields; ZN, Ziehl–Neelsen.
*Record the actual no. of bacilli seen in 100 fields, e.g., "Scanty 8".

Kinyoun's Cold Acid-fast Staining

It differs from ZN stain in that—(i) heating is not required, (ii) phenol concentration in carbol fuchsin is increased, and (iii) duration of carbol fuchsin staining is more.

Fluorescence Staining

It is a fluorescent staining technique, uses auramine-phenol solution (for 7-10 min) as primary stain, 0.5% acid alcohol (for 2 min, twice) as decolorizer and 0.1% potassium permanganate (for 30 sec) as counter stain. Then the slide is examined under fluorescent LED (light-emitting diode) microscope.
- The bacilli appear brilliant yellow against the dark background (Fig. 35.1B)
- Smears are screened by using 20X or 25X objective, hence can be screened faster (2 min for 100 fields)
- It is more sensitive than ZN staining and has been the recommended screening method by RNTCP
- However, artifacts may confound with the interpretation. Hence the reading should be taken by an expert.

Culture Methods

Culture is traditionally considered as the gold standard method of diagnosis of TB. It offers several advantages:
- It is more sensitive than microscopy with the detection limit of 10-100 viable bacilli
- Indicates viability: TB bacilli growing on culture indicates that they are viable
- Drug susceptibility testing can be performed.

RNTCP recommended culture media include both conventional solid media (Lowenstein–Jensen medium) and automated liquid culture, such as Mycobacteria Growth Indicator Tube (MGIT).

Conventional Solid Media (Lowenstein–Jensen Medium)

Lowenstein–Jensen (LJ) medium has been the most widely used and recommended by RNTCP.
- It is composed of coagulated hen's eggs, mineral salt solution, asparagine and malachite green (as a selective agent)
- Inoculated media are incubated for a prolonged duration of 6-8 weeks. This is because of the slow-growing nature of tubercle bacilli (long generation time of 10-15 hours)
- **Colonies:** *M. tuberculosis* produces typical rough, tough and buff-colored colonies (Fig. 35.2A). In contrast, *M. bovis* produces smooth, moist and white colored colonies that break up easily when touched.

Conventional liquid media are Kirchner's medium and Middlebrook 7H9 medium. They are not routinely used.

Automated Liquid Culture

Automated culture systems monitor the growth continuously and offer a faster turnaround time compared to conventional culture.
- Positive growth (99%) gets detected within 3-4 weeks. However, the negative result is reported after 6 weeks of incubation
- They use liquid broth such as Middlebrook 7H9 medium supplemented with enriched growth media and antibiotic mixture (to inhibit other organisms).

Various automated systems available are:
- **BACTEC MGIT** (**M**ycobacteria **g**rowth **i**ndicator **t**ube): This is the automated system endorsed by WHO and RNTCP (Figs 35.2B and C)

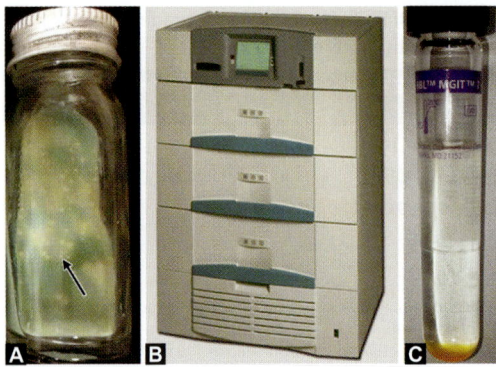

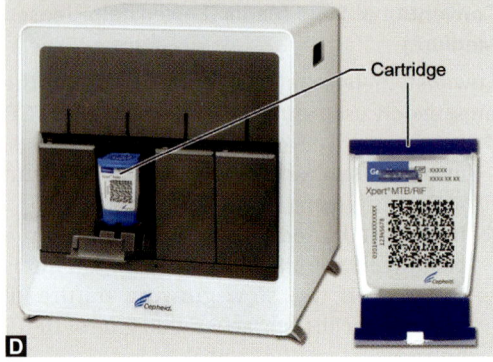

Figs 35.2A to D: Culture media/culture systems for *M. tuberculosis*: (A) Lowenstein–Jensen medium (arrow showing rough, tough and buff-colored colonies); (B) BACTEC MGIT; (C) MGIT liquid culture medium; (D) GeneXpert system with cartridge.

Source: Department of Microbiology, JIPMER, Puducherry (*with permission*).

- **Uses:** (i) It detects growth of mycobacteria, and (ii) also performs the drug susceptibility testing against first-line and second-line antitubercular drugs
- **Principle:** It uses an oxygen sensitive fluorescent compound, dissolved in the broth. Initially, the large amount of dissolved oxygen in the medium quenches emissions from the fluorescent compound. Later, actively respiring microorganisms consume the oxygen; the quenching effect is lost which allows the fluorescence to be detected.
❖ Other automated systems include BacT/ALERT systems.

Culture Identification

The colonies grown on LJ media and the broth from a positively flagged automated culture bottle are first subjected to acid-fast stain. If found AFB positive, then further tests are done for species identification.

❖ **MPT 64 antigen** detection by rapid immunochromatographic test: MPT64, a 28 Da antigen is specific for *M. tuberculosis* complex (*M. tuberculosis*, *M.bovis* and *M. africanum*) and negative for NTM (nontuberculous mycobacteria)
❖ **Automated identification system** such as MALDI-TOF
❖ **Biochemical tests** such as niacin test and **Rabbit pathogenicity tests** were in use in the past; now obsolete.

Molecular Methods

Molecular methods are extremely useful as:
❖ They take less time than culture
❖ They are more sensitive than culture. This is very much useful for extrapulmonary samples that are usually paucibacillary
❖ They can also detect the genes coding for drug resistance
❖ Used for epidemiological typing of strains.

There are several molecular methods available as described below.

Polymerase Chain Reaction

Nested polymerase chain reaction (PCR) targeting *IS6110* gene was the most common molecular test used earlier. Other genes which were targeted by using PCR—*MPT64* gene, *65 KDa* and *38 KDa* genes.

Automated Real Time PCR

With the advent of automated real time PCR systems, the diagnosis of TB has been completely revolutionized. In addition, these systems can be used for diagnosis of other diseases such as COVID-19. Methods available are:
❖ Cartridge-based nucleic acid amplification test (CBNAAT): GeneXpert
❖ Chip-based real-time PCR: Truenat.

GeneXpert (CBNAAT)

GeneXpert (Cepheid's) is the CBNAAT system endorsed by WHO and is used in India under RNTCP (Fig. 35.2D).
❖ **Rapid:** It has the lowest turnaround time (2 hours) among all the diagnostic methods currently available for TB

- **Principle:** It is based on real-time PCR technique; simultaneously detects: (i) MTB complex DNA, and (ii) rifampicin resistance (mutations of the *rpoB* gene). It uses five probes targeting various sequences of *rpoB* gene
- **EPTB:** WHO recommends GeneXpert as the initial test for diagnosis of EPTB; especially for CSF, lymph nodes and other tissue specimens
- **Diagnostic utility:** The detection limit of GeneXpert is about 131 bacilli/mL of specimen
- **Disadvantages:** (i) Very expensive, (ii) cannot further speciate MTB complex.

Chip-based NAAT (Truenat)

Truenat is a chip-based real-time PCR system, validated recently by Indian Council of Medical Research (ICMR), in 2017; also endorsed by WHO in 2019. It is used in India under RNTCP. It has been developed by the Indian firm Molbio Diagnostics.
- **Advantages:** It is an automated battery operated device; can be used at level of primary health center where GeneXpert cannot be used as it needs uninterrupted power supply and air conditioning. The turnaround time is around one hour
- **Disadvantages:** (i) Very expensive, (ii) cannot further speciate MTB complex, and (iii) it tests only limited samples (1–4) at a time.

Line Probe Assay (LPA)

Line probe assay involves probe-based detection of amplified DNA in the specimen.
- **Uses:** LPA in TB diagnostics has the following uses:
  - Identification of MTB complex
  - Detection of resistance to first-line antitubercular drugs (ATDs)
  - Speciation of MTB complex and NTM
  - Detection of resistance to second line ATDs.
- **Limitation:** LPA can be performed only on positive cultures or smear positive clinical specimens. It is not recommended for smear negative specimens as the sensitivity is low
- LPA is useful particularly in isoniazid mono-resistant cases of TB, which are not diagnosed by GeneXpert.

RNTCP Diagnostic Algorithm

RNTCP recommended diagnostic algorithm should be followed for the diagnosis and further management of tuberculosis.
- **For pulmonary TB in adult** (Flowchart 35.1): First sputum smear examination is performed
  - If smear positive—diagnosis is confirmed
  - If smear negative, but chest X-ray is suggestive or in presence of high clinical suspicion—CBNAAT is performed to confirm the diagnosis.
- **For pediatric pulmonary TB:** CBNAAT is directly performed
- **For EPTB:** EPTB specimens are paucibacillary, therefore, CBNAAT is directly performed. If not available, liquid culture (MGIT) is performed.

Diagnosis of Latent Tuberculosis

Latent tuberculosis is diagnosed by demonstration of delayed or type IV hypersensitivity reaction against the tubercle bacilli antigens. Two methods are available, (1) tuberculin skin test (also called Mantoux test), (2) IFN-γ release assay.

DST (Drug Susceptibility Testing)

Several methods of DST (drug susceptibility testing) are available which can be grouped into:

Phenotypic Methods

- **MGIT** (used for 1st and 2nd line drugs): Resistance is determined by growth of TB bacilli in drug containing tube as compared to the control tube (drug free) within 4–21 days of incubation
- **Proportion method** (used for 1st and 2nd line drugs): An isolate is considered resistant to a given drug when growth of 1% or more is observed in the drug containing LJ medium compared to the control LJ medium without drug after 42 days of incubation.

Genotypic Methods

- **GeneXpert:** It is used for detection of resistance to rifampicin, targeting five different sequences of *rpoB* gene. Turnaround time is <2 hours
- **Line probe assay (LPA):** It detects resistance to both first-line and second-line anti-

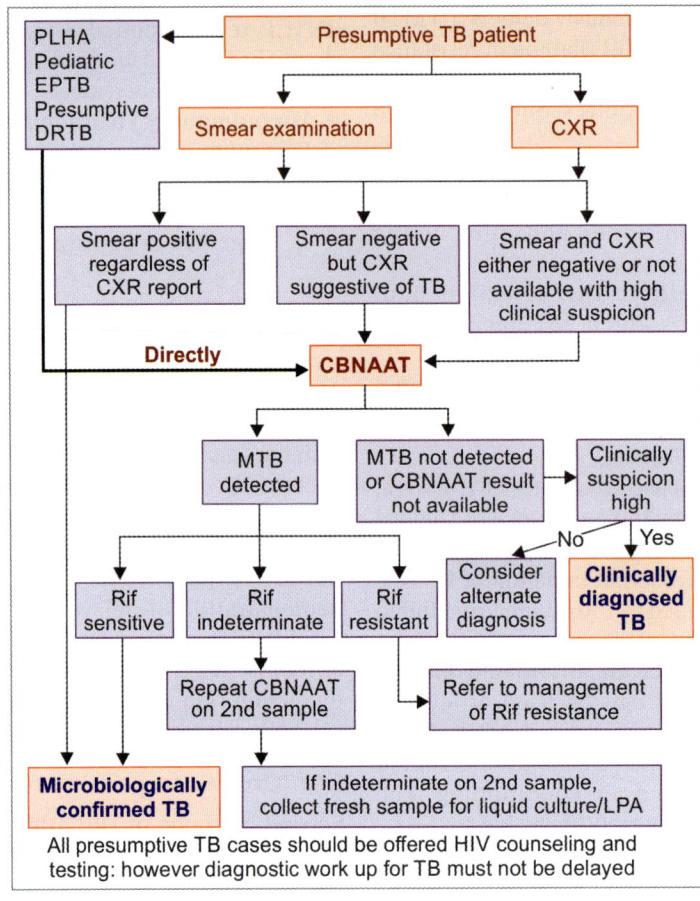

Flowchart 35.1: Diagnostic algorithm for pulmonary tuberculosis.

Source: Adapted from RNTCP guideline 2016.

Note: **Presumptive pulmonary TB** refers to a person with any of the following—(i) cough >2 weeks, (ii) fever >2 weeks, (iii) significant weight loss, (iv) hemoptysis, (v) any abnormalities in the chest X-ray.

Abbreviations: Rif, Rifampicin; CBNAAT, cartridge-based nucleic acid amplification test; PLHA, people living with HIV/AIDS; DRTB, drug resistant tuberculosis; CXR, chest X-ray; LPA, line probe assay.

tubercular drugs; with a turnaround time of 2–3 days.

U-DST
Universal-Drug Susceptibility Testing (U-DST) refers to testing all TB patients for resistance to at least rifampicin (by performing CBNAAT). U-DST program has been rolled out across India since January 2018.

Treatment
Multidrug therapy is recommended for tuberculosis, for rapid and effective killing of tubercle bacilli. The treatment should be planned only after the result of DST is available. The treatment regimens are of various types, depending upon the resistance pattern.

Standard regimen for drug sensitive-TB: It is a six-month course; comprises of two phases.
1. **Intensive phase**, with four drugs [HRZE-isoniazid (H), rifampicin (R), pyrazinamide (Z), ethambutol (E)] for two months; followed by
2. **Continuation phase**, with three drugs (HRE) for four months.

FDC: All drugs must be given in fixed dose combination (FDC) tablets as per appropriate weight bands. The FDC tablets should be taken orally, once in a day.

Drug Resistance

- ❖ **MDR-TB:** Multidrug-resistant tuberculosis (MDR-TB) is defined as resistance to both isoniazid and rifampicin with or without resistance to other first-line drugs
- ❖ **XDR-TB:** Extensively drug-resistant tuberculosis (XDR-TB) is defined as MDR-TB case which is also resistant to:
  - Fluoroquinolones (levofloxacin/moxifloxacin/gatifloxacin), and
  - At least one second-line injectable agents (amikacin/capreomycin/kanamycin).

Prevention

- ❖ **Infection control:** Airborne precautions need to be followed while giving care to a TB patient; various components include use of N95 respirator, negative pressure room and others (Refer Chapter 11, for detail)
- ❖ **BCG Vaccine:** Bacillus Calmette-Guerin (BCG) vaccine is available. It is a live-attenuated vaccine, made up of *Mycobacterium bovis* strain. It is given at birth, administered as single dose, intradermally.

Pseudomonas and Acinetobacter Infections

CHAPTER 36

■ INTRODUCTION

Non-fermenting gram-negative bacilli (NF-GNB) do not ferment any sugars, but they utilize the sugars oxidatively.

❖ Most of the NF-GNB exist as environmental commensals in hospitals that inhabit in moist environments, detergents and IV fluids. They are resistant to multiple antibiotics. However, they cause various infections in hospitalized patients, of which respiratory infections are noteworthy. Examples include:

- *Pseudomonas aeruginosa*
- *Burkholderia cepacia*
- *Acinetobacter baumannii*
- *Stenotrophomonas maltophilia*
- *Elizabethkingia meningosepticum.*

❖ However, there are some non-fermenters which are principally community associated pathogens. Classical example is *Burkholderia pseudomallei*, which causes **melioidosis**, characterized by infections of various systems, of which the notable are respiratory, skin and soft tissue, and bloodstream infections.

■ PSEUDOMONAS INFECTIONS

Problem Solving Exercise

A 32-year-old man with 30% burn injury developed burn wound infection after 5 days of hospitalization. Exudate specimen was sent for culture (Fig. 36.1B), biochemical reaction (Fig. 36.4) and AST (Fig. 36.5 and Table 36.1).
- What is the causative organism?
- List the clinical conditions caused by this organism.
- What are the various modalities of laboratory diagnosis?
- How will you treat this condition?
- How is this disease prevented in hospitals?

Explanation

Clinical Diagnosis

It is a case of burn wound surface infection. Nosocomial pathogens such as *Pseudomonas* and *Staphylococcus aureus,* etc. frequently colonize and cause infection on burn wound surface.

Identification

The causative organism is *Pseudomonas aeruginosa*. Points in favor are:

- Burn wound infection
- Hospitalized patient
- MacConkey agar showing blue green pigmented nonlactose fermenting (NLF) colonies with metallic sheen (Fig. 36.1B)
- Biochemical reactions are typical of *Pseudomonas* (Fig. 36.4): Indole test (negative), Citrate test (positive), Urease (negative), TSI test showing alkaline slant/alkaline butt (no change) with no gas and no H_2S, and Oxidase positive.

Antimicrobial Susceptibility Test

Antimicrobial susceptibility test on Muller–Hinton agar (Fig. 36.5 and Table 36.1) reveals the organism is sensitive to ceftazidime, amikacin, ciprofloxacin, piperacillin/tazobactam and meropenem. The drug of choice would be one of the narrow spectrum antibiotic such as ceftazidime, or ciprofloxacin.

(For answers to other questions, refer below).

Clinical Manifestations

Pseudomonas aeruginosa is notorious to cause infections at almost all sites, most common being lungs, skin and soft tissues. Most of the infections are encountered in hospitalized patients who get colonized with the organisms

either from heavily contaminated hospital environment or from the hospital staff (through contaminated hands). Colonized patients develop disease in the presence of underlying risk factors such as burn wounds, patients with immunosuppression and post-surgeries. The common infections are:
- Ventilator-associated pneumonia
- Chronic respiratory tract infections in patients with cystic fibrosis (mucoid strains)
- Ear infections: *Swimmer's ear* (in children) and *malignant otitis externa* (in elderly diabetics)
- Eye infections such as corneal ulcers (in contact lens wearers) and endophthalmitis
- Shanghai fever (typhoid like illness)
- Skin and soft tissue infections
- Wound infection in burns patients
- Ecthyma gangrenosum
- Cellulitis (characterized by *blue green pus*)
- Urinary tract infection in catheterized patients.

Laboratory Diagnosis

Specimen: Various specimens such as pus, wound swab, urine, sputum, blood or cerebrospinal fluid (CSF) are collected, depending upon the site infected.

Direct smear: Gram staining of the specimen shows plenty of pus cells and slender gram-negative bacilli, occasionally capsulated.

Culture

Pseudomonas is nonfastidious, can grow in ordinary media but it is obligate aerobe.
- **Nutrient agar:** It produces opaque, irregular colonies with a metallic sheen with greenish pigmentation (commonly) (Fig. 36.2)
  - Diffusible pigments are produced by most strains which produce blue green (pyocyanin) or yellow green (pyoverdin) pigmentation
  - Most colonies have a characteristic sweet ether or alcohol-like fruity odor
  - *Morphotypes*: Colonies show various morphological appearances such as large spreading type, mucoid type, small round type, minute type, etc.
- **Blood agar:** It produces hemolytic colonies on blood agar (Fig. 36.1A)
- **MacConkey agar:** Produce pale NLF colonies with metallic sheen (Fig. 36.1B)

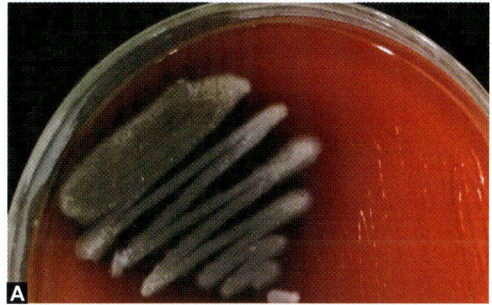
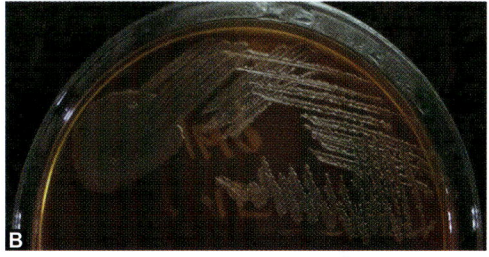

Figs 36.1A and B: *Pseudomonas aeruginosa* on: (A) Blood agar showing hemolytic colonies; (B) MacConkey agar showing NLF colonies with metallic sheen.
Source: Department of Microbiology, Pondicherry Institute of Medical sciences, Puducherry (*with permission*).

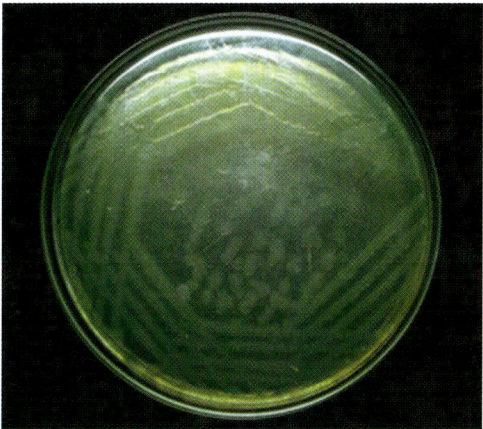

Fig. 36.2: Large, opaque, irregular colonies of *Pseudomonas aeruginosa* with a metallic sheen and green color pigmentation on nutrient agar.
Source: Department of Microbiology, Pondicherry Institute of Medical sciences, Puducherry (*with permission*).

- **Selective media** such as *cetrimide agar* can be used to isolate the organism from mixed growth in purulent specimens
- **Culture smear and motility testing:** Gram staining of the culture smear reveals gram-negative bacilli (Fig. 36.3). They are motile with single polar flagellum.

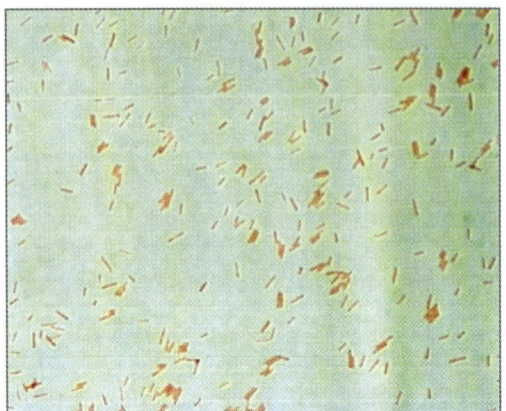

Fig. 36.3: Gram-stained culture smear of *Pseudomonas* showing gram-negative bacilli.
Source: Department of Microbiology, JIPMER, Puducherry (*with permission*).

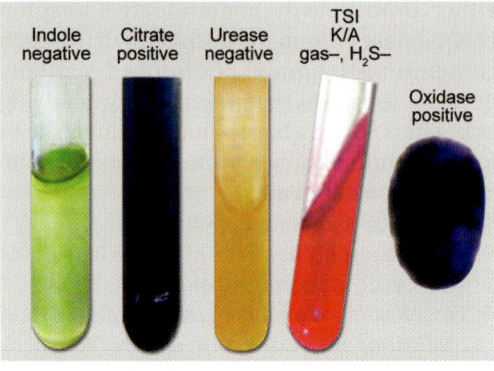

Fig. 36.4: Biochemical reactions of *Pseudomonas*.
Source: Department of Microbiology, JIPMER, Puducherry (*with permission*).

Biochemical Properties

Pseudomonas shows the following biochemical properties (Fig. 36.4):
- Oxidase and catalase—positive
- Nonfermenter—*OF test* (oxidative fermentative test) shows oxidative pattern
- Indole test—negative
- Citrate test—variable
- Urease—negative
- TSI test shows alkaline slant/alkaline butt (no change) with no gas and no H_2S.

Identification of *Pseudomonas* from colonies can also be made by automated identification systems such as MALDI-TOF or VITEK.

Antimicrobial Susceptibility Testing (AST)

AST is essential to administer proper antibiotics. It is done on Mueller–Hinton agar by disk diffusion method (Fig. 36.5 and Table 36.1).

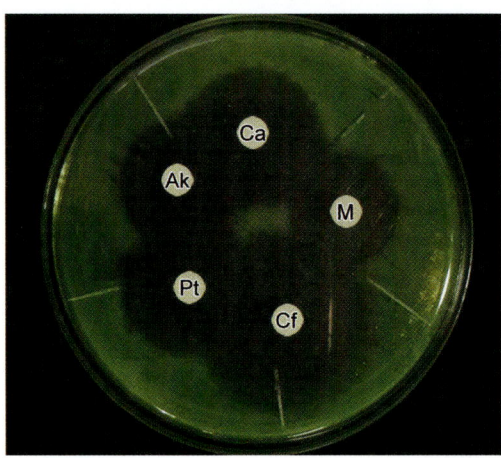

Fig. 36.5: Antimicrobial susceptibility testing on Mueller–Hinton Agar (*Pseudomonas*) (Refer Table 36.1 for CLSI zone interpretation).
Abbreviations: Cf, ciprofloxacin; Ca, ceftazidime; Ak, amikacin; Pt, piperacillin-tazobactam; M, meropenem; CLSI, Clinical and Laboratory Standards Institute.
Source: Department of Microbiology, Pondicherry Institute of Medical sciences, Puducherry (*with permission*).

Table 36.1: Interpretative categories (CLSI) and observed zone size diameter (mm) to various antimicrobial agents tested for *Pseudomonas aeruginosa*.

Antimicrobial agents	Disk strength (µg)	CLSI interpretative criteria for *Pseudomonas aeruginosa* (in mm)			Observed zone size (in mm) (Fig. 36.5)	Interpretation
		Resistant	Intermediate	Sensitive		
Ceftazidime (Ca)	30	≤14	15–17	≥18	26	Sensitive
Amikacin (Ak)	30	≤14	15–16	≥17	22	Sensitive
Ciprofloxacin (Cf)	5	≤18	19–24	≥25	30	Sensitive
Piperacillin/Tazobactam (Pt)	100/10	≤14	15–20	≥21	26	Sensitive
Meropenem (M)	10	≤15	16–18	≥19	21	Sensitive

Abbreviation: CLSI, Clinical and Laboratory Standards Institute.

Treatment

Pseudomonas species are widely distributed and inherently resistant to most of the antibiotics. Only limited antimicrobial agents have antipseudomonal action such as:
- Penicillins: Piperacillin, mezlocillin and ticarcillin
- Cephalosporins: Ceftazidime, cefoperazone and cefepime
- Carbapenems: Imipenem and meropenem
- Monobactam: Aztreonam
- Aminoglycoside: Tobramycin, gentamicin and amikacin
- Quinolones: Ciprofloxacin and levofloxacin
- Polymyxins: Polymyxin B and colistin.

Drug Resistance

Pseudomonas possesses a number of drug-resistant plasmids which confer multiple drug resistance. Many strains are producers of β-lactamases such as extended spectrum β-lactamases, carbapenemases and AmpC β-lactamases. Many strains are resistant to aminoglycosides and quinolones.

Prevention

Infection control measures such as contact isolation precautions and improved hand hygiene are essential to prevent nosocomial infections (Refer Chapter 11).

ACINETOBACTER INFECTIONS

Acinetobacter baumannii is another non-fermenter like *Pseudomonas* which has attracted attention recent days as nosocomial pathogen. Hospital environment is heavily contaminated with these organisms. They are also commensals in skin, oral cavity and intestine of hospitalized patients. They are resistant to most of the available antibiotics; pose a huge challenge for treatment.

Clinical Manifestations

A. baumannii causes widespread hospital infections such as:
- Ventilator associated pneumonia

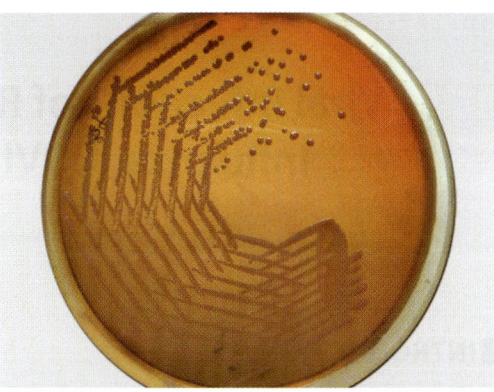

Fig. 36.6: Lactose non-fermenting colonies (with faint pink tint) of *Acinetobacter* on MacConkey agar.
Source: Department of Microbiology, JIPMER, Puducherry (*with permission*).

- Central line associated bloodstream infection
- Post-neurosurgical meningitis
- Catheter- associated UTI
- Wound and soft tissue infections
- Infections in burn patients.

Laboratory Diagnosis

It is an obligate aerobe, grows well on ordinary medium. Specimens can be inoculated onto blood agar (non-hemolytic colonies) and MacConkey agar (lactose non-fermenting colonies with faint pink tint) (Fig. 36.6).

Important identification features of *A. baumannii* include:
- **Gram staining:** They are gram-negative coccobacilli
- Non-motile
- Oxidase negative and catalase positive
- Non-fermenter of sugars
- **ICUT tests** (Fig. 36.4): Indole test (negative), citrate test (positive), urease test (negative) and TSI (triple sugar iron agar) test shows alkaline slant/alkaline butt with no gas and no H_2S
- **Automation:** Species identification can also be made by automated identification systems such as MALDI-TOF or VITEK.

Treatment for *Acinetobacter* infections is similar to that of *Pseudomonas* infections.

CHAPTER 37

Viral Infections of Respiratory Tract: Influenza, COVID-19 and Others

■ INTRODUCTION

Viruses account for vast majority of respiratory illness. Common respiratory viruses include:
- ❖ **Myxoviruses:** Influenza viruses, parainfluenza viruses, respiratory syncytial virus (RSV) and mumps
- ❖ **Coronaviruses** including the virus causing COVID-19
- ❖ **Epstein–Barr virus:** Causes infectious mononucleosis

- ❖ **Other respiratory viruses include:**
  - Enteroviruses: Coxsackie A virus (causes vesicular pharyngitis or herpangina), echoviruses, enterovirus 71
  - Adenoviruses: Cause upper respiratory tract infection in children and pneumonia
  - Rhinoviruses: Cause common cold syndrome
  - Herpes simplex virus
  - HIV (as acute retroviral syndrome).

■ INFLUENZA

Problem Solving Exercise 1

In month of December, a 53-year-old man from Puducherry presented with fever with chills, myalgia, dry cough and sore throat and running nose. A clinical diagnosis of influenza-like illness (ILI) was made. The treating physician revealed that always there has been an increase in number of such cases during winter season. A nasopharyngeal swab was collected, sent for real-time polymerase chain reaction (PCR) and result is shown here (Fig. 37.1).

1. Mention the ideal method of specimen collection and transport.
2. What is the reason behind repeated outbreaks of this clinical condition?
3. What are the precautions to be taken to prevent the spread of the disease?
4. What are the different modalities of laboratory diagnosis?

Explanation

Clinical Diagnosis

The symptoms of cough, sore throat, myalgia, etc., in a winter season is suggestive of influenza-like illness.

Etiological Diagnosis

Real-time PCR (Fig. 37.1) revealed that there is emission of fluorescence during the cycles for Influenza A (matrix gene), H1N1 (HA gene) and the internal control RNP (ribonucleoprotein) gene. But there is no emission of fluorescence for H3N2 (HA gene) and Influenza B (HA gene). Therefore, it is identified as Influenza A/H1N1.
(For answers to other questions, refer below).

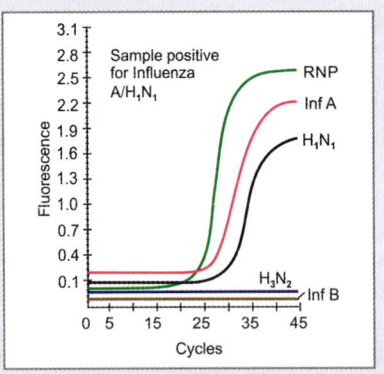

Fig. 37.1: Real-time RT-PCR showing the result (amplification curves) of specimen tested for Influenza types A/H1N1, A/H3N2 and B.

CHAPTER 37 ◆ Viral Infections of Respiratory Tract

Introduction

Influenza viruses are the members of Orthomyxoviridae family. They are one of the major causes of morbidity and mortality and have been responsible for several epidemics and pandemics of respiratory diseases in the last two centuries. It has four types—A, B, C and D. Influenza type A can be further subtyped based on hemagglutinin (HA) and neuraminidase (NA) peplomer antigens present in its envelope.

Antigenic Variation

Antigenic variation is an unique property of influenza viruses, which is responsible for causing epidemics and pandemics. Antigenic variation is due to the result of antigenic changes occurring in HA and NA antigens. It is of two types.

Antigenic Variations

1. Antigenic Drift

It is a minor change occurring due to **point mutations** in the HA/NA gene, resulting in alteration of amino acid sequence of the antigenic sites on HA/NA, such that virus can partially escape recognition by the host's immune system. The new variant must sustain two or more mutations to become epidemiologically significant.
- Seen in both influenza virus type—A and B
- Results in outbreaks and minor periodic epidemics
- Antigenic drift occurs more frequently, every 2–3 years.

2. Antigenic Shift

It is an abrupt, major drastic, discontinuous variation in the sequence of a viral surface protein (HA/NA), that occurs due to **genetic reassortment** between genomes of two or more influenza viruses infecting the same host cells; resulting in a new virus strain, unrelated antigenically to the predecessor strains. Thus, antibodies developed against previous strain (due to infection or vaccination) become ineffective.
- Occurs only in influenza A virus
- Results in pandemics and major epidemics, e.g., H1N1 pandemics of 2009
- Antigenic shift occurs less frequently every 10–20 years.

Clinical Manifestations

Transmission

Influenza is transmitted by (i) **inhalation of respiratory droplets** generated by coughing and sneezing. This mode can infect only those people who are within 1-meter distance, (ii) **via direct contact** (e.g., touching the droplets) **or indirect contact with surfaces or fomites** infected with respiratory droplets and then touching nose, eyes or mouth

Uncomplicated Influenza (Flu Syndrome)

Incubation period is about 18–72 hours. Majority of the individuals are either asymptomatic or develop minor upper respiratory symptoms such as chills, headache, and dry cough, followed by high-grade fever, myalgia and anorexia. It is a self-limiting condition, indistinguishable from the infections caused by other upper respiratory tract pathogens.

Complications

Occasionally, patient may develop complications.
- ❖ **Pneumonia:** It occurs either as a result of secondary bacterial infection (most common) or as a primary influenza pneumonia
- ❖ **Other respiratory tract complications** include worsening of chronic obstructive pulmonary disease, exacerbation of chronic bronchitis, etc.

Influenza A (H1N1) pdm09

It has caused the most recent pandemic of influenza in 2009, affecting several countries including India. However, thereafter it is circulating in the community and has been causing sporadic infection and periodic outbreaks of seasonal flu.

Seasonal Flu

Influenza viruses cause outbreaks of seasonal flu worldwide during winter season almost every year, however, they differ widely in severity and the extent of spread. The common serotypes currently circulating in India to cause seasonal influenza include influenza A/H1N1, influenza A/H3N2 and influenza B.

Laboratory Diagnosis

Specimen Collection

- ❖ **Ideal specimens** are nasopharyngeal swab or lavage fluid, nasal aspirate or to a less extent throat swab

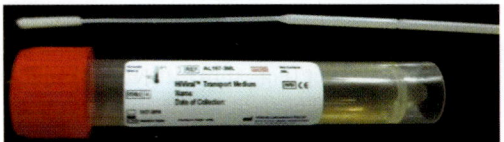

Fig. 37.2: Viral transport medium and swab.
Source: Department of Microbiology, JIPMER, Puducherry (with permission).

- **Swabs** with a synthetic tip (e.g., polyester or Dacron swabs) are best for specimen collection (Fig. 37.2). Cotton or alginate swabs are unsatisfactory
- **Transport:** Swabs are immediately put inside the viral transport media, kept at 4°C during transport up to 4 days, thereafter at –70°C.

Isolation of Virus

Embryonated eggs (amniotic cavity) and primary monkey kidney cell lines have been used (in past); viral growth was detected by hemadsorption or hemagglutination test.

Direct Immunofluorescence Test

Viral antigens coated onto epithelial cells can be directly detected in nasal aspirates by using fluorescent tagged antibodies. This is rapid, but less sensitive than viral isolation.

Molecular Methods

Molecular methods have revolutionized the diagnosis of influenza.
- **RT-PCR** (reverse transcriptase polymerase chain reaction): It is highly sensitive, specific and rapid (turnaround time of <1 day). It can also detect the specific type and subtype of influenza virus
- **Real-time RT-PCR:** It is currently the gold standard method for influenza diagnosis. It has higher sensitivity and specificity than RT-PCR with turnaround time of 2–3 hours. It simultaneously detects the three common seasonal flu strains (A/H1N1, A/H3N2 and type B). The result is expressed as the emission of fluorescence during the cycles as described in Figure 37.3 and Table 37.1
- **BioFire FilmArray Respiratory Panel (RP)** tests simultaneously 20 respiratory pathogens, including Influenza A, Influenza A/H1, Influenza A/H3, Influenza A/H1-2009 and Influenza B.

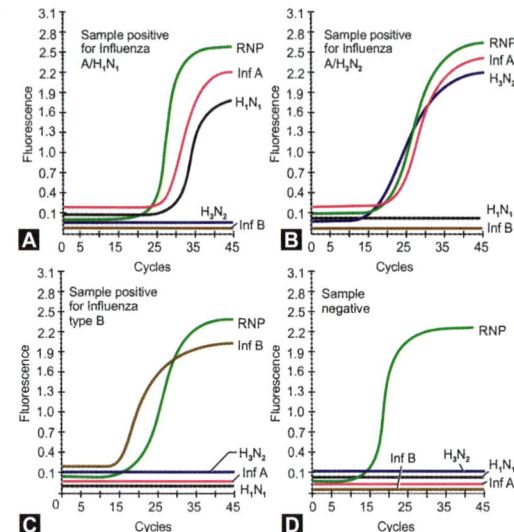

Figs 37.3A to D: Real-time RT-PCR showing the result (amplification curves) of specimen(s) tested positive for Influenza type: (A) A/H_1N_1; (B) A/H_3N_2; (C) Type B; (D) Negative (Refer Table 37.1).
Source: Department of Microbiology, JIPMER, Puducherry (with permission).

Antibody Detection (Serology)

Various assays are available such as ELISA, neutralization test, and previously used HAI (hemagglutination inhibition) test, to detect subtype specific serum antibodies by using specific influenza antigens. It is mainly useful for sero-epidemiology purpose, not for clinical diagnosis.

Table 37.1: Real-time RT-PCR for seasonal influenza types.

Simultaneously detects five genes	Specimens positive with influenza type			Influenza negative
	A/H1N1	A/H3N2	Type B	
Influenza A (matrix gene)	+	+	–	–
H1N1 (HA gene)	+	–	–	–
H3N2 (HA gene)	–	+	–	–
Influenza B (HA gene)	–	–	+	–
RNP (ribonucleoprotein)*	+	+	+	+

*RNP (ribonucleoprotein) is used as internal control in real-time RT-PCR; if it is not detected, then the test is considered invalid.

Treatment

Neuraminidase inhibitors (such as zanamivir or oseltamivir) are effective for influenza.
* It is the drug of choice for A/H1N1 2009 flu, A/H5N1 avian flu and influenza-B
* **Oseltamivir** (75 mg tablets): Given twice a day for 5 days (for treatment) or once daily for 7 days (for chemoprophylaxis).

Vaccine

Both injectable (inactivated) and nasal spray (live attenuated) vaccines are available.

* **Serotypes:** Vaccines contain the common influenza types/subtypes currently circulating—A/H1N1, A/H3N2 and influenza B
* **Indication:** Given annually (once in a year) to people at higher risk of infection.

Prevention

Infection control measures such as droplet precautions and contact precautions need to be followed while giving care to patients with influenza (Refer Chapter 11, for detail).

COVID-19

Problem Solving Exercise 2

Laboratory Diagnosis of COVID-19
A 72-year-old patient with complaints of dry cough, sore throat and fever visited a hospital. He was kept in an isolation room. His throat swab was sent for COVID-19 testing by real-time RT-PCR. The result is shown Fig. 37.4.
1. Interpret the test result.
2. Discuss the method of specimen collection.
3. Discuss the laboratory diagnosis of this disease.

Explanation

Clinical diagnosis
Dry cough, sore throat and fever suggests that it is a case of Influenza like illness (ILI).

Interpretation of test
Throat swab was subjected to COVID-19 testing by real-time RT-PCR. Fig. 37.4 shows the following findings.
❑ There is emission of fluorescence during the cycles for:
  ➢ Envelope (E) gene (for screening, specific for beta coronavirus)
  ➢ RdRp gene (for confirmation, specific to SARS-CoV-2) and
  ➢ The internal control RNP (ribonucleoprotein) gene.
❑ The threshold (Ct value) of the run (the point at which the fluorescence starts emitting) is found to be satisfactory; 25th cycle (for E gene) and 30th cycle (for *RdRP* gene).

Therefore, the serotype is identified as SARS-CoV-2. Refer text below, for answer to other questions.

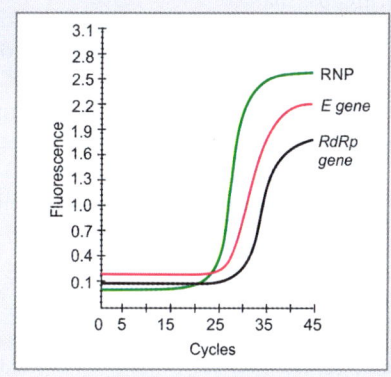

Fig. 37.4: Real-time RT-PCR showing the result (amplification curves) of specimen tested for SARS-CoV-2.

Clinical Manifestations

COVID-19 (Coronavirus disease-2019) is caused by severe acute respiratory syndrome coronavirus 2 (SARS-CoV-2). It is primarily transmitted via respiratory droplets and contact routes (same, as discussed for influenza). The incubation period for COVID-19 is on an average of 5–6 days, but can be as long as 14 days. COVID-19 patients may present with following signs and symptoms:

* **Common features:** Fever, cough with expectoration, fatigue, shortness of breath, myalgia, rhinorrhea, sore throat, diarrhea. Loss of smell or taste sensation may occasionally occur preceding the onset of respiratory symptoms
* **Atypical symptoms:** Particularly seen in older people and immune-suppressed patients—such as fatigue, reduced alertness, reduced mobility, diarrhea, loss of appetite, delirium,

and absence of fever. Children might not develop fever or cough as frequently as adults
- ❖ **Clinical severity:** Based on the clinical severity, the disease may be classified into the three clinical stages
    1. **Mild disease** (ILI or influenza-like illness)
    2. **Moderate disease:** Pneumonia with no signs of severe disease
    3. **Severe disease:** Called as severe acute respiratory illness (SARI), characterized by severe pneumonia, acute respiratory distress, sepsis or septic shock.

Laboratory Diagnosis

Specimen Collection and Transport

- ❖ **Preferred specimens:** Throat (i.e., oropharyngeal) and nasal swabs are the preferred specimens. Dacron or polyester flocked swabs are used, dipped in viral transport media (VTM) after collection
- ❖ **Alternative specimens include:** Nasopharyngeal swab, bronchoalveolar lavage (BAL) or endotracheal aspirate (in ventilated patients)
- ❖ **PPE:** Appropriate PPE should be used for specimen collection such as gloves, gown, N95 respirator and face shield
- ❖ **Specimen transport and packing:** Samples collected should be properly labelled, packed in three layers (triple packaging method) and transported to the laboratory maintaining an adequate cold chain.

Nucleic Acid Amplification Testing (NAAT)

Real-time RT-PCR

Real-time reverse transcriptase PCR is the gold standard test for diagnosis of COVID-19.
- ❖ The average time taken is around 4–5 hours from receipt of sample to generation of the result
- ❖ The advantage of this platform lies in its accuracy of detection as well as the ability to run up to 90 samples in a single run. Therefore, if available, this platform should be used as a frontline test for the diagnosis of SARS-CoV-2
- ❖ **Gene targets:** Most of the commercial kits target two genes, performed in a single reaction—one for screening and other for confirmatory

Gene targets for screening are genus specific; i.e., specific for *Sarbecovirus* (*Betacoronavirus*):
- ☐ Spike protein (S)
- ☐ Envelope protein (E)
- ☐ Membrane protein (M)
- ☐ Nucleocapsid protein (N).

Gene targets for confirmation are species specific; i.e., specific for SARS-CoV-2
- ☐ RNA-dependent RNA polymerase (*RdRp*)
- ☐ Open reading frames (ORF1a/b)
- ☐ N2 nucleocapsid.

- ❖ **Principle:** Most commercial kits available are based on qualitative real-time PCR
    - The target gene/s in the specimen is amplified in the thermocycler
    - When the amplicon binds with the probe, a fluorescence is generated. The point at which the fluorescence starts is the cycle threshold (Ct) of the run
    - A sample is considered positive when both screening, as well as confirmatory genes, are detected with a Ct value ≤40 cycles (Fig. 37.4)
    - **Detectable:** NAAT becomes positive as early as day 1 of onset of symptom (usually after 5 days of infection) and starts to decline by 3rd week and subsequently becomes undetectable (Fig. 37.5).

Automated Real-time RT-PCR

Several automated real-time PCR are commercially available such as—Truenat and CBNAAT (cartridge-based nucleic acid amplification test, e.g., GeneXpert). Both these

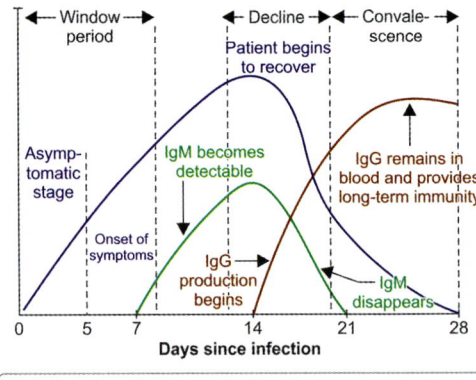

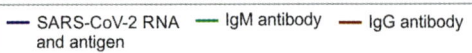

Fig. 37.5: Course of the diagnostic markers in COVID-19.

systems are already in use for the diagnosis of tuberculosis.
- ❖ **Advantages** of these systems include:
  - These platforms have widespread availability even at district and primary health center level as these systems are already in use for the diagnosis of tuberculosis and other infectious diseases
  - They have a quick turnaround time (30–60 minutes)
  - Fully-automated, involves minimal handling; therefore poses minimum biosafety hazard. Safety is further augmented by the closed nature of these platforms.
- ❖ **Gene targets used are:**
  - **CBNAAT**: Two targets are used; *E* gene for screening and *N2* gene for confirmation
  - **Truenat:** Two targets are used; *E* gene for screening and *RdRp* gene for confirmation.
- ❖ However, **disadvantages** of these systems include: Only 1–4 samples can be tested in one run, therefore, suitable only for laboratories with less sample load (24–48 samples/day).

Antigen Detection

A rapid chromatographic immunoassay is commercially available (SD Biosensor) for qualitative detection of specific antigens (nucleocapsid protein) to SARS-CoV-2.
- ❖ **Nasopharyngeal swab,** after collection should be immersed and squeezed in the viral extraction buffer, provided with the kit. This buffer inactivates the virus, releasing the antigen
- ❖ It is a **point-of-care test**, conducted at the bedside within one hour, as the antigen in the extracted buffer is stable only for an hour
- ❖ **Performance:** It is highly specific (99–100%), with moderate sensitivity (50–84%). Therefore, symptomatic but negative patients should be essentially referred for a real-time RT-PCR test (Fig. 37.6).

There are various other antigen detection kits under validation, which may be marketed in near future.

Antibody Detection

IgG antibodies start appearing after two weeks of the onset of infection, after recovery

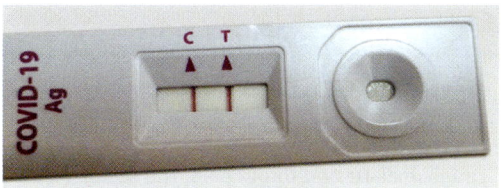

Fig. 37.6: Antigen detection test for COVID.
Source: Department of Microbiology, JIPMER, Puducherry (with permission).

and last for several months. Therefore, IgG test should not be used for clinical diagnosis. ELISA, chemiluminescence and ICT formats are available. They may be useful for sero-surveillance purpose and to conduct survey among high-risk or vulnerable populations.

Nonspecific Tests

- ❖ **Prognostic markers:** There are several prognostic markers which can be used in the setting of ARDS, include:
  - Elevated IL-6 level: Indicates cytokine storm
  - Elevated D-dimer: Indicates the presence of high level of fibrin degradation products, thus suggesting an underlying coagulopathy
  - Elevated serum ferritin: Indicates inflammation
  - Severe lymphopenia
  - Elevated C-reactive protein: Marker of acute inflammation.
- ❖ **CT scan** of lungs shows *ground glass appearance* (Fig. 37.7) and/or consolidation.

Treatment

Currently, there is no definitive therapy available for COVID-19; however many drugs are under research such as remdesivir, favipiravir, lopinavir/ritonavir, hydroxychloroquine, plasma therapy and anti-cytokines such as tocilizumab (IL-6 receptor blocker).

Prevention of COVID-19

Infection prevention and control (IPC) is the most effective method currently available for the prevention of COVID-19. The following are the key IPC measures need to be strictlyfollowed.

Problem Solving Exercise 3

Prevention of COVID-19

A 72-year-old patient (without wearing any mask) presented to casualty with complaints of fever, dry cough, malaise and throat pain. The security guard (without mask) guided him to go to the casualty. The resident doctor (without mask) took history, examined the patient. His throat swab was sent for COVID-19 testing which came positive. Subsequently the security staff and the resident doctor were also turned positive for COVID-19.
1. Identify the infection control breaches
2. What are the personal protective equipment (PPE) need to be worn while giving care to this patient?
3. What is the correct sequence of donning and doffing of PPE
4. Discuss the infection control measures to prevent the transmission.

Explanation

Influenza like illness (fever, dry cough, malaise and throat pain) with throat swab confirmed for COVID-19, suggests that it is case of COVID-19
- **Infection control breaches:** Patient was not wearing mask. Security staff and resident doctor were not wearing mask or any other PPE. Patient was not kept in isolation room. No hand hygiene was performed
- **PPE:** 3-ply mask, pair of gloves, gown and eye protection (goggle or face shield) need to be worn while giving care to this patient
- **Donning (wearing) sequence:** Gown first → Mask or respirator → Goggles or face shield → Gloves
- **Doffing (removing) sequence:** Gloves first → Face shield or goggles → Gown → Mask or respirator.

Refer text below, for answer to other questions.

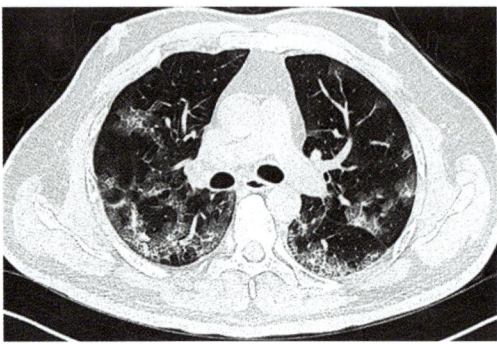

Fig. 37.7: A case of COVID-19 pneumonia with CT scan lungs showing ground-glass opacity seen in both lungs, predominantly subpleural in distribution. Ground-glass opacity is a feature of interstitial pneumonia.
Source: Dr Sunitha V, Department of Radiology, JIPMER, Puducherry (*with permission*).

IPC Measures at Healthcare Facility

IPC measures of droplet and contact precautions need to be followed by the healthcare workers while handling COVID-19 cases, except for aerosol-generating procedures (AGPs) when airborne precautions need to be followed (Refer Chapter 11).

Hand Hygiene

As contact mode appears to be an important mode of transmission, absolute hand hygiene is probably the most effective method for the prevention of COVID-19.

- Hand hygiene needs to be performed when opportunity arises (as per WHO's 'my five moments of hand hygiene', refer Chapter 10)
- Hand hygiene must be performed by the correct technique, and for appropriate duration (20–30 sec for hand rub).

Personal Protective Equipment

The following are the current recommendations:
- **HCWs giving care to the COVID-19 suspects:** Should wear a medical (3-ply) mask, a pair of gloves, gown, and a face shield. Medical mask should be replaced by a N95 respirator if AGPs are carried out (Fig. 37.8)
- **HCWs working in non-COVID areas:** Should wear a medical (3-ply) mask. This referred to as '*targeted continuous medical mask use*'
  - Should wear masks during all routine activities throughout the entire shift
  - Masks are only changed if they become soiled, wet or damaged, or at the end of shift
  - Front part of the mask should never be touched
  - Mask should never be hanged around the neck.
- **Anyone entering into a healthcare facility:** Must wear a face mask (e.g., cloth/fabric mask), regardless of the activities he is involved in. This is referred to as '*universal masking*' in healthcare facilities.

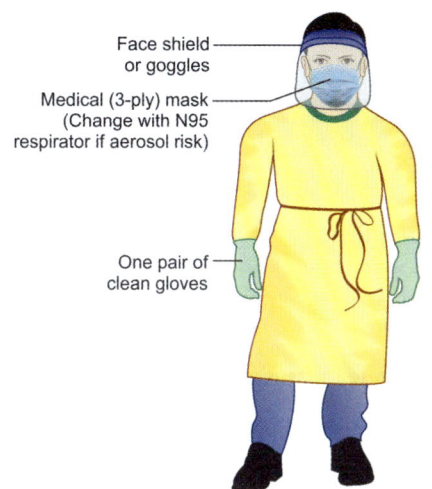

Fig. 37.8: Personal protective equipment recommended for healthcare workers when giving care to COVID-19 patients.

Environmental Cleaning

SARS-CoV-2 may survive on surface and floor for a variable period, ranging from few hours to as long as 9 days. This may be a potential source of transmission by indirect contact. Therefore, the following measures need to be followed.

- ❖ **Floor and surfaces:** Should be cleaned with a detergent, followed by disinfected with sodium hypochlorite (0.5%)
- ❖ **Cleaning of equipment** or patient care items such as stethoscope, BP apparatus, etc. should be done by using alcohol (70%)
- ❖ **High touch surfaces** such as lift button, rail of the staircase, patient trolley, bed rails, bed frames, bedside tables, door handles, etc. should be frequently disinfected with alcohol
- ❖ **Terminal disinfection** in patient care room after discharge/transfer of patients.

Other IPC Measures

- ❖ **Respiratory hygiene and cough etiquette** such as wearing a medical mask by all individuals who are symptomatic, hand wash immediately after sneezing or coughing, etc. (Refer Chapter 11)
- ❖ **Biomedical waste management** should be carried out as per the 2016 guideline (Refer Chapter 13). However, additional precautions are taken such as use of double bag, use of dedicated trolley and collection bins, label as "COVID-19 waste", and disinfecting outer bag with hypochlorite before handing over
- ❖ **Laundry:** All linens used for COVID-19 patients should be washed at 60–90°C with laundry detergent followed by soaking in 0.1% sodium hypochlorite for approximately 30 minutes and dried.

IPC Measures for General Public

Handwash

Frequent handwash is necessary after contact with other individuals, high-touch area, public places, after receipt of any items, or after blowing nose, coughing, or sneezing. Touching of eyes, nose, and mouth with unwashed hands must be avoided.

Social Distancing

Ideally, people should stay at home as much as possible. If not possible, 1 meter (2 arms) distance should be strictly maintained from other people at all times. As droplets can travel a maximum of 1-meter distance, therefore, the social distance of 1 meter would prevent the droplet transmission.

Environmental Cleaning

Frequently touched surfaces should be disinfected daily. This includes tables, doorknobs, light switches, countertops, handles, desks, phones, keyboards, toilets, faucets, and sinks. If surfaces are dirty, then it should be cleaned with detergent or soap and water prior to disinfection.

Cloth Mask (Non-medical Masks)

Everyone should wear a cloth face mask when they have to go out in public, e.g., for the grocery store. It primarily aims at **source control**, i.e., preventing transmission from the wearers to others).

- ❖ Cloth masks are made from a variety of fabrics, such as polypropylene. It should comprise of at least two layers:
  - Internal layers are made up of water-absorbing (hydrophilic) fabrics to readily absorb droplets
  - An external synthetic material (hydrophobic), which does not easily absorb liquid.
- ❖ They should not be used in hospital settings, as there is no filter used
- ❖ They can be washed and reused
- ❖ Should not be shared between individuals.

INFECTIOUS MONONUCLEOSIS

Problem Solving Exercise 4

An 18-year-old young boy presented with headache, fever, malaise, pharyngitis and rashes. On examination, he was found to have hepatosplenomegaly and enlarged cervical lymph nodes. Peripheral blood examination shows presence of atypical lymphocytes.
1. What is the clinical diagnosis and the most common causative organism?
2. What is the next investigation you would like to advise?
3. List the clinical conditions caused by this organism.
4. What are the different modalities of laboratory diagnosis?

Explanation
Clinical Diagnosis
It is a case of infectious mononucleosis (IM). Points in favor are:

- Young patient with pharyngitis, rashes, hepatosplenomegaly and enlarged cervical lymph nodes.
- Atypical lymphocytes in peripheral smear.

Identification
Infectious mononucleosis (IM) is caused by **Epstein–Barr virus**. However, IM-like syndrome may be seen in various infections such as CMV following blood transfusion, toxplasmosis, HIV infection, etc.
Paul–Bunnell test is the next investigation to be done as it can differentiate IM (Paul–Bunnell test positive) from mononucleosis like syndrome (PB test negative).
For answers to other questions, refer below.

Clinical Manifestations of EBV

Infectious Mononucleosis

It is also called as kissing disease (transmitted through salivary contact) or glandular disease, affecting young adults. It is characterized by:
- Headache, fever, malaise and pharyngitis
- Cervical lymphadenopathy
- Hepatosplenomegaly
- Rashes following ampicillin therapy
- Atypical lymphocytosis (CD8 T cells)
- Autoantibodies reactive to sheep RBC antigens (detected by Paul–Bunnell test).

EBV Associated Malignancies

Epstein–Barr virus is associated with several malignancies such as Burkitt's lymphoma, nasopharyngeal carcinoma, Hodgkin's and non-Hodgkin's lymphoma.

Laboratory Diagnosis

Heterophile Agglutination Test

Paul-Bunnell test is a tube agglutination test that uses sheep RBCs to detect heterophile antibodies in patient's serum. Agglutination titer of >256 is considered as significant. It is a heterophile agglutination test; false positive test results (normal individuals, following serum therapy) can be confirmed by **differential absorption test** (e.g., monospot test).

Other Tests

Other tests for diagnosis of EBV include:
- Specific antibody detection such as:
    - Antibody to viral capsid antigen (VCA)
    - Antibodies to early antigen
    - Antibodies to EBNA (Epstein–Barr nuclear antigen).
- EBV antigen detection by immunofluorescence
- EBV DNA (by PCR) detection
- EBER RNA (EBV encoded small RNAs, by reverse transcriptase PCR)
- Real-time PCR.

Treatment

Acyclovir is not useful for IM cases; symptomatic treatment is needed.

Parasitic and Fungal Infections of Respiratory Tract

CHAPTER 38

INTRODUCTION

Parasitic infections of respiratory tract include:
- *Paragonimus westermani:* This human parasite is a primary pathogen of lungs
- Parasites that pass through lungs during their life cycle, e.g., intestinal nematodes, such as *Ascaris*, hookworm, and *Strongyloides*
- Parasites causing hypersensitivity in lungs: Filarial nematodes causing tropical pulmonary eosinophilia (TPE)
- Parasites that infect elsewhere, rarely infect lungs: *E. histolytica, Toxoplasma, Balantidium coli, Cryptosporidium parvum* and *Echinococcus granulosus*.

Fungal infections of respiratory tract include:
- **Opportunistic fungal agents:** They are major fungal agents that cause respiratory infections:
  - Zygomycoses
  - Aspergillosis
  - Penicillosis
- *Pneumocystis jirovecii* pneumonia.
- **Fungi causing systemic mycoses:** They involve multiple organs. They are saprophytic fungi present in the environment. Human infection occurs by inhalation of spores leading to pulmonary infection. From lungs, they disseminate to cause various systemic manifestations (discussed in detail in Chapter 21). There are four agents of systemic mycoses, all are dimorphic fungi:
  1. *Blastomyces dermatitidis*
  2. *Histoplasma capsulatum*
  3. *Paracoccidioides brasiliensis*
  4. *Coccidioides immitis*.
- **Yeast:** *Cryptococcus neoformans:* It also causes meningitis, (Refer Chapter 41).

Note: Isolation of *Candida* species in sputum culture is a common finding; but it represents colonization. It is almost never indicative of underlying pulmonary candidiasis and therefore does not warrant antifungal treatment.

PARAGONIMIASIS

Problem Solving Exercise 1

Paragonimiasis

A 12-year-old girl from Manipur presented with productive cough with blood-tinged, rusty sputum with offensive fishy odor. Sputum specimen was sent for microscopic examination (Fig. 38.1).
1. Identify the causative agent based on sputum microscopy.
2. Which is the infective stage for man?
3. Mention two complications caused by the adult worm.

Explanation

The causative agent is *Paragonimus westermani*. Points in favor are:
- From Manipur—area endemic for paragonimiasis
- Productive cough with blood-tinged, rusty sputum with offensive fishy odor

- Sputum microscopy reveals large operculated oval eggs, golden-brown in color, measuring 80–120 µm × 45–65 µm in size (Fig. 38.1).
For further details, refer Table 38.1.

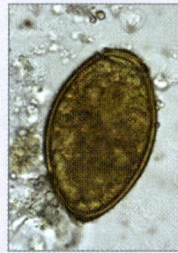

Fig. 38.1: *Paragonimus westermani* (egg).
Source: DPDx Image Library, Centers for Disease Control and Prevention (CDC), Atlanta (*with permission*).

Table 38.1: Features of paragonimiasis.

Properties	*Paragonimus westermani*
Definitive host	Man
Intermediate hosts	1st—Snail 2nd—Cray fish/carb
Infective form	Metacercaria larva
Transmission	Ingestion of cray fish/carb containing metacercaria
Habitat	Lungs
Manifestations	**Endemic hemoptysis:** • Granuloma formation in lungs and extrapulmonary sites, such as liver, spleen, brain • Blood tinged rusty sputum with offensive fishy odour
Diagnostic form	Eggs (operculated) in sputum (Fig. 38.1) • Large oval eggs • Operculated • Measures 80–120 μm long and 45–65 μm in breadth • Golden brown in color
Treatment	Praziquantel

ZYGOMYCOSIS

Zygomycosis represents group of life-threatening infections caused by aseptate fungi called as zygomycetes. The important causative agents of zygomycosis are *Rhizopus*, *Mucor* and *Absidia*. Zygomycosis caused due to these agents is known as Mucormycosis.

Risk Factors

Agents of mucormycosis require iron as growth factor. Hence, conditions with increased iron load are at higher risk of developing invasive mucormycosis, such as:
❖ Diabetic ketoacidosis (DKA) is the most important risk factor. Acidosis causes release of iron from the sequestered proteins in serum
❖ End-stage renal disease
❖ Patients taking iron therapy or deferoxamine (iron chelator)
❖ Defects in phagocytic functions.

Clinical Manifestations

Agents of mucormycosis are angioinvasive in nature.
❖ **Rhinocerebral mucormycosis:** Occurs commonly in patients with DKA. It starts as eye and facial pain, may progress to cause orbital cellulitis, proptosis and vision loss
❖ Pulmonary mucormycosis
❖ Cutaneous mucormycosis
❖ Gastrointestinal mucormycosis
❖ Disseminated mucormycosis.

Laboratory Diagnosis

❖ **Histopathological staining** of tissue biopsies shows broad aseptate hyaline hyphae with wide angle branching (Fig. 38.2)

Problem Solving Exercise 2

Mucormycosis

A 40-year-old female with uncontrolled diabetes mellitus was referred to a teaching hospital with severe eye pain and facial rash for 4 days. Facial rash progressed to extensive ulceration of the midface and bilateral loss of vision. She had nasal bridge collapse, with black eschars on the nasal mucosa and markedly elevated fasting blood sugar. She had surgical debridement and tissue was sent for histopathological examination (Fig. 38.2) and fungal culture (Fig. 38.3A and C).
1. What is the clinical diagnosis and the likely etiological agent based on the histopathological finding?
2. How can you confirm the diagnosis in the laboratory?
3. What are the other clinical manifestations caused by this organism?
4. Mention the treatment option for this clinical condition.

Explanation

Clinical Diagnosis

Female patient with *uncontrolled diabetes,* with acute presentation of progressive facial ulceration, nasal bridge collapse with black eschars on nasal mucosa and bilateral loss of vision give clue to the diagnosis of "Rhinocerebral mucormycosis".

Identification

Histopathological examination also showed broad aseptate hyaline hyphae with wide angle branching, gives presumptive identification of one of the agents causing mucormycosis (Fig. 38.2).

Culture of the tissue (nasal mucosa) on Sabouraud's dextrose agar (SDA) grew cottony woolly brown-black colonies with tube filling growth (Fig. 38.3A) and lactophenol cotton blue (LPCB) tease mount (Fig. 38.3C) of the colony revealed broad aseptate hyaline hyphae, from which sporangiophore arise which ends at sporangium-containing numerous sporangiospores, which are characteristic identification features of fungi *Rhizopus*.

For answers to the other questions, refer below.

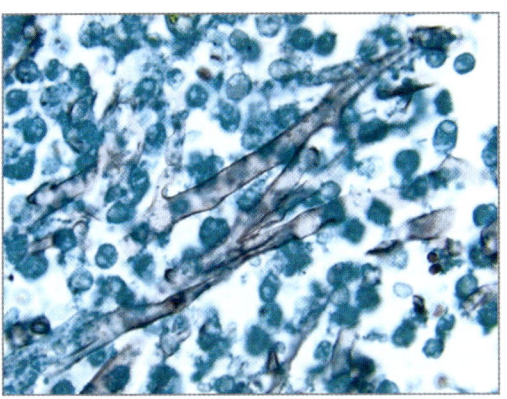

Fig. 38.2: Zygomycosis—histopathology of tissue section shows aseptate broad hyphae.
Source: Public Health Image Library, Centers for Disease Control and Prevention (CDC), Atlanta; Dr Libero Ajello, ID #4234 (*with permission*).

- ❖ **Culture on SDA** at 25°C reveals characteristic cottony woolly colonies with tube filling growth
  - White cottony colonies initially, later turn to brown-black due to sporulation giving rise to *salt and pepper* appearance seen in *Rhizopus* (Fig. 38.3A)
  - White cottony colony seen in *Mucor* (Fig. 38.3B).
- ❖ **Microscopic appearance:** LPCB mount of the colonies reveals broad aseptate hyaline hyphae, from which sporangiophore arise which ends at sporangium-containing numerous sporangiospores (Figs 38.3C and D)
- ❖ **Rhizoid:** Some species bear a unique root like growth arising from hyphae called rhizoid, which provides initial clue for identification of the fungus. Species can be differentiated depending on the position of the rhizoids with respect to sporangiophore (Figs 38.4A to C)
  - *Rhizopus* bears nodal rhizoids (Fig. 38.3C, 38.4A)
  - *Lichtheimia* bears internodal rhizoids (Fig. 38.4B)
  - *Mucor*: Rhizoids are typically absent (Fig. 38.3D and 38.4C).

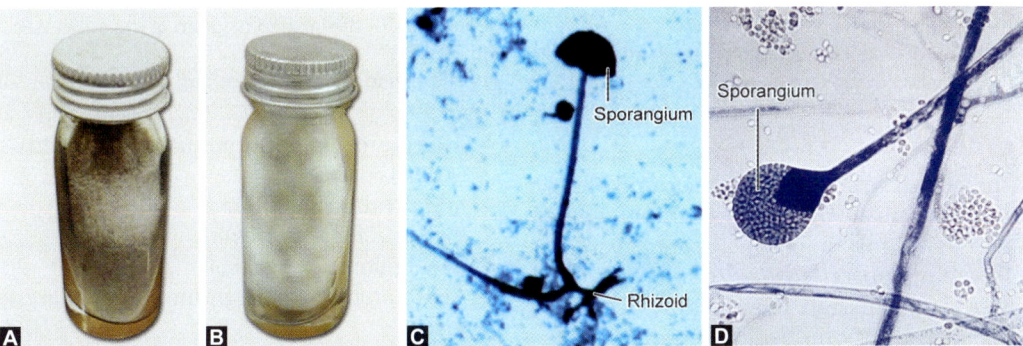

Figs 38.3A to D: (A) *Rhizopus* colony on SDA shows white cottony woolly colonies with black spores (salt and pepper appearance); (B) *Mucor* on SDA—white cottony woolly colonies; (C) LPCB mount of colonies of *Rhizopus* shows sporangium with rhizoid present; (D) LPCB mount of colonies of *Mucor* shows sporangium (absence of rhizoid).
Source: (A to C) Department of Microbiology, Pondicherry Institute of Medical Sciences, Puducherry; (D) Public Health Image Library/Dr Lucille K Georg, ID#:3960/Centers for Disease Control and Prevention (CDC), Atlanta (*with permission*).

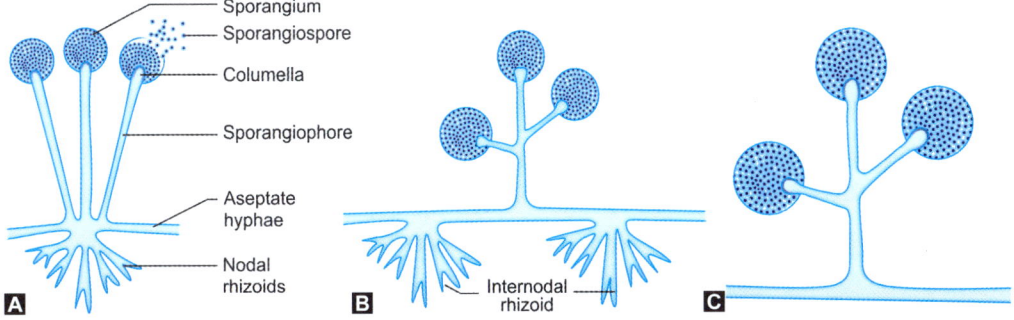

Figs 38.4A to C: Microscopic schematic diagram: (A) *Rhizopus;* (B) *Lichtheimia;* (C) *Mucor*.

Treatment

Amphotericin B remains the drug of choice for all forms of mucormycosis, except the mild localized skin lesions in immunocompetent patients, which can be removed surgically. Azoles are usually ineffective, except posaconazole.

ASPERGILLOSIS

Problem Solving Exercise 3

Aspergillosis

A 46-year-old lady complaints of hemoptysis for 2–3 episodes in 2 days and cough for 1 month.

She gave past history of pulmonary tuberculosis 10 years back. On chest examination, bilateral breath sounds were reduced. Chest X-ray revealed fungal ball in previous cavitary lesion in right upper lobe of lung. Sputum and lung biopsy were sent for fungal culture and identification (Figs 38.5, 38.7A and 38.8A).
1. What is the clinical diagnosis and the likely etiological agent based on the chest X-ray finding?
2. How can you confirm the diagnosis in the laboratory?
3. What are the other clinical manifestations caused by this organism?
4. Mention the treatment option for this clinical condition.
5. Draw a neat labeled diagram of microscopic appearance in LPCB mount?

Explanation

Clinical Diagnosis

History of hemoptysis, chronic cough, past history of pulmonary tuberculosis and chest X-ray showing fungal ball in previous cavitary lesion suggests fungal invasion into previously formed cavitary lesions in the lung. These clues suggest fungal ball due to *Aspergillus* infection in lung (Aspergilloma).

Identification

Histopathological staining reveals narrow septate hyphae (Fig. 38.5). Sputum culture on SDA showed smoky green, velvety to powdery colonies (Fig. 38.7A), and LPCB mount of the colonies showed conical-shaped vesicle, uniseriate phialides, and conidia arise from upper third of vesicle; hence, final identification of the causative agent is *Aspergillus fumigatus* (Fig. 38.8A) and for the labeled diagram of the agent (see Fig. 38.6A).

For answers to the other questions, refer below.

Introduction

Aspergillosis refers to the invasive and allergic diseases caused by a hyaline mold named *Aspergillus*. Important species are *Aspergillus fumigatus, Aspergillus flavus* and *Aspergillus niger*. Transmission of infection occurs by inhalation of airborne conidia.

Risk Factors

Risk factors for invasive aspergillosis are:
- Glucocorticoid use
- Profound neutropenia
- Neutrophil dysfunction
- Underlying pneumonia or chronic obstructive pulmonary disease, tuberculosis or sarcoidosis
- Antitumor necrosis factor therapy.

Clinical Manifestations

Pulmonary Aspergillosis

It is the most common form; appears in various forms, such as:

- Allergic bronchopulmonary aspergillosis (ABPA)
- Severe bronchial asthma
- Extrinsic allergic alveolitis
- Aspergilloma (fungal ball)
- Acute angioinvasive pulmonary aspergillosis
- Chronic cavitary pulmonary aspergillosis.

Other Types of Aspergillosis

- Invasive sinusitis
  - Invasive sinusitis (acute and chronic from)
  - Chronic granulomatous sinusitis
  - Allergic fungal sinusitis
- Cardiac aspergillosis
- Cerebral aspergillosis
- Ocular aspergillosis—keratitis and endophthalmitis
- Ear infection—otitis externa
- Cutaneous aspergillosis
- Nail bed infection—onychomycosis.

Clinical manifestations also depend on the species involved:

- *A. fumigatus* causes commonly—acute pulmonary and allergic aspergillosis
- *A. flavus* causes more commonly sinus, skin and ocular infections
- *A. niger* can cause invasive infection and causes otitis externa.

Laboratory Diagnosis
Specimens, such as sputum and tissue biopsies may be collected.

Direct Examination
Ten percent KOH mount or histopathological staining of specimens reveal characteristic narrow septate hyaline hyphae with acute angle branching (Fig. 38.5).

Culture
Specimens are inoculated onto SDA and incubated at 25°C. Species identification is done based on macroscopic and microscopic (LPCB mount) appearance of the colonies (Table 38.2).
- Colonies consist of hyaline septate hyphae from which conidiophores arise which end at vesicles. Vesicles are either tubular or globular in shape
- From the vesicle, finger-like projections of conidia-producing cells arise called as phialides or sterigmata. Phialides are arranged either in one or two rows, the first row is called as metulae

Table 38.2: Identification features of *Aspergillus* species.

Aspergillus	Macroscopic appearance of colony	Microscopic appearance (LPCB mount)
A. fumigatus (Figs 38.6A and 38.7A and 38.8A)	Colonies: Smoky green, velvety to powdery, reverse is white	Vesicle is conical-shaped Phialides are arranged in single row Conidia arise from upper third of vesicle Conidia are hyaline
A. flavus (Figs 38.6B and 38.7B and 38.8B)	Colonies: Yellow green, velvety, reverse is white	Vesicle is globular-shaped Phialides in one or two rows Conidia arise from upper two-third to entire vesicle Conidia are hyaline
A. niger (Figs 38.6C and 38.7C and 38.8C)	Colonies: Black, cottony type, reverse is white	Vesicle is globular shaped Phialides in two rows Conidia arise from entire vesicle Conidia are black

- Conidia arise from the vesicles either on their entire surface or only on the upper half (Figs 38.6A to C, 38.8A to C, Table 38.2).

Antigen Detection
- **β-d-Glucan antigen assay:** It is a marker of invasive fungal infections, raised in most invasive fungal infection including invasive aspergillosis
- **Galactomannan antigen:** This is an *Aspergillus* specific antigen, can be detected by ELISA in patient's sera or urine. It is useful for establishing early diagnosis.

Antibody Detection
- Detection of serum antibodies is very useful for chronic invasive aspergillosis and aspergilloma, where the culture is usually negative. Titer falls rapidly following clinical improvement
- In allergic syndromes such as ABPA and severe asthma, specific serum IgE levels are elevated.

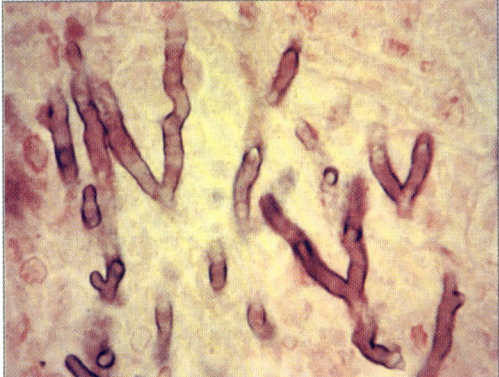

Fig. 38.5: Hematoxylin-eosin stained (H&E) lung section shows septate narrow hyphae—confirms invasive aspergillosis.
Source: Public Health Image Library/Armed Forces Institute of Pathology, Centers for Disease Control and Prevention (CDC), Atlanta; Dr Hardin, ID #15630 (*with permission*).

Treatment
- For invasive aspergillosis, voriconazole is the drug of choice
- For ABPA, itraconazole is the drug of choice

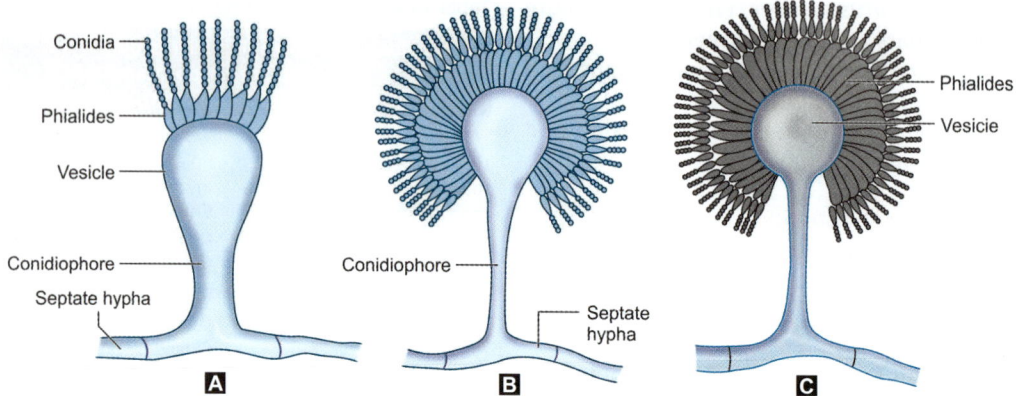

Figs 38.6A to C: Conidiation of various *Aspergillus* species (schematic diagram): (A) *A. fumigatus;* (B) *A. flavus;* (C) *A. niger.*

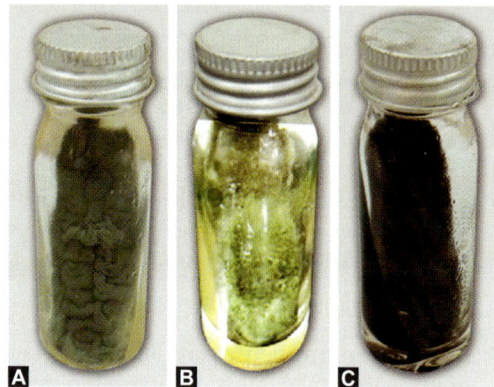

Figs 38.7A to C: *Aspergillus* (colonies on Sabouraud's dextrose agar): (A) *Aspergillus fumigatus;* (B) *Aspergillus flavus;* (C) *Aspergillus niger.*
Source: Department of Microbiology, Pondicherry Institute of Medical Sciences, Puducherry (*with permission*).

- For chronic pulmonary aspergillosis, itraconazole or voriconazole is the drug of choice
- For prophylaxis, posaconazole is indicated.

PENICILLIOSIS

Penicilliosis denotes the group of infections caused by pathogenic *Penicillium* species.

Clinical Disease

Penicillium species are most often environmental contaminants. Occasionally, they cause human infections.

Penicillium marneffei (a dimorphic fungus): Produces skin lesions

- Mycotoxicoses is caused by *Penicillium cyclopium, Penicillium verrucosum* and *Penicillium puberulum*

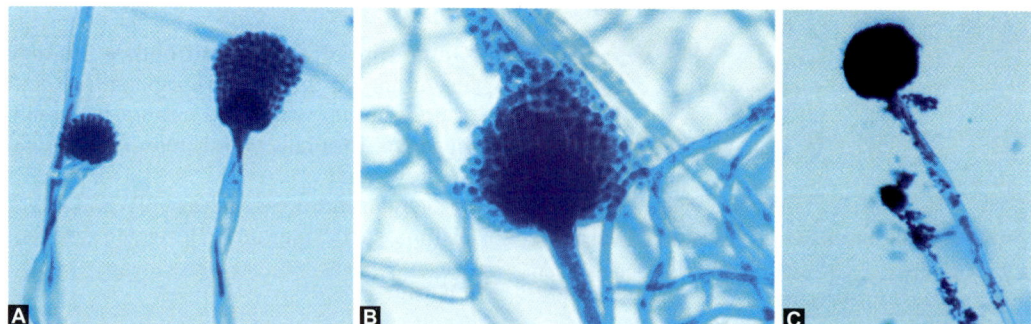

Figs 38.8A to C: *Aspergillus* microscopic picture (LPCB mount): (A) *Aspergillus fumigatus;* (B) *Aspergillus flavus;* (C) *Aspergillus niger.*
Source: Department of Microbiology, Pondicherry Institute of Medical Sciences, Puducherry (*with permission*).

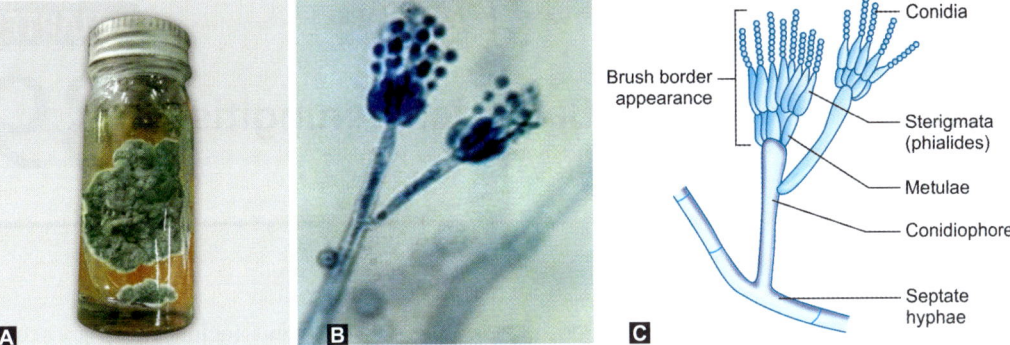

Figs 38.9A to C: *Penicillium* species: (A) Colonies on SDA; (B) Microscopic picture (LPCB mount); (C) Schematic microscopic picture.
Source: (A) Department of Microbiology, Pondicherry Institute of Medical Sciences, Puducherry; (B) Public Health Image Library/Lucille Georg, ID#:8398/Centers for Disease Control and Prevention (CDC), Atlanta (*with permission*).

- Endophthalmitis and endocarditis
- Otomycosis, keratitis and onychomycosis
- Allergic disease—asthma and allergic pneumonitis.

Laboratory Diagnosis

- *Penicillium* species occur as molds on SDA at 25°C (except for *P. marneffei* which is a dimorphic fungus)
- **Colonies** are rapid growing, flat with velvety to powdery texture and greenish in color (Fig. 38.9A)
- **Microscopic appearance:** LPCB mount of the colonies reveal hyaline thin septate hyphae, vesicles are absent, and conidiophore directly divides into elongated metulae, from which flask-shaped phialides originate which bear chain of conidia. Such an arrangement is called as *brush border appearance* (Figs 38.9B and C).

PNEUMOCYSTIS PNEUMONIA

Pneumocystis pneumonia (PcP) has been increasingly reported after the discovery of human immunodeficiency virus (HIV) or AIDS. Causative agent is *Pneumocystis jirovecii*.

Pathogenesis

- *Pneumocystis* exists in cyst and trophozoite forms
- Cysts are inhaled, carried to the lungs, transformed into trophozoite which induces an inflammatory response that leads to recruitment of plasma cells resulting in formation of *frothy exudate* filling the alveoli.

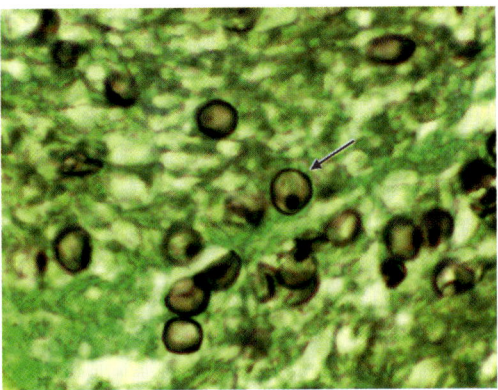

Fig. 38.10: Cysts of *Pneumocystis jirovecii* in an AIDS patient (methenamine silver stain).
Source: Public Health Image Library, Centers for Disease Control and Prevention (CDC), Atlanta; Dr Edwin P Ewing, Jr., ID #960 (*with permission*).

Laboratory Diagnosis

- Histopathological examination of lung tissue or fluids or open lung biopsy reveals *cysts*
- Gomori's methenamine silver (GMS) staining demonstrates the cysts of *P. jirovecii* (Fig. 38.10). The cysts resemble black-colored *crushed ping-pong balls*, against the green background
- *Pneumocystis* is not cultivable and there is no serological test available
- Polymerase chain reaction assays have been developed for detection of *P. jirovecii* specific genes.

Treatment

Cotrimoxazole is the drug of choice for *Pneumocystis* pneumonia.

CHAPTER 39
Bacterial Meningitis

ACUTE BACTERIAL MENINGITIS

Acute bacterial meningitis (also called as pyogenic meningitis), is an acute purulent infection within the subarachnoid space. It is characterized by elevated polymorphonuclear cells in CSF.

The agents implicated in pyogenic meningitis may vary according to the age.

- ❖ **Overall:** *Streptococcus pneumoniae* is the most common cause of pyogenic meningitis (~50%). Other agents include meningococcus (~25%), *Streptococcus agalactiae* (~15%), *Listeria* (~10%) and *Haemophilus influenzae* (<10%)
- ❖ **Neonates:** The common agents of neonatal meningitis include *Streptococcus agalactiae*, gram-negative bacilli, such as *Escherichia coli* and *Klebsiella,* and *Listeria monocytogenes*
- ❖ **Elderly (>60 years):** Common agents are *Streptococcus agalactiae* and *Listeria monocytogenes.*

Problem Solving Exercise 1

Meningococcal meningitis

A 7-year-old girl was admitted to the hospital with complaints of high-grade fever, headache, vomiting, altered mental status, seizure and neck rigidity. CSF sample was collected by lumbar puncture in a sterile container and sent to the laboratory for Gram staining (Fig. 39.1). Biochemical analysis of CSF revealed CSF pressure (200 mm of water), protein (260 mg/dL) and glucose (20 mg/dL). Cytological analysis of CSF revealed the total leukocyte count (2000 per mm³) which is predominantly neutrophilic.

1. What is the probable clinical diagnosis and the etiological agent?
2. Describe the laboratory diagnosis in detail.
3. What is the preferred treatment of choice in this case?

Explanation

Clinical Diagnosis

History of high-grade fever, headache, vomiting, altered mental status, seizure and neck rigidity is suggestive of meningitis.
CSF analysis is characteristic of pyogenic (acute bacterial) meningitis.
- ❑ **Biochemical analysis:** Elevated CSF pressure (>180 mm of water), markedly elevated protein (>250 mg/dL) and decreased glucose (<40 mg/dL)
- ❑ **Cytological analysis:** Increased total leukocyte count which is predominantly neutrophilic.

Etiological Diagnosis

Gram staining of CSF (Fig. 39.1) reveals capsulated gram-negative diplococci, with adjacent sides flattened. This is suggestive of presumptive identification as meningococcal meningitis (*Neisseria meningitidis*).

Treatment

Third-generation cephalosporins, such as ceftriaxone or cefotaxime is the drug of choice for meningococcal meningitis; given for 7 days. Penicillin can also be given; however, reduced meningococcal sensitivity to penicillin has been reported from few countries. For answers to the other questions, refer text.

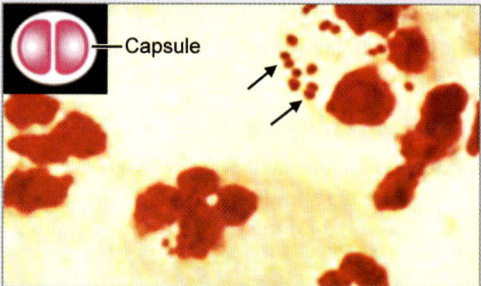

Fig. 39.1: Meningococci in CSF smear (gram-negative diplococci, lens-shaped) (arrows showing).
Source: Centers for Disease Control and Prevention (CDC), Atlanta (*with permission*).

Problem Solving Exercise 2

Pneumococcal meningitis

A 24-year-female was brought to the emergency room by her parents due to an acute onset of fever, neck rigidity and altered sensorium for the past 2 days. Physical examination showed that when her neck was passively flexed, her legs also flexed. Direct examination of the CSF is depicted in Figure 39.2.
1. Identify the clinical diagnosis of this condition and the most likely etiologic agent?
2. How will you confirm the etiological diagnosis in the laboratory?
3. What is the preferred treatment of choice in this case?

Explanation
Clinical Diagnosis
History of fever, neck rigidity and altered sensorium along with positive Brudzinski's sign (flexion of legs when neck was passively flexed) is suggestive of meningitis.

Etiological Diagnosis
Gram staining of CSF (Fig. 39.2) showed gram-positive, lanceolate-shaped diplococci surrounded by a clear halo (capsule). This is suggestive of presumptive identification as pneumococcal meningitis (*Streptococcus pneumoniae*).

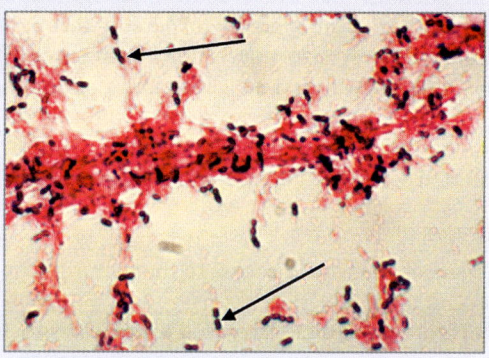

Fig. 39.2: Pneumococci in gram-stained smear of sputum [lanceolate-shaped gram-positive cocci in pair surrounded by clear halo (capsule)].
Source: Public Health Image Library, ID#/2896/Dr Mike Miller/ Centers for Disease Control and Prevention (CDC), Atlanta (*with permission*).

Treatment
As mortality is very high (~ 20%) in pneumococcal meningitis, treatment should be initiated as early as possible. Ceftriaxone ± vancomycin is given for 10–14 days.
For answers to the other questions, refer text.

Problem Solving Exercise 3

H. influenzae meningitis

A 7-year-old girl was admitted to the hospital with complaints of high-grade fever, altered mental status and neck rigidity. On examination, it was found that there was inability to straighten the leg when the hip is flexed to 90°. CSF sample was collected by lumbar puncture in a sterile container and sent to the laboratory for culture (Fig. 39.3).

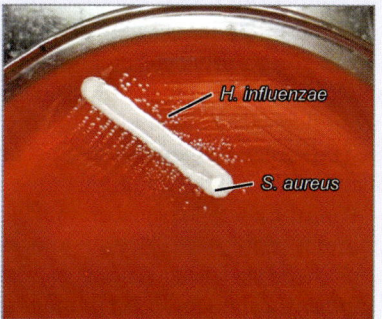

Fig. 39.3: Satellitism of *H. influenzae* around *S. aureus* streak line.
Source: Department of Microbiology, Pondicherry Institute of Medical Sciences, Puducherry (*with permission*).

1. What is the probable clinical diagnosis and the etiological agent?
2. What are the various tests you will perform from the CSF specimen for this case?
3. What is the preferred treatment of choice in this case?

Explanation
Clinical Diagnosis
History of fever, neck rigidity and altered sensorium along with positive Kernig's sign (severe stiffness of the hamstrings causes an inability to straighten the leg when the hip is flexed to 90°) is suggestive of meningitis.

Etiological Diagnosis
Culture on blood agar (Fig. 39.3). reveals larger colonies formed adjacent to *S. aureus* streak line and the size of the colonies decreased gradually away from the *S. aureus* streak line. This property is known as satellitism, which is a feature of *Haemophilus influenzae*.

Treatment
Third-generation cephalosporins, such as ceftriaxone or cefotaxime is the drug of choice.
For answers to the other questions, refer text.

Pathogenesis

The bacteria that cause acute meningitis are transmitted from person-to-person through droplets of respiratory secretions from cases or nasopharyngeal carriers. Close and prolonged contact—kissing, sneezing or coughing on someone, or living in close quarters with an infected person facilitate the spread of the disease.

Routes of Infection

Organisms may gain access to the meninges by several routes:
- **Hematogenous spread:** This is the most common route, where entry into the subarachnoid space is gained through the choroid plexus or through other blood vessels of the brain
- **Direct spread from an infected site** present close to meninges—otitis media, mastoiditis, sinusitis, etc.
- **Anatomical defect in central nervous system (CNS):** It may occur as a result of surgery, trauma, congenital defects, which can allow organisms for ready and easy access to CNS.

Clinical Manifestations

The average incubation period is 4 days but can range between 2 and 10 days. Patients with meningitis develop various manifestations, such as:
- **Important symptoms** include fever, vomiting, intense headache, altered consciousness and occasionally photophobia
- **Signs of meningism** (meningeal irritation), such as:
    - **Nuchal rigidity** ("stiff neck") is the pathognomonic sign of meningeal irritation and is present when the neck resists passive flexion
    - **Kernig's sign**: Severe stiffness of the hamstrings causes an inability to straighten the leg when the hip is flexed to 90° (Fig. 39.4A)
    - **Brudzinski's sign:** When the neck is passively flexed, results in spontaneous flexion of the hips and knees (Fig. 39.4B).
- **In infants:** Pyogenic meningitis in infants may have a slower onset, signs may be nonspecific, and neck stiffness may not be present.

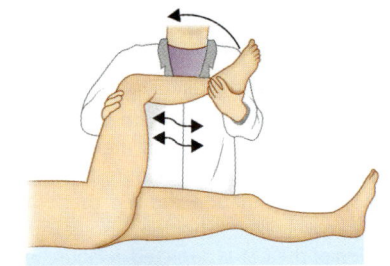
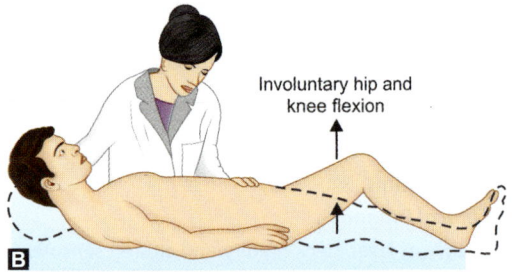

Figs 39.4A and B: Signs seen in meningitis: (A) Kernig's sign; (B) Brudzinski's sign.

Babies usually present with fever, irritability and bulging fontanelle
- **Complications:** In due course, the disease may involve brain parenchyma leading to meningoencephalitis—that may result in decreased consciousness, seizures, raised intracranial pressure, and stroke
- **Organism specific finding**, e.g., purpuric rashes seen in meningococcal meningitis.

Laboratory Diagnosis

Specimen Collection and Transport

CSF is the most ideal specimen for pyogenic meningitis. Blood culture is another useful specimen for culture.
- **CSF collection:** CSF is obtained by lumbar puncture under strict aseptic conditions. It is divided into three sterile containers; one each for cell count, biochemical analysis and bacteriological examination
- **CSF transport:** CSF being the most precious specimen should be examined immediately
    - When the bacteriological examination (culture) is required, CSF should never be refrigerated as delicate pathogens, such as *H. influenzae*, pneumococci or meningococci may die. Therefore if a delay is expected, it may be kept in an incubator at 37°C

CHAPTER 39 ◆ Bacterial Meningitis

Table 39.1: Cytological and biochemical parameters in CSF of normal individuals and in different types of meningitis.

Characteristics	Normal individual	Pyogenic meningitis	Tuberculous meningitis	Viral meningitis
CSF pressure (mm of water)	Normal (50–150)	Highly elevated (>180)	Moderately elevated	Slightly elevated/normal
Total leukocyte count (per mm³)	0–5	100–10,000	10–500	25–500
Predominant cell type	Lymphocytes	Neutrophils	Lymphocytes	Lymphocytes
Glucose (mg%)	40–70	<40 mg/dL (decreased to absent)	20–40 mg/dL (slightly decreased)	Normal
Total proteins (mg%)	15–45	>45 mg/dL (usually >250; markedly increased)	100–500 mg/dL (moderate to markedly increased)	20–80 mg/dL (normal or slightly elevated)

- However for molecular diagnosis, CSF can be kept inside the freezer.

Other useful specimens for isolation of etiological agents of pyogenic meningitis are:
- ❖ **Blood culture:** Blood should be collected in automated blood culture bottles, such as BacT/ALERT
- ❖ **For suspected meningococcal meningitis:** Other useful specimens are nasopharyngeal swabs, pus or scrapings from rashes; which should be carried in transport media (such as Stuart's medium). These specimens are inoculated onto selective media, such as Thayer Martin medium or New York City medium, to suppress the growth of normal flora.

Cytological and Biochemical Analysis

Biochemical analysis and cell count of CSF give a preliminary clue about the type of meningitis (Table 39.1)
In acute bacterial (pyogenic) meningitis:
- ❖ CSF usually contains >1000 leukocytes/μL and predominantly neutrophils (90-95%). However in *Listeria* meningitis, there is increased lymphocyte count in CSF
- ❖ The total protein content is elevated and the glucose level is markedly diminished or even absent
- ❖ CSF pressure is highly elevated.

CSF Microscopy (Gram Staining)

Microscopic examination of gram-stained smear may give a preliminary clue about the etiological agent of pyogenic meningitis based on the morphology of the bacteria (Table 39.2).

Table 39.2: Preliminary clue about the etiological agents of pyogenic meningitis based on CSF Gram stain.

Appearance in CSF Gram stain	Suggestive of
Gram-positive diplococci, flame or lanceolate-shaped with clear halo (capsulated) (Fig. 39.2)	*Streptococcus pneumoniae*
Gram-negative diplococci, capsulated, with adjacent sides flattened (lens or half-moon shaped) (Fig. 39.1)	*Neisseria meningitidis*
Pleomorphic gram-negative coccobacilli (Fig. 34.5A)	*Haemophilus influenzae*
Gram-negative bacilli, arranged singly	*Escherichia coli* or others
Gram-positive cocci in short chain	*Streptococcus agalactiae*
Gram-positive short bacilli, often confused with diphtheroids	*Listeria monocytogenes*

- ❖ This helps in early initiation of appropriate empirical antimicrobial therapy
- ❖ **Heaped smear:** As the bacterial load in CSF may be very low, to increase the sensitivity, several drops of CSF should be placed at the same spot on the slide, each drop being allowed to air dry before the next is added
- ❖ **Centrifugation:** Alternatively, CSF can be centrifuged (by cytospin) and the deposit is examined for Gram staining.

Direct Antigen Detection

From CSF: After centrifugation of CSF, the supernatant can be used for antigen detection. Latex agglutination test is performed using latex beads coated with anti-capsular antibodies.

- It is available for detection of capsular antigens of common agents of meningitis, such as *S. pneumoniae, S. agalactiae, N. meningitidis, H. influenzae* or *E. coli*
- Detection of capsular antigens in CSF is more sensitive than CSF microscopy.

From urine: Antigen detection in urine is useful for pneumococcal meningitis. Immunochromatographic test (ICT) is available to detect the C-polysaccharide antigen of *S. pneumoniae* in urine.

Culture

Ideal media for bacteriological culture of CSF are enriched media, such as chocolate agar and blood agar, and differential media, such as MacConkey agar
- **Enriching:** As the bacterial load is very low, a part of the CSF can be inoculated into enriched media, such as blood culture bottles at the bed side (preferred) or brain heart infusion (BHI) broth in the laboratory
- **Blood culture** can be collected in conventional blood culture bottles, such as BHI broth/agar or preferably in automated blood cultures (e.g., BacT/ALERT)
- **Culture plates** (blood agar and chocolate agar) are incubated at 37°C, preferably in candle jar (provides 5% CO_2) for 48 hours
- **Identification:** Colonies grown on solid media are processed for identification of the organism either by automated identification system, such as MALDI-TOF or VITEK, or by conventional biochemical tests (Table 39.3)
- **Antimicrobial susceptibility test** should be done to initiate definitive antimicrobial therapy. It is carried out by disk diffusion test or preferably by automated MIC-based methods, such as VITEK
- **Sensitivity:** CSF and blood cultures may take >48 hours for organism identification and are positive in 70–85% of patients with bacterial meningitis. However, sensitivity drops rapidly in case of prior antimicrobial therapy or delay in processing

Table 39.3: Culture and identification properties of common bacterial agents of pyogenic meningitis.

Common bacterial agents of pyogenic meningitis and their culture and identification properties
Streptococcus pneumoniae (Chapter 34)
• **Culture:** It produces α-hemolytic colonies on blood agar, described as draughtsman-shaped or carrom coin appearance
• **Biochemical identification:** It shows bile soluble, ferments inulin and sensitive to optochin
Neisseria meningitidis
It produces non-hemolytic colonies on blood agar, which on smear shows gram-negative diplococci (Fig. 39.1)
• **Biochemical identification:** Meningococci are catalase and oxidase positive. They ferment glucose and maltose but not sucrose
• **Serogrouping:** Slide agglutination serogrouping (SASG) test is done to identify the serogroups of meningococci isolates by using appropriate antisera
Haemophilus influenzae (Chapter 34)
• **Culture:** Blood agar with *S. aureus* streak line shows satellitism.
• **Biochemical identification:** Disk test for X and V factor requirement shows growth surrounding combined XV disk
Streptococcus agalactiae (Chapter 29)
• **Culture:** It produces β-hemolytic colonies on blood agar, which on smear shows gram-positive cocci in short chain
• **Biochemical identification:** It shows CAMP test positive and resistance to bacitracin
• **Serogrouping** with group specific antisera shows Lancefield group B
Gram-negative bacilli meningitis
• *Escherichia coli* and *Klebsiella* produce lactose-fermenting colonies on MacConkey agar; identified by ICUT tests
• Non-fermenters: *Pseudomonas* is oxidase positive, whereas *Acinetobacter* is oxidase negative. They produce non-lactose fermenting colonies; identified by ICUT tests (Chapter 36)
Listeria monocytogenes
• **Motility:** It shows **tumbling type of motility** at 25°C but non-motile at 37°C (called **differential motility,** which is due to temperature dependent flagella expression)
• **Culture:** It grows on blood agar (β-hemolytic colonies), and chocolate agar.
Note: Selective media, such as **PALCAM agar** (containing mixture of antibiotics) may be useful for isolation of *Listeria* from specimens, such as food and environmental samples.
Abbreviations: ICUT tests, indole, citrate, urease and triple sugar iron agar test; CAMP, Christie, Atkins, and Munch-Peterson test.

- Therefore, **rapid diagnostic tests**, such as antigen detection or molecular test should be considered to determine the bacterial etiology of pyogenic meningitis.

Serology

Antibodies to capsular antigens of meningococci can be detected in patient's serum by ELISA. This is useful to study seroprevalence and to know the response to vaccination; not for diagnosis.

Molecular Methods

Molecular tests are highly sensitive, detect even few bacteria in CSF with less turnaround time than culture and also help in serogroup identification.
- **Formats:** Multiplex PCR and multiplex real-time PCR can be used for simultaneous detection of common agents of pyogenic meningitis
- **BioFire FilmArray** is an automated nested multiplex PCR commercially available, which can simultaneously detect 14 common agents of meningitis (both pyogenic and viral) in CSF, with a turnaround time of 1 hour
- **Common genes** targeted include:
  - For meningococcus: *ctrA* (capsule transport gene) and *sodC* (Cu-Zn superoxide dismutase gene)
  - For pneumococcus: *lytA* (autolysin gene), *ply* (pneumolysin) and *psaA* (pneumococcus surface antigen A)
  - For *H. influenzae*: Conserved capsular gene *bexA*.

Treatment of Pyogenic Meningitis

The mortality of pyogenic meningitis is very high (~20% for pneumococci) and among the survivors, up to 50% develop complications. Therefore, treatment should be initiated as early as possible.

The choice of antimicrobial agent is based on the type of organism suspected and good CSF penetration ability of the agent.

Empirical therapy comprises of:
- **Adult:** IV cefotaxime or ceftriaxone and vancomycin is the recommended regimen. If *Listeria* is suspected, IV ampicillin can be added to the regimen
- **For neonates:** IV ampicillin plus gentamicin is the recommended regimen
- **IV dexamethasone** is added to the regimen to reduce intracranial pressure.

Definitive therapy: After the culture report is available, the empirical therapy is modified based on the organism isolated and its antimicrobial susceptibility pattern.

CHRONIC BACTERIAL MENINGITIS

Several bacterial meningitis present as chronic stage, characterized by persistence of signs and symptoms as well as the CSF abnormality for >4 weeks. The bacterial agents causing chronic meningitis include the following.
- Partially treated pyogenic meningitis
- Parameningeal infections (e.g., otitis media)
- *Mycobacterium tuberculosis*
- *Borrelia burgdorferi* (Lyme disease)
- *Treponema pallidum* (tertiary syphilis)
- Rare bacterial agents, such as *Nocardia*, *Actinomyces*, *Tropheryma whipplei*, *Leptospira* and *Brucella*.

Tuberculous Meningitis (TBM)

TBM results from the hematogenous spread of primary or post-primary pulmonary TB. Typically, the disease evolves over 1–2 weeks or longer, which differentiates it from bacterial meningitis.

Clinical Features

TBM often presents subtly as headache, slight mental changes, low-grade fever, malaise, night sweat, anorexia, and irritability.
- Subsequently, it may evolve acutely with severe headache, confusion, lethargy, altered sensorium, and neck rigidity
- Cranial nerves paresis (ocular nerves in particular) is a frequent finding. Stroke may occur due to involvement of cerebral arteritis
- Ultimately, it progresses towards coma, with hydrocephalus and intracranial hypertension.

Laboratory Diagnosis

- **CSF analysis:** Examination of CSF reveals (Table 39.1):

- High leukocyte count (up to 1,000/μL), mostly lymphocytic. However, neutrophils may be elevated in the early stage
- Protein content of 100–800 mg/dL
- Low glucose concentration.

However, it should be noted that any of these three parameters can be within the normal range.

❖ **Cobweb coagulum:** When CSF is kept in a tube for 12 hours, a coagulum forms in the form of a cobweb due to higher fibrin content in the fluid

❖ **Acid-fast staining of CSF:** Direct smear of CSF sediment may reveal long slender beaded acid-fast bacilli
  - However, the sensitivity of acid-fast stain is very low (10–40%) and may require repeated lumbar punctures to increase the yield
  - Acid-fast staining of cobweb may give better yield as TB bacilli may be trapped in the cobweb. However, fibrin strands in the cobweb may be mistaken as fungi.

❖ **Culture of CSF** is diagnostic in up to 80% of cases and remains as the gold standard test. However, culture is time consuming, takes 4–8 weeks by Lowenstein-Jensen medium and 2–3 weeks by automated liquid culture, such as Mycobacteria Growth Indicator Tube (MGIT)

❖ **GeneXpert assay:** It is an automated real-time PCR, has a sensitivity of up to 80% and is the preferred initial diagnostic option. In addition to detection of *M. tuberculosis,* it can also detect resistance to rifampicin

❖ **Imaging studies** (CT and MRI) may show hydrocephalus and abnormal enhancement of basal cisterns. In more than half of cases, evidence of old pulmonary lesions or a miliary pattern is found on chest X-ray.

Treatment

If unrecognized, TBM is invariably fatal. Treatment should be initiated immediately upon a positive GeneXpert MTB/RIF result. It responds well to anti-tubercular therapy, if started early.

CHAPTER 40

Viral Meningitis and Viral Encephalitis

■ VIRAL MENINGITIS

Problem Solving Exercise 1

Viral Meningitis

A 12-year-old girl was admitted to the hospital with complaints of high-grade fever, headache, vomiting, altered mental status, seizure and neck rigidity. Biochemical and cytological analysis of CSF sample revealed glucose level (40 mg/dL), CSF pressure (100 mm H_2O), protein (60 mg/dL) and cell count (25/μL), which is predominantly lymphocytic. No organisms were detected in Gram staining and Indian ink staining of CSF.

1. What is the probable clinical diagnosis and the probable etiological agent(s)?
2. Describe the laboratory diagnosis in detail.
3. What is the preferred treatment of choice in this case?

Explanation

Clinical Diagnosis

History of high-grade fever, headache, vomiting, altered mental status, seizure and neck rigidity is suggestive of meningitis.

- **Biochemical and cytological analysis** of CSF sample is suggestive of viral meningitis.
  - *Biochemical analysis:* Normal glucose level (40 mg/dL), mildly elevated CSF pressure (100 mm H_2O) and slightly elevated protein (60 mg/dL)
  - *Cytological analysis:* Mildly increased cell count (25/μL), which is predominantly lymphocytic. This is suggestive of viral meningitis
  - No organisms were detected on Gram staining and Indian ink staining of CSF.
- **Etiological agents** of viral meningitis include enteroviruses (most common cause, accounting for >85% of cases), herpes simplex and arboviruses
- **Molecular methods:** Multiplex PCR and multiplex real-time PCR can be used for simultaneous detection of common agents of viral meningitis.

For answers to the other questions, refer text.

Viral meningitis, inflammation of subarachnoid space due to viral etiology. It is the second most common type of meningitis, next to acute bacterial meningitis. However, it is often less severe than bacterial meningitis and has a better prognosis.

Epidemiology

- ❖ **People at risk:** Although people of any age can get viral meningitis, some have a higher risk of acquiring the disease, including:
  - Children (<5 years old) and old age
  - Immunocompromised individuals, chemotherapy or transplant recipients.
- ❖ **Transmission:** Close contacts with infected patients is necessary for the transmission to set in
- ❖ **Seasonality:** Most cases of viral meningitis occur from nonwinter months (from late spring to fall), the time when enteroviruses and arbovirus spread most often.

Clinical Manifestations

Common symptoms in children and adults include fever, headache (frontal or retro-orbital), stiff neck (milder than bacterial meningitis), photophobia, sleepiness or trouble in waking up from sleep, nausea, irritability, vomiting, lack of appetite (poor eating in babies), and lethargy.

Note: Seizures or focal neurologic signs, or profound alterations in consciousness, such as coma, or marked confusion does not occur in viral meningitis and suggest the presence of encephalitis or other alternative diagnoses.

Laboratory Diagnosis

Laboratory diagnosis of viral meningitis includes the following investigations.

CSF Analysis (Cytological and Biochemical)

Examination of CSF reveals the following (Table 39.1, Chapter 39).
- Normal or slightly elevated protein level (20–80 mg/dL)
- Normal glucose level (rarely low glucose level may occur, as in cytomegalovirus meningitis)
- Normal or mildly elevated CSF pressure (100–350 mm H_2O)
- **Cell count** is typically 25–500/µL, although in some viral meningitis (e.g., LCM virus and mumps) the cell counts of several thousands/µL may be seen
- **Pleocytosis:** Lymphocytes are typically the predominant cell type, although neutrophils may predominate in the first 48 h of illness in some viral meningitis (e.g., West Nile virus)
- Organisms are not seen on Gram staining of CSF.

Molecular Methods

Molecular methods have become the gold standard method for diagnosing viral meningitis, appears to be more sensitive than viral cultures.
- Amplification of specific viral DNA or RNA from CSF by PCR-based method provides definitive diagnosis
- PCR of throat washings or stool specimen may assist in the diagnosis of enterovirus infections
- **Formats:** Multiplex PCR and multiplex real-time PCR can be used for simultaneous detection of common agents of viral meningitis
- **BioFire FilmArray** is an automated nested multiplex PCR commercially available that can simultaneously detect 14 common agents of meningitis in CSF, which include agents of pyogenic and viral meningitis. It is extremely sensitive and specific, with a turnaround time of 1 hour.

Viral Culture

The sensitivity of CSF cultures for the diagnosis of viral meningitis is generally poor.
- In addition to CSF, specific viruses may also be isolated from throat swabs, stool, blood, and urine
- However, isolation of enteroviruses from stool is not diagnostic as it may also result from residual fecal shedding from a previous infection.

Antibody Detection

Antibody detection is important for the diagnosis of less prevalent arboviruses, such as West Nile virus, however, it is of less useful for viruses that have a high seroprevalence in the general population, such as HSV and VZV.

Treatment of Viral Meningitis

Treatment of almost all cases of viral meningitis is **primarily symptomatic**, which includes use of analgesics, antipyretics, antiemetics and fluid and electrolyte replacement. Antivirals may be useful for certain viral agents.
- Oral or intravenous acyclovir may be of benefit in patients with meningitis caused by HSV-1 or 2 and in cases of severe EBV or VZV infection
- Patients with HIV meningitis should receive highly active antiretroviral therapy.

Agents Causing Viral Meningitis

Non-polio Enterovirus Infections

Non-polio enteroviruses are the most common cause of viral meningitis, accounting for >85% of cases in which a specific etiology can be identified.
- Cases may either be sporadic or occur in clusters
- Although cases can occur throughout the year, affecting any age, but majority occur in the summer and rainfall, especially in children
- Examples include Coxsackieviruses, echoviruses, parechoviruses and Enterovirus 71.

HSV Meningitis

Herpes simplex viruses (HSV) are the second most common cause of viral meningitis, next to enteroviruses; accounting for 5% of cases. Adults are commonly affected than children.

- HSV-2 is a more frequent cause of meningitis than HSV-1; in contrast to HSV encephalitis, where HSV-1 accounts for >90% of cases
- **History of genital herpes** may be an important clue as HSV meningitis can occur in ~25–35% of women and ~10–15% of men at the time of an initial (primary) episode of genital herpes.

Mollaret Meningitis

HSV typically produces a chronic recurrent lymphocytic meningitis, called as **Mollaret meningitis**; characterized by repeated episodes of meningitis, typically lasting two to five days; occurring weeks to years apart. It can also be caused by EBV.

■ VIRAL ENCEPHALITIS

Encephalitis is an acute inflammation of the brain parenchyma, caused by invasion of infectious agents—most often viruses; rarely by parasites. The common etiological agents of viral encephalitis is enlisted in Table 40.1. The parasitic causes of encephalitis (e.g., *Toxoplasma*) is discussed in Chapter 41.

Clinical Manifestations

In addition to the acute febrile illness, the patients with encephalitis commonly present with the following features depending upon the site of involved:
- Altered level of consciousness (confusion) or a depressed level of consciousness ranging from mild lethargy to coma
- Seizures: Focal or generalized seizures
- Neuropsychiatric manifestations, such as hallucinations, agitation, personality change, behavioral disorders, and, at times, a frankly psychotic state
- Focal or diffuse neurologic signs: The common focal findings are:
  - Aphasia, ataxia, upper or lower motor neuron patterns of weakness
  - Involuntary movements (e.g., myoclonic jerks, tremor)
  - Cranial nerve deficits (e.g., ocular palsies, facial weakness).
- Features of meningitis (if involved), such as neck rigidity
- Involvement of the hypothalamic-pituitary axis may result in temperature dysregulation, diabetes insipidus, etc.

Table 40.1: Agents of viral encephalitis and encephalopathy.

Viral encephalitis
Herpesviruses   • Herpes simplex virus (HSV-1>HSV-2): The most common cause of sporadic encephalitis   • Cytomegalovirus (in immunocompromised host)   • Human herpesvirus 6   • Varicella-zoster virus   • Epstein-Barr virus
Arboviruses: Important ones in India are: • Japanese encephalitis virus (the most common cause of epidemic encephalitis in India)   • West Nile virus (the most common cause of epidemic encephalitis in USA)
Rabies virus: Causes encephalitis following dog bite
Nipah and **Hendra** viruses
Rare causes: Enteroviruses and mumps virus

CSF analysis: The characteristic CSF profile in encephalitis is indistinguishable from that of viral meningitis; typically consists of a lymphocytic pleocytosis, a mildly elevated protein level, and a normal glucose level.

Problem Solving Exercise 2

HSV Encephalitis

A 7-year-old boy presented with high-grade fever, vomiting altered consciousness (confusion), seizures, personality change, aphasia, ataxia, and tremor for 3 days. Cerebrospinal fluid (CSF) specimen collected by lumbar puncture was sent for a multiplex polymerase chain reaction (PCR) for vial etiology (see below) (Fig. 40.1).

1. What is the clinical diagnosis?
2. Identify the causative organism based on the test result.
3. List the clinical conditions caused by this organism.

4. How this clinical condition can be diagnosed in the laboratory?
5. How will you treat this condition?

Explanation

Clinical Diagnosis

History of high-grade fever, altered consciousness (confusion), seizures, personality change, and focal or diffuse neurologic signs (aphasia, ataxia, and tremor)—suggestive of encephalitis.

Etiological Diagnosis

The multiplex PCR done here (Fig. 40.1) is for herpes simplex virus (HSV)-1 and 2. Band of 391 bp appeared for test region which coincides with HSV-1 band in positive control. This confirms the diagnosis as HSV-1 infection.
For answers to other questions, refer below.

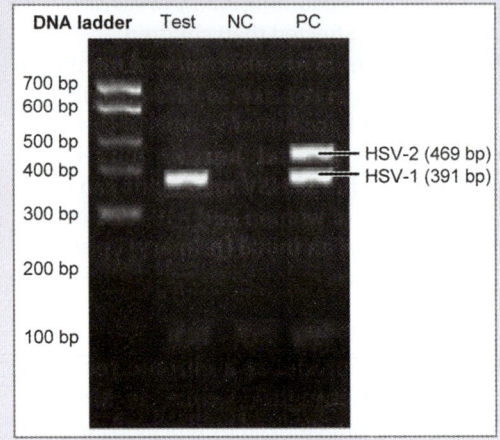

Fig. 40.1: Multiplex PCR for herpes meningitis.
Abbreviations: HSV, herpes simplex virus; NC, negative control; PC, positive control.

Problem Solving Exercise 3

Japanese Encephalitis

A 10-year-old boy is presented to causality with fever, mental confusion, disorientation, delirium and seizures. The CSF specimen collected was sent to microbiology laboratory for molecular diagnosis by real time PCR, which detected JE virus specific envelope (E) gene.
1. What is the clinical diagnosis and the etiological agent?
2. What is the mode of transmission and amplifier host?
3. Which district of India reported highest endemicity for this disease?
4. What are the vaccines available?

Explanation

Clinical and Etiological Diagnosis

History of fever, mental confusion, disorientation, delirium, seizures in a 10-year-old boy is suggestive of acute encephalitis syndrome.
Real time PCR detected JE virus specific envelope (E) gene in CSF; confirms the etiology to be Japanese encephalitis virus.
For answers to other questions, refer below.

HSV Encephalitis

HSV is the most common cause (10–20%) of acute sporadic viral encephalitis, most frequently involving temporal lobe. HSV-1 is more common (95%) than HSV-2.
- Children generally get primary HSV infection, acquired exogenously and invades CNS via the olfactory bulb; whereas adults get recurrent infections due to reactivation of HSV in trigeminal nerve
- Clinical manifestation is same as for viral encephalitis described earlier
- **Laboratory diagnosis:** Detection of viral DNA in CSF remains the mainstay of diagnosis
- **Treatment:** IV acyclovir (10 mg/kg q8h) is given for 10 days or until HSV DNA is no longer detected in CSF.

Japanese Encephalitis

Japanese encephalitis virus is the leading cause of vaccine preventable viral encephalitis in Asia, including India. It is an arbovirus, belongs to family Flaviviridae. It is an enveloped virus, containing ssRNA.
- **Vector:** JE virus is transmitted by bite of *Culex* mosquito. *C. tritaeniorhynchus* is the major vector worldwide including India. *C. vishnui* is the next common vector found in India
- **Animal hosts:** JE virus has several animal hosts. **Pigs** have been incriminated as the major vertebrate host; considered as the **amplifier host** for JE. Cattle and buffaloes may act as mosquito attractants
- **Geographical distribution:** Currently, JE is endemic in Southeast Asian region. **In India,**

JE is endemic in 15 states; Uttar Pradesh (Gorakhpur district) accounted for the largest burden in past.

Clinical Manifestations

JE is the most common cause of epidemic encephalitis. The incubation period is 5–15 days. Majority of infections are asymptomatic (iceberg phenomenon). **Clinical course** of the disease can be divided into three stages:
1. **Prodromal stage** of febrile illness
2. **Acute encephalitis stage:** JE is the most common cause of acute encephalitis syndrome (AES) in India; characterized by an acute onset of fever, mental confusion, disorientation, delirium, seizures (among children), or coma
3. **Late stage and sequelae:** It is the convalescent stage in which the patient may be recovered fully or retain some neurological deficits permanently (up to 50%).

Laboratory Diagnosis

- **IgM capture antibody (MAC) ELISA** supplied by NIV, Pune has been the recommended method for diagnosis of JE. It is a two-step sandwich ELISA, uses JERA (JE recombinant antigen) to detect JE-specific IgM antibody in serum. Refer Figure 8.4B (Chapter 8) for detail
- **Molecular methods:** Reverse-transcriptase (RT) PCR and real time RT-PCR have been developed to detect JE virus specific envelope (E) gene in blood.

Treatment of JE is only by supportive measures; no specific antiviral drugs are available.

Vaccine Prophylaxis

The following JE vaccines are licensed in India.
- **Live attenuated SA 14-14-2 vaccine** (prepared from SA 14-14-2 strain of JE virus)
  - It is cell line-derived; primary hamster kidney cell lines are commonly used
  - Under National Immunization Program, it is given to 231 endemic districts of states, such as—UP, Bihar, Assam, West Bengal and Karnataka
  - Schedule: Two doses; 1st at 9 completed months-12 months of age and 2 nd at 16–24 months.
- **Inactivated JE vaccine:** It is inactivated, Vero cell culture-derived vaccine.

RABIES ENCEPHALITIS

Problem Solving Exercise 4

Rabies Encephalitis

A 25-year-old man is bitten by a street dog, which was barking excessively and very agitated in behavior. Four days later, the dog was found dead. Brain biopsy of the dog was done and sent for histopathological staining (Fig. 40.2A). The electron micrograph of the causative agent is also shown in Figures 40.4A and B.
- What is the most probable diagnosis based on histopathology and electron micrograph given in Fig. 40.2B.
- What are the various modalities of diagnosis of this disease?
- How will you manage this case of dog bite?

Explanation

Clinical Diagnosis

This is proven case of Rabies. Points in favor are:
- History of dog bite (dog bite without provocation) with abnormal behavior and dog died within 4 days.

- *Dog brain biopsy*: Showed Negri bodies (Fig. 40.2A)
- *Electron micrograph*: Showed bullet-shaped rabies virus (Fig. 40.2B).

(For answers to other questions, refer below).

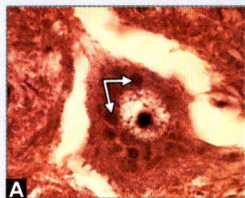 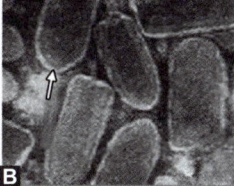

Figs 40.2A and B: (A) Histopathological biopsy from brain and (B) Electron micrograph of the causative agent.
Source: Public Health Image Library, (A) ID# 3377; (B) ID# 5611; Centers for Disease Control and Prevention, Atlanta (*with permission*).

Clinical Manifestations of Rabies

Rabies is transmitted by—(1) animal bite (mainly dog, but can be any animals); (2) exposure to bat (inhalation); and (3) corneal transplantation. Symptoms appear after an incubation period of 1-12 weeks; categorized into two types.
1. **Encephalitic rabies**: Most common (80%); characterized by—
   - Hyperexcitability and agitation
   - Autonomic dysfunction features
   - Hydrophobia (fear of water) or aerophobia.
2. **Paralytic or dumb rabies**: Occurs in 20% of cases. Hydrophobia will be absent. Paralytic features predominate.

Laboratory Diagnosis

Rabies Antigen Detection

Direct immunofluorescence test is performed to detect rabies nucleoprotein antigens in specimens (hair follicle of nape of neck or corneal impression smear) by using specific monoclonal antibodies tagged with fluorescent dye.

Viral Isolation

- Intracerebral inoculation into suckling mice
- **Cell lines**: Mouse neuroblastoma cell lines and baby hamster kidney cell lines are the preferred cell lines.

Antibody Detection

Detection of cerebrospinal fluid antibodies is more significant than serum antibodies. Various antibody detection tests include:
- Mouse neutralization test (MNT)
- Rapid fluorescent focus inhibition test (RFFIT)
- Fluorescent antibody virus neutralization (FAVN)
- Indirect fluorescence assay (IFA).

Viral RNA Detection

Reverse transcriptase PCR can be used to amplify genes of rabies virus RNA from fixed or unfixed brain tissue. It is the most sensitive and specific assay available presently.

Negri Body Detection

It is useful for postmortem diagnosis of rabies.
- They are intracytoplasmic eosinophilic inclusions with characteristic basophilic inner granules
- Sharply demarcated, spherical to oval, and about 2–10 μm in size (Fig. 40.2A)
- Most common sites of Negri bodies are neurons of cerebellum and hippocampus; however, they can also be less frequently seen in cortical and brainstem neurons
- Commonly used stains are: Histological stains, such as hematoxylin and eosin and Sellers stains (basic fuchsin and methylene blue in methanol)
- Negri body is pathognomonic of rabies. However, it may not be detected in 20% of cases. Therefore, the absence of Negri bodies does not rule out the diagnosis of rabies.

Prevention of Human Rabies (WHO Guideline 2018)

Rabies is prevented by providing prophylactic measures, such as post-exposure prophylaxis (PEP) and pre-exposure prophylaxis (PrEP).

PEP For Individuals not Received Vaccine

Post-exposure prophylaxis (PEP) consists of three components—local wound care, rabies vaccine and rabies immunoglobulin (RIG). Inclusion of these components in PEP depends upon the risk of exposure. WHO has classified the exposures into three categories (Table 40.2).
- **For category I exposures:** Require only wound care. Vaccine or RIG are not required
- **For category II exposures:** Require local wound care and rabies vaccine. RIG is not required except for immunodeficient individuals who need RIG in addition
- **For category III exposures:** All three components of PEP are required, such as local wound care, rabies vaccine and RIG.

Local Wound Care

It consists of the following measures:
- **Physical cleansing** of bite wounds with soap and water, followed by antiseptics, such as povidone iodine or alcohol

Table 40.2: Risk categorization and recommended anti-rabies prophylaxis (WHO, 2018).

Category of risk	Type of exposure	Recommended prophylaxis (WHO**)
Category I (No risk)	• Touching, or feeding of animal • Licks on intact skin	• No treatment needed if history is reliable
Category II (Minor risk)	Minor scratches or abrasions without bleeding or nibbling of uncovered skin	• Wound management • Rabies vaccine • Observe the dog for 10 days*
Category III (Major risk)	• Single or multiple transdermal bites with oozing of blood • Licks on broken skin (fresh wounds) or mucous membrane • Direct contact with bats or wild animals	• Wound management • Rabies immunoglobulin • Rabies vaccine • Observe the dog for 10 days*

*Vaccine may be discontinued if animal (dogs and cats) is healthy after 10 days of bite. Other animals are humanely killed and tissue is examined for detection of rabies antigen/Negri body in brain biopsies.
**In India post-exposure prophylaxis is indicated following exposure to any animal bite except rodents and bat bite.

- **Suturing:** To be avoided as it causes local tissue damage, which may help in spreading of the virus
- **Debridement** of devitalized tissues
- Tetanus prophylaxis.

Rabies Vaccine

A series of rabies vaccine injections should be administered promptly after the exposure.
- **Type of vaccines:** Cell line derived non-neural vaccines are recommended. Three vaccines are available
    1. Purified chick embryo cell (PCEC) vaccine: It is prepared from chicken fibroblast cell line
    2. Purified Vero cell (PVC) vaccine: It is prepared from Vero cell line
    3. Human diploid cell (HDC) vaccine: It is derived from WI-38 (human embryonic lung fibroblast cell line).
- **Schedule of PEP regimen:** Intradermal (ID) regimens are cost-effective; dose-sparing and time-sparing and therefore are preferred over intramuscular (IM) regimens. 2-site ID vaccine (six doses) is given on days 0, 3 and 7.

Rabies Immunoglobulin (RIG)

RIG provides passive immunization, by neutralizing the virus.
- **Preparations:** It is available in two forms; human RIG (hRIG) and equine RIG (eRIG)
- **Dose:** The maximum dose is 20 IU (hRIG) or 40 IU (eRIG) per kg body weight. There is no minimum dose.

PEP for Individuals Previously Vaccinated

For individuals who previously received rabies vaccine (either PEP or PrEP), RIG is not necessary regardless of exposure category. They need local wound care and an accelerated vaccine regimen; consisting of one of the following schedules.
- 1-site ID vaccine given on days 0 and 3 or
- 4-site ID vaccine given on day 0 only (left and right deltoids, thigh and suprascapular areas).

Pre-exposure Prophylaxis (PrEP)

PrEP is recommended in two conditions.
- **For individuals at higher occupational risk,** such as laboratory staff handling the virus and infected material, clinicians attending to human rabies cases, veterinarians, animal handlers and travelers to endemic areas
- **For sub-populations in remote endemic areas,** which have limited access to PEP and if annual dog bite incidence is > 5% or vampire bat exposures prevail
- **Schedule:** 2-site ID vaccine (four doses) is given on days 0 and 7. Boosters are usually not necessary as the protection is long-term.

CHAPTER 41

Parasitic and Fungal Infections of Central Nervous System

▌INTRODUCTION

A number of parasites and fungi can infect central nervous system (CNS).
* **Major parasitic infections of CNS include:**
    - Free-living amoebae
    - Toxoplasmosis
    - Neurocysticercosis
    - Cerebral malaria
* **Major fungal infections of CNS include:** Cryptococcal Meningitis.

▌FREE-LIVING AMOEBAE INFECTIONS

Free-living amoebae are small, freely living, widely distributed in soil and water and can cause opportunistic infections in humans. Among the many free-living amoebae that exist in nature, only four genera have an association with human disease.
1. *Naegleria fowleri:* It is a causative agent of primary amoebic meningoencephalitis (PAM)
2. *Acanthamoeba* species: It causes granulomatous amoebic encephalitis (GAE) in patients with HIV/AIDS and amoebic keratitis in contact lens wearers
3. *Balamuthia mandrillaris*: It causes granulomatous amoebic encephalitis (GAE)
4. *Sappinia* species: Causes encephalitis.

▌TOXOPLASMOSIS

Problem Solving Exercise 1

Toxoplasma Encephalitis

A 55-year-old person reactive for HIV, presented with altered mental status, seizures, sensory abnormalities. The bone marrow aspirate collected was sent for Giemsa stain (Fig. 41.1).
- Identify the etiological agent and diagnose the clinical condition based on the smear focused.
- What is the host, infective form, pathogenic form, diagnostic form and modes of transmission of the parasite?
- What are the various diagnostic modalities?
- How will you treat this condition?

Explanation

This is a case of *Toxoplasma* encephalitis. Points in favor are:
- HIV infected patient
- Presented with altered mental status, seizures, sensory abnormalities—encephalitis

- Giemsa stained smear showing crescent-shaped tachyzoites (6 × 2 μm in size)—confirms the etiological agent to be *Toxoplasma gondii* (Fig. 41.1).
- *Treatment*: Cotrimoxazole is drug of choice in HIV infected patients.

For answers to the other questions, refer Tables 41.1 and 41.2.

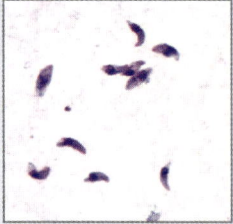

Fig. 41.1: Giemsa stained smear showing comma-shaped tachyzoites of *Toxoplasma gondii*.
Source: DPDx Image Library, Centers for Disease Control and Prevention (CDC), Atlanta.

Table 41.1: Features or characteristics of *Toxoplasma*.

Properties	Characteristics of *Toxoplasma*
Host	• Definitive host—cat and other feline animals • Intermediate host—man and other mammals (sheep, goat)
Morphological forms	• Tachyzoites in blood (man) • Tissue cyst containing bradyzoites in organs (man) • Oocyst found in cat (feces)
Infective form	All the three morphological forms
Transmission	• Ingestion of tissue cyst from undercooked meat (most common route) • Ingestion of sporulated oocysts from contaminated soil, food, or water • By blood transfusion, organ transplantation, or mother-to-fetus: Tachyzoites are the infective form
Habitat	Reticuloendothelial cells of spleen, bone marrow, lymph node, liver and peripheral blood
Pathogenic form	Tachyzoites
Manifestations (Adult)	• Asymptomatic—most common • Cervical lymphadenopathy
Manifestations (congenital toxoplasmosis)	• 1st trimester: More severe infection • 3rd trimester: More chance of transmission of infection • Manifestation: chorioretinitis, cerebral calcification, convulsion, microcephaly and mental retardation
Manifestations in HIV	• Encephalitis, pulmonary infections and chorioretinitis • Occurs if CD4 T-cell count <100/μL
Diagnostic form	• Tachyzoites in blood • Tissue cyst containing bradyzoites in organs
Treatment	• Immunocompetent adults—no treatment required • Toxoplasmosis during pregnancy—spiramycin • In HIV infected patients—cotrimoxazole

Table 41.2: Laboratory diagnosis of *Toxoplasma gondii*.

Methods	Salient features
Direct microscopy (Giemsa stain)	**Blood smear**—Crescent- or comma-shaped tachyzoites (indicates acute infection) (Fig. 41.1). **Smear from biopsy from organs**—tissue cyst with bradyzoites (indicates chronic or past infection)

Antibody detection	Antibody detection remains the most widely used method for diagnosis of acute toxoplasmosis in immunocompetent individuals.
	• **Capture ELISA** and immunosorbent agglutination assay (ISAGA). Acute toxoplasmosis is diagnosed by:
	  ➢ Four-fold rise in IgG titer, low IgG avidity
	  ➢ Detecton of IgM or IgA
	• **Sabin-Feldman dye test:** This is the gold standard antibody detection method, usually done in the reference laboratories. As it is technically difficult, seldom used nowadays in routine diagnostics

PCR	Detects *T. gondii* specific genes
Animal inoculation	Intraperitoneal inoculation into mice
Imaging	CT and MRI scan for encephalitis

CEREBRAL MALARIA

Cerebral malaria occurs as a complication of *Plasmodium falciparum* infection, not by any other *Plasmodium* species (Chapter 20).

❖ **Pathogenesis:** *P. falciparum* exhibit unique property of being sequestered inside the brain capillaries by:
  ▪ Expressing a protein called PfEMP (*P. falciparum* erythrocyte membrane protein-1), by virtue of which, the parasitized RBCs adhere to vascular endothelium and also adhere to non-parasitized RBCs
  ▪ This results in plugging of brain capillaries by the rosettes of sequestered parasitized RBCs leading to vascular occlusion and cerebral anoxia.

❖ **Clinical manifestations**: Cerebral malaria manifests as diffuse symmetric encephalopathy characterized by repeated

seizures, reduced muscle tone and tendon reflexes
- Seizures are more common in children (up to 50%) than in adults (10%)
- Other defects are retinal hemorrhages, neurologic sequelae, and rarely deep coma
- Signs of focal neurologic and meningeal irritations are absent
- Associated with high mortality rate of 15–20%.
❖ **Laboratory diagnosis:** The various diagnostic methods include (Chapter 20):

- Peripheral blood smear examination is the gold standard method to identify *P. falciparum*
  - Banana-shaped gametocytes
  - Ring forms-multiple ring forms, accole forms and head-phone shaped ring forms
  - Schizonts are not seen.
- Quantitative buffy coat examination
- Rapid diagnostic tests: ICT detecting *P. falciparum* specific HRP-II antigen.

❖ **Treatment:** Artesunate, artemether, arteether and quinine are the drugs used for treatment of cerebral malaria (Chapter 20).

CYSTICERCOSIS

Problem Solving Exercise 2

Cysticercosis

A 32-year-old vegetarian male presented with recurrent episodes of seizure, headache vomiting and vertigo. MRI scan of brain was done (Fig. 41.2A), following which surgery was performed. The surgically removed cysts have been focused in Figure 41.2B, which were subjected to histopathological examination (Fig. 41.2C).
1. Identify the etiological agent and the clinical condition based on the investigations done.
2. What is the host, infective form, pathogenic form, diagnostic form and mode of transmission of the parasite?
3. What are the various diagnostic modalities?
4. How will you treat this condition?

Explanation

This is a case of neurocysticercosis. Points in favor are:

- *Vegetarian diet* (cysticercosis can also occur among vegetarians, in contrast to intestinal taeniasis which occurs only to beef/pork eaters).
- CNS involvement: Presented with recurrent episodes of seizure, headache, vomiting and vertigo.
- MRI scan shows cystic lesion in subarachnoid space (arrow) (Fig. 41.2A).
- Figure 41.2B shows cysticercus cellulosae (surgically removed):
  ➢ Yellowish white, 0.5–1.5 cm size, slightly oval
  ➢ Bladder-like sac filled with vesicular fluid
  ➢ White spot which represents the future growing scolex.
- Histopathological biopsy from the brain (hematoxylin and eosin stain) shows entire cysticercus seen within the bladder walls. Arrow showing the extensive folding of the spiral canal and one sucker of the scolex (Fig. 41.2C).

For answer to the other questions, refer Table 41.3.

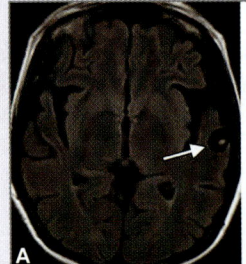 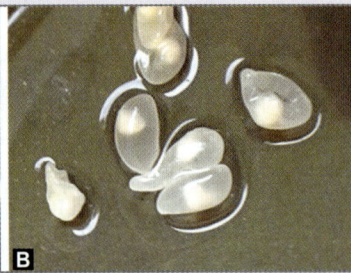 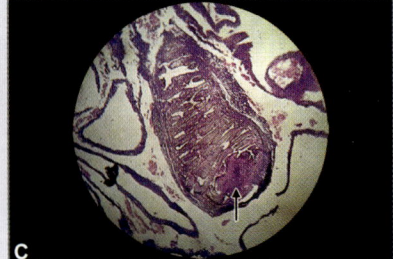

Figs 41.2A and B: (A) MRI of brain—arrow shows cystic lesion in subarachnoid space; (B) Cysticercus cellulosae (surgically removed). *Source:* (A) Dr A Subathra. Department of Radiodiagnosis, JIPMER, Puducherry (*with permission*); (B) Head of Department (Microbiology), Meenakshi Medical College, Chennai (*with permission*).

Fig. 41.2C: Cysticercus cellulosae in biopsy from the brain (hematoxylin and eosin stain). *Source:* Head of Department (Pathology), Meenakshi Medical College, Chennai (*with permission*).

Table 41.3: Differences between intestinal taeniasis and cysticercosis.

Properties	Intestinal taeniasis	Cysticercosis
Agent	*Taenia saginata, T. solium*	*Taenia solium*
Definitive host	Man	Man
Intermediate host	T. saginata-cattle T. solium-pig	Man
Infective form	Larva (cysticercus bovis or cysticercus cellulosae)	Eggs of *T. solium*
Transmission by ingestion of	Contaminated beef or pork meat (partially /uncooked)	1. Contaminated food and water 2. Autoinfection (contaminated fingers)
Habitat	Intestine	Tissue (CNS, eye, muscle)
Pathogenic form	Adult	Larva (Cysticercus cellulosae)
Manifestations	Intestinal symptoms only	CNS- Seizure, hydrocephalus, pressure effect etc
Diagnostic form	Demonstration of eggs in feces	Demonstration of larvae in tissues—by CT or MRI scan Antibody detection—ELISA or Western blot- detecting antibody against highly specific 50–13 kDa lentil lectin-purified seven glycoprotein (LLGP) antigenic fractions
Treatment	Praziquantel (DOC), Niclosamide	Drugs: Albendazole, Praziquantel Surgery

CRYPTOCOCCAL MENINGITIS

Problem Solving Exercise 3

Cryptococcal Meningitis

A 45-year-old HIV-infected male presented to the emergency department with on and off fever and severe headache for 1 month duration. On examination, he had signs of meningeal irritation. His cerebrospinal fluid (CSF) sample was collected by lumbar puncture and sent for microbiological investigation, such as CSF smear (India ink preparation) (Fig. 41.3A) and culture on SDA (Fig. 41.3B).

1. Identify the etiological agent based on the tests done.
2. What is the clinical diagnosis?
3. Name the virulence factors responsible for this clinical condition.
4. Describe the various modalities of laboratory diagnosis of this clinical condition.
5. Mention the treatment of choice in this clinical condition.

Explanation

Clinical diagnosis

HIV-infected adult patient with intermittent fever and chronic headache (1 month) gives clue that probably the patient is suffering from chronic meningitis.

Identification

India ink staining showed clear refractile capsules surrounding spherical budding yeast cells (Fig. 41.3A) and creamy-to-white mucoid colonies on SDA (Fig. 41.3B), hence the final identification is *C. neoformans*.

Cryptococcosis is caused by capsulated yeast called *Cryptococcus neoformans*.

Pathogenesis

Virulence Factors

Cryptococcus has ability to cross blood-brain barrier and can cause fatal meningitis with help of various virulence factors, such as:

- **Polysaccharide capsule:** It is the principal virulence factor, antiphagocytic and also inhibits the host's local immune responses
- Ability to make melanin by producing
- Production of other enzymes, such as phospholipase, urease and phenyl oxidase enzyme (help in melanin synthesis).

Risk Factors

Individuals at high risk for cryptococcosis include:
- Patients with advanced HIV infection with CD4 T cell counts less than 200/µL
- Patients with hematologic malignancies
- Transplant recipients
- Patients on immunosuppressive therapy.

Clinical Manifestation

Various clinical manifestations of cryptococcosis include:
- **Pulmonary cryptococcosis:** It is the first and the most common presentation
- **Cryptococcal meningitis:** It presents as chronic meningitis, with headache, fever, sensory and memory loss, cranial nerve paresis and loss of vision (due to optic nerve involvement)
- Skin lesions and osteolytic bone lesions.

Laboratory Diagnosis

Specimens such as CSF, blood or skin scrapings can be collected in cryptococcosis, depending upon the site affected.

Direct Detection Methods

- **Negative staining** by modified India ink stain (added with 2% mercurochrome) and nigrosin stain are used to demonstrate the capsule, which appears as refractile clear space surrounding the spherical budding yeast cells against black background (Fig. 41.3A). India ink stain is less sensitive (60–70%)
- Other stains that can be used are:
  - Mucicarmine stain
  - Masson-Fontana stain
  - Alcian blue stain (to demonstrate the capsule).
- **Capsular antigen detection** from CSF or serum by latex agglutination test is a rapid, sensitive and specific method.

Culture

Cerebrospinal fluid is inoculated onto SDA without antibiotics, blood agar or chocolate agar and incubated at 37°C. Colonies appear as mucoid creamy-white yeast-like colonies (Fig. 41.3B).

Confirmation of *Cryptococcus* species is made by:
- Niger seed agar and bird seed agar is used to demonstrate melanin production (brown-colored colonies)
- Growth at 37°C
- Urease test positive.

Treatment

- Cryptococcosis without central nervous system (CNS) involvement—fluconazole is the drug of choice
- HIV-infected patients with CNS involvement, the recommended regimen is *induction phase* for 2 weeks (Amphotericin B ± flucytosine) followed by lifelong *maintenance therapy* with fluconazole.

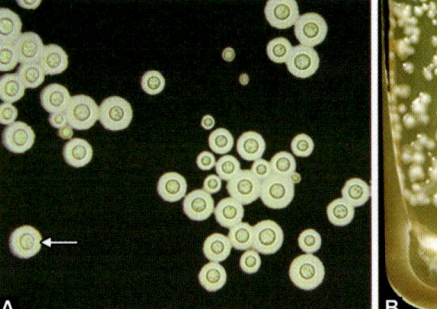

Figs 41.3A and B: *Cryptococcus neoformans*: (A) India ink staining shows clear refractile capsules surrounding round budding yeast cells (arrow showing); (B) Growth on SDA at 37°C—shows creamy white mucoid colonies.

Source: Public Health Image Library/(A) Dr Leanor Haley, ID#:3771; (B) Dr William Kaplan, ID#:3199/Centers for Disease Control and Prevention (CDC), Atlanta (*with permission*).

CHAPTER 42

Urinary Tract Infections

■ INTRODUCTION

Urinary tract infection (UTI) is defined as a disease caused by microbial invasion of the urinary tract that extends from the renal cortex of the kidney to the urethral meatus. UTI is the leading cause of morbidity and healthcare expenditures in persons of all ages.

Classification

- UTIs may be broadly classified into two types—lower UTI and upper UTI (Table 42.1) depending upon the anatomical sites involved
- Depending upon the source of infection, UTI can be of two types: healthcare-associated (e.g., catheter-associated UTI) and community-acquired.

Predisposing Factors

- **Prevalence:** About 10% of humans develop UTI in some part of their life
- **Gender:** UTI is predominantly a disease of females. The higher prevalence in females is due to the anatomical structure of female urogenital system—(1) short urethra, and (2) close proximity of urethral meatus to anus; so that there is more chance of introduction of endogenous bacteria into the urinary tract
- **Age:** UTI is common during adult life (10–20% in females)
- **Pregnancy:** Anatomical and hormonal changes in pregnancy favor the development of UTIs. Most females develop asymptomatic bacteriuria during pregnancy. In some cases, it can lead to serious infections in both mother and fetus
- **Structural and functional abnormality** of urinary tract may obstruct the urine flow, that can lead to urinary stasis; which predisposes to infection
- **Bacterial virulence**, such as expression of pili helps in bacterial adhesion to uroepithelium
- **Vesicoureteral reflux:** If the normal valve-like mechanism at the vesicoureteric junction is weakened, it allows urine to flow from the bladder up into the ureters and sometimes into the renal pelvis
- **Genetic factors:** Genetically determined receptors present on uroepithelial cells may help in bacterial attachment.

Etiology

Escherichia coli (uropathogenic *E. coli*) is by far the most common cause of all forms of UTIs (i.e., community-acquired and healthcare-associated UTI and upper and lower UTI); accounting for 70% of total cases.

- The endogenous flora, such as gram-negative bacilli (e.g., *E. coli, Klebsiella, Proteus,* etc.) and enterococci are the important agents
- In healthcare-associated UTIs, the agents are often multidrug resistant. In addition to the members of Enterobacteriaceae, other organisms, such as staphylococci, *Pseudomonas, Acinetobacter* are also increasingly reported.

Table 42.1: Comparison between lower and upper UTIs.

	Lower UTI	Upper UTI
Sites involved	Urethra, and bladder	Kidney and ureter
Symptoms	Local manifestations: dysuria, urgency, frequency	Local and systemic manifestations (fever, vomiting, abdominal pain)
Route of spread	Ascending route	Both ascending (common) and descending route
Occurrence	More common	Less common

Table 42.2: Common microorganisms causing UTIs.

Bacterial agents	Other agents
Gram-negative bacilli: Enterobacteriaceae • *Escherichia coli:* Most common (70%) • *Klebsiella pneumoniae* • *Enterobacter* species • *Proteus* species • *Serratia* species **Non-fermenters** • *Pseudomonas aeruginosa* • *Acinetobacter* species	**Fungus:** *Candida albicans* **Parasites:** • *Schistosoma haematobium* • *Trichomonas vaginalis* • *Dioctophyme renale*
Gram-positive cocci: • *Enterococcus* species • *Staphylococcus saprophyticus** • *Staphylococcus aureus* • *Staphylococcus epidermidis* • *Streptococcus agalactiae*	**Viruses:** • BK virus • Adenovirus types–11 and 21

Abbreviation: UTI, Urinary tract infection.
*Common in sexually active females.

Bacterial pathogens are the major cause of UTI. In general, viruses, parasites and fungi infrequently infect the urinary tract; discussed subsequently in this chapter (Table 42.2).

Laboratory Diagnosis

Specimen Collection

Urine should be collected in a wide mouth screw capped sterile container by various methods.
- **Clean voided midstream urine:** It is the most common specimen for UTI; collected after properly cleaning the urethral meatus or glans
- **Suprapubic aspiration** of urine from the bladder: It is the most ideal specimen. It is recommended for patients in coma or infants
- **In catheterized patients,** urine should be collected from the catheter tube (after clamping distally and disinfecting); but not from the uro bag.

Transport

Urine sample should be processed immediately. If delay is expected for more than 1–2 hours, then it can be stored in refrigerator or stored by adding boric acid for maximum 24 hours.

Direct Examination

The screening tests done are as follows:
- **Wet mount examination:** It is done to demonstrate the pus cells in urine. Pyuria of more than 8 pus cells/mm^3 is taken as significant
- **Leukocyte esterase test:** It is a rapid and cheaper method that detects leukocyte esterases secreted by pus cells present in urine
- **Nitrate reduction test (Griess test):** Nitrate reducing bacteria, such as *E. coli* gives a positive result
- **Gram staining** of urine is not a reliable indicator as—(1) the bacterial count in urine is usually low, (2) pus cells rapidly deteriorate in urine and may not be seen well. Gram staining may be limited to pyelonephritis and invasive UTI cases and a count of ≥1 bacteria/oil immersion field is taken as significant.

Culture

- **Culture media:** Urine sample should be inoculated onto CLED agar (cysteine lactose electrolyte deficient agar) or combination of MacConkey agar and blood agar. CLED agar is preferred in laboratories with higher sample load
- **Kass concept of significant bacteriuria:** This is based on the fact that, though the normal urine is sterile, it may get contaminated during voiding, with normal urethral flora. However, the bacterial count in contaminated urine would be lower than that caused by an infection

> **Significant bacteriuria**
> ❑ A count of ≥**10^5 colony forming units (CFU)/mL** of urine is considered as significant—indicates infection (referred as 'significant bacteriuria' developed by Kass)
> ❑ **Count between 10^4 to 10^5 CFU/mL** indicates doubtful significance; should be clinically correlated
> ❑ **Low count of** <10^4 CFU/mL is due to presence of commensal bacteria (due to contamination during voiding) and is of no significance. However, low counts can be significant in the following conditions:
> ➤ Patient on antibiotic or on diuretic treatment
> ➤ Infection with some gram-positive organisms, such as *S. aureus*
> ➤ Pyelonephritis and acute urethral syndrome
>
> *Contd...*

Contd...

> - Sample taken by suprapubic aspiration
> - In catheterized patients: If the patient is symptomatic, then a count of ≥10^3 CFU/mL is considered significant

- **Quantitative culture:** This is done to count the number of colonies. Each colony on plate corresponds to one bacterium in urine sample. Quantitation is done by:
  - Semi-quantitative method, such as standardized loop technique
  - Quantitative method, such as pour plate method.
- **Colony appearance**: It depends upon the organism grown. For example, lactose fermenters, such as *E. coli* and *Klebsiella* produce pink colonies on MacConkey agar and yellow colonies on CLED agar; whereas non-lactose fermenters, such as *Proteus, Pseudomonas* and *Acinetobacter* produce pale colonies
- **Identification**: The colonies grown are identified either by automated identification systems, such as MALDI-TOF or VITEK, or by conventional biochemical tests
- **AST:** Antimicrobial susceptibility test is essential to guide the appropriate treatment. It is performed conventionally by disk diffusion test (on Mueller-Hinton agar) or by automated MIC-based methods, such as VITEK.

Treatment

Treatment of UTI should be based on antimicrobial susceptibility testing report. Quinolones (e.g., norfloxacin), nitrofurantoin, cephalosporins, and aminoglycosides are among the preferred drugs.

Higher antibiotics, such as carbapenem (e.g., meropenem), β-lactam/β-lactamase inhibitor combinations (e.g., piperacillin/tazobactam) or fosfomycin are used for treatment of healthcare-associated UTIs caused by multidrug resistant gram-negative bacilli.

▮COMMON AGENTS OF UTI

Escherichia coli UTI

Escherichia coli is a commensal harbored in intestine. At the same time, it is also one of the most common organism associated with human infections and also commonly isolated from various hospital-acquired infections.

Clinical Manifestations

Escherichia coli is associated with the following manifestations:
- **Urinary tract infection**—caused by uropathogenic *E. coli* (UPEC)
- **Diarrhea**—caused by six types diarrheagenic *E. coli* (Chapter 22)
- **Other infective syndromes include:**
  - *Abdominal infections*—bacterial peritonitis occurs secondary to intestinal perforation leading to spillage of commensal *E. coli* from intestine
  - *Pneumonia* (especially in hospitalized patients—ventilator-associated pneumonia)
  - *Meningitis* (especially *neonatal meningitis*)
  - *Wound and soft tissue infections*, such as cellulitis and infection of ulcers and wounds especially in diabetic foot
  - Osteomyelitis
  - Endovascular infection and bacteremia.
- It is responsible for severe lobar pneumonia, UTIs, meningitis (neonates), septicemia and pyogenic infections, such as abscesses and wound infections
- It frequently colonizes the oropharynx of hospitalized patients and is a common cause of nosocomial infections. Most of the hospital strains are multidrugresistant.

Klebsiella pneumoniae UTI

Klebsiella pneumoniae is usually found as commensal in human intestines; causes infections similar to *E. coli* such as urinary tract infections, meningitis (neonates), septicemia and pyogenic infections such as abscesses and wound infections. Detail is discussed in Chapter 34.

Proteus UTI

Proteus mirabilis and *P. vulgaris* are the most commonly encountered species from the clinical specimens.
- *Proteus* species are widely distributed in nature and also commensal of human intestine
- They are opportunistic pathogens, commonly responsible for urinary, wound and soft tissue infections and septicemia

Problem Solving Exercise 1

Urinary Tract Infections (*E. coli/Klebsiella/ Proteus*)

A 24-year-old female was admitted with fever, dysuria and frequency of micturition for the past 3 days. Urine microscopy revealed pyuria. Urine specimen was further subjected to cculture, Gram staining of culture smear and biochemical reactions. Result of antimicrobial susceptibility test (AST) is demonstrated in Figure 42.4 and Table 42.3.
Exercise 1: Figures 42.1 to 42.3
Exercise 2: Figures 42.5 to 42.7
Exercise 3: Figures 42.8 to 42.11

1. What is the clinical diagnosis and its causative organism in all three exercises?
2. List the clinical conditions caused by this organism.
- What are the various modalities of laboratory diagnosis?
- How will you treat this condition?

Explanation

Clinical Diagnosis

The history of fever, dysuria and frequency of micturition in a female of reproductive age is suggestive of urinary tract infection (UTI). The common agents of UTI are the gram-negative bacilli, such as *E. coli* (most common), *K. pneumoniae* and *Proteus* and gram-positive cocci, such as enterococci.

Identification

Based on the culture on MacConkey agar, Gram staining of culture smear and biochemical reactions, the identification in all three exercises is as follows:

Exercise 1: Figures 42.1 to 42.3 (*Escherichia coli*)

The identification is *Escherichia coli*, as it shows the following properties:
- **Figs 42.1A to C:** (A) Blood agar shows moist colonies; (B) MacConkey agar shows flat lactose fermenting (LF) colonies; (C) Semi quantitative urine culture on cysteine lactose electrolyte deficient agar showing significant growth of flat LF colonies
- **Fig. 42.2:** Gram-stained culture smear showing gram-negative bacilli
- **Biochemical tests (ICUT tests, Fig. 42.3):**
  - Indole test—positive (cherry red ring is formed)
  - Citrate test—negative (citrate is not utilized)
  - Urease test—negative (urea is not hydrolyzed)
  - TSI (triple sugar iron test)—shows acid slant/ acid butt, gas present, H_2S absent.

Exercise 2: Figures 42.5 to 42.7 (*Klebsiella pneumoniae*)

The identification is *Klebsiella pneumoniae*, as it shows the following properties:
- **Fig. 42.6:** Mucoid dome-shaped pink-colored colonies on MacConkey agar
- **Fig. 42.5:** Gram-stained smear showing short stout gram-negative bacilli (*Klebsiella*)
- **Biochemical tests (ICUT tests, Fig. 42.7):**
  - Indole test—negative
  - Citrate test—positive (citrate is utilized)
  - Urease test—positive (urea is hydrolyzed)
  - TSI (triple sugar iron test)—shows acid slant/ acid butt, gas present, H_2S absent.

Exercise 3: Figures 42.8 to 42.1 (*Proteus*)

The identification is *Proteus mirabilis*, as it shows the following properties:
- **Fig. 42.9:** Swarming growth on blood agar
- **Fig. 42.10:** Non-lactose fermenting colonies on MacConkey agar
- **Fig. 42.8:** Gram-stained smear showing pleomorphic gram-negative bacilli (*Proteus*)
- **Biochemical tests (ICUT tests, Fig. 42.11):**
  - Indole test—negative (therefore, *P. mirabilis*) (*P. vulgaris* gives positive reaction)
  - Citrate positive (citrate is utilized)
  - Urease positive (urea is hydrolyzed)

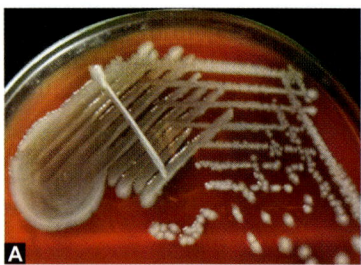 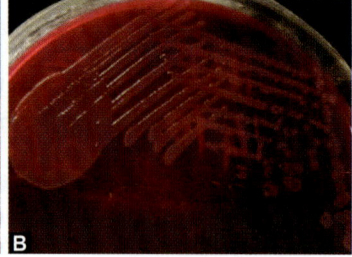 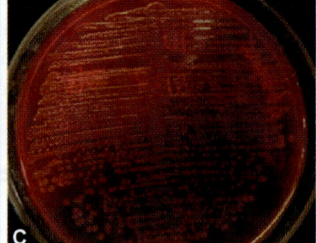

Figs 42.1A to C: *Escherichia coli* on (A) Blood agar (moist colonies); (B) MacConkey agar [flat lactose fermenting (LF) colonies]; (C) Semiquantitative urine culture on cysteine lactose electrolyte deficient agar showing significant growth of flat LF colonies.

Source: Department of Microbiology, Pondicherry Institute of Medical Sciences, Puducherry (*with permission*).

- TSI shows alkaline slant/acid butt, gas present and H_2S present

Antimicrobial Susceptibility Test and Treatment

Antimicrobial susceptibility test on Muller Hinton agar (Fig. 42.4) with zone interpretation chart (Table 42.3) shows that the causative urinary pathogen is resistant to ceftriaxone, gentamicin, ciprofloxacin and sensitive to amikacin, meropenem, piperacillin or tazobactam and nitrofurantoin; hence one of the sensitive drug would be the antibiotic of choice. However, nitrofurantoin is not given for *Proteus* infections as it is intrinsic resistant.

(For answers to other questions, refer below).

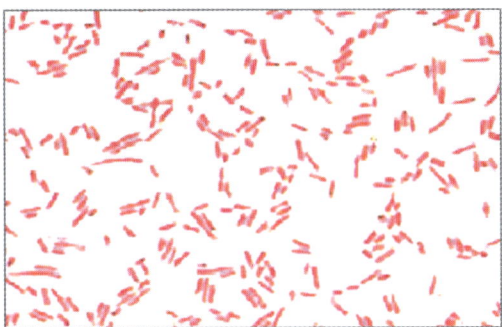

Fig. 42.2: Gram-stained culture smear showing gram-negative bacilli *(Escherichia coli)*.
Source: Department of Microbiology, JIPMER, Puducherry *(with permission)*.

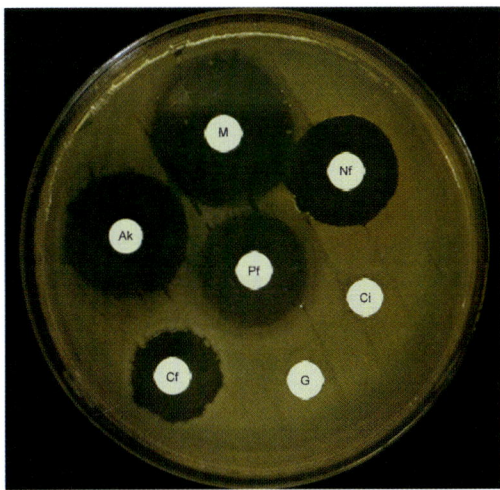

Fig. 42.4: Antimicrobial susceptibility testing on Mueller-Hinton Agar for *Escherichia coli/Klebsiella/Proteus* (observed zone size diameter (mm) and zone interpretation to various antimicrobial agents tested are given in Table 42.3).

Abbreviations: Cf, ciprofloxacin; Ak, amikacin; G, gentamicin; Ci, ceftriaxone; Pt, piperacillin/tazobactam; M, meropenem; Nf, nitrofurantoin.

Source: Department of Microbiology, Pondicherry Institute of Medical Sciences, Puducherry *(with permission)*.

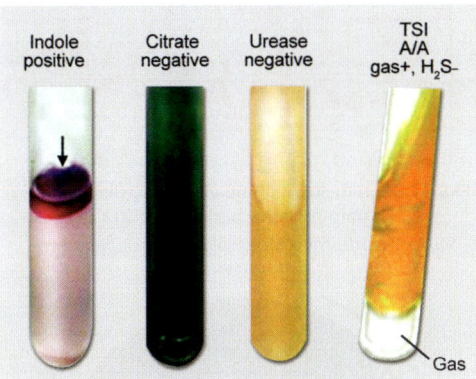

Fig. 42.3: Biochemical reactions of *Escherichia coli*.
Source: Department of Microbiology, JIPMER, Puducherry *(with permission)*.

- *Proteus* species are often involved in nosocomial outbreaks
- They can cause *Struvite stones in bladder* in alkaline urine
- Basis of *Weil-Felix reaction*: Certain *Proteus* antigens cross react with antigen of some *Rickettsia* species and hence are used to detect antibodies in various rickettsial diseases.

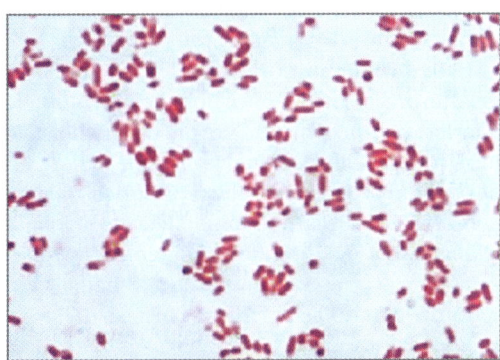

Fig. 42.5: Gram-stained smear showing short stout gram-negative bacilli *(Klebsiella)*.
Source: Department of Microbiology, JIPMER, Puducherry *(with permission)*.

Table 42.3: Interpretative categories (CLSI) and observed zone size diameter (mm) to various antimicrobial agents tested for Enterobacteriaceae.

Antimicrobial agents	Disk strength (µg)	CLSI interpretative criteria for Enterobacteriaceae (in mm)*			Observed zone size (in mm) (Fig. 42.4)	Interpretation
		Resistant	Intermediate	Sensitive		
Ciprofloxacin (Cf)	5	≤21	22–25	≥26	16	Resistant
Amikacin (Ak)	30	≤14	15–16	≥17	24	Sensitive
Gentamicin (G)	10	≤12	13–14	≥15	6	Resistant
Ceftriaxone (Ci)	30	≤19	20–22	≥23	6	Resistant
Piperacillin/Tazobactam (Pt)	100/10	≤17	18–20	≥21	22	Sensitive
Meropenem (M)	10	≤19	20–22	≥23	28	Sensitive
Nitrofurantoin (Nf)**	300	≤14	15–16	≥17	21	Sensitive

Abbreviations: CLSI, Clinical and Laboratory Standards Institute.
Note*: CLSI interpretative categories and zone size diameter (mm) to various antimicrobial agents tested for *Klebsiella* and *Proteus* are same as that for *E. coli*.
**Proteus species are intrinsically resistant to nitrofurantoin.

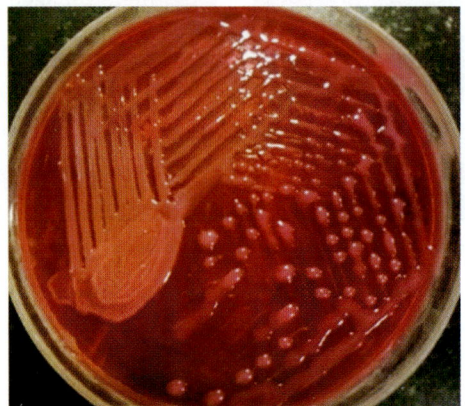

Fig. 42.6: *Klebsiella* species on MacConkey agar (Mucoid dome-shaped pink-colored lactose-fermenting colonies).
Source: Department of Microbiology, Pondicherry Institute of Medical Sciences, Puducherry (*with permission*).

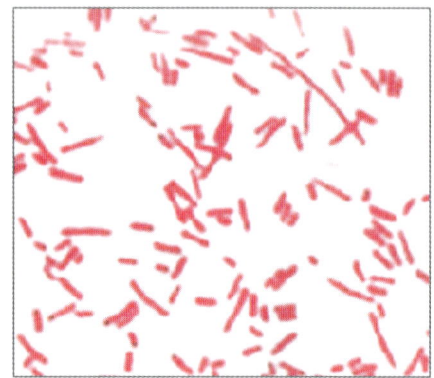

Fig. 42.8: Gram-stained smear showing pleomorphic gram-negative bacilli (*Proteus*).
Source: Department of Microbiology, JIPMER, Puducherry (*with permission*).

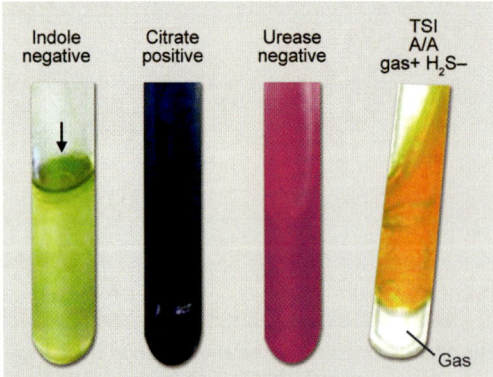

Fig. 42.7: Biochemical reactions of *Klebsiella* species.
Source: Department of Microbiology, JIPMER, Puducherry (*with permission*).

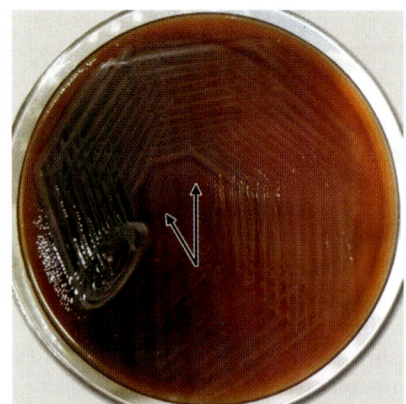

Fig. 42.9: *Proteus* on blood agar, showing swarming growth (arrow showing).
Source: Department of Microbiology, JIPMER, Puducherry (*with permission*).

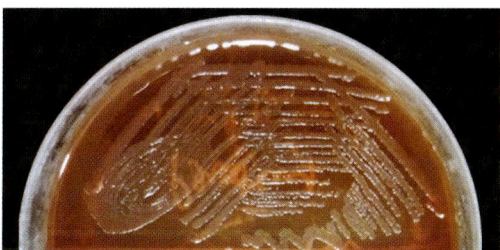

Fig. 42.10: *Proteus* species on MacConkey agar (nonlactose fermenting colonies).
Source: Department of Microbiology, Pondicherry Institute of Medical Sciences, Puducherry (*with permission*).

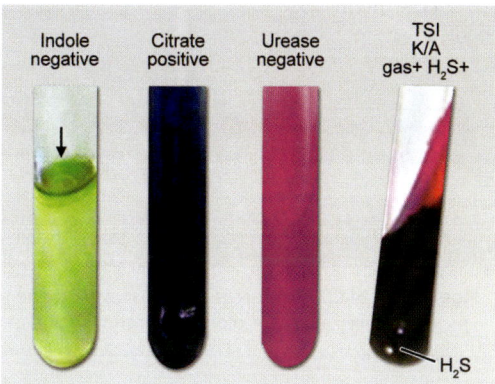

Fig. 42.11: Biochemical reactions of *Proteus mirabilis*.
Source: Department of Microbiology, JIPMER, Puducherry (*with permission*).

Enterococcal UTI

Clinical Manifestations

Enterococci produce various manifestations:
- Urinary tract infections (cystitis, urethritis, pyelonephritis and prostatitis)
- Bacteremia and mitral valve endocarditis (in intravenous drug abusers)
- Intra-abdominal, pelvic and soft tissue infections
- Late-onset neonatal sepsis and meningitis.

Laboratory Diagnosis

They show the following characteristics that help in the identification:
- Blood agar: It produces nonhemolytic, translucent colonies (rarely produces α or β-hemolysis) (Fig. 42.12A)
- MacConkey agar: It produces minute magenta pink colonies (Fig. 42.12B)
- Enterococci are gram-positive oval cocci arranged in pairs (spectacle eyed appearance)—both in direct smear and colony smear (Fig. 42.12C)
- Bile esculin hydrolysis test is positive (Fig. 42.13A)
- Growth occurs in presence of 6.5% NaCl, 40% bile, pH 9.6, and at 45°C and 10°C
- Heat tolerance test: They are relatively heat resistant, can survive 60°C for 30 minutes
- Pathogenic species are two: *E. faecium* and *E. faecalis*. They can be differentiated based

---

Problem Solving Exercise 2

Enterococcal UTI

A 25-year-old female admitted to the hospital with complaints of burning micturition, fever, vomiting and abdominal pain. Urine specimen was collected and sent to microbiology laboratory for culture identification (Figs 42.12 and 42.13) and AST (Fig. 42.14 and Table 42.4).
1. What is the clinical diagnosis and its causative organism?
2. List the infections caused by this organism.
3. Briefly discuss the laboratory diagnosis.
4. Interpret the AST.
5. What antibiotic you would like to prescribe?

Explanation

Clinical Diagnosis

Burning micturition, fever, vomiting and abdominal pain in a patient are clinically suggestive of urinary tract infection (UTI).

Identification

Translucent nonhemolytic colonies on blood agar (Fig. 42.12A), magenta pink colonies on MacConkey agar (Fig. 42.12B), gram-positive oval cocci in pair (Fig. 42.12C), positive bile esculin hydrolysis tests (Fig. 42.13A) and arabinose nonfermentation (Fig. 42.13B) together reveal the identification as *Enterococcus faecalis*.

Antimicrobial Susceptibility Testing and Treatment

Antimicrobial susceptibility testing on Mueller Hinton agar (Fig. 42.14 and Table 42.4) showed resistant to ampicillin, high level gentamicin, nitrofurantoin and sensitive to ciprofloxacin, linezolid and vancomycin. So any of the sensitive antibiotics should be given for treatment.
(For answers to other questions, refer below).

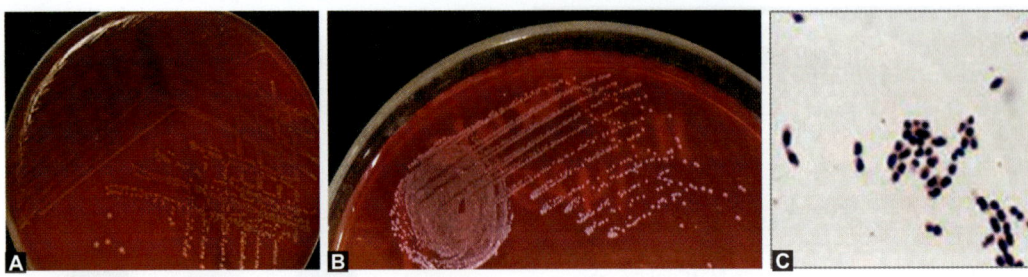

Figs 42.12A to C: *Enterococcus*: (A) Translucent nonhemolytic colonies on blood agar; (B) Magenta pink colonies on MacConkey agar; (C) Colony smear showing gram-shaped oval cocci in pair (spectacle-eyed appearance).
Source: Department of Microbiology, Pondicherry Institute of Medical Sciences, Puducherry (*with permission*).

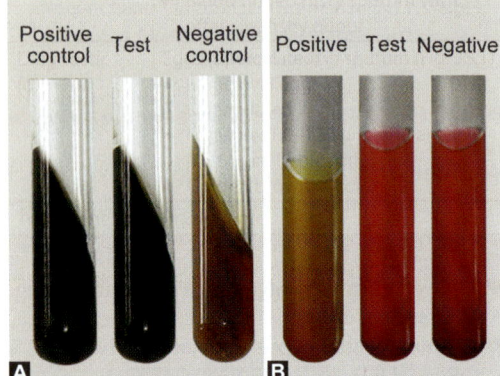

Figs 42.13A and B: *Enterococcus faecalis*: (A) Bile esculin agar test (test-positive); (B) Arabinose fermentation (test not fermented).
Source: Department of Microbiology, JIPMER, Puducherry (*with permission*).

on arabinose fermentation (Fig. 42.13B); *E. faecium* ferments arabinose and *E. faecalis* is arabinose nonfermenter.

Antimicrobial Susceptibility Test

It is carried out on MHBA by disk diffusion test (Fig. 42.14) and reported as per CLSI zone interpretation criteria (Table 42.4).

Treatment

Most strains of enterococci are resistant to penicillins, aminoglycosides and sulfonamides. They show intrinsic resistance to cephalosporins and cotrimoxazole.

❖ For UTI, monotherapy with ampicillin or nitrofurantoin is sufficient, if isolate is sensitive
❖ Life-threatening infections—combination therapy with penicillin and aminoglycoside (due to synergistic effect). Resistance to this combination therapy may also be developed
❖ Vancomycin is usually indicated in resistant cases; but resistance to vancomycin has also been reported.

Table 42.4: Interpretative categories (CLSI) and observed zone size diameter (mm) to various antimicrobial agents tested for Enterococcus faecalis isolates.

Antimicrobial agents	Disk strength (µg)	CLSI interpretative criteria for *Enterococcus* (in mm)			Observed zone size (in mm) (Fig. 42.14)	Interpretation
		Resistant	Intermediate	Sensitive		
Ampicillin (A)	10	≤16	-	≥17	6	Resistant
High level gentamicin (HLG)	120	6	7–9	≥10	6	Resistant
Nitrofurantoin (Nf)	300	≤14	15–16	≥17	6	Resistant
Ciprofloxacin (Cf)	5	≤15	16–20	≥21	22	Sensitive
Linezolid (Lz)	30	≤20	21–22	≥23	25	Sensitive
Vancomycin (Va)	30	≤14	15–16	≥17	17	Sensitive

Abbreviation: CLSI, Clinical and Laboratory Standards Institute.

CHAPTER 42 ♦ Urinary Tract Infections

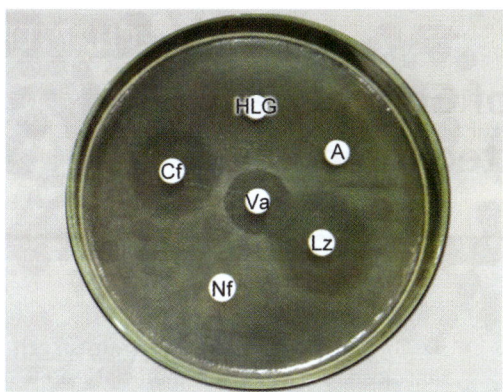

Fig. 42.14: Antimicrobial susceptibility testing on Mueller Hinton agar for *Enterococcus faecalis* (Refer Table 42.4 for CLSI zone interpretation).

Abbreviations: A; ampicillin; HLG, high level gentamicin; Nf, nitrofurantoin; Cf, ciprofloxacin; Lz, linezolid; Va, vancomycin; CLSI, Clinical and Laboratory Standards Institute.

Source: Department of Microbiology, PIMS, Puducherry (with permission).

Table 42.5: *Schistosoma haematobium* infection.

Properties	*Schistosoma haematobium*
Definitive host	Man
Intermediate host	Snail
Infective form	Cercaria larva
Transmission	Skin penetration
Habitat	Blood vessels of bladder
Manifestations	Dysuria, hematuria Hydroureter, hydronephrosis Bladder carcinoma
Laboratory diagnosis	
Diagnostic form (in urine)	Elliptical, non-operculated eggs of 112–170 × 40–70 µm in size, with a sharp terminal spine
Antibody detection (in serum)	By HAMA-FAST-ELISA; uses *S. hematobium* microsomal antigen
Antigen detection (in urine and serum)	Antigens such as CCA and CAA can be detected by ELISA or dip stick assays
Treatment	Praziquantel

Abbreviations: HAMA-FAST-ELISA, *S. haematobium* microsomal antigen-Falcon assay screening test-ELISA; CCA, Circulating cathodic antigen; CAA, circulating anodic antigen.

Problem Solving Exercise 3

Schistosoma haematobium Infection

A traveler from Africa came to the OPD with abdominal pain, hematuria and dysuria. Urine culture was sterile. Urine was collected and sent for wet mount examination (Fig. 42.15A). The adult form of the same parasite has been focused in Figure 42.15B.
1. Identify the causative agent based on the microscopic findings.
2. How will you collect and process urine specimen?
3. Which is the infective stage, host and mode of transmission of the parasite?
4. Mention two complications produced by infection with this parasite.

Explanation

Clinical Diagnosis and Identification

The causative agent is *Schistosoma haematobium*. Points in favor are:
- From Africa—endemic for schistosomiasis
- Presented with abdominal pain, hematuria and dysuria
- Bacterial UTI can be ruled out as urine culture is sterile
- Urine microscopy reveals oval nonoperculated elongated eggs with terminal spine (Fig. 42.15A)
- Figure 42.15B shows the adult worms of schistosomes. The thin female worm resides in the gynecophoric canal of the thicker male.

Urine Collection

The terminal hematuria portion of urine should be collected and concentrated by centrifugation or by membrane filtration. Refer Table 42.5 for details.

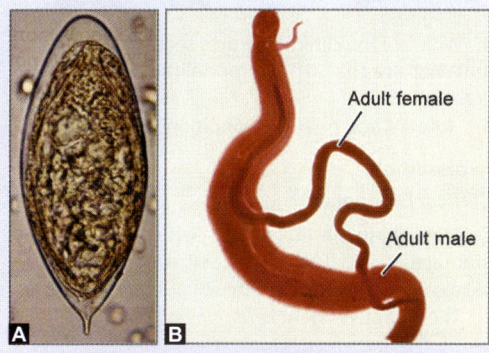

Figs 42.15A and B: (A) *Schistosoma haematobium* (egg); (B) Adult worms of schistosomes.

Source: (A) ID# 4843. Public Health Image Library; (B) DPDx Image Library, CDC, Atlanta (with permission).

Infective Syndromes of Genital Tract (Sexually-transmitted Infections)

CHAPTER 43

▮ INTRODUCTION

The sexually transmitted infections (STIs) are a group of communicable diseases which are transmitted by sexual contact. Causative agents of STIs may be classified into two groups (Table 43.1):
1. **Agents causing local manifestations**—called genital tract infections
   - Lesions common to both sexes:, such as genital ulcers, urethritis, and anorectal lesions
   - Female genital tract infections:, such as vulvovaginitis, cervicitis and others
   - Male genital tract infections:, such as prostatitis, epididymitis, and orchitis.
2. **Agents causing systemic manifestations** without producing local manifestations (e.g., HIV, hepatitis B and C).

▮ SYPHILIS

Problem Solving Exercise 1

A 35-year-old male with a history of extramarital sexual contact presented with localized, painless indolent ulcers with hard base on the penis. On examination, the inguinal lymph nodes were found to be enlarged, hard, and nontender. The serum collected from patient was subjected to a serological test given below (Fig. 43.1):
1. Identify the test and interpret the result.
2. What is the clinical diagnosis and its causative organism?
3. What tests do you recommend to confirm this diagnosis?
4. What are the clinical features seen in this disease?
5. What are the various modalities of laboratory diagnosis?
6. How will you treat this condition?

Explanation

Clinical Diagnosis
Painless, hard genital ulcers with painless non-indurated inguinal lymph nodes in a man with history of sexual contact is suggestive of primary syphilis.
The causative agent is *Treponema pallidum*.

Serological Test (VDRL)
The serological test shown in the picture is venereal disease research laboratory (VDRL) test (Fig. 43.1). The test serum is weakly reactive. Quantitative VDRL test should be repeated on serial dilution of the test serum with saline to know the titer. As VDRL is a nonspecific test, the result has to be confirmed by a specific/treponemal test, such as TPHA (*T. pallidum* hemagglutination test).
(For answers to other questions, refer below).

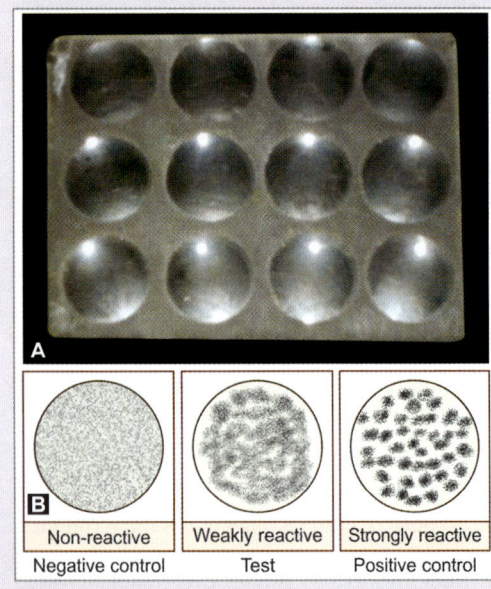

Figs 43.1A and B: (A) VDRL slide; (B) VDRL test done on a test sample with positive and negative controls.

CHAPTER 43 ◆ Infective Syndromes of Genital Tract (Sexually-transmitted Infections)

Table 43.1: Causative agents of sexually transmitted infections.

Agents causing local manifestations (genital tract infections)
In both sexes:
I. Genito-ulcerative disease: • **Syphilis:** Caused by *Treponema pallidum*   • **Chancroid:** Caused by *Haemophilus ducreyi*   • **Genital herpes**: Caused by herpes simplex viruses   • **Lymphogranuloma venereum:** Caused by *Chlamydia trachomatis*   • **Donovanosis:** Caused by *Klebsiella granulomatis*   The above genito-ulcerative diseases can be differentiated from each other by several properties (Table 43.2).   **II. Urethritis:**   • **Gonococcal urethritis:** Caused by *Neisseria gonorrhoeae*   • **Non-gonococcal urethritis (NGU)**: Caused by   ➢ *Chlamydia trachomatis* (D-K)   ➢ Genital mycoplasmas: *Ureaplasma urealyticum, Mycoplasma genitalium, M. hominis*   ➢ Herpes simplex virus   ➢ *Candida albicans*   ➢ *Trichomonas vaginalis*   **III. Other genital tract infections common to both sexes**   • **Genital tuberculosis:** Caused by *M. tuberculosis*   • Anorectal lesions: ➢ Proctitis: Caused by HSV, gonococcus, *C. trachomatis*   ➢ Anogenital warts: Caused by human papilloma virus
In females only:
• **Vulvovaginitis:** Bacterial vaginosis, trichomoniasis and candidiasis   • **Mucopurulent cervicitis** caused by gonococcus, *C. trachomatis*   • **Pelvic inflammatory disease**
In males only:
Prostatitis, epididymitis, and orchitis

Note: Agents sexually-transmitted, but cause only systemic manifestations—HIV, Hepatitis B virus, Hepatitis C virus.

Clinical Manifestations of Syphilis

Syphilis is a sexually transmitted disease caused by *T. pallidum*.
- ❖ **Primary syphilis** develops after incubation period of 9–90 days and is characterized by painless hard chancre (genital ulcer) and painless indurated lymphadenopathy
- ❖ **Secondary syphilis** usually develops 4–8 weeks later, characterized by skin rashes, condylomata lata (mucocutaneous papules) and mucosal patches
- ❖ **Late or tertiary syphilis** develops several decades after, characterized by:
  - Skin lesions called gumma
  - Neurosyphilis—general paresis of insane and tabes dorsalis
  - Cardiovascular syphilis—such as aneurysm of ascending aorta and aortic regurgitation.

Laboratory Diagnosis of Syphilis

Microscopy

- ❖ **Specimen collection:** Surface of the chancre is cleaned with saline, gentle pressure is applied at the base of the lesion, and a drop of exudate is collected on a slide
- ❖ **Dark-ground microscopy:** *T. pallidum* appears as slender, flexible, spirally coiled bacilli with tapering ends (Fig. 43.2A)
- ❖ **DFA-TP:** Direct fluorescent antibody staining for *T. pallidum* (Fig. 43.2B)
- ❖ **Silver impregnation** method, such as Levaditi stain (for tissue section) and Fontana stain (for smear) (Fig. 43.2C).

Serological Test (Antibody Detection)

Serological tests are grouped into treponemal and nontreponemal tests.

Nontreponemal or Nonspecific Tests

These are also called as standard tests for syphilis. Here, the reagin antibodies are detected by using nonspecific cardiolipin antigen derived from bovine heart muscle. Examples include:
- ❖ Venereal disease research laboratory (VDRL)
- ❖ Rapid plasma reagin (RPR) test.

1. Venereal disease research laboratory

This test was named after Venereal Disease Research Laboratory, New York, where the test was developed. It is the most widely used, simple and rapid serological test. VDRL antigen is a cardiolipin antigen to which cholesterol and lecithin are added.

Procedure:
1. **VDRL antigen** is reconstituted by mixing with a buffer. Then the patient's serum is heat inactivated at 56°C for 30 minutes to remove the nonspecific inhibitors

Table 43.2: Comparison of manifestations of genito-ulcerative diseases.

Features	Syphilis	Genital herpes	Chancroid	LGV	Donovanosis
Incubation period	9–90 days	2–7 days	1–14 days	3 days–6 weeks	1–4 weeks (up to 6 months)
Genital ulcer	Painless, single, indurated	Painful, multiple, bilateral, tiny vesicular ulcers	Painful, soft, usually multiple, purulent, bleeds easily	Painless, firm single lesion	Painless, single/multiple, beefy-red ulcer, bleeds readily
Lymphadenopathy	Painless, non-indurated (firm), bilateral	Painful, firm, often bilateral with initial episode	Painful, soft, marked swelling leads to bubo formation, unilateral	Painful and soft, unilateral	Absent (pseudobubo may be present due to subcutaneous swelling)
Treatment	Penicillin (single dose)	Acyclovir (7–14 days)	Azithromycin (single dose)	Doxycycline (21 days)	Azithromycin (7 days)

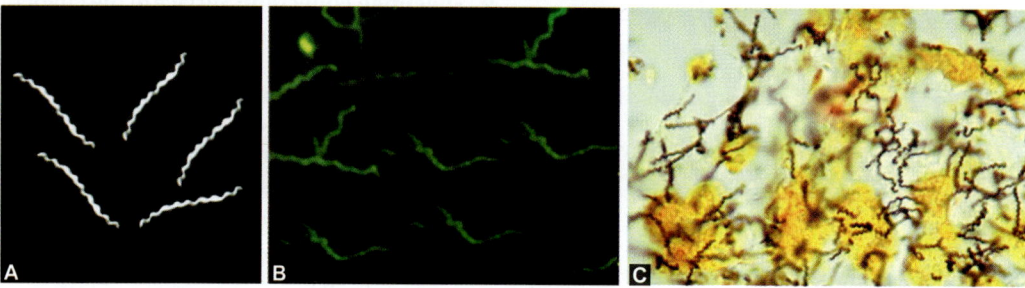

Figs 43.2A to C: Direct microscopy of *T. pallidum*. (A) Dark-ground microscope; (B) Direct fluorescent antibody staining (DFA-TP); (C) Silver impregnation method.
Source: Public Health Image Library, (A) ID# 2043; (B) ID# 14967/Dr Russell; (C) ID# 836, Centers for Disease Control and Prevention (CDC), Atlanta (*with permission*).

2. **VDRL slide** containing 12 concave rings is used (Fig. 43.1A)
3. **Qualitative test:** 50 µL of inactivated serum is mixed with a drop of VDRL antigen and the slide is rotated at 180 revolutions per minute for 4 minutes in a VDRL rotator and examined under microscope (10X). The results are read as follows:
   - *Nonreactive:* Uniformly distributed fusiform crystals represent the presence of VDRL antigen only, which indicates a negative result
   - *Reactive:* Presence of medium to large clumps signifies antigen antibody complexes, hence indicates a positive result (Fig. 43.1B).
4. **Quantitative test:** If the test is found reactive, antibody titer is determined by performing the test with serial dilutions with saline.

2. Rapid plasma reagin test
A drop of RPR reagent is added to a drop of the test serum, positive and negative controls onto separate reaction circles of the disposable slide. The slide is rotated either manually or on a mechanical rotor at 180 rpm for at least 8 minutes (Table 43.3).
- *Reactive:* Indicated by aggregates in the center or the periphery of the test circle (Fig. 43.3)
- *Nonreactive:* Indicated by a smooth, even light grey appearance with no aggregates visible.

Advantages of nontreponemal tests
- Used to monitor the response to treatment
- Neurosyphilis: VDRL can also be used to detect cerebrospinal fluid (CSF) antibodies.

Disadvantages of nontreponemal tests
- **Biological false positive (BFP) reactions:**
  - Biological false positive reactions are defined as positive results in non-treponemal tests, with negative results in treponemal tests, in the absence of syphilis and not caused by technical faults

Table 43.3: Differences between venereal disease research laboratory (VDRL) and rapid plasma reagin (RPR).

VDRL	RPR
Results read microscopically as clumps are smaller in size	Results read macroscopically. Finely divided carbon particles coated cardiolipin antigens are used so that larger visible clumps are formed
Preheating of serum is required	Preheating of serum is not required
Blood, plasma, serum, and cerebrospinal fluid can be tested	Blood, plasma and serum can be tested but not cerebrospinal fluid
Rotation of slide is done for 4 minutes	Rotation of card is done for 8 minutes
Sensitivity (78%)	More sensitive (86%)
It is cheaper. It is preferred when sample load is high	RPR is expensive than VDRL. It is preferred when sample load is less

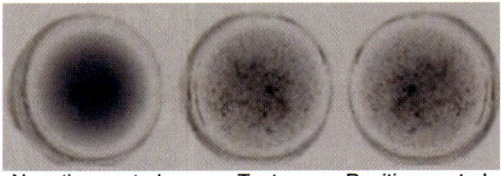

Negative control   Test   Positive control

Fig. 43.3: Rapid plasma reagin test done on a test sample with positive and negative control.

- Cardiolipin antigen being nonspecific may react with the sera of patients suffering from unrelated diseases but not having syphilis
- Biological false positive antibody is usually of IgM type, while reagin antibody in syphilis is mainly IgG
- *Types of BFP:* Conditions in which BFP reactions occur can be classified into:
  - *Acute BFP reactions* persist for less than 6 months and are usually associated with acute infections, injuries or inflammatory conditions
  - *Chronic BFP reactions* last for more than 6 months and are typically seen in systemic lupus erythematosus (SLE) and other collagen diseases, such as rheumatoid arthritis.

- ❖ **Prozone phenomenon:** If antibody titer in patient's sera is high, it may lead to false negative result; hence, it is essential to test sera in dilutions.

Specific/Treponemal Serological Test

As the nontreponemal tests are nonspecific, the result has to be confirmed by a specific/treponemal test which detects antibodies by using *T. pallidum* antigens.
- ❖ FTA-ABS (Fluorescent treponemal antibody absorption test)
- ❖ TPHA (*T. pallidum* hemagglutination test)
- ❖ TPPA (*T. pallidum* particle agglutination test)
- ❖ Western blot
- ❖ Enzyme immunoassay (EIA)
- ❖ TPI (*T. pallidum* immobilization test).

Testing Algorithm

CDC recommends to use a **testing algorithm** comprising of non-treponemal test (as screening test), followed by treponemal test (for confirmation) for serodiagnosis of syphilis.

Testing for syphilis in pregnancy: Every pregnant woman should undergo a non-treponemal screening test at her first antenatal visit and, if there is high-risk of exposure, again retested at the third trimester and at delivery.

Treatment of Syphilis

- ❖ Penicillin is the drug of choice for all the stages of syphilis
- ❖ Alternate drug is used in patients with penicillin allergy:
  - Primary, secondary, latent, cardiovascular system or benign tertiary syphilis—tetracycline is recommended
  - Neurosyphilis or pregnancy or associated human immunodeficiency virus infection—desensitization to penicillin has to be done following which penicillin is administered.

GONORRHOEA

Clinical Manifestations

Gonorrhea is a venereal disease, caused by *Neisseria gonorrhoeae*.

Problem Solving Exercise 2

A 32-year-old male with history of frequent sexual contact with a commercial sex worker presented with urethral discharge. Gram staining of the urethral discharge is shown in Figure 43.4.
1. What is the clinical diagnosis and its causative organism?
2. List the infections caused by this organism.
3. What are the various modalities of laboratory diagnosis?
4. What antibiotic you would like to prescribe?

Explanation

Clinical Diagnosis
History of urethral discharge from a male who has a relationship with sex worker is suggestive of sexually transmitted disease, such as gonorrhea or *Chlamydia* infection.

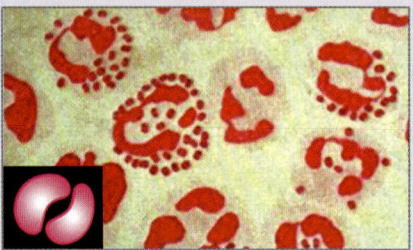

Fig. 43.4: Gram staining of the urethral discharge.
Source: Public Health Image Library, ID# /2108, Centers for Disease Control and Prevention (CDC), Atlanta (*with permission*).

Identification
Direct Gram staining of urethral discharge (Fig. 43.4) shows gram-negative cocci in pair (kidney shaped). This is suggestive of *Neisseria gonorrhoeae*.
(For answers to other questions, refer below).

- Males present as acute urethritis, epididymitis and abscess in periurethral region with sinus formation (known as *water-can perineum*)
- In females, infection is less severe; more asymptomatic carriage than males. Symptomatic females present with mucopurulent cervicitis and pelvic inflammatory disease
- In pregnant women, it causes premature delivery, chorioamnionitis and sepsis in the infant
- In neonates (ophthalmia neonatorum)
- Disseminated gonococcal infection (DGI).

Laboratory Diagnosis

Specimen Collection
Urethral swab in men and cervical swab in women are the preferred specimens. Vaginal and supravaginal swabs are not satisfactory.
- The urethral meatus is cleaned with gauze soaked in saline. The purulent discharge is expressed out by pressing at the base of the penis and collected directly on to slides or swabs
- *Dacron or rayon swabs* are preferred, as cotton and alginate swabs are inhibitory to gonococci
- *In chronic urethritis*—as discharge is minimal, prostatic massage is done to collect the secretion; alternatively the morning drop of secretion may be collected
- Blood and synovial fluid in DGI cases.

Transport Media
Specimens should be transported immediately. If not possible, then urethral discharge should be collected in charcoal coated swabs kept in Stuart's transport medium or alternatively, charcoal-containing medium (Amies medium) can be used.

Gram-staining of Urethral Exudates
It reveals gram-negative intracellular kidney-shaped diplococci (Fig. 43.4). Gram staining is more useful in males than in females because of the presence of commensal *Neisseria* species in female genital tract confound with interpretation. Hence, culture is recommended for diagnosis of gonorrhea in women.

Culture
As cervical swabs contain normal flora, hence *selective media* are preferred, such as:
- Thayer Martin medium

CHAPTER 43 ◆ Infective Syndromes of Genital Tract (Sexually-transmitted Infections)

- Modified New York City medium
- Martin Lewis medium.

Colonies on Thayer Martin media are gray, convex, with crenated margin and raised opaque center.

Biochemical Tests

- Gonococci are catalase and oxidase positive
- They ferment only glucose, but not maltose and sucrose.

Treatment

- Drug of choice: Third generation cephalosporins:
    - Ceftriaxone (250 mg given intramuscularly, single dose)
    - Cefixime (400 mg given orally, single dose).
- Both the sexual partners should be treated
- Azithromycin is added if coexisting chlamydial infection is suspected.

NON-GONOCOCCAL URETHRITIS (NGU)

Chronic urethritis where gonococci cannot be demonstrated has been labeled as non-gonococcal urethritis. NGU is more common than gonococcal urethritis. Several agents are implicated in NGU, such as:

- **Bacteria:** These agents are discussed below:
    - *Chlamydia trachomatis*: Most common agent of NGU
    - Urogenital *Mycoplasma*: *Ureaplasma urealyticum* and *Mycoplasma hominis*.
- **Viruses:** Herpes simplex virus
- **Fungi:** *Candida albicans*
- **Parasites:** *Trichomonas vaginalis*.

Differences between gonococcal and non-gonococcal urethritis are given in Table 43.4.

VULVOVAGINITIS

Vulvovaginitis refers to inflammation of the vaginal mucosa (called vaginitis) and the external genitalia vulva (called vulvitis). It is the most common genital tract infection in females.

- Women present with vaginal symptoms, such as abnormal discharge with/without offensive odor or itching
- The three most common causes of vaginitis in premenopausal women are trichomoniasis, bacterial vaginosis and vaginal candidiasis; can be differentiated from each other as given in Table 43.5.

TRICHOMONIASIS

Trichomonas vaginalis is a genital flagellate, causes trichomoniasis; the only parasitic sexually transmitted disease (Table 43.6 and Fig. 43.5).

Table 43.4: Differences between gonococcal and non-gonococcal urethritis.

Features	Gonococcal urethritis	Non-gonococcal urethritis
Onset	48 hours	Longer (>1 week)
Urethral discharge	Purulent (flow of seed-resembling semen)	Mucous to mucopurulent
Complication	DGI (polyarthritis and endocarditis) Water-can perineum	**Reiter's syndrome:** Characterized by conjunctivitis, urethritis, arthritis and mucosal lesions
Diagnosis	• Gram stain • Culture on Thayer Martin media	• For *Chlamydia* (most common agent): Culture on McCoy and HeLa cell lines • For *Trichomonas*—detection of trophozoite • For *Candida*—detection of budding yeast cells in discharge • For PCR—can be done for HSV or *Chlamydia*
Treatment	Ceftriaxone	• For *Chlamydia*—Doxycycline • For *Trichomonas*—Metronidazole • For *Candida*—Clotrimazole (as vaginal cream or tablet)

Abbreviations: DGI, disseminated gonococcal infection; HSV, herpes simplex virus; PCR, polymerase chain reaction.

Problem Solving Exercise 3

Trichomoniasis

A 28-year-old female sex worker presents to the STD clinic with history of thin profuse foul smelling purulent vaginal discharge, dysuria and lower abdominal pain. The wet mount examination of vaginal discharge is depicted in Figure 43.5B. What is the etiologial diagnosis and how will you treat this case?

Explanation

Clinical Diagnosis

History of thin profuse foul smelling purulent vaginal discharge, dysuria and lower abdominal pain is suggestive of vulvovaginitis.

Etiology

Figure 43.5B reveales permanent staining of vaginal discharge showing trophozoites of *Trichomonas vaginalis*.
- Pear-shaped, measures 7–23 μm, possesses one nucleus, axostyle and five flagella:
- Four anterior flagella
- One posterior recurrent flagellum supported by undulating membrane and costa

Treatment

Treatment of *Trichomonas vaginalis* includes metronidazole 2 g, single dose; given to both sexual partners

Table 43.5: Differential diagnosis of vulvovaginitis.

Feature	Vulvovaginal candidiasis	Trichomonal vaginitis	Bacterial vaginosis
Etiology	*Candida albicans*	*Trichomonas vaginalis*	*Gardnerella vaginalis*, various anaerobic bacteria
Typical symptoms	Vulvar itching and/or irritation	Profuse purulent discharge; vulvar itching	Malodorous, slightly increased discharge
Discharge	Scanty, white, thick and cheesy	Profuse, white or yellow	Moderate, thin, white to gray
pH of vaginal fluid	Usually ≤4.5	Usually ≥5	Usually >4.5
Fishy odor with 10% KOH	None	May be present	Present
Vaginal inflammation (erythema)	May be present	Colpitis macularis (strawberry appearance)	None
Microscopy of vaginal discharge	↑ Leukocytes, epithelial cells; budding yeast cell with pseudohyphae	↑ Leukocytes; trophozoites seen in 80–90% of symptomatic patients	Clue cells, few leukocytes, no/few lactobacilli (Nugent's score ≥7)
Other laboratory findings	Isolation of *Candida* spp.	Antigen detection or PCR	Culture, broad-range PCR
Treatment of the patient	Azole cream, tablet	Metronidazole or tinidazole	Metronidazole (tablet) and clindamycin cream
Treatment of sexual partner	None; topical treatment needed in case of *Candida* dermatitis of penis	Usually treatment needed	None

Table 43.6: Features of *Trichomonas vaginalis*.

Properties	Characteristics of *Trichomonas vaginalis*
Host	Humans are the only host
Infective form	Trophozoites
Transmission	Sexually transmitted
Habitat	Vagina
Pathogenic form	Trophozoites
Major manifestations (trichomoniasis)	Vulvovaginitis—characterized by: • Vaginal discharge with profuse foul smelling, increases by adding 10% KOH (Whiff test) • Raised pH (>4.5) • Strawberry appearance of vaginal mucosa (colpitis macularis)

Contd...

Contd...

Properties	Characteristics of *Trichomonas vaginalis*

Diagnostic form (Fig. 43.5)	• Trophozoites detected by wet mount or permanent staining of vaginal discharge
	• Pear-shaped, measures 7–23 μm, possesses one nucleus, axostyle and five flagella:
	  ➢ Four anterior flagella
	  ➢ One posterior recurrent flagellum supported by undulating membrane and costa

Other methods of diagnosis	• Antigen detection (ICT) • PCR detecting tubulin gene
Treatment	Metronidazole 2 g, single dose; given to both sexual partners

Abbreviations: ICT, immunochromatographic test; PCR, polymerase chain reaction.

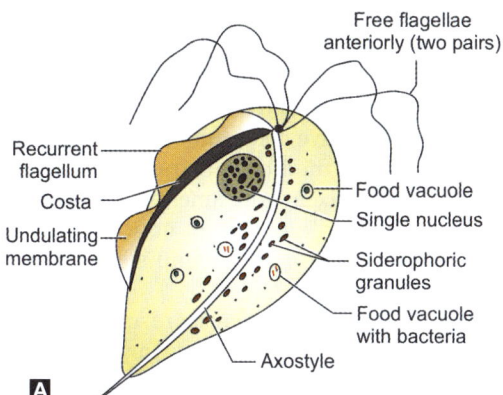 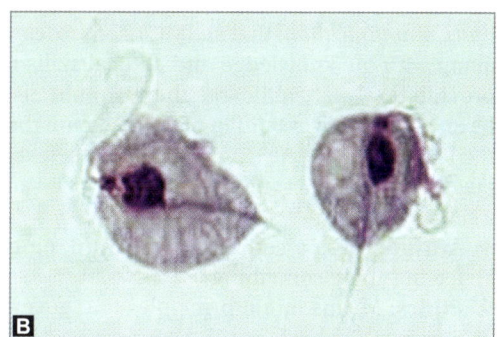

Figs 43.5A and B: *Trichomonas vaginalis* trophozoite: (A) Schematic diagram; (B) Giemsa staining.
Source: DPDx Image Library, CDC, Atlanta (*with permission*).

VAGINAL CANDIDIASIS

Problem Solving Exercise 4

A 32-year-old female sex worker presents to the STD clinic with complain of vulvar itching and/or irritation and scanty, white, thick and cheesy vaginal discharge. Vaginal discharge was sent for Gram staining and culture (Figs 43.6A and B). What is the etiological diagnosis and what further tests are needed for accurate species identification.

Explanation

Clinical Diagnosis
History of vulvar itching and/or irritation and scanty, white, thick and cheesy vaginal discharge is suggestive of vulvovaginitis, probably candidiasis.

Etiology
Gram staining (Fig. 43.6A) vaginal discharge reveals gram-positive oval budding yeast cells with pseudohyphae and culture on Sabouraud's dextrose agar (Fig. 43.6B) showed dry creamy white colonies. The genus identification is *Candida* species. Species identification can be made by conventional (e.g., germ tube test, growth on CHROM agar, cornmeal agar, etc.) or automated methods (VITEK or MALDI-TOF).

For, answer to other questions, refer Chapter 21.

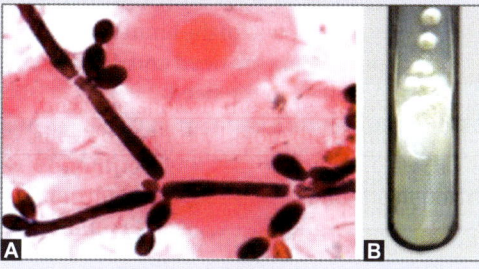

Figs 43.6A and B: *Candida albicans:* (A) Gram-positive oval budding yeast cells with pseudohyphae; (B) On SDA shows creamy-white colonies.
Source: (A) Public Health Image Library, Centers for Disease Control and Prevention (CDC), Atlanta; ID #2934; (B) Pondicherry Institute of Medical Sciences, Puducherry (*with permission*).

CHAPTER 44

AETCOM in Microbiology

AETCOM

AETCOM refers to the **soft skills** '*Attitude, Ethics and Communication*,' that an IMG needs to learn along with the knowledge and clinical skills to provide holistic healthcare. There should also be an assessment system in place to ensure that the learning about AETCOM has actually taken place. The essential components of AETCOM are as follows.

- ❖ **Attitude:** It is a settled way of thinking or feeling about something
- ❖ **Ethics:** Means moral principles that govern a person's behavior or the conducting of an activity. Ethics in MBBS curriculum basically means bioethics or more specifically medical ethics, which has the 4 pillars—
  1. **Patient autonomy**: Allowing a capable person to exercise the right to make own decisions and only facilitating in such decision-making, e.g., informed consent
  2. **Beneficence:** Patients' right to improvement or restoration of their health
  3. **Non-maleficence**: An obligation not to inflict harm on others
  4. **Social justice:** Fair and non-discriminatory distribution of the limited resources and, prioritising the need and distribution proportionate to the need.
- ❖ **Communication:** It is imparting or exchanging of information by speaking, writing, or using some other medium.

Need for AETCOM Competencies

Patients and members of the healthcare team value AETCOM skills as much as the clinical skills.
- ❖ Proficiency in AETCOM competencies is very much essential in carrying out routine healthcare activities including doctor-patient interactions, practicing informed decision making, breaking bad news (new diagnosis of chronic disease, malignancy, death, etc.), communication and documentation
- ❖ Lack of effective communication has direct bearing on medical errors, mistakes in diagnosis, inaccurate treatment, compromised patient safety, and patient noncompliance leading to stressful legal and sociocultural issues
- ❖ AETCOM competencies are essential to address issues, such as growing distrust in healthcare, violence on doctors, litigations on doctors, etc.

AETCOM Learning in Current vs Previous Curriculum

AETOM in earlier MBBS curriculum: Before CBME was introduced, medical education focussed mainly on gaining knowledge and clinical skills. AETCOM competencies were neither formally taught nor assessed. Some learning used to happen by observing seniors (role modelling) or with self-experience.

AETCOM in current curriculum: AETCOM modules in current MBBS curriculum aim at acquisition of minimum essential skills, such as communicating effectively and sympathetically with patients and their relatives by all the IMGs uniformly.
- ❖ **Longitudinally spread:** AETCOM competencies relevant to each subject are defined in the CBME and will be taught longitudinally spread over all the phases of MBBS
- ❖ **Increasing complexity:** The topics/competencies are interlinked and are of increasing complexity as one moves from the first year to the final professional year of MBBS.

Teaching-Learning Methods for AETCOM Competencies

Similar to gaining subject knowledge and learning clinical skills, AETCOM competencies can also be taught and learnt, though the approach needs appropriate modifications. Teaching-Learning sessions are planned in such a way that the students are provided with opportunities to learn the basic essential background knowledge, opportunities to learn by experiencing (mostly simulated) and reflect on the experiences. Innovative teaching-learning (TL) methods can be used for AETCOM competencies which will be more engaging and effective.

Problem-based Learning (PBL)

Problem-based learning (PBL) is suggested by the MCI as the main TL method for AETCOM. PBL helps students explore the various facets of "real life issues" that will confront them in their careers, develop problem solving skills. **Case discussions** promote collaborative learning and team work, reflection and self-directed learning.

- In this, first a case scenario is introduced to the students and they are guided to explore ethical, legal and sociocultural aspects involved in that case and prepare learning objectives
- Then the students are divided into groups and assignments are given for self-directed learning (SDL) by using various teacher-suggested or self-explored resources. Student learning may also be helped by an anchoring learning activity to increase relevant background knowledge (e.g., lecture, panel discussion) or experience (e.g., visit to hospital/laboratory, observation of working pattern of different types of healthcare workers, discussion with patients or their family members, etc.)
- After some days of learning time through SDL, the same case or another related case is discussed. The students provide suggestions and alternatives on the approach for doctors to follow and conclusions are drawn
- Finally the students write narrative about their learning experience which is expected to help

themselves to develop the following essential skills:
- To elicit, observe and record data
- To reflect on the data at a higher level of thinking and derive opinions and conclusions
- To communicate the observations and conclusions in a written and verbal form and expand on and defend the conclusions with colleagues and teachers, and
- To form new experiences and conclusions based on this discussion.

Assessment of AETCOM Competencies

In the CBME, AETCOM competencies will be assessed formatively as well as summatively.

Formative Assessment

Formative assessment is done during and along with day-to-day TL sessions and its purpose is to provide feedback to the students and help them improve. Formative assessment is done based on the student participation in small group discussions, performance in assignments or internal assessment tests, etc.

Summative Assessment

Summative assessment is qualifying examination which decides pass or fail status.
- There will be questions on AETCOM competencies in the theory and practical examinations conducted at the end of each professional year
- Student needs to maintain a logbook as a record of his performance and acquisition of essential competencies
- Objective structured clinical/practical examination (OSCE/OSPE) or Kalamazoo skill rating scale may be used to make the assessment less subjective and to include all relevant aspects in the assessment.

Communications Skill Rating Scale

It is adapted from Kalamazoo consensus. The parameters assessed are: (i) builds relationship, (ii) opens the discussion, (iii) gathers information, (iv) understands the patient's perspective, (v) shares information, (vi) manages flow, (vii) overall rating. Rating: 1–3 Poor, 4–6 Satisfactory, 6–10 Superior.

SUGGESTED AETCOM TOPICS IN MICROBIOLOGY

MCI has specified 8 AETCOM modules and 37 TL hours in the second professional year for all the subjects concerned. Following 2 competencies are specified in the Microbiology subject.

1. Demonstration of **confidentiality pertaining** to patient identity on laboratory results
2. Demonstration of **respect for patient samples** sent to the laboratory for performance of laboratory tests in the detection of microbial agents causing infectious diseases.

COMPETENCY-1
DEMONSTRATE CONFIDENTIALITY PERTAINING TO PATIENT IDENTITY ON LABORATORY RESULTS

Competency: Demonstrate confidentiality pertaining to patient identity on laboratory results
Domain: Attitude
Level of learning: Knows how

Sample Case Scenarios

Case scenario 1 (Disclosing HIV result)
A lady aged 20 years admitted for fever and breathlessness jumps from the 4th floor of the hospital and dies. On enquiry, it was revealed that she was recently diagnosed to be HIV reactive (one week ago) and "Retro positive" labels were put on her case file and bed. Her family members had come to know about her HIV status when they had enquired with a junior resident about the "Retro positive" label. They became stressed out and shouted at the patient. Except for her mother, all other family members had stopped visiting her then onwards.

Case scenario 2 (Not disclosing HIV result)
A 33-year-old man is admitted to the emergency ward with multiple limb fractures. With ongoing medical treatment, his vitals are stabilized, he is conscious and oriented. Emergency surgery is planned. His relative comes to the laboratory to collect the investigation reports, he is given all the reports except HIV results. He is suspicious and is specifically asking if the laboratory is not issuing only HIV report because it is reactive. Technician gets a call from the ward asking for the HIV report immediately over the phone, as the patient is being shifted to the operating room.

Case scenario 3 (Patient refuses to provide samples)
A nurse caring for an admitted patient gets a needle stick injury with a syringe used for the patient. The patient's HIV and HBV infection status unknown. To decide the need for post-exposure prophylaxis the nurse wants to get patient tested. The patient asks the nurse not to worry, refuses saying he has no such infection, hence no need to test and has financial constrain for performing the tests. The nurse is anxious. The nurse decides to use the patient's blood sample collected for some other tests for testing for HIV and HBsAg and bear the cost by herself.

Case scenario 4 (Social stigma in COVID-19)
A patient with influenza, such as illness (ILI) has come to the screening OPD. He had exposure to a confirmed COVID-19 case five days back. He wants to get tested and treated, as he is anxious. However, he does not want to be quarantined or discriminated, and has a fear of social stigma and losing the job. He is also the only caretaker of old parents at home.

Case scenario 5 (Occupational exposure)
A medical intern comes to the infection control division with a history of needle stick injury 1 hour back. The source patient's blood sample is collected and tested for HIV, hepatitis B and C. The intern is waiting in the reception of the infection control division to know about the test result of source sample. The test result shows it is reactive for HIV but negative for hepatitis B and C. The infection control officer discloses the source result to the intern immediately and provides appropriate counseling and post-exposure prophylaxis. He also forwards the source result to ICTC. The ICTC calls the source patient on next day and informs about the test result after providing counseling.

Essential Background Knowledge

1. Principles of medical ethics
2. Medicolegal aspects of confidentiality
3. Confidentiality and privileged communication related to laboratory results
4. Modes of transmission and diagnostic approach for HIV or COVID-19, etc.
5. Sociocultural issues related to sensitive infections, such as HIV or COVID-19 or needle stick injury
6. Post-exposure prophylaxis for needle stick injury when the source turns out to be positive for HIV or hepatitis B.

CHAPTER 44 ◈ AETCOM in Microbiology

Specific Learning Objectives
1. Discuss the rights and responsibilities of patients (or healthcare worker in case scenario 5)
2. Discuss the rights and responsibilities of the laboratory with respect to the confidentiality of laboratory results
3. Analyze the ethical issues involved in confidentiality pertaining to patient identity
4. Describe the medicolegal consequences of a breach in confidentiality
5. Demonstration of sympathy when breaking through of result to healthcare workers, providing counseling and maintaining confidentiality pertaining to occupational hazards, such as needle stick injury (in case scenario 5).

Teaching-Learning Method
1. **Introductory session:** Introduction of paper case in small group discussion, identification of various aspects involved, framing learning objectives and deciding assignments along with learning resources
2. **SDL:** Self-directed learning by the students
3. **Anchoring learning sessions:** This involves one or more of the following depending upon the case scenario:
    ➢ Interaction with laboratory technician and counselor of Integrated Counseling and Testing Center (ICTC)
    ➢ Interaction with Microbiology laboratory technician involved in HIV/COVID-19 testing and report dispatch
    ➢ Interaction with infection control officer involved in management of needle stick injury.
4. **Concluding session:** Small group discussion of various possible approaches for the case, their pros and cons, and justification for the best approach selected by each student. However, it may be possible that there may not be single best approach.
5. **Writing narratives** by the students about their learning experiences.

Resources: Standard medical microbiology and forensic medicine textbooks, NACO guidelines.

Assessment
Formative: Participation in the group discussion, assignments, reflection writing, MCQs to assess relevant background knowledge, OSPE, etc.
Summative (Theory): Short notes and short answer questions.
Summative (Practical): Includes OSPE with a simulated patient–HIV pre-test/post-test counseling, counseling following needle stick injury, informing positive COVID-19 report to the patient and informing needle stick injury test result to the healthcare worker.

Key Learning Points
1. **Confidentiality:** It is part of the professional secrecy, where a patient's personal/health information (history, clinical diagnosis, lab results, etc.) is not shared with others, including close relatives and employers, without the patient's consent. The person with HIV has the right to privacy, and the right to exercise informed consent in all decisions about disclosure of his/her HIV status except in circumstances when disclosure to another person is required by law or ethical or health considerations
2. **Informed consent:** The patient gives written permission to carry out HIV testing after understanding the potential implications, risks and advantages of the possible test results
3. **Counseling** is confidential communication limited to the patient and a counselor with the purpose of understanding the risk of HIV infection, to help cope with the stress and to make personal decisions related to HIV/AIDS
4. **Privileged communication:** It is the unbiased, bonafide communication by a doctor (bypassing confidentiality) to an individual or an authority who has corresponding legal, social and moral obligations. The doctor first tries to convince the patient to disclose the information himself to the person(s) at risk and to avoid risky behavior and, informs the potentially affected/authority directly when in doubt. Such disclosures are made to the people at risk, such as the spouse, healthcare workers involved in patient care, etc.
5. **The method followed in ICTC for HIV testing:** Only the counselor interacts with the patient with privacy. Pre-test counseling is done and written informed consent is taken before sample collection and testing. Report will not have the patient's name written, instead will have identification marks (moles, scars, etc.), age and gender mentioned for patient identification. Irrespective of the result, the counselor does the post-test counseling and hands over the report directly to the patient. Confidentiality regarding patient identity and HIV infection status is maintained throughout
6. **Method followed for other STDs (Syphilis, Gonorrhea):** Confidentiality is maintained regarding patient identity and laboratory results. Patient is counseled to avoid risky behavior, get partner also tested and both advised to get treated simultaneously if required

7. **Method followed for COVID-19**: Patient is identified with an alphanumeric code instead of the name. Details are released in the media by the Government authorities with the code and not disclosing the patient identity. Labels are put on the patient house to identify and alert other people.

COMPETENCY-2
DEMONSTRATION OF RESPECT FOR PATIENT SAMPLES

Competency: Demonstration of respect for patient samples sent to the laboratory for performance of laboratory tests in the detection of microbial agents causing infectious diseases
Domain: Attitude
Level of learning: Shows how

Sample Case Scenarios

Case scenario 1 (Rejection due to improper transport)
Sequestrum from a chronic osteomyelitis case was debrided and sent for culture and sensitivity. The sample was rejected by the laboratory mentioning that it was received in formalin, hence unsuitable for culture. There is no more sample available for culture now.

Case scenario 2 (Specimen did not reach laboratory)
A critically ill 5-year-old child's CSF report is awaited for 3 days. On enquiry, laboratory says it did not receive the sample. On further probing, it was found that the nursing staff had kept the small bottle with the sample in his pocket and mistakenly taken it outside the hospital and had dropped it somewhere, and did not submit it to the laboratory for testing. Now, the baby needs to undergo lumbar puncture again, results may not be the same as antibiotics are given and need to wait for some more days for the culture report.

Case scenario 3 (Misguided report due to inadequate information in requisition form)
Urologist calls up the laboratory to discuss about "Insignificant bacteriuria" culture report of a pyelonephritis patient. He says it was a percutaneous nephrostomy sample and asks for the organism and antimicrobial sensitivity. Microbiologist says it was written as urine sample on the request form, some gram-negative bacillus had grown and the count was less than 10,000 CFU/mL, so it was thought to be a periurethral commensal and the isolate was discarded, and hence further testing cannot be done.

Case scenario 4 (Specimen kept at wrong place)
Junior resident gets angry and yells at the patient on noticing a stool sample kept on the bedside table. The patient's attendant tries to explain that the container is covered in a plastic cover and all these days the junior resident herself used to keep collected blood and swab samples in that very same place, and he was not informed that stool sample was not to be kept on the side table.

Case scenario 5 (Rejection due to improper collection)
A suspected pulmonary tuberculosis patient, who would travel 30 km from his village to the private hospital with the attached laboratory in the city, had submitted spot sputum sample the previous day and an early morning sample today for acid-fast staining. Reports of both the samples mentioned "many epithelial cells suggestive of excessive salivary contamination. Repeat with the proper sample". Blood culture was also collected from the patient by the clinical team, the result of which came as contaminated blood culture specimen with patient's skin flora.
The doctor found it very difficult to convince the patient to submit proper samples again and pay for them too.

Case scenario 6 (Sample collected for culture and sensitivity in unsterile container)
Paired blood specimen (5 mL each) was sent to the laboratory in two vacutainers for blood culture. The laboratory rejected the specimen. The patient screams that he cannot allow to draw another set of blood specimen for investigation.

Case scenario 7 (Rejection due to lack of patient informations)
Microbiology laboratory rejects a bunch of specimens because one or the other relevant informations were missing in those specimens—patient's name, age or gender, ward, hospital number, sample type, clinical diagnosis, or treatment history. The clinical team screams at the laboratory that they could have called the ward or the patient's attendant and verified the details instead of rejecting.

Case scenario 8 (Rejection due to mismatch of name)
Microbiology laboratory rejects a blood culture specimen collected in BacT/ALERT bottle because the patient's name written on the bottle did not match with that of the requisition form. The clinical team asks the patient to pay again

for a repeat blood culture investigation. The patient complains that he cannot afford the price for another test and neither he can give consent to draw another specimen.
Case scenario 9 (Prioritising a sample requiring immediate processing and reporting over the others)
In the midnight, the Microbiology laboratory receives three specimens (urine, sputum, CSF) from a patient for culture. The technician was already processing a huge load of investigations, therefore he informed the clinical team that these specimens can only be processed on the next day.

Essential Background Knowledge

1. Appropriate sample for the test planned: Sample type, amount, collection procedure, preservative if any, container type used—and its transportation and storage
2. Appropriate labeling for correct sample identification
3. Accompanying clinical information for correlation
4. Possible medicolegal issues following incomplete/incorrect sample identification
5. Sociocultural issues following incomplete/incorrect sample identification, relevant clinical information for correlation, improper storage or transportation
6. Ethical issues following incomplete/incorrect sample identification, relevant clinical information for correlation, improper storage or transportation.

Specific Learning Objectives

1. Choose an appropriate container for sample collection
2. Demonstrate an appropriate procedure for temporary storage and transportation of clinical sample
3. Discuss the information that shall be written in the request form and the sample container, completely and legibly
4. Discuss the judicious application of sample rejection criteria in the best interest of patient care
5. Discuss the importance of prioritising the specimen as relevant to the clinical situation
6. Discuss medical, ethical and socio-economical considerations of errors in sample collection and submission process.

Teaching-Learning Methods

1. **Introduction of scenarios** with the help of paper case/role plays/videos
2. **Small group discussion**: Identification of clinical, medicolegal, sociocultural and ethical issues involved
3. **Writing learning objectives**
4. **Writing narratives** by the students about their learning experiences
5. **Anchoring lecture** and demonstration of appropriate procedure of sample collection, transportation and reception at the laboratory. Discussion with nursing staff, phlebotomist, laboratory technicians to gather first-hand information
6. **Closing session** with small group discussion
7. **Writing narratives** by the students about their learning experiences.

Resources: Sample collection (refer in this book), Textbook of Forensic Medicine, Communicate-care-Cure by Dr Alexander Thomas.

Assessment

Formative: Participation in the group discussion, Assignments, reflection writing, MCQs to assess relevant background knowledge and OSPE.
Summative (Theory): Short notes and short answer questions.
Summative (Practical): OSPE can be conducted covering the following aspects
- Sample collection with care and empathy, instructing patients on appropriate sample collection (e.g., urine, sputum, blood culture, etc.)
- Labeling sample containers and filling request form for the clinical scenario provided.

Key Learning Points

The method of collection and transport of various specimens for Microbiology investigations, the various specimen rejection criteria and the criteria for prioritizing the specimen for processing have been discussed in detail in Chapter 3.2.

CHAPTER 45

University Practical Examination

■ PRACTICAL ASSESSMENT PATTERN

The Competency-based Medical Education has been implemented in MBBS since 2019. The salient features of university practical examination according to this new MBBS curriculum is as follows.
- ❖ Total mark allotted for practical examination is 100, which is divided into:
  - Practical (80 marks) and
  - Viva voce (20 marks): Viva voce marks are to be added to practical, not to theory
- ❖ Topic distribution under practical assessment is up to the department to decide
- ❖ Departments are advised to have OSPE stations for assessment of practical skills.

■ AUTHOR'S SUGGESTION

Authors suggest the following model of topic distribution as given below in the Table 45.1.
- ❖ **Sample collection and transport**: Authors have suggested to keep ''Sample collection and transport' as a separate exercise as this

Table 45.1: Practical assessment pattern.

Practical	Marks
Practical	**80 marks**
Problem-based exercise on Gram-staining (Smears made from clinical specimens-Pus, sputum, body fluids, etc.) • Staining quality (5) • Microscopic finding with report writing (5) • Knowledge testing particularly application part (5)	15
Problem-based exercise on acid-fast staining of sputum smears • Staining quality (5) • Microscopic finding with report writing (5) • Knowledge testing particularly application part (5)	15
Sample collection and transport	10
Hospital infection control	10
Clinical Microbiology Applied Exercise (Based on clinical infective syndromes)	10 marks x 3 exercises= 30
Viva voce	**20 marks**
Viva voce-I: General Microbiology, immunology, infections of bloodstream and cardiovascular system, gastrointestinal tract and hepatobiliary system	10 marks
Viva voce-II: Infections of skin, soft tissue and musculoskeletal system, respiratory system, central nervous system, genitourinary and sexually-transmitted infections, hospital infection and control, and miscellaneous	10 marks
Overall total in practical assessment (including Viva)	100

Note: This is just an author's suggestion. Medical colleges can use this as a template and modify according to the departmental consensus and university policy.

is the most important part of microbiology that an Indian medical graduate should know
- ❖ **Hospital infection control**: Authors have suggested to keep 'Hospital infection control' as a separate exercise. In lieu of COVID-19 pandemic, MCI has implemented a pandemic module and has made it mandatory for every Indian medical graduate to know the detail of infection control practices
- ❖ **Stool examination** for parasites need not be kept as a separate exercise, but can be asked as problem based exercise under applied exercise.

Exercises included in practical assessment and chapter in which the topics are discussed are enlisted in Table 45.2.

Table 45.2: Exercises included in practical assessment and chapter in which the topics are discussed.

	Exercises included in practical assessment and chapter in which the topics are discussed
1	**Problem-based exercise on Gram staining (Chapter 3.4)**
	(Smears made from clinical specimens—pus, sputum, body fluids, etc.) • Staining quality • Microscopic finding with report writing • Knowledge testing particularly application part
2	**Problem-based exercise on acid-fast staining of sputum smears (Chapter 3.5)**
	• Staining quality • Microscopic finding with report writing • Knowledge testing particularly application part
3	**Sample collection and transport** (Any one of the following exercise)
	• Urine specimen for microscopy and culture (Chapters 3.2 and 42) • Blood specimen for culture (Chapters 3.2 and 17) • Blood specimen for serology • Stool specimen for microscopy (for parasites) and bacteriological culture (Chapters 3.2, 5 and 22) • Sterile body fluid specimens for microscopy and culture (Chapter 3.2) • Pus and wound swab specimens for microscopy and culture (Chapter 3.2) • Respiratory specimens for microscopy, culture or for molecular test (Chapter 3.2) • Anaerobic specimens for microscopy and culture (Chapters 3.2 and 30)
4	**Hospital infection control** (Any one of the following exercise)
	• Hand hygiene (methods and indications) (Chapter 10) • Personal protective equipment (donning and doffing of PPE and indications of their use) (Chapter 10) • Biomedical waste (segregation compliance) (Chapter 13) • Needle stick injuries (post-exposure prophylaxis for HIV and hepatitis B) (Chapter 14)
5	**Clinical Microbiology Applied Exercise** (Any three of the following exercise)
	Bloodstream and cardiovascular system infections • Infective endocarditis (Chapter 16) • Acute rheumatic fever (Chapter 16) • Bloodstream infections (sepsis) (Chapter 17) • Enteric fever (Chapter 18) • Scrub typhus (Chapter 18) • Brucellosis (Chapter 18) • Leptospirosis (Chapter 18) • HIV/AIDS (Chapter 19) • Dengue (Chapter 19) • Malaria (Chapter 20) • Visceral leishmaniasis (Chapter 20) • Lymphatic filariasis (Chapter 20) • Systemic candidiasis (Chapter 21)	**Gastrointestinal tract infections** • Shigellosis (Chapter 22) • Cholera (Chapter 22) • *Clostridioides difficile* diarrhea (Chapter 22) • Rotavirus diarrhea (Chapter 23) • Intestinal amoebiasis (Chapter 24) • Giardiasis (Chapter 24) • Cryptosporidiosis (Chapter 24) • Intestinal taeniasis (Chapter 25) • Hymenolepiasis (Chapter 25) • *Schistosoma mansoni* infection (Chapter 25) • Trichuriasis (Chapter 25) • Enterobiasis (Chapter 25) • Ascariasis (Chapter 25) • Hookworm infection (Chapter 25) • Strongyloidiasis (Chapter 25)

Contd...

Contd...

Exercises included in practical assessment and chapter in which the topics are discussed	
Hepatobiliary system infections • Viral hepatitis (Chapter 26) • Amoebic liver abscess (Chapter 27) • Hydatid disease (Chapter 27)	**Respiratory tract infections** • Streptococcal pharyngitis (Chapter 33) • Diphtheria (Chapter 33) • Pneumococcal pneumonia (Chapter 34) • *Haemophilus influenzae* pneumonia (Chapter 34) • *Klebsiella pneumoniae* pneumonia (Chapter 34) • Pulmonary tuberculosis (Chapter 35) • *Pseudomonas* infections (Chapter 36) • Influenza (Chapter 37) • COVID-19 (Chapter 37) • Infectious mononucleosis (Chapter 37) • Paragonimiasis (Chapter 38) • Zygomycosis (Chapter 38) • Aspergillosis (Chapter 38) • Pneumocystosis (Chapter 38)
Skin, soft tissue and musculoskeletal system infections • Staphylococcal skin and soft tissue infections (Chapter 28) • Streptococcal skin and soft tissue infections (Chapter 29) • Gas gangrene (Chapter 30) • Leprosy (Chapter 30) • Cutaneous anthrax (Chapter 30) • Herpes simplex (cutaneous and mucocutaneous) (Chapter 31) • Measles (Chapter 31) • Rubella (Chapter 31) • Dermatophytoses (Chapter 32) • Mycetoma (Chapter 32)	
Central nervous system infections • Pneumococcal meningitis (Chapter 39) • *Haemophilus influenzae* meningitis (Chapter 39) • Meningococcal meningitis (Chapter 39) • Viral meningitis (Chapter 40) • Hsv encephalitis (Chapter 40) • Japanese encephalitis (Chapter 40) • Rabies encephalitis (Chapter 40) • Neurocysticercosis (Chapter 41) • *Toxoplasma* encephalitis (Chapter 41) • Cryptococcal meningitis (Chapter 41)	**Genitourinary system infections** • Urinary tract infection (*Escherichia coli*) (Chapter 42) • Urinary tract infection (*Klebsiella pneumoniae*) (Chapter 42) • Urinary tract infection (*Proteus mirabilis*) (Chapter 42) • Urinary schistosomiasis (Chapter 42) • Syphilis (Chapter 43) • Gonorrhea (Chapter 43) • Non-gonococcal urethritis (Chapter 43) • Trichomoniasis (Chapter 43) • Vaginal candidiasis (Chapter 43)

Index

Page numbers followed by *f* refer to figure and *t* refer to table.

A

Acanthamoeba 302
Acid-fast stain 28, 191*f*, 262
Acinetobacter baumannii 271
Acquired immunodeficiency syndrome 153
Adenovirus 61*f*
AETCOM 324
Agar dilution method 53
Agglutination reaction 80
Air surveillance 128
Albert stain 28, 30, 245*f*, 247
Amoebic liver abscess 208
Amoebic meningoencephalitis, primary 302
Anaerobic culture 21, 22
Anaerobic glove box 40
Animal inoculation 65, 247
Anoxomat system 220
Anthrax 225
Antigen-antibody reactions, types of 78*t*
Antigenic variation 273
Antimicrobial susceptibility test 17, 48*f*, 49, 54
Anti-rabies prophylaxis 301*t*
Antiretroviral therapy 123, 159
Antistreptolysin O 217
Ascaris lumbricoides 198
Aspergillosis 105, 281, 284
Automated blood culture techniques 35
Automated identification system 247, 264

B

Bacillus cereus 176
Bacitracin sensitivity testing 217
Bacterial agglutination test 145*f*, 178*f*
Bacterial growth curve 14, 15
Bacterial meningitis 288
Bacterial motility 43
Bacterial pharyngitis 243
Bacterial pneumonia 250
Bacterial vaginosis 322
Balantidium coli 186, 281

Beta-hemolytic streptococcal infections 215
Bile esculin agar test 314*f*
Bile solubility test 252, 252*f*
Biomedical waste management 117, 119*t*, 279
Bloodstream infection 18, 138
Bordetella pertussis 20
Bright-field microscope 7*f*
Broth dilution method 52
Brown and Brenn modification 27
Brucellosis 148
Brugiya malayi 170, 170*f*
Burkholderia cepacia 258, 268
Burkholderia pseudomallei 268

C

Candida albicans 172, 173*f*, 321, 323*f*
Cellophane tape technique 198*f*
Central sterile services department 109, 109*f*
Cerebral malaria 303
Cerebrospinal fluid analysis 293, 296, 297
Cestode 192*f*
Chancroid 317, 318
Chemiluminescence-linked immunoassay 91
Chickenpox 230
Chlamydia trachomatis 321
Chlamydophila psittaci 135
Chocolate agar 33*f*, 252, 255*f*
Cholera 180
Citrate utilization test 45, 46*f*
Clonorchis 210, 210*f*
Clostridioides difficile 176
Clostridium perfringens 126, 176, 221
Coagulase negative *Staphylococcus* 214
Coccidian parasitic infections 190
Coccidioides immitis 174, 281
Congenital rubella syndrome 235
Corona virus 61*f*, 272
Corynebacterium diphtheria 30, 33, 43, 79, 243, 245, 245*f*
COVID-19 272, 275, 276*f*

Cryptococcal meningitis 306
Cryptosporidium 186, 190
Cyclospora 186, 190, 190*f*
Cystic echinococcosis 210*t*
Cystoisospora 186, 190, 190*f*

D

Dalmau plate culture 174
Dark-ground microscopy 31, 317
Dengue 153, 159, 160
Diarrheagenic *Escherichia coli* infections 176, 179
Dimorphic fungi 74
Diphtheria 102, 243-247
Diphyllobothriasis 194
Direct immunofluorescence assay 87, 274
Donovanosis 317, 318
Duke criteria, modified 134, 135*t*

E

Echinococcus granulosus 281
Eijkman test 127
Elek's gel precipitation test 78, 79, 79*f*, 248
Entamoeba histolytica 125, 186, 187*t*, 188*f*, 191, 208
Enteric fever 142
Enterobiasis 197
Enterococcus faecalis 314*f*
Entero-test 189
Enzyme-linked immunosorbent assay 59, 83, 84, 84*f*, 86, 156
Epstein-Barr virus 272, 280
Escherichia coli 14*f*, 34, 45, 126, 139, 258, 288, 307-310
Ethylene oxide sterilizer 108
Extrapulmonary tuberculosis 260

F

Fasciola hepatica 194, 208, 210, 210*f*
Fasciolopsis buski 192, 194, 196*f*
Flotation technique 71, 71*f*
Fluorescence microscope 9, 62
Formol-ether technique 71*f*
Free-living amoebae infections 302

G

Gas gangrene 220-222
GeneXpert 264, 265
Genito-ulcerative disease 317
Giardia lamblia 186, 189*f*
Giemsa stain 169*f*, 175*f*, 302
Gonococcal urethritis 317, 321
Gram-staining 25, 75, 247, 255, 271, 291, 291*t*, 308
Group A *Streptococcus* 136, 216

H

Haemophilus ducreyi 65
Haemophilus influenzae 14*f*, 250, 256*f*, 288, 292
Hand hygiene 92, 93, 96, 102
Hand-foot-and-mouth disease 235, 235*f*
Hanging drop method 44, 44*f*
Helicobacter pylori 22
Hepatitis viruses 203, 205, 206
Herpes simplex virus 227, 296
Heterophile agglutination test 81, 280
Histoplasmosis 174
Hookworm infections 200
Hospital infection control 331
Hot air oven 111
Human echinococcosis 208
Human immunodeficiency virus 153, 158
Human papillomavirus 231
Hydatid cyst 209*f*
Hymenolepiasis 193

I

ICUT tests 178, 258, 271
Immunochromatographic test 59, 90, 90*f*, 151, 169, 171, 187
Immunoelectron microscopy 184
Immunofluorescence assay 9, 59, 87, 87*f*, 191
Impregnation methods 23, 30
Inclusion bodies 62
Indole test 45, 45*f*
Infectious mononucleosis 280
Infective endocarditis 133, 135
Influenza 272, 273
Intestinal cestode infections 192
Intestinal coccidian parasites, laboratory diagnosis of 191*t*
Intestinal flukes 194
Intestinal taeniasis 193, 305*t*
Intestinal trematode 192
Invasive aspergillosis 285*f*
Invasive pneumococcal disease 251
Iodine mount 70

J

Japanese encephalitis 298
Jones criteria 137

K

Kinyoun's cold acid-fast staining 263
Kirby-Bauer's disk diffusion test 49, 50
Klebsiella 310
Kopeloff and Beerman's modification 27

L

Lactophenol cotton blue 75
Latex agglutination test 81, 82, 151
Leishmania donovani 168
Lepromin test 225
Leprosy 220, 224
Leptospira 151
Listeria monocytogenes 176, 288, 292
Loeffler's serum slope 37, 247
Lowenstein-Jensen medium 33, 34*f*, 263, 264*f*
Lung flukes 194
Lyme disease 293
Lymphatic filariasis 162, 170
Lymphogranuloma venereum 317

M

Malaria 162
McCrady statistical table 127*t*
McFadyean's reaction 226*f*
McIntosh and Filde's anaerobic jar 40*f*, 220
Measles 232
Melioidosis 268
Membrane filtration method 127
Meningitis 18, 172, 254, 290*f*
Meningococcal meningitis 288
Metachromatic granules 246
Microsporidia 186
Microsporum canis 236*f*, 237
Molecular test 148, 244
Molluscum bodies 63*f*, 232
Motility, types of 44, 44*t*
Mucormycosis 282
Mucosal candidiasis 238
Mueller-Hinton agar 50, 179*f*
Multiple tube method 126, 127*f*
Mycetoma 239
Mycobacterium tuberculosis 29, 33, 36, 104, 105, 260, 293
Mycoplasma pneumonia 81, 103, 243
Myxoviruses 272

N

Naegleria fowleri 302
Nagler's reaction 223, 223*f*
National AIDS Control Organization 120, 123, 153
Needle stick injury 121, 122
Negri body 63*f*, 300
Neisseria gonorrhoeae 243
Neisseria meningitidis 102, 292
Nipah virus 297
Nitrate reduction test 308
Nocardia 240
Non-gonococcal urethritis 317, 321, 321*t*
Nontreponemal tests 317
Non-typhoidal salmonellosis 179
Norwalk virus 185
Nutrient agar 33, 213*f*, 269

O

Optochin sensitivity 252
Orientia tsutsugamushi 148
Oxidase test 45, 45*f*, 178

P

Paracoccidioides brasiliensis 174, 175, 281
Paragonimiasis 281, 282*t*
Passive agglutination test 81
Paul-Bunnell test 280
Penicilliosis 281, 286
Peptone water 33*f*
Periodic acid-Schiff stain 75
Peripheral blood smear 163, 170*f*
Personal protective equipment 94, 95, 96*f*, 102, 103, 120, 278
Pertussis 102
Plasma sterilization 110
Plasmodium falciparum 165*f*, 166*f*, 303
Plasmodium vivax 162, 165*f*
Pneumococcal meningitis 250, 289
Pneumocystis pneumonia 287
Pneumonic plague 102
Polymerase chain reaction 56, 59*f*, 64, 147, 152, 169, 171
Post-exposure prophylaxis 122, 123, 124*t*, 248
Post-streptococcal glomerulonephritis 217, 244
Pour plate technique 38
Poxvirus 61*f*
Proteus 45, 147, 309
Pseudomonas 126, 258, 268, 269*f*, 270*t*
Psychrophiles 16*f*

Index

Pulmonary tuberculosis, primary 261, 261*t*
Pyogenic meningitis 291

Q

Quellung reaction 253, 255
Quick SOFA criteria 139

R

Rabies 299, 300, 301
Rapid diagnostic test 166, 293
Rapid plasma reagin test 318, 319*f*, 319*t*
Revised National Tuberculosis Control Program 260
Rheumatic fever 133, 136, 244
Rhinosporidiosis 241
Robertson cooked meat broth 35, 41, 220, 221*f*
Rotavirus 11*f*, 61*f*, 125, 184
Rubella 234

S

Sabin-Feldman dye test 303
Sabouraud's dextrose agar 75, 76*f*, 236*f*, 286*f*
Salmonella 45, 143*f*
Saturated salt solution technique 71, 71*f*
Schistosomiasis 194, 195*f*
Scrub typhus 142, 147, 148
Sedimentation technique 71
Sexually transmitted infections 60, 316
Shigella 144, 176
Silver impregnation method 31*f*, 317
Slide agglutination test 80*f*, 144
Slide coagulase test 212, 213*t*
Slide culture technique 76*f*
Specimen 163, 180, 220, 222
Sporothrix schenckii 240, 241*f*
Sporotrichosis 240
Sporulated oocysts 190*f*
Staphylococcal infections 211

Staphylococcal pneumonia 257
Staphylococcus aureus 53*f*, 53*t*, 82, 102, 133
Steam sterilizer 109, 110*f*
Sterile universal container 19
Sterilization 108
Streptococcus agalactiae 217*t*, 218, 219*f*, 219*t*, 288, 292
Streptococcus gallolyticus 133
Streptococcus pneumoniae 16, 250, 250*t*, 288, 292
Streptococcus pyogenes 215, 216, 216*f*, 216*t*, 217*t*, 243
String test 182*f*, 189
Strongyloides 192
Strongyloidiasis 200
Syphilis 78, 316-318

T

Taenia 192
Thayer Martin medium 320
Tissue culture 65
Toxocara 208
Toxoplasmosis 302
Transmission electron microscope 10, 10*f*
Treponema pallidum 31, 293
Treponemal serological test 319
Trichomonas vaginalis 321, 322*t*
Trichomoniasis 321, 322
Trichophyton mentagrophyte 237, 238*f*
Trichophyton schoenleinii 237
Trichuris 192, 197
Triple sugar iron agar test 46, 46*f*, 292
Tube coagulase test 212, 213*f*
Tuberculosis 18, 260
Tuberculous meningitis 291
Typhoid fever 147
Tzanck smear 63*f*, 228*f*

U

Ultraviolet radiation 114
Urea hydrolysis test 45, 46*f*

Urease test 46, 237
Urethritis 21, 313, 317, 320
Urinary tract infection 18, 172, 211, 307-310, 313

V

Vaginal candidiasis 323
Varicella-zoster virus 230
Vector-borne diseases 60
Venereal disease research laboratory 78, 316*f*, 317, 319*t*
Venkatraman-Ramakrishnan medium 34, 180
Vibrio cholerae 14*f*, 16, 33, 34, 45, 176, 180, 181, 181*f*, 182
Viral encephalitis 60, 295, 297
Viral exanthems 227
Viral hemorrhagic fevers 160
Viral isolation 300
Viral meningitis 291, 295, 296
Viral transport medium 61, 274
Viridans streptococci 250*t*
Visceral leishmaniasis 162, 168
Voges-Proskauer test 182
Vulvovaginal candidiasis 322

W

Water surveillance 125
Weigert's modification 27
Weil's disease 151
Weil-Felix test 147, 311
Western blot 88, 89*f*, 156
Whooping cough 102
Widal test 80, 81, 81*f*, 145
Wood's lamp examination 237
Wool Sorter's disease 225
Wuchereria bancrofti 170*f*

Z

Ziehl-Neelsen technique 28, 29, 29*f*, 262
Zygomycoses 281, 282, 283*f*